2023 ICD-10-CM
Coding for Chiropractic

Diagnosis Coding Essentials | Common Diagnosis Codes & Tips | Alphabetic Index
Tabular List | Provider Documentation Guides | ICD-10-CM Abridged Official Guidelines

ChiroCode
Insurance Reimbursement Solutions
62 East 300 North Spanish Fork, UT 84660 USA
(602) 944-9877 | ChiroCode.com

Copyright Notice and Disclaimer

This publication is distributed with the understanding that the publisher is not engaged in rendering legal or accounting or medical services. If legal advice or other expert assistance is required, the services of a competent professional person should be sought.

innoviHealth assumes no liability for data contained or not contained herein. It does not directly nor indirectly practice law or give legal opinions. It assumes no responsibility for the consequences attributable to or related to any use or interpretation of any information or views contained in or not contained in this publication. Absolute accuracy cannot be guaranteed. innoviHealth is not responsible for informing the purchaser of any updates. Unless noted, the views expressed herein are that of the innoviHealth and should not be construed as policy for any entity or insurance company.

Printed in the U.S.A.

ISBN: 978-1-64072-206-4

innoviHealth
62 East 300 North
Spanish Fork, UT 84660 USA
Phone (801) 528-6876

Visit innoviHealth.com for more information.

Acknowledgments

Development of this annual edition requires extensive review and input. The contributions over many years from numerous physicians, assistants, consultants, and attorneys have made this book possible. Their efforts and professional input are sincerely appreciated but they are too numerous to list here. Special thanks also goes to all of the hardworking ChiroCode, Inc. support staff.

President / Chief Executive Officer
LaMont Leavitt

Vice President / Chief Information Officer
David D. Berky

Chief Operations Officer
Tracy Young

Chief Financial Officer
John Davis

Chief Revenue Officer
Michael Hanahan

VP of Sales
Alan Crop

Director of Content
Wyn Staheli

Content, Design, Editorial, & Delivery
Alan Albright
Brandon Herman
Christine Woolstenhulme
David Lewis
DeVin Orton
Izzy Morris
Jan Anderson
Jason Boogert
Jeff Lewis
Jonathan Mitchell
Justin Lewis
Kristy Ritchie
Melissa Baker
Raquel Shumway
Reed Larson

Special thanks to our third-party partners and reviewers

2023 ICD-10-CM Coding for Chiropractic

The *2023 ICD-10-CM Coding for Chiropractic* continues the ChiroCode tradition of providing helpful tools and resources for healthcare providers. This unique compilation of coding essentials makes it easier to get the job done.

When used properly, this book can not only save valuable staff and doctor time, but it can also build confidence and compliance in your practice's coding, documentation, reimbursement, and more.

Our Commitment is to provide current information in a manner that is easy to understand and implement in a healthcare setting.

Our Mission is to support healthcare providers seeking to navigate the complex and ever-changing world of insurance reimbursement through high quality products, services, and education.

Our Pledge is to help your practice survive and thrive with greater assurance.

We encourage you to take advantage of our free newsletter, sent by email. These alerts include the latest industry and coding news, notifications of helpful webinars, coding and reimbursement tips, and more. To register, visit www.ChiroCode.com/#news. Your information privacy is assured – it is never shared with others.

Your opinions and suggestions are welcome and appreciated. With your feedback, we continue to improve year after year. Please send your comments and suggestions to support@ChiroCode.com.

Thank you for your continuing support.

LaMont J. Leavitt, President/CEO

Table of Contents

Icon Legend

The following icons are referenced throughout the book. Use this legend to understand how they are used.

Resources

Website/Book: This icon will direct you to online or print resources containing more information on a topic. Some resources are only accessible with a Find-A-Code subscription.

Tips/Notes

Tip: This icon is used to point out useful tips, notes or special instructions. These are things that your office needs to review and include in your office policies and procedures where applicable.

Alerts

Alert: This icon indicates a warning or other important information that we really want to make sure you notice. These alerts could save you time, money and frustration.

Store

Store: This icon indicates helpful resources which may be purchased from our online store at ChiroCode.com.

Example

Example:
This icon highlights an example that will help you better understand a concept.

This page is intentionally left blank

This page is intentionally left blank

Notes

Ch1

1. Diagnosis Coding Essentials

1. Diagnosis Coding Essentials

About ICD-10-CM

On October 1, 2015, ICD-10-CM replaced ICD-9-CM as the official Health Information Portability and Accountability Act (HIPAA) approved code set for diagnostic reporting. ICD-10-CM codes impact medical records and nearly every type of document used within a practice for reimbursement by third party payers. The International Classification of Diseases, Tenth Revision, Clinical Modification (ICD-10-CM) is the United States' adaptation of the World Health Organization's (WHO) ICD-10-CM codes. This "clinical modification" makes the codes (which are required for use on healthcare claims in the U.S.) useful for classifying morbidity data.

ICD-10-PCS (Procedure Classification System) is the replacement code set for reporting procedures performed in a facility or inpatient setting. There may be ICD-10-PCS codes describing services for chiropractic, but they are only to be used when the service is performed in a facility/inpatient setting. This publication does not cover ICD-10-PCS coding.

Note: ICD-10-PCS codes are the same length (seven characters), but have an entirely differently structure than ICD-10-CM codes. See FindACode.com for more information and the entire ICD-10-PCS code set.

Book: Due to space limitations, this book does not contain the complete ICD-10-CM code set, which includes nearly 71,500 codes. About 8,000 are found in Chapter 5 - The Tabular List, and shorter, more focused lists are found in Chapter 3 - Common Diagnosis Codes & Tips. While every effort has been made to make sure chiropractors can find the codes they need in this book, it is possible that providers may need to search the complete code set to find the code that most accurately represents their patient(s). The full code set can be searched at FindACode.com (with subscription).

Updates

New, revised, and deleted codes are implemented annually on October 1st. Depending on the year, some specialties may be impacted dramatically while others may not see any changes.

Book: New and revised codes will be flagged in Chapter 5 - The Tabular List and Chapter 3 - Common Diagnosis Codes & Tips.

Website: Go to FindACode.com (with subscription) to search the updated code set.

The WHO released ICD-11 in May of 2018, but it takes years to develop a clinical modification and then even more time to get it approved as the new HIPAA-compliant code set. Therefore, it is possible that it may take another decade before ICD-11-CM is implemented in the U.S.

Website: Go to ChiroCode.com and search on "ICD-11" for further information.

ICD-10-CM Basics

The ICD-10-CM code set is comprised of two parts:

1. The Alphabetic Index: Begin your search in this index by searching the key/main term to locate an ICD-10-CM code.

2. The Tabular List: Comprised of the 21 chapters below, enabling you to confirm the selected code.

Chapter	Description
1	Certain Infectious and Parasitic Diseases (AØØ-B99)
2	Neoplasms (CØØ-D49)
3	Diseases of the Blood and Blood-Forming Organs and Certain Disorders Involving the Immune Mechanism (D5Ø-D89)
4	Endocrine, Nutritional and Metabolic Diseases (EØØ-E89)
5	Mental, Behavioral and Neurodevelopmental Disorders (FØ1-F99)
6	Diseases of the Nervous System (GØØ-G99)
7	Diseases of the Eye and Adnexa (HØØ-H59)
8	Diseases of the Ear and Mastoid Process (H6Ø-H95)
9	Diseases of the Circulatory System (IØØ-I99)
10	Diseases of the Respiratory System (JØØ-J99)
11	Diseases of the Digestive System (KØØ-K95)
12	Diseases of the Skin and Subcutaneous Tissue (LØØ-L99)
13	Diseases of the Musculoskeletal System and Connective Tissue (MØØ-M99)
14	Diseases of the Genitourinary System (NØØ-N99)
15	Pregnancy, Childbirth and the Puerperium (OØØ-O9A)
16	Certain Conditions Originating in the Perinatal Period (PØØ-P96)
17	Congenital Malformations, Deformations and Chromosomal Abnormalities (QØØ-Q99)
18	Symptoms, Signs and Abnormal Clinical and Laboratory Findings, Not Elsewhere Classified (RØØ-R99)
19	Injury, Poisoning and Certain other Consequences of External Causes (SØØ-T88)
20	External Causes of Morbidity (VØØ-Y99)
21	Factors Influencing Health Status and Contact with Health Services (ZØØ-Z99)
22	Codes for Special Purposes (U00-U85)

The ICD-10-CM classification system includes up to seven alphanumeric characters in each code. The use of letters in addition to numbers allows for dozens of choices in each character position. Because of this, ICD-10-CM has the ability to describe conditions with great detail. For example, a broken bone code may include which bone is broken, which side of the body, what part of the bone, the episode of care for the encounter, and the status of the break.

The first character in an ICD-10-CM code is always a letter, and the second character is always a number. Characters three through seven may be either letters or numbers. There is always a decimal after, and only after, the third character, unless it is only a three character code. It is essential to understand that some codes are complete with only three characters, while others require up to seven.

The format of codes presented in this codebook set will indicate whether it is an incomplete or invalid code, meaning the code is not yet at the highest level of specificity. If a hyphen (-) is present at the end of a category or subcategory, it is an indicator that additional specificity is required. If an underscore (_) is present, it indicates the need for a seventh character extension. When a code is complete, it will be shown in a bold font or a bold font followed by an underscore (_) to indicate the need for a seventh character selection. See the segment "Structure of the Tabular List" on page 12 for additional information.

Examples:

M5Ø.1- "Cervical disc disorder with radiculopathy"

M5Ø.1Ø "Cervical disc disorder with radiculopathy, unspecified cervical region"

M5Ø.11 "Cervical disc disorder with radiculopathy, high cervical region"

M5Ø.12- "Cervical disc disorder with radiculopathy, mid-cervical region"

M5Ø.13 "Cervical disc disorder with radiculopathy, cervicothoracic region"

S13.4xx_ "Sprain of ligaments of cervical spine"

S13.4xxA "Sprain of ligaments of cervical spine, initial encounter"

S13.4xxD "Sprain of ligaments of cervical spine, subsequent encounter"

S13.4xxS "Sprain of ligaments of cervical spine, sequela"

In this example, M5Ø.1- requires further characters before it is complete, as indicated by the hyphen. **M5Ø.11** is complete, but M5Ø.12- requires another character. **S13.4xx_** needs a seventh character which is indicated by the underscore, rather than a hyphen.

Tip: Digits Ø through 9 and every letter of the English alphabet, except "U," are used in ICD-10-CM codes. The letter "U" is used for research purposes and for new diagnoses whose etiology is uncertain. If and when the etiology is confirmed, that diagnosis will be assigned to its proper location in the code set with the annual ICD-10-CM update. Generally, these codes will not be reported by providers.

Tip: When writing ICD-10-CM codes, consider using the slashed zero "Ø" so that it is not confused with the letter "O." Also, consider saying the word "zero," rather than "oh," when describing the number verbally.

Features of ICD-10-CM

The Clinical Modification of ICD-10 required a thorough evaluation which included input from technical advisors, physician groups, clinical coders, and other relevant organizations. This was done in an effort to ensure that users would experience consistency and accuracy in diagnostic coding. Some significant ICD-10-CM enhancements over previous code sets include:

- More combination codes, which reduced the number of codes needed to describe certain conditions;
- An expanded set of injury codes, with code extensions allowing for greater detail;
- Placeholders (designated by use of an "x") allowing for future expansion;
- Longer codes (up to seven characters) allowing for more detail;
- Laterality to indicate which side of the body is affected;
- The use of alphanumeric, rather than strictly numeric, characters;
- Additional codes relevant to ambulatory and managed care encounters;
- Additional alcohol and substance abuse codes;
- A greatly expanded set of external cause codes; and
- Greater overall specificity in code assignment.

These differences help to address quality concerns such as medical errors, poor documentation, a lack of support in establishing medical necessity, and fragmented care. With the greater ability of providers to accurately code a patient's condition, payers should be able to properly review claims with increased accuracy. Providers whose documentation fully supports accurate ICD-10-CM codes should get paid properly and avoid denials.

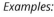

Structure of the Tabular List

The Tabular List in ICD-10-CM is divided into chapters, followed by blocks, categories, subcategories, and finally individual codes. ICD-10-CM can accommodate approximately 155,000 classifications.

Book: See *Figure 1.1* for a breakdown of the structure of a complete code.

Note: Many categories and subcategories were created with gaps in the alphanumeric sequence which will allow for the addition of new diagnoses without interrupting the established groupings. For example, there are categories from M4Ø to M43, and M45 to M49, but M44 was skipped. It is possible that future ICD-10-CM updates will make use of these empty categories.

Chapters

ICD-10-CM has 21 chapters. The first 17 chapters correspond to a body system or condition, Chapter 18 is for signs and symptoms, and Chapter 19 is for injuries and poisonings. Filling the roles of the E and V codes of ICD-9-CM, Chapter 20 is the chapter for external cause codes and Chapter 22 includes codes that report health status.

Example:
13. Diseases of the Musculoskeletal System and Connective Tissue (MØØ-M99)

Blocks

Chapters are divided into blocks, which are groups of categories.

Example:
M4Ø-M54 is the block for dorsopathies, or diseases of the spine. It is broken into three smaller blocks, which are slightly more specific:

- M4Ø-M43 "Deforming Dorsopathies"
- M45-M49 "Spondylopathies"
- M5Ø-M54 "Other Dorsopathies"

Providers and billers who are familiar with the code set could, theoretically, simply browse these blocks until they arrive at the desired code. However, the Alphabetic Index and other tools have been added to this codebook to make the code selection process easier.

Categories

Categories consist of three alphanumeric characters which further narrow the code possibilities to a more specific condition.

Example:

M47- "Spondylosis" is a category which includes 55 possible codes. Most of these require five or six characters to appropriately represent a valid code.

Note: Code **I1Ø** "Essential (primary) hypertension" is an example of a code that is complete with only three characters. Complete codes in this codebook, which may be from three to seven characters, will always be in bold type and will not include a hyphen. For claims reporting purposes, only complete codes of the highest level of specificity are permissible – not categories or subcategories; unless, of course, a complete code is its own category or subcategory. **Remember, in this publication, to pay attention to whether or not a code in bold text, rather than the number of characters it contains!**

Subcategories

Subcategories are at the level of the fourth and fifth characters. They begin to narrow down the category with greater specificity about the condition.

Example:
M47- "Spondylosis" has four fourth character subcategories and four fifth character subcategories, along with one complete code.

M47.Ø- "Anterior spinal and vertebral artery compression syndromes"

M47.Ø1- "Anterior spinal artery compression syndromes"
M47.Ø2- "Vertebral artery compression syndromes"

M47.1- "Other spondylosis with myelopathy"

M47.2- "Other spondylosis with radiculopathy"

M47.8- "Other spondylosis"

M47.81- "Spondylosis without myelopathy or radiculopathy"
M47.89- "Other spondylosis"

M47.9 "Spondylosis, unspecified"

Codes

At the sixth and seventh character level, codes are simply designated as "codes," but remember that a valid, complete code may be anything from 3-7 characters in length and will be shown in a bold font. In this codebook, if a code requires a seventh character to be valid, it is shown with an underscore (_) in the seventh character position. The seventh character choices are listed in a shaded box within the Tabular List at the level of either the category or subcategory.

A - initial encounter for fracture
D - subsequent encounter for fracture with routine healing
S - sequela of fracture

Examples:
M47.81- "Spondylosis without myelopathy or radiculopathy" has nine options for the sixth and final character, which identifies the location. These codes do not require a seventh character extension. If a seventh character extension is added to a six character code, it is invalid and will be denied by payers.

M47.811 "Occipito-atlanto-axial"

M47.812 "Cervical"

M47.813 "Cervicothoracic"

M47.814 "Thoracic"

M47.815 "Thoracolumbar"

M47.816 "Lumbar"

M47.817 "Lumbosacral"

M47.818 "Sacral and sacrococcygeal"

M47.819 "Site unspecified"

S33.5xx_ "Sprain of ligaments of lumbar spine" needs a seventh character extension to complete the code.

S33.5xxA "Sprain of ligaments of lumbar spine, initial encounter"

S33.5xxD "Sprain of ligaments of lumbar spine, subsequent encounter"

S33.5xxS "Sprain of ligaments of lumbar spine, sequela"

Book: For more information on seventh character extensions, see *Figure 1.3* on page 15 titled "7th Character Extensions in ICD-10-CM."

Figure 1.1

Tabular List Layout

Chapter	Block	Categories	Subcategories	Codes
21 of them from A to Z (body system or condition)	Ranges of categories (related conditions)	3 characters (more specific condition)	4th or 5th characters (etiology, location, etc.)	6th or 7th characters (laterality, encounter, etc.)
Chapter 19: S = Injury	S3Ø - S39 = Lower back and lumbar spine	S39 = Other injury of lower back	Ø = Muscle, fascia, tendon 1 = Strain	2 = Lower back A = Initial encounter

Example: S39.Ø12A Strain of muscle, fascia, and tendon of lower back, initial encounter

Tip: Although three (3) character codes exist, in most cases, additional characters are needed. The highest specificity codes may require up to seven (7) characters. Carefully read all applicable coding notes and guidelines before making final code selections.

Coding Conventions

The following selected coding conventions for the Alphabetic Index and the Tabular List are found in Section *I.A* of the *ICD-10-CM Official Guidelines for Coding and Reporting*. An abridged version of the guidelines is found in Appendix B, and the complete guidelines can be viewed at FindACode.com (with subscription).

If ICD-10-CM were a language, these conventions would be the "rules of grammar." They identify and define how terms, abbreviations, and punctuation are used throughout the code set.

Placeholder Character

The letter "x" is used as a placeholder in certain codes to leave room for future expansion and preserve the format of ICD-10-CM codes (e.g., to ensure that seventh character extensions are indeed the seventh character). The placeholder does not add to the code description, it just (as the name states) holds a place. It is important to note that there can be more than one placeholder in a code. Officially, it is *not* case sensitive and thus may be either upper or lowercase; however, be aware of individual payer policies which may differ from this standard.

Example:
XØØ.ØxxA "Exposure to flames in uncontrolled fire in building, initial encounter"

Alert — Do not add additional placeholder characters to codes that do not require them. It is incorrect to force every code to be seven characters long.

7th Characters

Instructional notes within the Tabular List will indicate whether a seventh character (also known as an extension) is required. The possible extensions will be listed in a shaded box at the level of either the category or subcategory. Seventh characters are currently only used for certain codes within the chapters listed in *Figure 1.2*. In *Figure 1.3* it provides more detail regarding the codes requiring a seventh character.

Figure 1.2

Chapters with 7th Character Extensions	
4	Endocrine, Nutritional and Metabolic Diseases (EØØ-E89)
7	Diseases of the Eye and Adnexa (HØØ-H59)
13	Diseases of the Musculoskeletal System and Connective Tissue (MØØ-M99)
15	Pregnancy, Childbirth and the Puerperium (OØØ-O9A)
18	Symptoms, Signs, and Abnormal Clinical and Laboratory Findings (RØØ-R99)
19	Injury, Poisoning, and Certain other Consequences of External Causes (SØØ-T88)
20	External Causes of Morbidity (VØ1-Y99)

Figure 1.3

7th Character Extensions in ICD-10-CM

Chapter	Affected Codes	Seventh Character Extension Options
Chapter 4 **Endocrine, Nutritional, and Metabolic Diseases**	**Ophthalmologic Complications in Diabetes** EØ8.32- EØ9.32- E1Ø.32- E11.32- E13.32-	**Laterality** 1 right 2 left 3 bilateral 9 unspecified
Chapter 7 **Diseases of the Eye and Adnexa**	**Retinal vein occlusion** H34.81- H34.83-	**Complications** Ø with macular edema 1 with retinal neovascularization 2 stable
	Nonexudative age-related macular degeneration H35.31-	**Stage** Ø unspecified 1 early dry stage 2 intermediate dry stage 3 advanced atrophic without subfoveal involvement 4 advanced atrophic with subfoveal involvement
	Exudative age-related macular degeneration H35.32-	**Stage** Ø unspecified 1 with active choroidal neovascularization 2 with inactive choroidal neovascularization 3 with inactive scar
	Glaucoma H4Ø.1Ø- H4Ø.2Ø- H4Ø.3Ø- H4Ø.4Ø- H4Ø.5Ø- H4Ø.6Ø-	**Stage** Ø unspecified 1 mild 2 moderate 3 severe 4 indeterminate
	Blindness H54-	**Level of Blindness** See the *ChiroCode Online Library*
Chapter 13 **Diseases of the Musculoskeletal System**	**Spondylopathies** M48.4-	**Episode of Care** A initial encounter for fracture (fx) care D subsequent encounter for fx care G subsequent encounter for fx care with delayed healing S sequela
	Disorder of bone density and structure M8Ø.Ø- M84.3-	**Episode of Care** A initial encounter for fracture (fx) care D subsequent encounter for fx care with routine healing G subsequent encounter for fx care with delayed healing K subsequent encounter for fx with nonunion P subsequent encounter for fx with malunion S sequela
	Periprosthetic fracture around internal prosthetic joint M97-	**Episode of Care** A initial encounter D subsequent encounter S sequela

7th Character Extensions in ICD-10-CM

Chapter	Affected Codes	Seventh Character Extension Options
Chapter 13 (continued) **Diseases of the Musculoskeletal System**	**Chronic gout** M1A-	**Presence of Tophus** Ø without tophus (tophi) 1 with tophus (tophi)
Chapter 15 **Pregnancy, Childbirth, and the Puerperium**	**Pregnancy Complications** O31- O32- O33.3- 036-	**Fetus** Ø not applicable or unspecified 1 fetus 1 2 fetus 2 3 fetus 3 4 fetus 4 5 fetus 5 9 other fetus
Chapter 18 **Symptoms, Signs, and Abnormal Findings**	**Coma Scale** R4Ø.2-	**Time of Score** Ø unspecified time 1 in the field [EMT or ambulance] 2 at arrival to emergency department 3 at hospital admission 4 24 hours or more after hospital admission
Chapter 19 **Injury, Poisoning, and Certain other Consequences of External Causes**	**Non-Fracture Injuries and Poisonings**	**Episode of Care** A initial encounter D subsequent encounter S sequela
	Fracture Injuries Not all fracture codes will use every option listed here as a seventh character extension. Consult the Tabular List to ensure accurate reporting.	**Episode of Care** A initial encounter OR, when applicable: A initial encounter for closed fracture (fx) B initial encounter for open fx D subsequent encounter for fx with routine healing G subsequent encounter for fx with delayed healing K subsequent encounter for fx with nonunion P subsequent encounter for fx with malunion S sequela
	Fractures of S52- Forearm S72- Femur S82- Lower leg, including ankle Note that there may be subcategories within the categories above that require different seventh character extension options. Consult the Tabular List to ensure accurate reporting.	**Episode of Care and Fracture (fx) Type** A initial, closed fx B initial, open fx type I, II, or NOS C initial, open fx type IIIA, IIIB, or IIIC D subsequent, closed fx with routine healing E subsequent, open fx type I or II with routine healing F subsequent, open fx type IIIA, IIIB, or IIIC with routine healing G subsequent, closed fx with delayed healing H subsequent, open fx type I or II with delayed healing J subsequent, open fx type IIIA, IIIB, or IIIC with delayed healing K subsequent, closed fx with nonunion M subsequent, open fx type I or II with nonunion N subsequent, open fx type IIIA, IIIB, or IIIC with nonunion P subsequent, closed fx with malunion Q subsequent, open fx type I or II with malunion R subsequent, open fx type IIIA, IIIB, or IIIC with malunion S sequela
Chapter 20 **External Causes of Morbidity**	Most codes in this chapter require a seventh character extension.	**Episode of Care** A initial encounter D subsequent encounter S sequela

Abbreviations

NEC (Not Elsewhere Classifiable)

This abbreviation, whether found in the Alphabetic Index or the Tabular List, represents "other specified." It is appropriate to use these codes when the information in the medical record provides detail for which a specific code does not exist. It may be helpful to think of NEC as "other." These codes are often indicated with the number "8" as the last or next to last character.

Example:

M53.86 "Other specified dorsopathies, lumbar region"

If a patient is presenting with the condition above, but in a manner that excludes it from classification in a category that currently exists, such as others in the "Dorsopathies" (M4Ø-M54) block, this NEC code could be used.

Tip: Instructional notes will often provide indication as to whether there are more specific codes that could be reported in place of the NEC code.

NOS (Not Otherwise Specified)

This abbreviation, whether found in the Alphabetic Index or the Tabular List, represents "unspecified." These codes might be selected when the record does not contain enough detail to choose a more specific code. If the category has no "unspecified" option, the "other specified" code (see "NEC" above) may be used. NOS codes often end with a "9" or "Ø."

Example:

M54.9 "Dorsalgia, unspecified"

Tip: Reporting unspecified codes may result in denial from a payer. However, the first priority for any biller or coder is to report what was documented. If the documentation does not provide enough information to select a more specific code, query the provider for clarity or better detail, but do not report a more specific code if the documentation does not support it.

Book: In order to avoid reporting unspecified codes, ensure that the provider knows what needs to be documented in patient encounters. See Appendix C - Provider Documentation Guides for more help.

Punctuation

Brackets [ ]

Brackets enclose words that are synonyms, alternative wordings, or explanatory phrases in the Tabular List. In the Alphabetic Index they enclose manifestation codes.

Tabular Example: M48.1- "Ankylosing hyperostosis [Forestier]"

This could be documented as "Forestier's" or "Ankylosing hyperostosis."

Alphabetic Example: Arthropathy, gouty in (due to) Lesch-Nyhan syndrome **E79.1** [M14.8-]

M14.8- "Arthropathies in other specified diseases classified elsewhere" instructs, via the "Code first" instructional note, to sequence the underlying disease first. See the segment "Etiology/Manifestation and Proper Code Sequencing" on page 20.

Parentheses ( )

Parentheses enclose supplementary words. The terms within the parentheses are nonessential modifiers.

Example:
M62.Ø11 "Separation of muscle (nontraumatic), right shoulder"
This would be properly documented with or without the word "nontraumatic."

And

The word "and" should be interpreted to mean "and" or "or" when it appears in a title.

Example:
S33- "Dislocation and Sprain of Joints and Ligaments of Lumbar Spine and Pelvis"
This category can be more correctly read as "dislocation AND/OR sprain of joints AND/OR ligaments of lumbar spine AND/OR pelvis."

With

The word "with" should be interpreted to mean "associated with" or "due to" when it appears anywhere in ICD-10-CM. Note that when the documentation does not specify the "with" information, the default code should be used.

Book: See the segment "Default Code" on page 26 for more information.

Example:
G43.1- "Migraine with aura" could be read as "migraine associated with aura."

See and See Also

When using the Alphabetic Index, the "see" instruction means that another term *should* be referenced, while "see also" means that another term *can* be referenced, but it is not necessary.

Examples:
Strain, postural - *see also* Disorder, soft tissue, due to use
Jaccoud's syndrome - *see* Arthropathy, postrheumatic, chronic

Inclusion Terms

Some codes may include a list of terms following the official code title. In some cases, these inclusion terms are synonyms of the code title. In the case of a code title with a description that is not specific, these terms are a listing of conditions assigned to that code. These terms are not necessarily exhaustive. Additional terms can also be found in the Alphabetic Index. They can be helpful when a provider is working on clinical documentation improvement as it pertains to diagnosis codes. To assist in identifying inclusion terms in the Tabular List, after the main description we have added the word, "Including:" before the inclusion terms.

Examples:
M54.1- "Radiculopathy"

Brachial neuritis or radiculitis NOS
Lumbar neuritis or radiculitis NOS
Lumbosacral neuritis or radiculitis NOS
Thoracic neuritis or radiculitis NOS
Radiculitis NOS neuritis or radiculitis NOS

This means that radiculitis, though technically different from radiculopathy, is designated by the same code.

Tabular List Instructional Notes and Terms

Alert — The instructional notes described in this section can appear at the chapter, block, category, subcategory, and code levels. When reporting codes, it is essential to be aware of the instructions at each level (block, category, subcategory, and code). Instructional notes appearing at any level within the block pertain to all codes beneath them, unless otherwise specified. To make sure all pertinent information is gathered, work backward. Find the instructions at the code level, then subcategory, category, and so on to ensure compliance at all levels.

Book: Searching through the dense *ICD-10-CM Official Guidelines for Coding and Reporting* to find all the needed instructions and guidelines can be time-consuming. To make this task easier, this book contains *Provider Documentation Guides*™ for common diagnoses which summarize all the applicable instructions and guidelines for that diagnosis. See Appendix C - Provider Documentation Guides.

Includes Notes

These instructional notes appear immediately under a three-character code title to further define, or give examples of, the content of the category. Most commonly, this is a list of similar conditions or different names for the conditions which are covered by the code. It is not the same thing as an "inclusion term," which is explained in the previous section.

Example:
M41- "Scoliosis"

Includes:
kyphoscolosis

There is no need to search for a code for "kyphoscoliosis;" it is included in this category.

Excludes Notes

ICD-10-CM has two types of excludes notes that are not interchangeable, with each performing a specific function.

Excludes1

An "Excludes1" note is used when two conditions cannot occur together. For instance, a condition can be either congenital or acquired, but cannot be both. This type of note conforms to the typical notion of what the word "excludes" means. Another way of saying this is "NOT CODED HERE!" An "Excludes1" note indicates codes that should *not* be used at the same time as the code located directly above the "Excludes1" notation. When this term appears, think, "consider these codes instead" or "only one code can apply." The codes are mutually exclusive. The one exception, according to the official guidelines is when "the two conditions are unrelated to each other." (See the Alert that follows for more information).

Example:
M43.Ø- "Spondylolysis"
Excludes1:
congenital spondylolysis (Q76.2)
M43.Ø- is for acquired spondylolysis, while **Q76.2** is for congenital spondylolysis so the two should never appear together on the same claim.

Alert — Exclude1 Payer Edits

Some payers may deny a claim when two codes are reported together that have an Excludes1 instructional note. Be sure to review the Tabular List or FindACode.com for the applicable year to understand what codes are being excluded from being reported together. However, it is important to note that there is an exception to Excludes1 edits as long as the two conditions are NOT related. As long as the documentation supports that exception, be sure to appeal the claim.

Website: See findacode.com/articles/excludes1 for more information.

Book: For more information on the two examples given in the CDC memo, see the segments in this chapter titled "Signs and Symptoms" on page 23 and "Sequela (Late Effects)" on page 25.

Excludes2

An "Excludes2" note means "not included here." A patient could have both conditions at the same time, but another code is required to describe both of them. Think, "consider these codes in addition." The diagnoses do not include each other so the Excludes2, if applicable, should also be coded.

Example:
S33- "Dislocation and Sprain of Joints and Ligaments of Lumbar Spine and Pelvis"
Excludes2:
islocation and sprain of joints and ligaments of hip (S73-)
strain of muscle of lower back and pelvis (S39.Ø1-)
This means that hip sprain or lower back strain would need to be coded in addition to the S33- code because it does not include them.

Tip: There are two types of "Excludes" notes used in ICD-10-CM to help identify situations where a different code might be better or if another code could be added.
Excludes1: Consider these codes instead.
Excludes2: Consider these codes in addition.

Etiology/Manifestation and Proper Code Sequencing

For certain codes, the underlying condition (etiology) should be sequenced (reported) first, followed by the manifestation. Other types of codes sometimes have sequencing rules as well. In either case, "Code First" or "Use additional code" will appear within the Tabular List to provide guidance. The order of sequencing is not optional; payers can and will deny a claim that does not follow proper sequencing guidelines.

Code First

The "Code First" instructional note is often attached to a manifestation code, which often includes the phrase "in diseases classified elsewhere" in the title. This notation points to an etiology code, which should appear first on a claim.

Example:
MØ2- "Postinfective and Reactive Arthropathies"
Code First:
underlying disease, such as:
congenital syphilis [Clutton's joints] (A5Ø.5)
enteritis due to Yersinia enterocolitica (AØ4.6)
infective endocarditis (I33.Ø)
viral hepatitis (B15-B19)
If a patient is presenting with with any of these underlying diseases, that disease must be reported first on the claim.

Use Additional Code

The etiology code will have an instructional note that says "Use additional code" to direct the coder to a manifestation code. The manifestation code cannot be listed as a primary diagnosis, but must always follow the etiology code.

Often, "use additional code" rules state that the manifestation code will be reported "if applicable." If the code is not applicable, do not report it. It is permissible to use etiology codes without a manifestation code, but do not report a manifestation code without its correctly sequenced etiology code.

Example:
Chapter 19: "Injury, Poisoning, and certain other Consequences of External Causes"
Use additional code to identify:
any retained foreign body, if applicable (Z18.-)
If a patient is presenting with a retained foreign body, the Z code would be sequenced after the code from Chapter 19.

Code Also

The "Code Also" instructional note indicates that two codes may be required to fully describe a condition, but unlike "Code First" or "Use additional code," the sequence depends on whichever condition is the primary reason for the encounter. If the "Code Also" information is not applicable, it is not required that it be reported.

Example:
M41.4- "Neuromuscular scoliosis"
Code Also
underlying condition

Notes

Notes are generally added under a chapter or a block, providing additional information necessary to understanding the codes in the chapter and their use. These notes are different than the instructional notations listed previously.

Example:
G43- "Migraine"
Notes:
the following terms are to be considered equivalent to intractable: pharmacoresistant (pharmacologically resistant), treatment resistant, refractory (medically) and poorly controlled

ChiroCode Enhancements to the Tabular List

To further assist in accurate coding, ChiroCode created two additional instructional notes which are found in this publication's presentation of the Tabular List.

See Guidelines

In the Tabular List of this codebook, "See guidelines" indicates that the referenced section of the *ICD-10-CM Official Guidelines for Coding and Reporting* contains information necessary to correctly code a condition. Make sure to review those guidelines before selecting a code.

Example:
E11- "Type 2 Diabetes Mellitus"
See guidelines:
1;C.4.a.2

ICD-10-CM Indicators

Special ICD-10-CM edits are included in this publication to assist with accurate ICD-10-CM code selection and reporting. These edits have been identified as "indicators." Appropriately employing them may improve coding accuracy and reduce claim denials. Automatic payer edits can identify and deny claims that fail to meet the basic edits identified here. Become familiar with the edits that affect your organization to avoid unnecessary claim denials.

Figure A.1 in Appendix A — Coding Reference Tables explains the indicators listed in the Tabular List. Familiarize yourself with them to identify situations in which proper sequencing, age, gender, or other indicators play a primary role in proper code reporting and reimbursement.

Some common outpatient denials include:

- Reporting a manifestation code as the first-listed diagnosis
- Coding a newborn-specific code for infants over 28 days of age
- Reporting specific Z codes as first-listed primary diagnoses
- Leaving off CCs and MCCs that could otherwise increase reimbursement.

These indicators will appear in the Tabular List, in their abbreviated format, below the codes they apply to. Some codes will have multiple indicators while others may have non. Below is an example of how a code will look with the indicators.

Example:
M42.1- "Adult osteochondrosis of spine"
Alerts:
Adult Dx, Age: 15-124

Notes

Ch1

1. Diagnosis Coding Essentials

General Coding Guidelines

General coding guidelines or rules are found in Section *I.B.* of the *ICD-10-CM Official Guidelines for Coding and Reporting*. These rules apply to the entire code set. Abridged official guidelines, relevant to chiropractic, are found in Appendix B, and the complete guidelines can be accessed at FindACode.com (with subscription) or in the *ICD-10-CM Comprehensive CodeBook*. Like the conventions of the preceding section, they provide a framework which, if followed, makes ICD-10-CM more logical and thus easier to use.

Locating a Code

The proper way to find the correct code(s) for a clinical scenario begins by first identifying the main term(s) in the provider documentation. If the provider is familiar with the terminology preferred by ICD-10-CM, it will be easier to locate the term in the Alphabetic Index. Once the Index indicates a code or codes, they should be verified using the Tabular List. Then, the instructional notations should be followed to ensure proper code selection.

Book: See Chapter 2 – Provider Documentation Training for more help with training your provider(s) on documentation as it pertains to ICD-10-CM.

Please note that the Alphabetic Index does not always provide the full code. Important coding information such as guidelines (e.g., Excludes1, Code First), laterality, or the seventh character may only be found in the Tabular List. Remember, in this codebook, incomplete codes will end with a hyphen (-) or, if the seventh character is required, an underscore (_). A code is invalid if it does not include the full number of characters required for that code.

Diagnosis codes must be used and reported with the highest number of characters available. Any reported code must be fully supported by the documentation. Three-character codes may only be used if there are no other subdivisions available.

Signs and Symptoms

Codes that describe symptoms and signs, as opposed to diagnoses, are acceptable for reporting purposes when a related definitive diagnosis has not been established (confirmed) by the provider. Chapter 18 of the Tabular List contains many, but not all, possible codes for reporting symptoms. Each healthcare encounter should be coded to the highest level of certainty known for that encounter.

Signs and symptoms that are associated routinely with a disease process should not be assigned as additional codes; however, they may be coded if they are not typically associated with the condition.

Example:

M54.2 "Cervicalgia" would not need to be coded with **S16.1xxA** "Strain of muscle, fascia, and tendon at neck level, initial encounter" because a neck muscle strain is routinely associated with neck pain. However, **R11.Ø** "Nausea" might be coded in addition because it is not routinely associated with neck muscle strain.

Acute and Chronic Conditions

If the same condition is described as both acute (subacute) and chronic (e.g., a flare up of a chronic condition), and separate subentries exist in the Alphabetic Index at the same indentation level, both conditions should be coded. However, it is necessary to sequence/report the acute (subacute) code first.

Example:

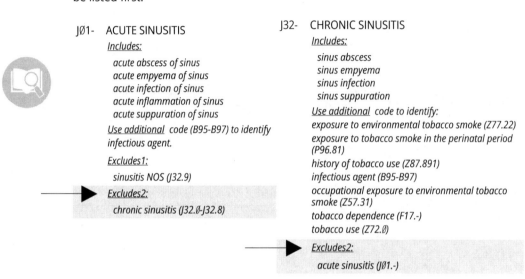

J32- is the category for chronic sinusitis, and JØ1- is the category for acute sinusitis. Each entry in the Tabular List includes an Excludes2 note for the other, indicating that both can be coded on the same claim. However, the acute code (from JØ1-) should be listed first.

JØ1- ACUTE SINUSITIS

Includes:

acute abscess of sinus
acute empyema of sinus
acute infection of sinus
acute inflammation of sinus
acute suppuration of sinus

Use additional code (B95-B97) to identify infectious agent.

Excludes1:

sinusitis NOS (J32.9)

Excludes2:

chronic sinusitis (J32.Ø-J32.8)

J32- CHRONIC SINUSITIS

Includes:

sinus abscess
sinus empyema
sinus infection
sinus suppuration

Use additional code to identify:

exposure to environmental tobacco smoke (Z77.22)
exposure to tobacco smoke in the perinatal period (P96.81)
history of tobacco use (Z87.891)
infectious agent (B95-B97)
occupational exposure to environmental tobacco smoke (Z57.31)
tobacco dependence (F17.-)
tobacco use (Z72.Ø)

Excludes2:

acute sinusitis (JØ1.-)

Combination Code

A combination code is a single code used to classify:

- Two diagnoses, or
- A diagnosis with an associated secondary process (manifestation), or
- A diagnosis with an associated complication.

These codes can be identified in the Alphabetic Index and by reading the inclusion and exclusion notes in the Tabular List. Multiple codes should not be used when a combination code is available that fully describes the condition. However, an additional code may also be used if the combination code lacks the specificity needed.

Example:
Even though there are codes for "lumbago" **(M54.50)** and for "sciatica, right" **(M54.31)**, if both have been documented in the clinical record, the correct code would be **M54.41** "Lumbago with sciatica, right."

Sequela (Late Effects)

A sequela is a residual effect, condition produced, or complication after the acute phase of an illness or injury has terminated. One example would be a scar formation as the sequela of a burn. There is no time limit on sequela; they may occur immediately (e.g., paralysis after a cerebral infarction) or months later (e.g., scar tissue following major trauma). The condition caused by the initial injury would be listed first. The second code, which ends with the letter "S" to indicate "sequela," would be the illness or injury that is no longer present, but led to the condition for which the patient is currently seeking treatment.

Example:
A patient presents with low back pain six months after being released from care for a low back sprain. The proper way to code this encounter, assuming that the sprain is resolved, but clearly documented as the cause of the current pain, would be:

M54.50 "Low back pain, unspecified"

followed by

S33.5xxS "Sprain of ligaments of lumbar spine, sequela"

Book: Please see Appendix B – ICD-10-CM Abridged Official Guidelines, Section *I.B.1Ø* for more information.

Note: A third party might deny payment based on the fact that they consider the sequela to be the liability of whoever is financially responsible for the initial condition.

Laterality

Many ICD-10-CM codes include the option to report the condition as occurring on the right side, left side, or bilaterally. When no bilateral code is available, but the condition is documented as bilateral, both codes for the right and left sides should be reported. If the side is not identified in the medical record, then an unspecified code must be used. Often, the number "1" is used to identify the right side and "2" is used to identify the left side, with "3" identifying the condition as occurring bilaterally (or unspecified if a bilateral code option was not created). Other conditions, however, may use different numbers to identify laterality so always confirm with the Tabular List before final code selection.

Note: Each unique ICD-10-CM code may be reported only once for an encounter, even if it is a bilateral condition and laterality choices are not available (i.e., there isn't a choice for right and/or left). For example, if a patient has a muscle spasm in the right and left calf, the code **M62.831** "Muscle spasm of calf," would only be reported once since there is no right, left, or bilateral code for this condition. The documentation will have to be relied upon to convey this information when the code(s) alone are not descriptive enough.

Syndromes

The Alphabetic Index will provide guidance for coding syndromes most of the time, but when it does not, code the documented manifestations of the syndrome. If there are manifestations that are not an integral part of the disease process, then additional codes may be assigned.

Unspecified Codes

There may be situations where an unspecified code is the appropriate code choice. These codes should be reported when they most accurately reflect what is known about the patient's condition at the time of that encounter. It would be inappropriate to select a specific code not supported by the medical record or to conduct medically unnecessary diagnostic testing in order to determine a more specific code.

Example:

The ICD-10-CM codes for ankle sprain specify the injured ligament, but in some cases, that may be difficult to determine. The mechanism of injury could be unclear and/or swelling of the ankle could make the examination inconclusive. Performing an MRI or a CT scan just for the sake of code selection would be inappropriate, therefore the right code might be: **S93.4Ø2A** "Sprain of unspecified ligament, left ankle, initial encounter."

There are three scenarios where reporting an unspecified code is the *incorrect* approach:

1. **The code set is not specific enough.** If a diagnosis is confirmed, but ICD-10-CM does not have a specific code that matches the diagnosis, the NEC code should be used, not the unspecified.
2. **The provider's documentation does not provide enough detail to select a more specific code.** If this is the case, query the provider for additional information about the encounter. Ensure that you are familiar with the guidelines and code options needed for complete and accurate documentation. See Appendix C – Provider Documentation Guides for a summarization of the guidelines and code options for common diagnoses.
3. **The diagnosis is unconfirmed.** If terms such as "rule out," "probable," "suspected," etc. are used, the guidelines pertaining to uncertain diagnoses must be adhered to. It is not as simple as reporting the unspecified code option. See the alert under "Uncertain Diagnosis" for information on coding these scenarios.

Tip: Always code to the highest level of certainty known for a given encounter.

Default Code

When a code is listed next to a main term in the Alphabetic Index, it represents the condition that is most commonly associated with the main term, or is the unspecified code for the condition. If the documentation provides the term, but not any additional information, the default code should be reported.

Example:

(Alphabetic Index) **Disorder disc (intervertebral) M51.9**
(Tabular List) **M51.9** "Unspecified thoracic, thoracolumbar, and lumbosacral disc disorder"

Typically, there are more specific options available for default codes. As long as the documentation provides the necessary information, the more specific code should always be used.

Book: Since the default code is often not specific, be sure to review other entries near it in either the Alphabetic Index or the Tabular List. Additionally, Chapter 2 – Provider Documentation Training and Appendix C – Provider Documentation Guides contain information on choosing the most specific code for a patient encounter.

Alert — The End of ICD-10-CM Flexibility on Unspecified Codes:

During the first year of ICD-10-CM implementation, CMS allowed the use of unspecified codes as long as they were done in an effort to smooth the transition process to an unfamiliar code set. As of October 1, 2016, providers must choose the highest specificity code, based on the documented encounter, if they want reimbursement for services provided.

Uncertain Diagnosis

Section *IV.H* of *ICD-10-CM Official Guidelines for Coding and Reporting* instructs that diagnoses documented as "probable," "suspected," "questionable," "rule out," "working diagnosis," or other similar terms indicating uncertainty should be coded differently depending on the setting.

Example:
M5Ø.121 "Cervical disc disorder at C4-C5 level with radiculopathy" might only be coded after an MRI has allowed the provider to be certain. Until then, a less specific diagnosis such as **M54.12** "Cervical radiculopathy" should be reported.

Alert — Coding an unconfirmed diagnosis is different depending on where the services are provided.

Professionals: In a professional setting, unconfirmed diagnoses (e.g., "possible," "rule out," "likely," "probable") should never be coded. For example, a patient presenting with lower right quadrant pain, nausea and vomiting, possible appendicitis should have the encounter coded with these symptoms until a confirmed diagnosis is documented. Make sure the symptoms are coded, not an unspecified code.

Facilities: In the facility setting, a patient who presents with the same symptoms and has an unconfirmed diagnosis of "possible appendicitis" would have the encounter coded as a confirmed diagnosis. Because the symptoms are explained by the condition, the symptoms would not be coded.

Code All Documented Coexisting Conditions

Section *IV.J* of the *ICD-10-CM Official Guidelines for Coding and Reporting* states that "all documented conditions that coexist at the time of the encounter/visit, and require or affect patient care, treatment, or management" should also be coded. Co-morbid conditions may affect the treatment plan and thus affect the patient care for that visit even if the patient receives no treatment for the co-morbid condition. Any co-morbidity considered when determining how the patient will be treated should be documented, even if the co-morbidity does not fall under the provider's specialty. However, conditions that were previously treated, no longer exist, and have no effect on the treatment of the current condition need not be coded.

Tip: As an example, in some circumstances a provider may treat a pregnant patient for a condition unrelated to, and not affecting, her pregnancy. In such a situation, assigning code **Z33.1** "Pregnant state, incidental" will allow the healthcare provider to acknowledge the pregnant state of the patient even if the treatment plan and condition are unaffected by the pregnancy. The codes found in Chapter 15 – Pregnancy, Childbirth, and the Puerperium of the Tabular List are reserved for conditions related to or aggravated by the pregnancy, childbirth, or by the puerperium. These codes can be reported by any type of provider as long as the obstetric condition is being managed by the provider or it affects patient care.

Chapter Specific Guidelines

Section *I.C* of the *ICD-10-CM Official Guidelines for Coding and Reporting* makes up about 80% of the official guidelines. There is a separate section for each of the 22 chapters. The portions of the guidelines that are likely to apply to chiropractic care are included in Appendix B – ICD-10-CM Abridged Official Guidelines.

Website: For the complete guidelines, including Sections II, III, and IV, visit FindACode.com.

Chiropractic Coding Tips

Diagnoses Code Hierarchy

According to Section *IV.G* of the *ICD-10-CM Official Guidelines for Coding and Reporting,* the first reported code should be the diagnosis, condition, problem or other reason for the encounter/visit shown in the medical record to be chiefly responsible for the services provided. Section *I.C.19.b* says that "The code for the most serious injury, as determined by the provider and the focus of treatment, is sequenced first." For chiropractic care, it should be noted that some Medicare Administrative Contractors (MACs) have lists of diagnosis codes which are grouped as warranting either short, moderate, or long term treatment based on severity. These three sources are the rationale for the sequencing suggestion provided here. Many payers require that the appropriate subluxation (or segmental dysfunction) code is listed first.

Alert: Consider the following hierarchy as a possible suggestion, but please remember that the provider's clinical judgment should always prevail when determining the order of reporting diagnoses.

- Nerve related disorders (e.g., radiculopathy)
- Acute injuries (e.g., sprains and strains)
- Structural diagnoses (e.g., degenerative disc disease)
- Functional diagnoses (e.g., difficulty with walking)
- Soft tissue problems (e.g., myalgia)
- Symptoms (e.g., neck pain)
- Complicating factors/comorbidities (e.g., diabetes)
- External causes (e.g., place and activity)

The "Subluxation"

Chiropractors use many of the same diagnosis codes as other healthcare providers who treat conditions of the nervous system, skeletal system, and muscular system. Yet, there is one diagnosis that is unique to doctors of chiropractic. It is the so-called vertebral "subluxation." It is the diagnosis that justifies the performance of a Chiropractic Manipulative Treatment, or adjustment; this is, by far, the most commonly performed procedure in a chiropractic setting.

Unfortunately, subluxation is defined differently by different groups. In a typical medical dictionary, it is simply a "partial dislocation," which implies some sort of torn ligaments and/or trauma. However, a different definition, such as the following from Medicare, should be considered by the chiropractic physician.

> *"A motion segment, in which alignment, movement integrity and/or physiological function of the spine are altered although contact between joint surfaces remains intact. For the purposes of Medicare, subluxation means an incomplete dislocation, off-centering, misalignment, fixation, or abnormal spacing of the vertebra anatomically."*

A recent OIG report about chiropractic claims says:

> *"Medicare requires that chiropractic claims have a primary diagnosis of "subluxation" for payment, but there is no diagnosis code that contains the word "subluxation." CMS has instructed chiropractors to use the diagnosis codes that indicate nonallopathic lesions of the spine."*

These codes were found in the 739- category in ICD-9-CM. The inclusion terms for the 739- category included "segmental and somatic dysfunction," but made no mention of the word "subluxation." Nonetheless, most private payers followed Medicare's lead and accepted the 739- category as a justification to provide Chiropractic Manipulative Treatment (the 9894X codes from the CPT codebook).

Store: See Chapter 6.3 – Common Procedure Codes & Tips in the *ChiroCode DeskBook* for more on 9894X procedure codes. It can be purchased at ChiroCode.com.

The ICD-10-CM code set brought a few new considerations, but not necessarily a solution. The clear replacement for 739- codes are the M99.Ø- codes, which are "segmental and somatic dysfunction." The word "subluxation" is still missing; nonetheless these are the codes that most Medicare contractors have instructed chiropractors to use, and private payers appear to have followed suit.

The next group of codes in the Tabular List are in the M99.1- subcategory, which is defined as "subluxation complex (vertebral)." These codes appear to use the verbiage many chiropractors are looking for, but unfortunately, they are **not** listed on most Medicare approved lists. This may be because the word "subluxation" in these codes still means "partial dislocation" to coders and payers which may be contraindicated for spinal manipulation. Therefore, they should not be used as justification for manipulation, despite the fact that they are valid codes.

The injury codes of Chapter 19 of ICD-10-CM also offer codes which use the term subluxation, which is commonly used by doctors of chiropractic: S13.1- for cervical subluxations, S23.1- for thoracic subluxations, and S33.1- for lumbar subluxations (with the sixth character "Ø"). There are several reasons why these codes are **not** the best option.

- They have been mapped (by GEMs) to the old 839- category, which was not payable by Medicare and considered by many to be contraindicated for CMT.
- Chapter 19 codes describe acute injuries, and the "Includes" list for each of these categories include sprains and other serious traumatic issues. Nonetheless there is no need to code sprains in addition to traumatic subluxations. Many chiropractic patients can have a chiropractic "subluxation" without this kind of trauma.
- The 5th character of these codes indicate a specific interspace, such as C2/C3 or L4/L5. If the patient encounter is not documented this way, then these codes should **not** be used. This differs from a classic chiropractic subluxation which is often listed as a specific segment (rather than the space between two segments) that is misaligned or fixated.
- There are no subluxation codes offered in these ranges for L5/S1 or the sacroiliac joints which are joints that are typically treated by chiropractors.
- These codes also require a seventh character to designate the episode of care, which may be confusing as it is forced into a recurring treatment model. See "Episode of Care" in the following segment for more information.

For these reasons, it is apparent that the injury codes (S13-, S23-, and S33-) do not match the chiropractic definition of a subluxation; nonetheless they are fine if the provider is trying to describe a partial dislocation which may need to be immobilized **rather** than manipulated.

The M99.Ø- codes remain the best option to code for a chiropractic subluxation and justify the need for chiropractic manipulation. Regardless of code selection, it is essential for the documentation to support the diagnosis code selected for a claim. If it is a traumatic subluxation which is more indicative of the general medical terminology of "subluxation," the most correct code would be from Chapter 19, the "S" injury codes. If it is a "subluxation complex," clinically supporting the need for spinal manipulation, then the M99.1- codes are the best match. Since both of these terms are potentially prone to misinterpretation, it may be best to document something like "segmental dysfunction (subluxation)" so that the M99.Ø- codes are the clear choice. Including the word "subluxation" in the documentation in parentheses lets the payer know that the provider is using the preferred code, while still documenting with common chiropractic terminology.

Book: See Chapter 3 – Common Diagnosis Codes & Tips for more information about subluxation codes.

Episode of Care

While chiropractic physicians primarily use the chronic and recurrent musculoskeletal conditions from Chapter 13 – Diseases of the Musculoskeletal System and Connective Tissue, in the Tabular List, the sprain and strain codes are found in Chapter 19 – Injury, Poisoning, and Certain other Consequences of External Causes. The Chapter 19 codes are easily identifiable because they begin with the letter "S." It is important to understand that sprain and strain codes require the addition of a 7th character extension that specifies the episode of care or encounter.

The three choices for most of the relevant ICD-10-CM codes used by chiropractors are:

A: Initial encounter
D: Subsequent encounter
S: Sequela

The following official guidelines below (with emphasis added), from Section *I.C.19.a,* for 7th characters provide more instruction on the proper use of these characters:

> While the patient may be seen by a new or different provider over the course of treatment for an injury, assignment of the 7th character is based on whether the patient is undergoing **active treatment** and not whether the provider is seeing the patient for the first time.
>
> 7th character "A" initial encounter, is used while the patient is receiving **active treatment** for a condition. Examples of active treatment are surgical treatment, emergency department encounters, and evaluation and **continuing treatment** by the same or a different physician.
>
> 7th character "D" subsequent encounter, is used for encounters after the patient has received active treatment of a condition and is receiving routine care for the condition during the **healing or recovery phase.** Examples of subsequent care are cast change or removal, an X-ray to check healing status of fracture, removal of external or internal fixation device, medication adjustment, other **aftercare, and follow-up** visits following treatment of the injury or condition.

Book: See "Sequela (Late Effects)" on page 25 for more information on the 7th character "S" sequela.

If it were assumed that "encounter" is synonymous with "visit," the "A" would be used for the first visit and the "D" for all other visits that follow. The "A" indicates "initial encounter," *but* it may be more clearly described as "active treatment" as outlined in the official guidelines. Upon further examination, since soft tissue injuries, such as sprains and strains, often require ongoing therapies, this makes the 7th character choice a little more confusing. The "D" should be used when active treatment ends rather than at the second visit.

Suppose a patient presents with **S16.1xxA** "Strain of muscles, fascia, and tendon at neck level, initial encounter." The code set does not define a point in time when it would be appropriate to begin using the "D" as the 7th character. Rather, it says is that this would be appropriate once the patient has entered the "healing or recovery phase of care" or once the patient is in "aftercare or follow-up." The clinician must decide when this transition occurs, whether it is two days, two weeks, or two months after care begins.

To further complicate matters, there is generally no reimbursement for chiropractic care once the patient is no longer progressing (maintenance care). The official guidelines define the "D" for subsequent encounter to be appropriate with "recovery" and "follow-up" which may be synonymous with maintenance care. Many Medicare Administrative Contractors provide lists of diagnosis codes that they allow chiropractors to use, and most of those lists include codes that end only in "A." This implies that chiropractors will only be reimbursed while the patient is in "active treatment."

Alert — Payers have indicated that "A" is the preferred option, therefore it may be prudent for doctors of chiropractic to use the "A" with injury codes for as long as they deem the patient to be receiving "active treatment" (that is, as long as the patient continues to progress). When the patient ceases to progress, but the provider wishes to continue treatment to facilitate healing, then the "D" should be used. Since it is possible that payers may not cover treatment when the "D" is used, providers need to ensure that the patient understands that they may need to pay out of pocket for these services.

Store: See Chapter 1.1 – Insurance & Reimbursement Essentials in the *ChiroCode DeskBook* for a more thorough discussion regarding how to appropriately establish patient financial responsibility. It can be purchased at ChiroCode.com.

External Cause Codes

Chapter 20 of the Tabular List includes codes from VØØ to Y99 which cover external causes of morbidity. These codes don't actually describe a condition, rather they just provide additional data, which can be useful for injury research and evaluation of injury prevention strategies. This is accomplished by identifying:

- how the injury or health condition happened (cause),
- the intent (unintentional or accidental; or intentional, such as suicide or assault),
- the place where the event occurred,
- the activity of the patient at the time of the event, and
- the person's status (e.g., civilian, military).

The chapter includes codes that begin with the letters V, W, X, and Y and they are divided into 29 blocks, such as water transport accidents V90-V94, slipping, tripping, stumbling and falls W00-W19, and exposure to animate mechanical forces W50-W64. Although there is no national requirement for mandatory external cause code reporting, voluntary reporting is encouraged. It may be helpful to review the chapter specific guidelines for external cause codes found in Section *I.C.20* in Appendix B. Several guidelines and definitions are also listed at the beginning of Chapter 20 within the Tabular List. A review of these rules is essential for a complete understanding of external cause code reporting.

Chiropractors may elect to add these codes to personal injury cases because they could potentially allow third parties to obtain information directly from the claim itself, without needing to review the medical records. Auto injury claims may use codes beginning with the letter "V," which are all transport accidents. There are 12 groups of transport accident types, and the first two characters identify the vehicle or type of transportation. The codes most likely to apply to common chiropractic cases begin with V4- for car occupants. The next character identifies the object that was struck. For example, the following code might be used on the claim for a passenger of a car who was injured when the car struck a pick-up truck in traffic.

V43.63xA "Car passenger injured in collision with pick-up truck in traffic accident, initial encounter"

When using these codes, it is essential for all of this information to be documented in the record because the claim must be a reflection of the documentation. Note that these codes should never be sequenced first since their only purpose is to provide additional data. The primary reason for the encounter should always be listed first. Place (Y92-) and activity (Y93-) codes only need to be reported on the first encounter.

Book: See Chapter 3 – Common Diagnosis Codes & Tips for some common external cause codes applicable to chiropractors.

Wellness Visits

Some diagnosis codes do not actually describe a condition, rather they simply explain the reason for an encounter with a health care provider. Classic medical examples include encounters for vaccines or health screenings. In other words, these patients have no complaints, therefore there is no condition to report. In this type of case, ICD-10 codes can still explain the reason for the encounter. These codes are found in Chapter 21 of the Tabular List. They are easy to identify because they all start with the letter "Z."

If a patient presents for an annual wellness exam (which would most appropriately be reported with Evaluation and Management codes from the range 99381-99397 Preventive Medicine Service), a few possible ICD-10 codes a healthcare provider might use are:

Z00.00 "Encounter for general adult medical examination without abnormal findings"

Z00.8 "Other encounter for general examination without complaint, suspected, or reported diagnosis"

The first code fits better for an annual general wellness check-up. The second might best describe an encounter for an annual exam for a patient receiving ongoing chiropractic wellness care. Keep in mind that most third-party payers do not reimburse chiropractors for these types of encounters, and the patient would be required to pay out-of-pocket. But it may be beneficial to use these codes so that a clinic can later pull reports that help track how many wellness exams are performed for a certain time period.

Wellness, or maintenance adjustments (HCPCS code S8990 Physical or manipulative therapy performed for maintenance rather than restoration) might work well with the following Z codes:

Z41.8 "Other encounter for procedure for purpose other than remedying health state"

Z51.5 "Encounter for palliative care"

These codes describe an encounter for a procedure, such as chiropractic manipulation, rather than an exam, like the ZØØ- codes suggested above. No health state is being remedied since the patient does not have any complaints. Palliative refers to alleviating a problem without remedying the underlying cause.

While these visits are also not likely to be reimbursed by third parties, it may be logical to assume that a patient would only receive an adjustment if a subluxation were found. Therefore, an additional code to consider for a wellness patient might be:

M99.1- Subluxation complex (vertebral)

The fifth character designates the anatomic region. These codes are not recognized as payable by many payers, but they seem to have been created just for chiropractors. The M99.Ø- Segmental and somatic dysfunction codes are those typically used for reimbursable encounters when Chiropractic Manipulative Treatment (CMT codes 98940-98942) is performed. M99.1- might be perfect to describe a wellness patient, along with, or in place of, **Z41.8.** In any case, these codes would likely only be used for internal purposes.

Store: See Chapter 6.3 – Common Procedure Codes & Tips in the *ChiroCode DeskBook* for coding and documentation tips on CMT codes. It can be purchased at ChiroCode.com.

Notes:

Notes:

Notes

2. Provider Documentation Training

Diagnosis codes provide valuable information which claims reviewers can use to determine if the care provided is medically necessary. However, the codes are only as good as the medical record which was used to select them. Documentation has many functions, but, for the provider, one of the most significant may be its relationship to reimbursement. This discussion is limited to the documentation necessary to support the diagnosis codes.

Store: Chapter 4 – Documentation, in the *ChiroCode DeskBook*, includes a more complete discussion of how to properly document the patient encounter in order to establish medical necessity. It contains several chapters dedicated to helping a doctor of chiropractic understand how to effectively communicate with third parties.

Figure 2.1

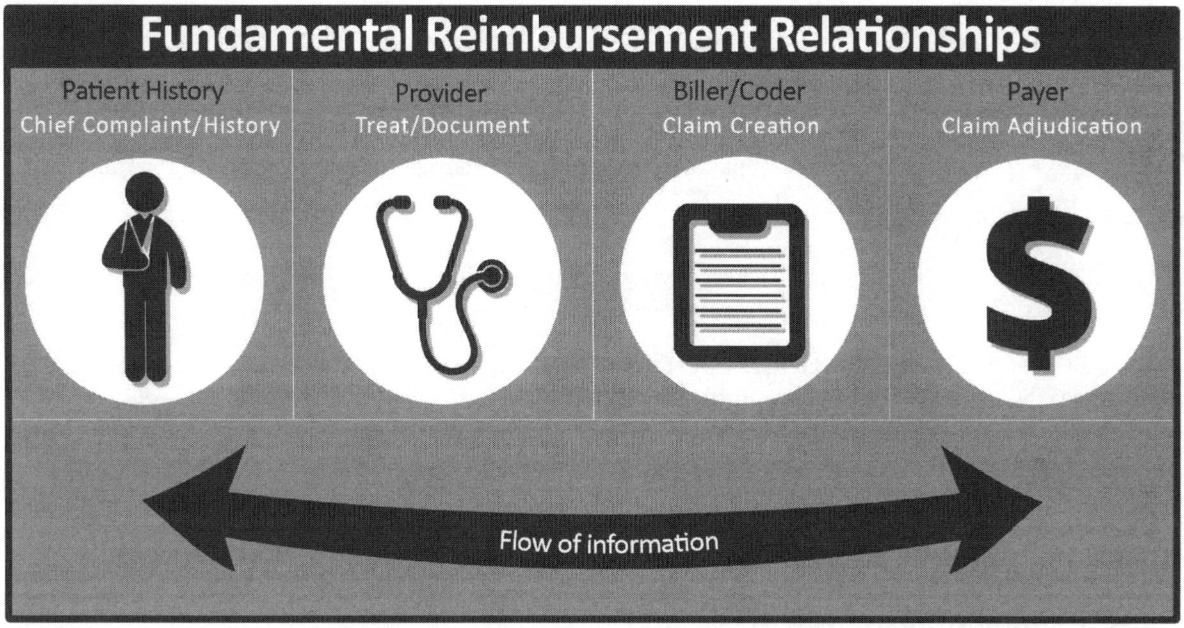

Figure 2.1 depicts the relationship between the parties involved in the healthcare reimbursement process. It all begins with an encounter, initiated by a patient who seeks care. The patient presents with a chief complaint and provides a health history. This information then becomes part of the healthcare record and the provider begins to document all relevant information regarding the patient and provide care. If someone were to review the record created by the provider, and interview the patient, the information should match.

Next, it is the responsibility of a biller and/or coder to translate the information from the medical record into a claim (paper or electronic). Ideally, the codes chosen will match exactly what was documented, which in turn matches what actually happened to the patient during the encounter. In order for this to happen, and the entire process to flow smoothly, both the provider and the biller must understand coding rules, descriptions, and documentation requirements. This publication was designed with that goal in mind. "*Provider Documentation Guides*™" and the "Diagnostic Statement," which are explained in this chapter, are two ways to accomplish that goal. Finally, the claim form with all the right codes goes to the payer. The payer then applies their payment policies, which ideally, are satisfied by the information found on the submitted claim. In some cases, the payer might request additional information from either the provider or the patient. With proper communication between all of these groups, additional requests for information should be minimal.

Building Provider Documentation Guides (PDGs)

ChiroCode formulated a method for helping providers become proficient with the ICD-10-CM documentation and coding requirements for the conditions they encounter most often. The process, which we call a *Provider Documentation Guide (PDG)*, is explained here and can be used with any ICD-10-CM code. It is a one to two page summary of all the components a provider and coder need to know about a condition. Each *PDG* is like a ready-made ten minute training which could be used in weekly office meetings to improve both ICD-10-CM documentation and code selection.

The following items are all included in each *Provider Documentation Guide:*

1. The condition (i.e., diagnosis), including the ICD-10-CM code or code range
2. Helpful information (e.g., terminology, what to document, list for the provider, and notes for the coder)
3. Applicable instructional notes/guidelines and indicator(s) at the chapter and block levels
4. Information conveyed by each character level with instructional notes, guidelines, and indicators applicable at the category and subcategory levels.

Once all of this information is gathered, it can be listed on a complete *Provider Documentation Guide (PDG).* When a patient presents with the condition, the *PDG* acts as a tool to help the provider ensure that all the necessary information is documented. It also assists the biller/coder by enabling them to quickly check relevant guidelines at a glance. Without a *PDG*, it would be necessary to thoroughly review multiple pages of the Tabular List and guidelines until all the correct information has been gathered. Providers may, of course, create their own *PDGs* using the steps outlined here. As an example, the following is a completed *PDG* for M54.4- "Lumbago with Sciatica," created by ChiroCode.

Item 1: Condition

The first item to identify is the condition, which serves as the title. The terms within the title can be based on common names for the condition, the exact medical term, or most often, the category of the codes this *PDG's* range covers.

Also included in the first item is the ICD-10-CM code or code range. Most *PDGs* cover several diagnoses, often grouping together laterality and anatomic site codes for more convenient access.

Lumbago with Sciatica

ICD-1Ø-CM: M54.4Ø - M54.42

Item 2: Helpful Information

Next is a summary of the other items to include in documentation. It can include relevant definitions, critical guidelines, and a brief description of what needs to be documented in order to support each character. *PDGs* help to clarify this information.

What to Document

3rd Character: Type of dorsopathy
4th Character: Type of dorsalgia
5th Character: Laterality

Document:
-Any external cause

Terminology:
Lumbago: Pain in the muscles and joints of the lower back.
Sciatica: Compression of a spinal nerve root, often due to intervertebral disc degeneration, causing pain in the back, hip, and leg.

For some conditions, this summary may be particularly useful, but in this instance, more information is needed if the provider wants to create a record that completely supports the diagnosis. Tips and definitions can be especially helpful for beginners or coders who lack sufficient training in anatomy or pathology.

Item 3: Applicable Guidelines at the Chapter and Block Level

The next piece of a *PDG* summarizes the relevant guidelines. In this case, there are important guidelines at the beginning of Chapter 13 of the Tabular List that apply to all "M" codes. There are also guidelines at the second block level.

3. Diseases of the musculoskeletal system and connective tissue (MØØ-M99)

Notes:

Use an external cause code following the code for the musculoskeletal condition, if applicable, to identify the cause of the musculoskeletal condition

Excludes2:

arthropathic psoriasis (L4Ø.5-)
certain conditions originating in the perinatal period (PØ4-P96)
certain infectious and parasitic diseases (AØØ-B99)
compartment syndrome (traumatic) (T79.A-)
complications of pregnancy, childbirth and the puerperium (OØØ-O9A)
congenital malformations, deformations, and chromosomal abnormalities (QØØ-Q99)
endocrine, nutritional and metabolic diseases (EØØ-E88)
injury, poisoning and certain other consequences of external causes (SØØ-T88)
neoplasms (CØØ-D49)
symptoms, signs and abnormal clinical and laboratory findings, not elsewhere classified (RØØ-R94)

DORSOPATHIES (M4Ø-M54)

OTHER DORSOPATHIES (M5Ø-M54)

Excludes1:

current injury - see injury of spine by body region
discitis NOS (M46.4-)

While most of the guidelines in this example may not pertain to typical chiropractic cases, it is important to be aware of them so they can be applied if necessary. For example, the Excludes1 note for the block (M5Ø-M54) states that M46.4- "Discitis, NOS" is mutually exclusive to every code within the block, and therefore, should not be used on the same date of service for the same patient.

Items 4–8: Third, Fourth, Fifth, Sixth, and Seventh Character Information

These remaining sections go into detail about each character in the code. Each of these sections will contain:

- A restatement of what needs to be documented.
- Any applicable instructional notes/guidelines. Remember that guidelines showing up at one level (i.e., category, subcategory, etc.) apply to all downstream codes. In other words, a guideline appearing at the category level applies at the subcategory and code levels as well.
- A list of all the possible categories, subcategories, or codes for a given character; the one that narrows the code choices toward the ICD-10-CM code for the condition will be highlighted.

If a seventh character exists for a given code or group of codes, highlighting may only occur to the fifth or sixth character, followed by a list of seventh character options to choose from. This allows the provider or individual using the *PDG* to see all the codes affected by the *PDG* in one area rather than spread across multiple *PDGs*.

Each *PDG* will have a section for all seven characters, even if they are not used, as a way to standardize the look of *PDGs* and help the provider ensure that all necessary information has been documented.

Third Character Information

3rd Character	
Document: Type of dorsopathy	
M5Ø-	Cervical disc disorders
M51-	Thoracic, thoracolumbar, and lumbosacral intervertebral disc disorders
M53-	Other and unspecified dorsopathies, not elsewhere classified
M54-	Dorsalgia

In this figure, the first thing shown is a reminder of what needs to be documented, followed by a listing of each option. M54- "Dorsalgia" is highlighted because that is the category where sciatica is found. If there were additional guidelines in the Tabular List at this level, they could be listed here.

Fourth Character Information

4th Character	
Document: Type and Anatomic site	
Excludes1: psychogenic dorsalgia (F45.41)	
M54.Ø-	Panniculitis affecting regions of neck and back
M54.1-	Radiculopathy
M54.2	Cervicalgia
M54.3-	Sciatica
M54.4-	Lumbago with sciatica
M54.5-	Low back pain
M54.6	Pain in thoracic spine
M54.8-	Other dorsalgia
M54.9	Dorsalgia, unspecified

What to document for the fourth character is listed first, followed by all of the options. The options in bold are complete, valid codes (the highest level of specificity). The ones with a hyphen (-) need more characters before they are complete. Also note that there is another Excludes1 note at this level. It means that code **F45.41** is mutually exclusive to any code that begins with M54- and should be considered instead of, but not in addition to, one of these codes. For this example, M54.4- "Lumbago with sciatica" is highlighted. The hyphen makes it clear that a fifth character is required.

Fifth Character Information

5th Character

Document: Laterality

Excludes1:
lumbago with sciatica due to intervertebral disc disorder (M51.1-)

M54.40	Lumbago with sciatica, unspecified side
M54.41	Lumbago with sciatica, right side
M54.42	Lumbago with sciatica, left side

The first thing listed is the "what to document" requirement, followed by the three code choices. Each one is in bold, so there is no need to go further, looking for a sixth or seventh character. Once again there is an Excludes1 note at this level which lets the provider and biller/coder know that lumbago with sciatica due to a disc problem would be coded in place of one of the options from the M54.4- subcategory. Documentation should provide the detail necessary to make that determination.

Sixth and Seventh Character Information

The *Provider Documentation Guides* published by ChiroCode list all seven characters as a way to standardize each *PDG*.

6th Character

N/A

7th Character

N/A

Notes

For this condition, the last two character positions do not apply. This *PDG* also includes a place for additional notes, which allows for further customization of the guide if necessary. Bringing all of these items together creates a single *PDG* for a single condition.

Book: Appendix C – Provider Documentation Guides contains a selection of *PDGs* for common diagnoses.

Diagnostic Statement

As indicated at the beginning of this chapter, using a Diagnostic Statement (sometimes called a Problem Statement, or Clinical Impression as part of an assessment) is another way to ensure a smooth flow of information between all parties involved in the Fundamental Reimbursement Relationships (*see Figure 2.1*).

Essentially, a Diagnostic Statement is a summary of the healthcare provider's impression of the patient history and exam findings, worded in a manner that anyone with an understanding of ICD-10-CM can easily find what they are looking for when auditing a record, regardless of their level of familiarity of terms and phrases used within the chiropractic specialty. The Diagnostic Statement, included in an initial report, clearly identifies which codes apply to the case.

A current issue arising from the use of electronic health records (EHRs) and electronic medical records (EMRs) is the replacement of the diagnostic statement with a bulleted diagnosis list and accompanying codes. The details of diagnosing the patient's condition and all the treatment options available to them is discussed in detail with the patient, but often, this information is not included in the documentation. The functionality of current EHR/EMR systems indirectly encourages the reporting of only a code and a diagnosis. The detail needed to show medical necessity and the provider's train of thought are lost in this process. The diagnostic statement (or clinical impression) identifies medical necessity and the provider's thought process in developing a diagnosis and treating it.

Note: It is a mistake to assume that a Diagnostic Statement includes *only* objective information. Many ICD-10-CM codes, such as symptom codes or external cause codes, are based on the patient history and other subjective information. The purpose of the Diagnostic Statement is to make the diagnosis code documentation easy to find and evaluate while still accurately representing the patient's condition.

The following Clinical Example provides a framework for understanding why a Diagnostic Statement is helpful. It is not intended to be a complete record, rather it only includes relevant information for the purpose of demonstrating the ICD-10-CM diagnosis code selection process and the creation of a Diagnostic Statement. It begins with "Relevant History" and "Relevant Exam Findings" for the six codes selected.

Figure 2.2

Clinical Example

Relevant History: Patient presents with generalized neck pain after the pick up truck she was driving was rear ended yesterday by a bus while waiting at a stop light. Patient reports pain and stiffness from C3 to C6 with extension and rotation. It improves throughout the day and with movement.

Relevant Exam Findings: Cervical paraspinal muscle pain is present during isometric muscle contraction, as well as during passive assisted motion. Cervical flexion/extension x-rays show increased anterior translation at C4, C5, and C6, but no other relevant findings. Tenderness and swelling is evident in the mid-cervical region. Chiropractic subluxation is found at C5, due to right spinous rotation palpated as well as visibility on AP x-ray. Trigger points are identified on the right from C4 to C6.

Codes that might be assigned to this case:

S13.4xxA	*Sprain of ligaments of cervical spine, initial encounter*
S16.1xxA	*Strain of muscle, fascia, and tendon at neck level, initial encounter*
M79.18	*Myalgia, other site*
M99.Ø1	*Segmental and somatic dysfunction, cervical region*
V54.5xxA	*Driver of pick-up truck or van in collision with heavy transport vehicle or bus in traffic accident, initial encounter*
Y92.41Ø	*Unspecified street and highway as the place of occurrence of the external cause*

Though the documentation provided in *Figure 2.2* is sufficient to support the selected codes, it does not necessarily use the same vocabulary as the ICD-10-CM code set. Consequently, if an auditor were reviewing this documentation, it would be an arduous task for them to sift through the history and the exam findings and then compare it to the codes selected. This might require someone with the clinical expertise of a doctor of chiropractic in order to correctly correlate the sample documentation with the codes assigned.

To avoid potential misunderstandings and a breakdown in the flow of information, the provider can make it easier for others to review his or her notes by creating a Diagnostic Statement that specifically states which codes the healthcare provider deems appropriate to the case. *Figure 2.3* is an example of a Diagnostic Statement for this clinical example:

Figure 2.3

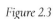

Diagnostic Statement: Patient suffers from segmental dysfunction in the cervical region with myofascial pain syndrome in the right cervical musculature. In addition, there is evidence of strain of the muscles at the neck level, as well as sprain of the ligaments of the cervical spine. Patient was the driver of a pick-up truck that was in a collision with a bus in a traffic accident on a paved roadway. Patient is now in active treatment.

If the diagnosis information in a record is audited, the last thing a provider wants to do is explain themselves to the reviewer. If the provider can give the auditor exactly what they want, as long as it is an accurate reflection of the patient encounter, there will be no need for clarification and denials will be far less likely. That is the purpose of a well designed Diagnostic Statement.

Alert: It is inappropriate to select diagnosis codes based solely on what will get the claim reimbursed. First and foremost, the diagnosis must be an accurate reflection of the patient's presentation, as depicted by *Figure 2.1 – Fundamental Reimbursement Relationships*. Medical necessity is the overarching criteria for claim payment. The Diagnostic Statement should accurately reflect the patient's condition and medical necessity for the treatment plan.

On the following pages, each code for this case will be reviewed one at a time. Compare the highlighted phrases from the History and Exam Findings to the highlighted phrases in the Diagnostic Statement. Note how they are converted into words that better match the code, but still reflect the patient presentation.

Ch2

2. Provider Documentation Training

S13.4xxA "Sprain of ligaments of cervical spine, initial encounter"

"Sprain of ligaments of the cervical spine" is used in the Diagnostic Statement because those are the words associated with **S13.4xxA**. The Relevant Exam Findings support a diagnosis of sprain of ligaments of the cervical spine, but they do not offer up any key terms to aid in code selection. Technically a phrase such as "neck sprain" might be insufficient because the code does not mention the "neck," rather it identifies the type of tissue that was injured and the bones involved. This Diagnostic Statement identifies both of those things. A competent auditor probably knows that the neck is the same thing as the cervical spine, but the provider can make the note easier for a coder/auditor to approve if the provider simply aligns his or her documentation with the terms that the coder/auditor expects to see.

Clinical Example

Relevant History:

Patient presents with generalized neck pain after the pick up truck she was driving was rear ended yesterday by a bus while waiting at a stop light. Patient reports pain and stiffness from C3 to C6 with extension and rotation. It improves throughout the day and with movement.

Relevant Exam Findings:

Cervical paraspinal muscle pain is present during isometric muscle contraction, as well as during passive assisted motion. Cervical flexion/extension x-rays show increased anterior translation at C4, C5, and C6, but no other relevant findings. Tenderness and swelling is evident in the mid-cervical region. Right spinous rotation at C5 is visible on AP cervical radiograph, indicating chiropractic subluxation. Trigger points are identified on the right from C4 to C6.

Codes that might be assigned to this case:

S13.4xxA	*Sprain of ligaments of cervical spine, initial encounter*
S16.1xxA	*Strain of muscle, fascia, and tendon at neck level, initial encounter*
M79.18	*Myalgia, other site*
M99.Ø1	*Segmental and somatic dysfunction, cervical region*
V54.5xxA	*Driver of pick-up truck or van in collision with heavy transport vehicle or bus in traffic accident, initial encounter*
Y92.41Ø	*Unspecified street and highway as the place of occurrence of the external cause*

versus

Diagnostic Statement:

Patient suffers from segmental dysfunction in the cervical region with myofascial pain syndrome in the right cervical musculature. In addition, there is evidence of strain of the muscles at the neck level, as well as sprain of the ligaments of the cervical spine. Patient was the driver of a pick-up truck that was in a collision with a bus in a traffic accident on a paved roadway. Patient is now in active treatment.

S16.1xxA "Strain of muscle, fascia, and tendon at neck level, initial encounter"

"Strain of the muscles at the neck level" is used in the Diagnostic Statement because it is consistent with the code description for **S16.1xxA.** Therefore it replaces the Relevant Exam Findings which are highlighted below. There might be other ways to describe this injury, but this is how it is done in the Tabular List, and that is why it is chosen for the Diagnostic Statement.

Clinical Example

Relevant History:

Patient presents with generalized neck pain after the pick up truck she was driving was rear ended yesterday by a bus while waiting at a stop light. Patient reports pain and stiffness from C3 to C6 with extension and rotation. It improves throughout the day and with movement.

Relevant Exam Findings:

Cervical paraspinal muscle pain is present during isometric muscle contraction, as well as during passive assisted motion. Cervical flexion/extension x-rays show increased anterior translation at C4, C5, and C6, but no other relevant findings. Tenderness and swelling is evident in the mid-cervical region. Right spinous rotation at C5 is visible on AP cervical radiograph, indicating chiropractic subluxation. Trigger points are identified on the right from C4 to C6.

Codes that might be assigned to this case:

S13.4xxA	*Sprain of ligaments of cervical spine, initial encounter*
S16.1xxA	*Strain of muscle, fascia, and tendon at neck level, initial encounter*
M79.18	*Myalgia, other site*
M99.Ø1	*Segmental and somatic dysfunction, cervical region*
V54.5xxA	*Driver of pick-up truck or van in collision with heavy transport vehicle or bus in traffic accident, initial encounter*
Y92.41Ø	*Unspecified street and highway as the place of occurrence of the external cause*

versus

Diagnostic Statement:

Patient suffers from segmental dysfunction in the cervical region with myofascial pain syndrome in the right cervical musculature. In addition, there is evidence of strain of the muscles at the neck level, as well as sprain of the ligaments of the cervical spine. Patient was the driver of a pick-up truck that was in a collision with a bus in a traffic accident on a paved roadway. Patient is now in active treatment.

Ch2

2. Provider Documentation Training

M79.18 "Myalgia, other site"

"Myofascial pain syndrome" is is a synonym for "trigger points" and it is used in the Diagnostic Statement because it is an inclusion term provided in the Tabular List with sub-category M79.1- "Myalgia." Inclusion terms are conditions for which a code is to be used. Therefore, M79.1- codes include both myofascial pain syndrome and myalgia.

Clinical Example

Relevant History:

Patient presents with generalized neck pain after the pick up truck she was driving was rear ended yesterday by a bus while waiting at a stop light. Patient reports pain and stiffness from C3 to C6 with extension and rotation. It improves throughout the day and with movement.

Relevant Exam Findings:

Cervical paraspinal muscle pain is present during isometric muscle contraction, as well as during passive assisted motion. Cervical flexion/extension x-rays show increased anterior translation at C4, C5, and C6, but no other relevant findings. Tenderness and swelling is evident in the mid-cervical region. Right spinous rotation at C5 is visible on AP cervical radiograph, indicating chiropractic subluxation. Trigger points are identified on the right from C4 to C6.

Codes that might be assigned to this case:

S13.4xxA	*Sprain of ligaments of cervical spine, initial encounter*
S16.1xxA	*Strain of muscle, fascia, and tendon at neck level, initial encounter*
M79.18	*Myalgia, other site*
M99.Ø1	*Segmental and somatic dysfunction, cervical region*
V54.5xxA	*Driver of pick-up truck or van in collision with heavy transport vehicle or bus in traffic accident, initial encounter*
Y92.41Ø	*Unspecified street and highway as the place of occurrence of the external cause*

versus

Diagnostic Statement:

Patient suffers from segmental dysfunction in the cervical region with myofascial pain syndrome in the right cervical musculature. In addition, there is evidence of strain of the muscles at the neck level, as well as sprain of the ligaments of the cervical spine. Patient was the driver of a pick-up truck that was in a collision with a bus in a traffic accident on a paved roadway. Patient is now in active treatment.

Notes

M99.Ø1 "Segmental and somatic dysfunction, cervical region"

The phrase "segmental dysfunction" and "cervical region" are both used in the Diagnostic Statement in place of "chiropractic subluxation" and "C5" from the exam findings. This is more in line with the M99.Ø- code selected, which does not use the phrase "subluxation." See Chapter 1 — Diagnosis Coding Essentials for more discussion on subluxations.

Clinical Example

Relevant History:

Patient presents with generalized neck pain after the pick up truck she was driving was rear ended yesterday by a bus while waiting at a stop light. Patient reports pain and stiffness from C3 to C6 with extension and rotation. It improves throughout the day and with movement.

Relevant Exam Findings:

Cervical paraspinal muscle pain is present during isometric muscle contraction, as well as during passive assisted motion. Cervical flexion/extension x-rays show increased anterior translation at C4, C5, and C6, but no other relevant findings. Tenderness and swelling is evident in the mid-cervical region. Right spinous rotation at C5 is visible on AP cervical radiograph, indicating chiropractic subluxation. Trigger points are identified on the right from C4 to C6.

Codes that might be assigned to this case:

S13.4xxA	*Sprain of ligaments of cervical spine, initial encounter*
S16.1xxA	*Strain of muscle, fascia, and tendon at neck level, initial encounter*
M79.18	*Myalgia, other site*
M99.Ø1	*Segmental and somatic dysfunction, cervical region*
V54.5xxA	*Driver of pick-up truck or van in collision with heavy transport vehicle or bus in traffic accident, initial encounter*
Y92.41Ø	*Unspecified street and highway as the place of occurrence of the external cause*

versus

Diagnostic Statement:

Patient suffers from segmental dysfunction in the cervical region with myofascial pain syndrome in the right cervical musculature. In addition, there is evidence of strain of the muscles at the neck level, as well as sprain of the ligaments of the cervical spine. Patient was the driver of a pick-up truck that was in a collision with a bus in a traffic accident on a paved roadway. Patient is now in active treatment.

V54.5xxA "Driver of pick-up truck or van in collision with heavy transport vehicle or bus in traffic accident, initial encounter"

The history uses words like "rear-ended," but the Diagnostic Statement uses words like "collision" and "traffic" because they are included in **V54.5xxA**. A competent coder probably knows that "rear-ended" implies the things found in the code. But why take that chance? It is better to spoon feed those who are looking for flaws in provider documentation.

Clinical Example

Relevant History:

Patient presents with generalized neck pain after the pick up truck she was driving was rear ended yesterday by a bus while waiting at a stop light. Patient reports pain and stiffness from C3 to C6 with extension and rotation. It improves throughout the day and with movement.

Relevant Exam Findings:

Cervical paraspinal muscle pain is present during isometric muscle contraction, as well as during passive assisted motion. Cervical flexion/extension x-rays show increased anterior translation at C4, C5, and C6, but no other relevant findings. Tenderness and swelling is evident in the mid-cervical region. Right spinous rotation at C5 is visible on AP cervical radiograph, indicating chiropractic subluxation. Trigger points are identified on the right from C4 to C6.

Codes that might be assigned to this case:

S13.4xxA	*Sprain of ligaments of cervical spine, initial encounter*
S16.1xxA	*Strain of muscle, fascia, and tendon at neck level, initial encounter*
M79.18	*Myalgia, other site*
M99.Ø1	*Segmental and somatic dysfunction, cervical region*
V54.5xxA	*Driver of pick-up truck or van in collision with heavy transport vehicle or bus in traffic accident, initial encounter*
Y92.41Ø	*Unspecified street and highway as the place of occurrence of the external cause*

versus

Diagnostic Statement:

Patient suffers from segmental dysfunction in the cervical region with myofascial pain syndrome in the right cervical musculature. In addition, there is evidence of strain of the muscles at the neck level, as well as sprain of the ligaments of the cervical spine. Patient was the driver of a pick-up truck that was in a collision with a bus in a traffic accident on a paved roadway. Patient is now in active treatment.

Y92.41Ø "Unspecified street and highway as the place of occurrence of the external cause"

The original history mentions a "stop light," so it is likely that this accident occurred on a paved roadway, but the Diagnostic Statement makes that more explicit. This supports code **Y92.41Ø**. An unspecified code is selected for the type of street because that is all that is documented. There are more detailed types of streets, but the record does not support the other codes.

Clinical Example

Relevant History:

Patient presents with generalized neck pain after the pick up truck she was driving was rear ended yesterday by a bus while waiting at a stop light. Patient reports pain and stiffness from C3 to C6 with extension and rotation. It improves throughout the day and with movement.

Relevant Exam Findings:

Cervical paraspinal muscle pain is present during isometric muscle contraction, as well as during passive assisted motion. Cervical flexion/extension x-rays show increased anterior translation at C4, C5, and C6, but no other relevant findings. Tenderness and swelling is evident in the mid-cervical region. Right spinous rotation at C5 is visible on AP cervical radiograph, indicating chiropractic subluxation. Trigger points are identified on the right from C4 to C6.

Codes that might be assigned to this case:

S13.4xxA	*Sprain of ligaments of cervical spine, initial encounter*
S16.1xxA	*Strain of muscle, fascia, and tendon at neck level, initial encounter*
M79.18	*Myalgia, other site*
M99.Ø1	*Segmental and somatic dysfunction, cervical region*
V54.5xxA	*Driver of pick-up truck or van in collision with heavy transport vehicle or bus in traffic accident, initial encounter*
Y92.41Ø	*Unspecified street and highway as the place of occurrence of the external cause*

versus

Diagnostic Statement:

Patient suffers from segmental dysfunction in the cervical region with myofascial pain syndrome in the right cervical musculature. In addition, there is evidence of strain of the muscles at the neck level, as well as sprain of the ligaments of the cervical spine. Patient was the driver of a pick-up truck that was in a collision with a bus in a traffic accident on a paved roadway. Patient is now in active treatment.

7th Character "A" Initial Encounter

All sprains, strains, and many external cause codes require the 7th character extension which indicates initial encounter, subsequent encounter, or sequela. "Active treatment" which is part of the definition of an "Initial Encounter," is a phrase included within the Diagnostic Statement to explain to a coder why the letter "A" is chosen as the 7th character for those codes which require it. This type of information is not typically found in the History or Exam Findings, but rather it might be included in the "Plan" of a SOAP note. This is an example of non-diagnostic information that is needed for diagnosis code selection. See Chapter 1 — Diagnosis Coding Essentials for a more complete discussion of episodes of care.

Clinical Example

Relevant History:

Patient presents with generalized neck pain after the pick up truck she was driving was rear ended yesterday by a bus while waiting at a stop light. Patient reports pain and stiffness from C3 to C6 with extension and rotation. It improves throughout the day and with movement.

Relevant Exam Findings:

Cervical paraspinal muscle pain is present during isometric muscle contraction, as well as during passive assisted motion. Cervical flexion/extension x-rays show increased anterior translation at C4, C5, and C6, but no other relevant findings. Tenderness and swelling is evident in the mid-cervical region. Right spinous rotation at C5 is visible on AP cervical radiograph, indicating chiropractic subluxation. Trigger points are identified on the right from C4 to C6.

Codes that might be assigned to this case:

S13.4xxA	*Sprain of ligaments of cervical spine, initial encounter*
S16.1xxA	*Strain of muscle, fascia, and tendon at neck level, initial encounter*
M79.18	*Myalgia, other site*
M99.Ø1	*Segmental and somatic dysfunction, cervical region*
V54.5xxA	*Driver of pick-up truck or van in collision with heavy transport vehicle or bus in traffic accident, initial encounter*
Y92.41Ø	*Unspecified street and highway as the place of occurrence of the external cause*

versus

Diagnostic Statement:

Patient suffers from segmental dysfunction in the cervical region with myofascial pain syndrome in the right cervical musculature. In addition, there is evidence of strain of the muscles at the neck level, as well as sprain of the ligaments of the cervical spine. Patient was the driver of a pick-up truck that was in a collision with a bus in a traffic accident on a paved roadway. Patient is now in active treatment.

Website: FindACode.com offers a tool (available by subscription) called Code-A-Note. Simply copy and paste the body of a note into this tool which then scans the note for potential code options in the ICD-10-CM, CPT, and HCPCS code sets. No Protected Health Information (PHI) is required or retained. It is a great tool when working with an unfamiliar specialty, or when trying to locate difficult codes.

Lessons from the Clinical Example

Provider Documentation Guides (*PDG*s)

The *Provider Documentation Guides (PDGs)* for the codes chosen for the Clinical Example can be helpful in determining if the codes are properly documented. For example, the *PDG* for segmental and somatic dysfunction makes it easy to see that the fifth character for M99.Ø- codes indicate the location of the dysfunction. The words in the documentation should list the spinal region to match up with the diagnosis code. It would not have been incorrect to state that the segmental dysfunction was at C5, but the diagnosis code does not require that level of detail, according to the *PDG*.

Symptom Codes

M54.2 "Cervicalgia" was not reported even though it is clearly documented in the history. Guideline *1.B.5* states that "symptoms that are associated routinely with a disease process should not be assigned as additional codes." Cervicalgia is routinely associated with **S16.1xxA** "Strain of muscle, fascia, and tendon at neck level, initial encounter," therefore it would be unnecessary and even incorrect to report cervicalgia in addition to a neck strain. However, after several weeks of treatment, the provider may determine that the the strain is resolved, despite the fact that neck pain is still present. It may then be appropriate to report **M54.2** "Cervicalgia" in place of the strain to indicate the need for ongoing care.

Excludes2 for Sprains and Strains

The PDGs for cervical sprain have many great tips. For example, at the 4th character level, it is clear that there is an Excludes2 note for S16.1- "Strain of muscle, fascia, and tendon at neck level." According to Guideline *1.A.12.b*, "Excludes2 indicates that the condition excluded is not part of the condition represented by the code, but a patient may have both conditions at the same time." Therefore, the strain code should be added to the sprain code since it was also documented. A clinician may argue that only one code described both the sprain and the strain in ICD-9-CM, and that these conditions always occur together, but the ICD-10-CM guidelines make it clear that two codes are now required to describe both conditions. As a result, the provider should document them distinctly.

Strains and the Word "and"

The strain code, **S16.1xxA**, lists several types of tissues: "muscle, fascia, <u>and</u> tendon." Only muscle was documented, which is acceptable because Guideline *1.A.14* states that "the word 'and' should be interpreted to mean either 'and' or 'or' when it appears in a title." Therefore, fascia and tendon are not required elements of this code. The same is true for M99.Ø- which lists segmental <u>and</u> somatic dysfunction. One or the other must be present, *but not necessarily both*. The Diagnostic Statement was designed with this guideline in mind.

Subluxations

Many would argue that the subluxation codes, commonly referred to as traumatic, would be more appropriate for a personal injury scenario such as the above Clinical Example. Could code **S13.16ØA** "Subluxation of C5/C6 cervical vertebrae, initial encounter" be reported instead of **M99.Ø1** "Segmental and somatic dysfunction, cervical region?" The traumatic subluxation codes do not support CMT; however, if no CMT is being performed at this time, it would be necessary to revise the Diagnostic Statement in order to support this code, which has different requirements than the M99.Ø- series. M99.Ø- codes need to specify a spinal region, but S13.1- codes are selected based on a specific vertebral interspace (C5/C6), and whether or not the injury is a dislocation or a subluxation (partial dislocation). The exam findings to support this type of subluxation should be clear as well. See "The Subluxation" in Chapter 1 — Diagnosis Coding Essentials for a more thorough discussion of subluxation code options.

External Cause Codes

The external cause codes included in the Clinical Example specify what kind of vehicle the patient was in, whether or not she was a passenger or the driver, whether or not it was in traffic, and the episode of care. Therefore all of that information must be clearly documented. Note that it all comes from the history, not the exam findings. It is a mistake to think that diagnosis codes are based only on objective information. External Cause codes are subjective; that is, reported by the patient, rather than observed by the clinician as with most other diagnosis codes.

The instructions for transport accidents (VØØ-V99) at the beginning of Chapter 20 in the Tabular List have the following guidelines:

Use additional code to identify:
Airbag injury (W22.1)
Type of street or road (Y92.4-)
Use of cellular telephone and other electronic equipment at the time of the transport accident (Y93.C-)

Only the type of street or road is documented; therefore, it is the only one of these additional codes reported even though the instructions ask for information about airbags and cell phone use. The chapter guidelines also define "traffic" versus "non-traffic." "Non-traffic" is any place other than a public highway. "Traffic" is assumed unless another place is specified.

Code Sequencing

Guideline *I.C.19.D* says "The code for the most serious injury, as determined by the provider and the focus of treatment, is sequenced first." In this scenario the sprain was deemed to be the most serious, followed by the strain and trigger point problem. The subluxation, or segmental dysfunction, might become the first listed diagnosis later in treatment as the other issues are resolved.

Guideline *I.C.20* says "The external causes of morbidity codes should never be sequenced as the first-listed or principal diagnosis." Therefore, in this example, they were listed last. Since there is no national requirement for external cause codes, they were provided here voluntarily.

Notes:

Notes:

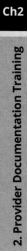

3. Common Diagnosis Codes & Tips

The codes in this chapter are grouped two ways: by anatomic location and by seven common conditions encountered in a chiropractic setting. The correct way to select a code is to look up the main term from the documentation in the Alphabetic Index and then confirm it with the Tabular List. These lists are just a supplemental reference rather than a replacement to the official code list. Comments and suggestions are welcome. Contact ChiroCode at support@ChiroCode.com.

Book:
See page 54 for the Anatomic Diagnosis Code List.
See page 67 for the Non-Musculoskeletal and Other Conditions List.
See page 70 for the Condition-Based Diagnosis Code List.

Website: See FindACode.com (with subscription) to review and search the complete ICD-10-CM code list. You can also download the free Find-A-Code app from the Google Play Store or the Apple Store for your smartphone, iPad, or tablet.

Codes found in this list that include all the necessary characters are in bold, but those that need additional characters will end with a hyphen (-). To identify the missing characters, search out the codes in the Tabular List. Some of the codes end with an underscore, (_) for example, **S16.1xx_** "Strain of muscle, fascia, and tendon at neck level." The underscore indicates that a seventh character is required. For the codes included in this list, the seventh character will be one of the three following options:

A - initial encounter (use for "active treatment")

D - subsequent encounter (use for "follow up" care)

S - sequela (use for "late effects")

Book: See Chapter 1 — Diagnosis Coding Essentials to learn more about the proper application of these characters.

Alert: Some of these codes include "x" placeholders. Do not delete them if they are included here and do not add them to codes that do not have them listed. For more on "x" placeholders, See Chapter 1 — Diagnosis Coding Essentials.

Subluxation codes are provided first in the "Anatomic List" because Medicare, and many private payers, require chiropractors to list them as the principal diagnosis, followed by a neuromusculoskeletal condition related to that region. However, many codes are included in this chapter that may not be Medicare approved.

Some Medicare Administrative Contractors (MACs) separate approved ICD-10-CM codes into groups for short, moderate, and long term treatment in prior years. Where possible, these have been identified in the anatomic list with the following designations:

[S] diagnoses that generally require short term treatment, perhaps 6 to 12 visits*

[M] diagnoses that generally require moderate term treatment, perhaps 12 to 24 visits*

[L] diagnoses that generally require long term treatment, perhaps more than 24 visits*

**note: number of visits should be based on clinical judgment.*

Note that new codes will not have these indications because at the time of printing, MAC guidance was not available for these codes.

Most of the codes marked with these designations in this list are found on a Medicare Article. Remember that Articles vary between MACs. Also, private payers may approve additional codes and have different guidelines regarding their standards for the appropriate length of treatment. Please use clinical judgment when determining the length of treatment for a patient. Longer term diagnoses should be listed first since they are generally more serious conditions than those that only require short term treatment. For more information about sequencing of diagnosis codes, see the segment "Diagnosis Code Hierarchy" at the end of Chapter 1.

Store: The *ChiroCode DeskBook*, available in the online store, includes additional guidance on setting up evidence-based care plans that are appropriate in duration.

You will see these icons below throughout Chapter 3 – Common Diagnosis Codes & Tips and Chapter 5 – The Tabular List.

N Signifies a code added this year.

R Signifies a code revised this year. *

* Revised codes may have had a change to their description, inclusion terms, and/or instructional notes.

Disclaimer: Some of the information in this chapter contains material that is the opinion of the authors. It should not be interpreted by providers/payers as official guidance. As such, this information should not be used for claim adjudication. Third party payers should utilize their own payment policies based on clinically sound guidelines.

Index

Anatomic Diagnosis Code List

Cervical and Head Diagnoses

Subluxations

M99.ØØ **Segmental and somatic dysfunction of head region** *(i.e., chiropractic subluxation)*
M99.Ø1 **Segmental and somatic dysfunction of cervical region** *(i.e., chiropractic subluxation)*
M99.1Ø **Subluxation complex (vertebral) of head region**
M99.11 **Subluxation complex (vertebral) of cervical region**

Notes

Headaches [G43-G44]

G43.ØØ1	**Migraine w/o aura, not intractable; w/status migrainosus**	
G43.ØØ9	**Migraine w/o aura, not intractable; w/o status migrainosus**	**[S]**
G43.Ø11	**Migraine w/o aura, intractable; w/status migrainosus**	
G43.Ø19	**Migraine w/o aura, intractable; w/o status migrainosus**	**[S]**
G43.1Ø1	**Migraine with aura, not intractable; with status migrainosus**	
G43.1Ø9	**Migraine with aura, not intractable; w/o status migrainosus**	**[S]**
G43.111	**Migraine with aura, intractable; with status migrainosus**	
G43.119	**Migraine with aura, intractable; w/o status migrainosus**	**[S]**
G43.909	**Migraine, unspecified, not intractable, w/o status migrainosus**	**[S]**
G43.919	**Migraine, unspecified, intractable, w/o status migrainosus**	**[S]**
G43.909	**Migraine, unspecified, not intractable, w/o status migrainosus**	**[S]**
G43.919	**Migraine, unspecified, intractable, w/o status migrainosus**	**[S]**
G44.Ø-	Cluster headaches	
G44.1	**Vascular headache, not elsewhere classified**	**[S]**
G44.2Ø1	**Tension-type headache, unspecified, intractable**	
G44.2Ø9	**Tension-type headache, unspecified, not intractable**	**[S]**
G44.211	**Episodic tension-type headache, intractable**	
G44.219	**Episodic tension-type headache, not intractable**	**[S]**
G44.221	**Chronic tension-type headache, intractable**	
G44.229	**Chronic tension-type headache, not intractable**	**[S]**
G44.3-	Post-traumatic headaches	
G44.4Ø	**Drug-induced headache, NEC, not intractable**	
G44.41	**Drug-induced headache, NEC, intractable**	
G44.86	**Cervicogenic headache**	
G54.Ø	**Brachial plexus disorders**	**[M]**
G54.2	**Cervical root disorders, NEC**	**[M]**

Dorsopathies [M4Ø-M43]

M4Ø.Ø3	**Postural kyphosis, postural, cervicothoracic region**	
M4Ø.292	**Other kyphosis, cervical region**	
M4Ø.293	**Other kyphosis, cervicothoracic region**	
M41.41	**Neuromuscular scoliosis, occipito-atlanto-axial region**	
M41.42	**Neuromuscular scoliosis, cervical region**	
M41.43	**Neuromuscular scoliosis, cervicothoracic region**	
M43.11	**Spondylolisthesis, occipito-atlanto-axial region**	**[M]**
M43.12	**Spondylolisthesis, cervical region**	**[M]**
M43.13	**Spondylolisthesis, cervicothoracic region**	**[M]**
M43.6	**Torticollis**	**[M]**

Spondylopathies [M45-M49]

M45.A1	**Non-radiographic axial spondyloarthritis of occipito-atlanto-axial region**	
M45.A2	**Non-radiographic axial spondyloarthritis of cervical region**	
M45.A3	**Non-radiographic axial spondyloarthritis of cervicothoracic region**	
M46.41	**Discitis, unspecified, occipito-atlanto-axial region**	**[M]**
M46.42	**Discitis, unspecified, cervical region**	**[M]**
M46.43	**Discitis, unspecified, cervicothoracic region**	**[M]**
M47.21	**Other spondylosis w/radiculopathy, occipito-atlanto-axial region**	**[S]**
M47.22	**Other spondylosis w/radiculopathy, cervical region**	**[S]**
M47.23	**Other spondylosis w/radiculopathy, cervicothoracic region**	**[S]**

M47.811	**Spondylosis w/o myelopathy or radiculopathy, occipito-atlanto-axial region**	**[S]**
M47.812	**Spondylosis w/o myelopathy or radiculopathy, cervical region**	**[S]**
M47.813	**Spondylosis w/o myelopathy or radiculopathy, cervicothoracic region**	**[S]**
M48.Ø1	**Spinal stenosis, occipito-atlanto-axial region**	**[L]**
M48.Ø2	**Spinal stenosis, cervical region**	**[L]**
M48.Ø3	**Spinal stenosis, cervicothoracic region**	**[L]**

Other Dorsopathies [M5Ø-M54]

M5Ø.Ø1	**Cervical disc disorder with myelopathy, high cervical region**	
M5Ø.Ø21	**Cervical disc disorder with myelopathy, C4-C5 level**	
M5Ø.Ø22	**Cervical disc disorder with myelopathy, C5-C6 level**	
M5Ø.Ø23	**Cervical disc disorder with myelopathy, C6-C7 level**	
M5Ø.Ø3	**Cervical disc disorder with myelopathy, cervicothoracic region**	
M5Ø.11	**Cervical disc disorder with radiculopathy, high cervical region**	**[M]**
M5Ø.121	**Cervical disc disorder with radiculopathy, C4-C5 level**	**[M]**
M5Ø.122	**Cervical disc disorder with radiculopathy, C5-C6 level**	**[M]**
M5Ø.123	**Cervical disc disorder with radiculopathy, C6-C7 level**	**[M]**
M5Ø.13	**Cervical disc disorder with radiculopathy, cervicothoracic region**	**[M]**
M5Ø.21	**Other cervical disc displacement, high cervical region**	**[L]**
M5Ø.221	**Other cervical disc displacement, C4-C5 level**	**[L]**
M5Ø.222	**Other cervical disc displacement, C5-C6 level**	**[L]**
M5Ø.223	**Other cervical disc displacement, C6-C7 level**	**[L]**
M5Ø.23	**Other cervical disc displacement, cervicothoracic region**	**[L]**
M5Ø.31	**Other cervical disc degeneration, high cervical region**	**[L]**
M5Ø.321	**Other cervical disc degeneration, C4-C5 level**	**[L]**
M5Ø.322	**Other cervical disc degeneration, C5-C6 level**	**[L]**
M5Ø.323	**Other cervical disc degeneration, C6-C7 level**	**[L]**
M5Ø.33	**Other cervical disc degeneration, cervicothoracic region**	**[L]**
M5Ø.81	**Other cervical disc disorders, high cervical region**	**[M]**
M5Ø.821	**Other cervical disc disorders, C4-C5 level**	**[M]**
M5Ø.822	**Other cervical disc disorders, C5-C6 level**	**[M]**
M5Ø.823	**Other cervical disc disorders, C6-C7 level**	**[M]**
M5Ø.83	**Other cervical disc disorders, cervicothoracic region**	**[L]**
M5Ø.91	**Cervical disc disorder, unspecified, high cervical**	**[M]**
M5Ø.921	**Cervical disc disorder, unspecified, C4-C5 level**	**[M]**
M5Ø.922	**Cervical disc disorder, unspecified, C5-C6 level**	**[M]**
M5Ø.923	**Cervical disc disorder, unspecified, C6-C7 level**	**[M]**
M5Ø.93	**Cervical disc disorder, unspecified, cervicothoracic**	**[M]**
M53.Ø	**Cervicocranial syndrome**	**[M]**
M53.1	**Cervicobrachial syndrome**	**[M]**
M53.82	**Other specified dorsopathies, cervical region**	
M54.11	**Radiculopathy, occipito-atlanto-axial region**	**[M]**
M54.12	**Radiculopathy, cervical region**	**[M]**
M54.13	**Radiculopathy, cervicothoracic region**	**[M]**
M54.2	**Cervicalgia**	**[S]**

Injuries [SØØ-S19]

SØ2-	Fracture of skull and face bones	
SØ3.4-	Sprain of jaw	
S12-	Fracture of cervical vertebrae and other parts of the neck	
S13.11Ø_	**Subluxation of CØ/C1 cervical vertebrae**	
S13.12Ø_	**Subluxation of C1/C2 cervical vertebrae**	
S13.13Ø_	**Subluxation of C2/C3 cervical vertebrae**	
S13.14Ø_	**Subluxation of C3/C4 cervical vertebrae**	
S13.15Ø_	**Subluxation of C4/C5 cervical vertebrae**	
S13.16Ø_	**Subluxation of C5/C6 cervical vertebrae**	
S13.17Ø_	**Subluxation of C6/C7 cervical vertebrae**	
S13.18Ø_	**Subluxation of C7/T1 cervical vertebrae**	
S13.4xx_	**Sprain of ligaments of cervical spine**	**[M]**
S13.8xx_	**Sprain of joints and ligaments of other parts of neck**	**[M]**
S16.1xx_	**Strain of muscles fascia, and tendon at neck level**	**[M]**

Other Conditions

M25.78	**Osteophyte, vertebrae**	
M26.611	**Adhesions and ankylosis of temporomandibular joint, right**	
M26.612	**Adhesions and ankylosis of temporomandibular joint, left**	
M26.613	**Adhesions and ankylosis of temporomandibular joint, bilateral**	
M26.621	**Arthralgia of temporomandibular joint, right**	
M26.622	**Arthralgia of temporomandibular joint, left**	
M26.623	**Arthralgia of temporomandibular joint, bilateral**	
M26.631	**Articular disc disorder of temporomandibular joint, right**	
M26.632	**Articular disc disorder of temporomandibular joint, left**	
M26.633	**Articular disc disorder of temporomandibular joint, bilateral**	
M26.69	**Other specified disorders of temporomandibular joint**	
M6Ø.88	**Other myositis, other site**	**[M]**
M62.838	**Other muscle spasm**	**[M]**
M79.12	**Myalgia of auxiliary muscles, head and neck**	**[M]**
M79.18	**Myalgia, other site**	**[M]**
M79.7	**Fibromyalgia**	**[M]**
M96.1	**Postlaminectomy syndrome, NEC**	**[L]**
N94.3	**Premenstrual tension syndrome**	
N95.1	**Menopausal and female climacteric states**	
QØ5.5	**Cervical spina bifida w/o hydrocephalus**	
R29.3	**Abnormal posture**	
R51.Ø	**Headache with orthostatic component, not elsewhere classified**	**[S]**
R51.9	**Headache, unspecified**	**[S]**

Thoracic / Rib Cage Diagnoses

Subluxation

M99.Ø2	**Segmental and somatic dysfunction of thoracic region** *(i.e., chiropractic subluxation)*
M99.Ø8	**Segmental and somatic dysfunction of rib cage**
M99.12	**Subluxation complex (vertebral) of thoracic region**
M99.18	**Subluxation complex (vertebral) of rib cage**

Dorsopathies [M4Ø-M43]

M4Ø.Ø4	Postural kyphosis, thoracic region	
M4Ø.Ø5	Postural kyphosis, thoracolumbar region	
M4Ø.14	Kyphosis, other secondary; thoracic region	
M4Ø.15	Kyphosis, other secondary; thoracolumbar region	
M4Ø.2Ø4	Kyphosis, unspecified; thoracic region	
M4Ø.2Ø5	Kyphosis, unspecified; thoracolumbar region	
M4Ø.294	Kyphosis, other; thoracic region	
M4Ø.295	Kyphosis, other; thoracolumbar region	
M4Ø.35	Flatback syndrome, thoracolumbar region	
M4Ø.45	Postural lordosis, thoracolumbar region	
M4Ø.55	Lordosis, unspecified; thoracolumbar region	
M41.Ø4	Scoliosis, idiopathic, infantile; thoracic region	
M41.Ø5	Scoliosis, idiopathic, infantile; thoracolumbar region	
M41.114	Scoliosis, idiopathic, juvenile; thoracic region	
M41.115	Scoliosis, idiopathic, juvenile; thoracolumbar region	
M41.124	Scoliosis, idiopathic, adolescent; thoracic region	
M41.125	Scoliosis, idiopathic, adolescent; thoracolumbar region	
M41.24	Scoliosis, idiopathic, other; thoracic region	
M41.25	Scoliosis, idiopathic, other; thoracolumbar region	
M41.34	Scoliosis, thoracogenic; thoracic region	
M41.35	Scoliosis, thoracogenic; thoracolumbar region	
M41.44	Scoliosis, neuromuscular; thoracic region	
M41.45	Scoliosis, neuromuscular; thoracolumbar region	
M43.Ø4	Spondylolysis, thoracic region	[M]
M43.Ø5	Spondylolysis, thoracolumbar region	[M]
M43.14	Spondylolisthesis, thoracic region	[M]
M43.15	Spondylolisthesis, thoracolumbar region	[M]
M43.8x4	Other specified deforming dorsopathies, thoracic region	
M43.8x5	Other specified deforming dorsopathies, thoracolumbar region	

Spondylopathies [M45-M49]

M45.4	Ankylosing spondylitis of thoracic region	
M45.5	Ankylosing spondylitis of thoracolumbar region	
M45.A4	Non-radiographic axial spondyloarthritis of thoracic region	
M45.A5	Non-radiographic axial spondyloarthritis of thoracolumbar region	
M46.44	Discitis, unspecified, thoracic region	[M]
M46.45	Discitis, unspecified, thoracolumbar region	[M]
M47.24	Other spondylosis with radiculopathy, thoracic region	[S]
M47.25	Other spondylosis with radiculopathy, thoracolumbar region	[S]
M47.814	Spondylosis without myelopathy or radiculopathy, thoracic region	[S]
M47.815	Spondylosis without myelopathy or radiculopathy, thoracolumbar region	[S]
M48.Ø4	Spinal stenosis, thoracic region	[L]
M48.Ø5	Spinal stenosis, thoracolumbar region	[L]
M48.24	Kissing spine, thoracic region	
M48.25	Kissing spine, thoracolumbar region	

Notes

Other Dorsopathies [M5Ø-M54]

M51.Ø4	**Intervertebral disc disorders with myelopathy, thoracic region**	
M51.Ø5	**Intervertebral disc disorders with myelopathy, thoracolumbar region**	
M51.14	**Intervertebral disc disorders with radiculopathy, thoracic region**	**[M]**
M51.15	**Intervertebral disc disorders with radiculopathy, thoracolumbar region**	**[M]**
M51.24	**Other intervertebral disc displacement, thoracic region**	**[L]**
M51.25	**Other intervertebral disc displacement, thoracolumbar region**	**[L]**
M51.34	**Other intervertebral disc degeneration, thoracic region**	**[L]**
M51.35	**Other intervertebral disc degeneration, thoracolumbar region**	**[L]**
M51.44	**Schmorl's nodes, thoracic region**	
M51.45	**Schmorl's nodes, thoracolumbar region**	
M51.84	**Other intervertebral disc disorders, thoracic region**	**[M]**
M51.85	**Other intervertebral disc disorders, thoracolumbar region**	**[M]**
M53.1	**Cervicobrachial syndrome**	**[M]**
M54.14	**Radiculopathy, thoracic region**	**[M]**
M54.15	**Radiculopathy, thoracolumbar region**	**[M]**
M54.6	**Pain in thoracic spine**	**[S]**

Injuries [S2Ø-S29]

S22-	Fracture of rib(s), sternum and thoracic spine	
S23.11Ø_	**Subluxation of T1/T2 thoracic vertebra**	
S23.12Ø_	**Subluxation of T2/T3 thoracic vertebra**	
S23.122_	**Subluxation of T3/T4 thoracic vertebra**	
S23.13Ø_	**Subluxation of T4/T5 thoracic vertebra**	
S23.132_	**Subluxation of T5/T6 thoracic vertebra**	
S23.14Ø_	**Subluxation of T6/T7 thoracic vertebra**	
S23.142_	**Subluxation of T7/T8 thoracic vertebra**	
S23.15Ø_	**Subluxation of T8/T9 thoracic vertebra**	
S23.152_	**Subluxation of T9/T1Ø thoracic vertebra**	
S23.16Ø_	**Subluxation of T1Ø/T11 thoracic vertebra**	
S23.162_	**Subluxation of T11/T12 thoracic vertebra**	
S23.17Ø_	**Subluxation of T12/L1 thoracic vertebra**	
S23.3xx_	**Sprain of ligaments of thoracic spine**	**[M]**
S23.41x_	**Sprain of ribs**	
S23.8xx_	**Sprain of other specified parts of thorax**	**[M]**
S29.ØØ1_	**Strain of muscle and tendon of front wall of thorax**	
S29.ØØ2_	**Strain of muscle and tendon of back wall of thorax**	

Other Conditions

G54.Ø	**Brachial plexus disorders**	**[M]**
G54.3	**Thoracic root disorders, NEC**	**[M]**
M25.78	**Osteophyte, vertebrae**	
M6Ø.88	**Other myositis, other site**	**[M]**
M62.83Ø	**Muscle spasm of back**	**[M]**
M79.18	**Myalgia, other site**	**[M]**
M79.7	**Fibromyalgia**	**[M]**
M96.1	**Postlaminectomy syndrome, NEC**	**[L]**
Q76.2	**Congenital spondylolisthesis**	**[M/L]**
R29.3	**Abnormal posture**	

Lumbar Diagnoses

Subluxation

M99.Ø3	**Segmental and somatic dysfunction of lumbar region** *(i.e., chiropractic subluxation)*	
M99.13	**Subluxation complex (vertebral) of lumbar region**	

Dorsopathies [M4Ø-M43]

M41.46	**Neuromuscular scoliosis, lumbar region**	
M41.47	**Neuromuscular scoliosis, lumbosacral region**	
M43.Ø6	**Spondylolysis, lumbar region**	**[M]**
M43.Ø7	**Spondylolysis, lumbosacral region**	**[M]**
M43.16	**Spondylolisthesis, lumbar region**	**[M]**
M43.17	**Spondylolisthesis, lumbosacral region**	**[M]**
M43.27	**Fusion of spine, lumbosacral region**	**[M]**

Spondylopathies [M45-M49]

M45.6	**Ankylosing spondylitis, lumbar region**	
M45.7	**Ankylosing spondylitis, lumbosacral region**	
M45.A6	**Non-radiographic axial spondyloarthritis of lumbar region**	
M45.A7	**Non-radiographic axial spondyloarthritis of lumbosacral region**	
M46.46	**Discitis, unspecified, lumbar region**	**[M]**
M46.47	**Discitis, unspecified, lumbosacral region**	**[M]**
M47.27	**Other spondylosis with radiculopathy, lumbosacral region**	**[S]**
M47.817	**Spondylosis w/o myelopathy or radiculopathy, lumbosacral region**	**[S]**
M48.Ø6-	Spinal stenosis, lumbar region	[L]
M48.Ø7	**Spinal stenosis, lumbosacral region**	**[L]**
M48.26	**Kissing spine, lumbar region**	
M48.27	**Kissing spine, lumbosacral region**	

Other Dorsopathies [M5Ø-M54]

M51.Ø6	**Intervertebral disc disorders with myelopathy, lumbar region**	
M51.16	**Intervertebral disc disorders with radiculopathy, lumbar region**	**[M]**
M51.17	**Intervertebral disc disorders with radiculopathy, lumbosacral region**	**[M]**
M51.26	**Other intervertebral disc displacement, lumbar region**	**[L]**
M51.27	**Other intervertebral disc displacement, lumbosacral region**	**[L]**
M51.36	**Other intervertebral disc degeneration, lumbar region**	**[L]**
M51.37	**Other intervertebral disc degeneration, lumbosacral region**	**[L]**
M51.86	**Other intervertebral disc disorders, lumbar region**	**[M]**
M51.87	**Other intervertebral disc disorders, lumbosacral region**	**[M]**
M53.2x7	**Spinal instabilities, lumbosacral region**	**[M]**
M53.86	**Other specified dorsopathies, lumbar region**	**[M]**
M53.87	**Other specified dorsopathies, lumbosacral region**	**[M]**
M54.15	**Radiculopathy, thoracolumbar region**	**[M]**
M54.16	**Radiculopathy, lumbar region**	**[M]**
M54.17	**Radiculopathy, lumbosacral region**	**[M]**
M54.31	**Sciatica, right side**	**[L]**
M54.32	**Sciatica, left side**	**[L]**
M54.41	**Lumbago with sciatica, right side**	**[L]**
M54.42	**Lumbago with sciatica, left side**	**[L]**
M54.50	**Low back pain, unspecified**	**[S]**
M54.51	**Vertebrogenic low back pain**	**[S]**
M54.59	**Other low back pain**	**[S]**
M54.89	**Other dorsalgia**	**[S]**

Injuries [S3Ø-S39]

S32-	Fracture of lumbar spine and pelvis	
S33.11Ø_	**Subluxation of L1/L2 lumbar vertebra**	
S33.12Ø_	**Subluxation of L2/L3 lumbar vertebra**	
S33.13Ø_	**Subluxation of L3/L4 lumbar vertebra**	
S33.14Ø_	**Subluxation of L4/L5 lumbar vertebra**	
S33.5xx_	**Sprain of ligaments of lumbar spine**	**[M]**
S33.8xx_	**Sprain of other parts of lumbar spine and pelvis**	**[M]**
S39.Ø11_	**Strain of muscle, fascia and tendon of abdomen**	
S39.Ø12_	**Strain of muscle, fascia and tendon of lower back**	**[M]**

Other Conditions

G54.1	**Lumbosacral plexus disorders**	**[M]**
G54.4	**Lumbosacral root disorders, NEC**	**[M]**
G54.8	**Other nerve root and plexus disorders**	**[M]**
M25.78	**Osteophyte, vertebrae**	
M6Ø.88	**Other myositis, other site**	**[M]**
M62.83Ø	**Muscle spasm of back**	**[M]**
M79.18	**Myalgia, other site**	**[M]**
M79.7	**Fibromyalgia**	**[M]**
M96.1	**Postlaminectomy syndrome, NEC**	**[L]**
QØ5.7	**Lumbar spina bifida w/o hydrocephalus**	
Q76.2	**Congenital spondylolisthesis**	**[M/L]**
R26.Ø	**Ataxic gait**	
R26.1	**Paralytic gait**	
R26.2	**Difficulty in walking, NEC**	**[M]**
R26.89	**Other abnormalities of gait and mobility**	
R29.3	**Abnormal posture**	

Sacral / Pelvic Diagnoses

Subluxation

M99.Ø4	**Segmental and somatic dysfunction of sacral region** *(i.e., chiropractic subluxation)*
M99.Ø5	**Segmental and somatic dysfunction of pelvic region** *(i.e., chiropractic subluxation)*
M99.14	**Subluxation complex (vertebral) of sacral region**
M99.15	**Subluxation complex (vertebral) of pelvic region**

Dorsopathies [M4Ø-M43]

M43.Ø8	**Spondylolysis, sacral and sacrococcygeal region**	**[M]**
M43.17	**Spondylolisthesis, lumbosacral region**	**[M]**
M43.18	**Spondylolisthesis, sacral and sacrococcygeal region**	**[M]**
M43.27	**Fusion of spine, lumbosacral region**	**[M]**
M43.28	**Fusion of spine, sacral and sacrococcygeal region**	**[M]**

Spondylopathies [M45-M49]

M45.8	**Ankylosing spondylitis sacral and sacrococcygeal region**	
M45.A8	**Non-radiographic axial spondyloarthritis of sacral and sacrococcygeal region**	
M46.1	**Sacroiliitis, NEC**	
M47.27	**Other spondylosis with radiculopathy, lumbosacral region**	**[S]**

M47.28	**Other spondylosis with radiculopathy, sacral and sacrococcygeal region**	**[S]**
M47.817	**Spondylosis w/o myelopathy or radiculopathy, lumbosacral region**	**[S]**
M47.818	**Spondylosis w/o myelopathy or radiculopathy, sacral and sacrococcygeal region**	**[S]**
M48.Ø8	**Spinal stenosis, sacral and sacrococcygeal region**	
M48.27	**Kissing spine, lumbosacral region**	

Other Dorsopathies [M5Ø-M54]

M53.2x7	**Spinal instabilities, lumbosacral region**	**[M]**
M53.2x8	**Spinal instabilities, sacral and sacrococcygeal region**	**[M]**
M53.3	**Sacrococcygeal disorders, NEC**	
M54.18	**Radiculopathy, sacral and sacrococcygeal region**	
M54.31	**Sciatica, right side**	**[L]**
M54.32	**Sciatica, left side**	**[L]**

Injuries [S3Ø-S39]

S32-	Fracture of lumbar spine and pelvis	
S33.6xx_	**Sprain of sacroiliac joint**	**[M]**
S33.8xx_	**Sprain of other parts of lumbar spine and pelvis**	**[M]**
S39.Ø13_	**Strain of muscles, fascia and tendon of pelvis**	**[M]**

Other Conditions

M6Ø.88	**Other myositis, other site**	**[M]**
M62.83Ø	**Muscle spasm of back**	**[M]**
M76.11	**Psoas tendinitis, right side**	
M76.12	**Psoas tendinitis, left side**	
M76.21	**Iliac crest spur, right side**	
M76.22	**Iliac crest spur, left side**	
QØ5.8	**Sacral spina bifida w/o hydrocephalus**	
Q76.2	**Congenital spondylolisthesis**	**[M/L]**
R26.Ø	**Ataxic gait**	
R26.1	**Paralytic gait**	
R26.2	**Difficulty in walking, NEC**	**[M/L]**
R26.89	**Other abnormalities of gait and mobility**	
R29.3	**Abnormal posture**	

Upper Extremity Diagnoses (Extra-Spinal)

Subluxation

M99.Ø7	**Segmental and somatic dysfunction of upper extremity** *(i.e., chiropractic subluxation)*
M99.17	**Subluxation complex (vertebral) of upper extremity**

Nerve, Nerve Root and Plexus Disorders [G5Ø-G59]

G56.Ø1	**Carpal tunnel syndrome, right upper limb**
G56.Ø2	**Carpal tunnel syndrome, left upper limb**
G56.Ø3	**Carpal tunnel syndrome, bilateral upper limbs**
G56.11	**Other lesions of median nerve, right upper limb**
G56.12	**Other lesions of median nerve, left upper limb**
G56.13	**Other lesions of median nerve, bilateral upper limbs**
G56.21	**Lesion of ulnar nerve, right upper limb**
G56.22	**Lesion of ulnar nerve, left upper limb**

G56.23	**Lesion of ulnar nerve, bilateral upper limbs**	
G56.31	**Lesion of radial nerve, right upper limb**	
G56.32	**Lesion of radial nerve, left upper limb**	
G56.33	**Lesion of radial nerve, bilateral upper limbs**	

Osteoarthritis [M15-M19]

M15.Ø	**Primary generalized (osteo)arthritis**	
M15.1	**Heberden's nodes (with arthropathy)**	
M15.2	**Bouchard's nodes (with arthropathy)**	
M15.3	**Secondary multiple arthritis**	
M15.4	**Erosive (osteo)arthritis**	
M18-	Osteoarthritis of first carpometacarpal joint	

Other Joint Disorders [M2Ø-M25]

M2Ø.Ø-	Deformity of finger(s)	
M21-	Other acquired deformities of limbs	
M24.Ø-	Loose body in joint	
M24.2-	Disorder of ligament	
M24.3-	Pathological dislocation of joint, NEC	
M24.4-	Recurrent dislocation of joint, NEC	
M24.5-	Contracture of joint	[S]
M24.6-	Ankylosis of joint	
M25.4-	Effusion of joint	[M]
M25.511	**Pain in right shoulder**	**[M]**
M25.512	**Pain in left shoulder**	**[M]**
M25.521	**Pain in right elbow**	**[M]**
M25.522	**Pain in left elbow**	**[M]**
M25.531	**Pain in right wrist**	**[M]**
M25.532	**Pain in left wrist**	**[M]**
M25.541	**Pain in joints of right hand**	
M25.542	**Pain in joints of left hand**	
M25.611	**Stiffness of right shoulder, NEC**	**[M]**
M25.612	**Stiffness of left shoulder, NEC**	**[M]**
M25.621	**Stiffness of right elbow, NEC**	
M25.622	**Stiffness of left elbow, NEC**	
M25.631	**Stiffness of right wrist, NEC**	
M25.632	**Stiffness of left wrist, NEC**	
M25.641	**Stiffness of right hand, NEC**	
M25.642	**Stiffness of left hand, NEC**	
M25.7-	Osteophyte	

Disorders of Muscles [M6Ø-M63]

M6Ø.8-	Other myositis	
M62.Ø-	Separation of muscle (nontraumatic)	
M62.4-	Contracture of muscle	
M62.5-	Muscle wasting and atrophy, NEC	
M62.81	**Muscle weakness, generalized**	
M62.838	**Other muscle spasm**	**[S]**

Other Soft Tissue Disorders [M7Ø-M79]

M7Ø.Ø-	Crepitant synovitis (acute) (chronic) of hand and wrist
M7Ø.11	**Bursitis, right hand**
M7Ø.12	**Bursitis, left hand**
M7Ø.21	**Olecranon bursitis, right elbow**
M7Ø.22	**Olecranon bursitis; left elbow**
M72.Ø	**Palmar fascial fibromatosis [Dupuytren]**
M75.Ø1	**Adhesive capsulitis of right shoulder**
M75.Ø2	**Adhesive capsulitis of left shoulder**
M75.1-	Rotator cuff tear or rupture, not specified as traumatic
M75.21	**Bicipital tendinitis, right shoulder**
M75.22	**Bicipital tendinitis, left shoulder**
M75.41	**Impingement syndrome of right shoulder**
M75.42	**Impingement syndrome of left shoulder**
M75.51	**Bursitis of right shoulder**
M75.52	**Bursitis of left shoulder**
M77.Ø1	**Medial epicondylitis, right elbow**
M77.Ø2	**Medial epicondylitis, left elbow**
M77.11	**Lateral epicondylitis, right elbow**
M77.12	**Lateral epicondylitis, left elbow**
M79.6Ø1	**Pain in right arm**
M79.6Ø2	**Pain in left arm**
M79.621	**Pain in right upper arm**
M79.622	**Pain in left upper arm**
M79.631	**Pain in right forearm**
M79.632	**Pain in left forearm**
M79.641	**Pain in right hand**
M79.642	**Pain in left hand**
M79.644	**Pain in right finger(s)**
M79.645	**Pain in left finger(s)**

Injuries [S4Ø-S69]

S43.Ø-	Subluxation and dislocation of shoulder joint
S43.1-	Subluxation and dislocation of acromioclavicular joint
S43.2-	Subluxation and dislocation of sternoclavicular joint
S43.3-	Subluxation and dislocation of other and unspecified parts of shoulder girdle
S43.4-	Sprain of shoulder joint
S43.5-	Sprain of acromioclavicular joint
S43.6-	Sprain of sternoclavicular joint
S44-	Injury of nerves at shoulder and upper arm level
S46-	Injury of muscle, fascia and tendon at shoulder and upper arm level
S53.Ø-	Subluxation and dislocation of radial head
S53.1-	Subluxation and dislocation of ulnohumeral joint
S53.4-	Sprain of elbow
S54-	Injury of nerves at forearm level
S63.Ø-	Subluxation and dislocation of wrist and hand joints
S63.1-	Subluxation and dislocation of thumb
S63.2-	Subluxation and dislocation of other finger(s)
S63.5-	Other and unspecified sprain of wrist
S63.6-	Other and unspecified sprain of finger(s)
S64-	Injury of nerves at wrist and hand level

Lower Extremity Diagnoses (Extra-Spinal)

Subluxation

M99.Ø6	**Segmental and somatic dysfunction of lower extremity** *(i.e., chiropractic subluxation)*	
M99.16	**Subluxation complex (vertebral) of lower extremity**	

Nerve, Nerve Root and Plexus Disorders [G5Ø-G59]

G57.Ø1	**Lesion of sciatic nerve, right lower limb**	**[M]**
G57.Ø2	**Lesion of sciatic nerve, left lower limb**	**[M]**
G57.Ø3	**Lesion of sciatic nerve, bilateral lower limbs**	**[M]**
G57.11	**Meralgia paresthetica, right lower limb**	
G57.12	**Meralgia paresthetica, left lower limb**	
G57.13	**Meralgia paresthetica, bilateral lower limbs**	
G57.21	**Lesion of femoral nerve, right lower limb**	**[M]**
G57.22	**Lesion of femoral nerve, left lower limb**	**[M]**
G57.23	**Lesion of femoral nerve, bilateral lower limbs**	**[M]**
G57.51	**Tarsal tunnel syndrome, right lower limb**	
G57.52	**Tarsal tunnel syndrome, left lower limb**	
G57.53	**Tarsal tunnel syndrome, bilateral lower limbs**	
G57.61	**Lesion of plantar nerve, right lower limb**	
G57.62	**Lesion of plantar nerve, left lower limb**	
G57.63	**Lesion of plantar nerve, bilateral lower limbs**	

Osteoarthritis [M15-M19]

M15.Ø	**Primary generalized (osteo)arthritis**	
M15.3	**Secondary multiple arthritis**	
M15.4	**Erosive (osteo)arthritis**	**[M]**
M16-	Osteoarthritis of hip	
M17-	Osteoarthritis of knee	

Other Joint Disorders [M2Ø-M25]

M2Ø.Ø-	Deformity of finger(s)	
M21-	Other acquired deformities of limbs	
M22-	Disorder of patella	
M23-	Internal derangement of knee	
M24.Ø-	Loose body in joint	
M24.2-	Disorder of ligament	
M24.3-	Pathological dislocation of joint, NEC	
M24.4-	Recurrent dislocation of joint, NEC	
M24.5-	Contracture of joint	[S]
M24.6-	Ankylosis of joint	
M25.4-	Effusion of joint	[M]
M25.551	**Pain in right hip**	**[M]**
M25.552	**Pain in left hip**	**[M]**
M25.561	**Pain in right knee**	**[M]**
M25.562	**Pain in left knee**	**[M]**
M25.571	**Pain in right ankle and joints of right foot**	**[M]**
M25.572	**Pain in left ankle and joints of left foot**	**[M]**
M25.651	**Stiffness of right hip, NEC**	**[M]**
M25.652	**Stiffness of left hip, NEC**	**[M]**

M25.661	**Stiffness of right knee, NEC**	**[M]**
M25.662	**Stiffness of left knee, NEC**	**[M]**
M25.671	**Stiffness of right ankle, NEC**	**[M]**
M25.672	**Stiffness of left ankle, NEC**	**[M]**
M25.674	**Stiffness of right foot, NEC**	**[M]**
M25.675	**Stiffness of left foot, NEC**	**[M]**
M25.7-	Osteophyte	

Disorders of Muscles [M6Ø-M63]

M6Ø.8-	Other myositis
M62.Ø-	Separation of muscle (nontraumatic)
M62.4-	Contracture of muscle
M62.5-	Muscle wasting and atrophy, NEC
M62.81	**Muscle weakness, generalized**
M62.838	**Other muscle spasm**

Other Soft Tissue Disorders [M7Ø-M79]

M7Ø.41	**Prepatellar bursitis, right knee**
M7Ø.42	**Prepatellar bursitis, left knee**
M7Ø.61	**Trochanteric bursitis, right hip**
M7Ø.62	**Trochanteric bursitis, left hip**
M72.2	**Plantar fascial fibromatosis**
M76-	Enthesiopathies, lower limb, excluding foot
M77.31	**Calcaneal spur, right foot**
M77.32	**Calcaneal spur, left foot**
M77.41	**Metatarsalgia, right foot**
M77.42	**Metatarsalgia, left foot**
M79.651	**Pain in right thigh**
M79.652	**Pain in left thigh**
M79.661	**Pain in right lower leg**
M79.662	**Pain in left lower leg**
M79.671	**Pain in right foot**
M79.672	**Pain in left foot**
M79.674	**Pain in right toe(s)**
M79.675	**Pain in left toe(s)**

Injuries [S7Ø-S99]

S73.Ø-	Subluxation and dislocation of hip
S73.1-	Sprain of hip
S74-	Injury of nerves at hip and thigh level
S76-	Injury of muscle, fascia and tendon at hip and thigh level
S83.Ø-	Subluxation and dislocation of patella
S83.1-	Subluxation and dislocation of knee
S83.2-	Tear of meniscus, current injury
S83.3-	Tear of articular cartilage of knee, current
S83.4-	Sprain of collateral ligament of knee
S83.5-	Sprain of cruciate ligament of knee
S84-	Injury of nerves at lower leg level
S86-	Injury of muscle, fascia and tendon at lower leg level
S93.Ø-	Subluxation and dislocation of ankle joint

S93.1-	Subluxation and dislocation of toe
S93.3-	Subluxation and dislocation of foot
S93.4-	Sprain of ankle
S93.5-	Sprain of toe
S93.6-	Sprain of foot
S94-	Injury of nerves at ankle and foot level
S96-	Injury of muscle and tendon at ankle and foot level

Non-Musculoskeletal and Other Conditions

This section includes other conditions which might also be used in a chiropractic setting. Many of them are systemic conditions and comorbidities. Most of the common codes from Chapters 6, 13, and 19 are found on the preceding pages. This section includes some codes from other chapters that did not fit into any previous category.

Website: See FindACode.com (with subscription) for the complete code set.

Chapter 1. Infectious diseases [AØØ-B99]

BØ2.2-	Zoster with other nervous system involvement
B91	**Sequelae of poliomyelitis**

Chapter 3. Diseases of the blood [D5Ø-D89]

D5Ø-	Anemia

Chapter 4. Endocrine diseases [EØØ-E89]

EØ8-	Diabetes mellitus due to underlying condition
EØ9-	Diabetes mellitus, drug or chemical induced
E1Ø-	Diabetes mellitus, type 1
E11-	Diabetes mellitus, type 2
E13-	Diabetes mellitus, other specified
E16.2	Hypoglycemia, unspecified
E55.9	**Vitamin D deficiency, unspecified**
E66-	Obesity

Chapter 6. Diseases of the nervous system [GØØ-G99]

G12-	Spinal muscular atrophy and related syndromes
G25-	Tremors
G4Ø.9-	Epilepsy, unspecified
G47.3-	Sleep apnea
G51-	Facial nerve disorders
G52-	Disorders of other cranial nerves
G54.6	**Phantom limb syndrome with pain**
G54.7	**Phantom limb syndrome w/o pain**
G7Ø-	Myasthenia Gravis
G81-	Hemiplegia and hemiparesis
G82-	Paraplegia and quadriplegia
G83-	Monoplegia
G83.4	**Cauda equina syndrome**
G89-	Pain, NEC

Chapter 8. Diseases of the ear [H6Ø-H95]

H6Ø-	Otitis externa
H61-	Impacted cerumen
H65-	Otitis media
H81-	Disorders of vestibular function
H83.Ø-	Labyrinthitis

Chapter 9. Diseases of the circulatory system [IØØ-I99]

I1Ø	**Essential (primary) hypertension**
I69.3-	Sequelae of cerebral infarction
I83-	Varicose veins of lower extremities

Chapter 1Ø. Diseases of the respiratory system [JØØ-J99]

JØ1-	Sinusitis, acute
J2Ø-	Bronchitis, acute
J3Ø-	Allergic rhinitis
J32-	Sinusitis, chronic
J4Ø	**Bronchitis, not specified as acute or chronic**
J44.9	**COPD, unspecified**

Chapter 12. Diseases of the skin [LØØ-L99]

L23-	Allergic contact dermatitis
L24-	Irritant contact dermatitis
L55-	Sunburn

Chapter 13. Diseases of the musculoskeletal system [MØØ-M99]

MØ5-	Rheumatoid arthritis with rheumatoid factor
MØ6.Ø-	Rheumatoid arthritis w/o rheumatoid factor
MØ6.2-	Rheumatoid bursitis
MØ6.3-	Rheumatoid nodule
MØ6.9	**Rheumatoid arthritis, unspecified**
MØ8-	Juvenile arthritis
M1Ø-	Idiopathic gout
M12.5-	Traumatic arthropathy
M1A-	Chronic gout

Chapter 14. Diseases of the genitourinary system [NØØ-N99]

N3Ø-	Cystitis
N4Ø-	Prostate disorders
N63-	Unspecified lump in breast
N94.3	**Premenstrual tension syndrome**

Chapter 15. Pregnancy, childbirth, and the puerperium [OØØ-O9A]

O12-	Gestational edema
O24-	Gestational diabetes
O26.7-	Subluxation of symphysis pubis

Chapter 17. Congenital malformations [QØØ-Q99]

QØ5-	Spina bifida

Q65-	Congenital dislocation
Q76.4-	Congenital malformations of spine
Q76.5	**Cervical rib**
Q77-	Osteochondrodysplasia

Chapter 18. Symptoms and signs [RØØ-R99]

RØ3.Ø	**Elevated blood-pressure reading, without diagnosis of hypertension**	
RØ5-	Cough	
RØ7.1	**Chest pain on breathing**	
RØ7.82	**Intercostal pain**	
R1Ø-	Abdominal and pelvic pain	
R11-	Nausea and vomiting	
R22-	Localized swelling	
R26.2	**Difficulty in walking, NEC**	**[M]**
R26.81	**Unsteadiness on feet**	
R27.Ø	**Ataxia, unspecified**	
R29.3	**Abnormal posture**	
R29.4	**Clicking hip**	**[M]**
R29.6	**Repeated falls**	
R42	**Dizziness and giddiness**	
R5Ø.9	**Fever, unspecified**	
R51.Ø	**Headache with orthostatic component, not elsewhere classified**	**[S]**
R51.9	**Headache, unspecified**	**[S]**
R53.1	**Weakness**	
R6Ø.Ø	**Localized edema**	

External Cause Codes

Transport Accidents [VØØ-V99]

VØØ.31-	Snowboard accident
VØØ.32-	Snow-ski accident
V18-	Pedal cycle rider injured in noncollision transport accident
V43-	Car occupant injured in collision with car, pick-up truck, or van
V53-	Occupant of pick-up truck or van injured in collision with car, pick-up truck, or van

Slipping, tripping, stumbling and falls [WØØ-W19]

WØØ-	Fall due to ice and snow
WØ1-	Fall on same level from slipping, tripping, and stumbling
W1Ø-	Fall on and from stairs and steps
W11-	Fall on and from ladder

Exposure to inanimate mechanical forces [W2Ø-W49]

W21-	Striking against or struck by sports equipment
W22.1-	Striking against or struck by automobile airbag

Place of occurrence of the external cause [Y92.-]

Y92.Ø-	Non-institutional (private) residence as the place of occurrence of the external cause
Y92.1-	Institutional (non private) residence as the place of occurrence of the external cause
Y92.2-	School, other institution and public administrative area as the place of occurence of the external cause
Y92.3-	Sports and athletics area as the place of occurrence of the external cause

Y92.4-	Street, highway and other paved roadways as the place of occurrence of the external cause
Y92.5-	Trade and service area as the place of occurrence of the external cause
Y92.6-	Industrial and construction area as the place of occurrence of the external cause
Y92.7-	Farm as the place of occurrence of the external cause
Y92.8-	Other places as the place of occurrence of the external cause

Activities [Y93.-]

Y93.Ø-	Activities involving walking and running
Y93.1-	Activities involving water and water craft
Y93.2-	Activities involving ice and snow
Y93.3-	Activities involving climbing, rappelling and jumping off
Y93.4-	Activities involving dancing and other rhythmic movement
Y93.5-	Activities involving other sports and athletics played individually
Y93.6-	Activities involving other sports and athletics played as a team or group
Y93.7-	Activities involving other specified sports and athletics
Y93.8-	Activities, other specified
Y93.A-	Activities involving other cardiorespiratory exercise
Y93.B-	Activities involving other muscle strengthening exercises
Y93.C-	Activities involving computer technology and other devices
Y93.D-	Activities involving arts and handicrafts
Y93.E-	Activities involving personal hygiene and interior property and clothing maintenance
Y93.F-	Activities involving caregiving
Y93.G-	Activities involving food preparation, cooking and grilling
Y93.H-	Activities involving exterior property and land maintenance, building and construction
Y93.I-	Activities involving roller coasters and other types of external motion
Y93.J-	Activities involving playing musical instrument

Condition-Based Diagnosis Code List

This section lists seven conditions commonly seen in a chiropractic practice. Four topics are discussed for each one:

1. Code options
2. Common diagnostic tests
3. Sample documentation
4. Coding considerations

The common codes included here are mostly incomplete to avoid repetition. Readers are encouraged to find the details from the *Provider Documentation Guides* in Appendix C or in the Tabular List. While the diagnostic tests are intended to be helpful, they are not all-inclusive. Clinical judgement should be applied to each individual patient. The sample documentation is just an example of subjective and objective findings for one code, and all documentation should reflect each unique patient encounter.

Disc Disorders (M5Ø-, M51-)

Code Options		
M5Ø-	Cervical Disc Disorders	
M5Ø.Ø-	With myelopathy	*Example*: Neurologic deficit to spinal cord
M5Ø.1-	With radiculopathy	*Example*: Neurologic deficit to nerve roots
M5Ø.2-	Other disc displacement	*Example*: No neurological complications
M5Ø.3-	Degeneration	*Example*: Only x-ray findings, no neurological complications
M5Ø.8-	Other disc disorders	*Example*: Documented detail does not match the other options
M5Ø.9-	Unspecified	*Example*: None of the above details are documented

Code Options		
M51-	Thoracic, Thoracolumbar, and Lumbosacral Intervertebral Disc Disorders	
M51.Ø-	With myelopathy	*Example*: Neurologic deficit to spinal cord
M51.1-	With radiculopathy	*Example*: Neurologic deficit to nerve roots
M51.2-	Other disc displacement	*Example*: No neurological complications
M51.3-	Degeneration	*Example*: Only x-ray findings, no neurological complications
M51.4-	Schmorl's nodes	*Example*: As seen on x-ray
M51.8-	Other disc disorders	*Example*: Documented detail does not match the other options
M51.9-	Unspecified	*Example*: None of the above details are documented

Common diagnostic tests for disc disorders include: deep tendon reflexes, muscle strength, pinwheel test, X-ray, MRI scan, CT scan with myelogram, and EMG.

Sample Documentation

M51.16 "Intervertebral disc disorders with radiculopathy, lumbar region"

Subjective: Patient complains of pain and numbness in the right buttock and posterior thigh. It shoots into the thigh when the patient coughs.

Objective: Symptoms are reproduced with right Straight Leg Raiser. Diminished right patellar reflex, muscle strength 4/5 right quadriceps. MRI shows right posterior disc bulge at L4/L5.

Coding Considerations

- The fifth character for all of these codes designates the specific anatomic location. See the Tabular List for details.
- **M54.2** "Cervicalgia" would not be coded along with M5Ø- "Cervical disc disorders" codes because it is already included.
- M54.5- "Low back pain" would not be coded along with M51.2- "Other disc displacement" because it is already included.
- M54.1- "Radiculopathy" would not be coded with M5Ø.1- or M51.1- "Disc disorders with radiculopathy" because it is already included.
- M54.3- or M54.4- "Sciatica" would not be coded with M51.1- "Disc disorder with radiculopathy" because it is already included.

Headaches(G43-, G44-)

Code Options		
G43-	Migraines	*Example*: Severe headaches, usually one side of head, with nausea, vomiting, and extreme sensitivity to light and sound
G43.Ø-	Migraine without aura	*Example*: No visual or other disturbance noticed before headache
G43.1-	Migraine with aura	*Example*: Visual or other disturbance noticed before headache
G43.7-	Chronic migraine without aura	*Example*: 15 or more days per month, for at least three months
G43.8-	Migraine, other	*Example*: Documented detail does not match the other options
G43.9-	Migraine, unspecified	*Example*: None of the above details are documented
G44-	Other Headaches	*Example*: Non-migraines
G44.Ø-	Cluster headaches	*Example*: Recurrent, cyclical severe headaches
G44.1	**Vascular headache, not elsewhere classified**	*Example*: Documented detail does not match the other options
G44.2-	Tension-type headache	*Example*: Hat-band pattern, often with muscle involvement
G44.3-	Post-traumatic headache	*Example*: Follows brain injury, such as concussion
G44.4-	Drug-induced headache	*Example*: Worsens with medication use
G44.86	**Cervicogenic headache**	*Example*: Caused by cervical disorders (e.g., arthritis, strained neck muscles)

Common diagnostic tests for headaches include: cranial nerve evaluation, MRI, and CT scan.

Sample Documentation

G44.221 "Chronic tension-type headache, intractable"

Subjective: Patient is a middle aged female who complains of dull ache and tightness in a hat band pattern, with muscle rigidity in the neck and shoulders. Headaches occur more than 15 days per month, for the last six months. It does not respond to over the counter medication.

Objective: Cranial nerve tests within normal limits, consider MRI or CT scan to rule out tumors.

Coding Considerations

- For most headache codes, the fifth or sixth character identifies whether or not the headache is intractable. This is defined in the code set as pharmacoresistant, treatment resistant, refractory, and poorly controlled.
- **R51.9** "Headache, unspecified" is the symptom code for headaches that do not have a definitive diagnosis. This would be used only when the provider has not documented one of the headaches from G43- or G44-.

Notes

Muscle Conditions

Code Options		
M6Ø.8-	Other myositis	*Example*: Inflammation of muscles, but documented detail does not match other myositis codes
M62.4-	Contracture of muscle	*Example*: Shortening and hardening of muscle, leading to rigitity
M62.81	**Muscle weakness (generalized)**	*Example*: Measurable loss of muscle function
M62.83-	Muscle spasm	*Example*: Involuntary muscle contractions
M79.1-	Myalgia, myofascial pain syndrome	*Example*: Pain in muscle, trigger points
M79.7	**Fibromyalgia**	*Example*: Disorder characterized by widespread musculoskeletal pain and fatigue, sleep, memory and mood issues

Common diagnostic tests for muscle conditions include: muscle strength, palpation, and algometry.

Sample Documentation

M62.83Ø "Muscle spasm of the back"

Subjective: Patient complains of hard, tight muscles in the mid back. He is a 55 year old sedentary male whose symptoms began after 36 holes of golf last weekend.

Objective: Palpation reveals tight and rigid fibers in the thoraco-lumbar paraspinals bilaterally. ROM limited 50% in all directions. Consider x-ray to evaluate for spinal arthritis.

Coding Considerations

- M6Ø.8- "Other myositis" documentation should include weakness and signs of inflammation: heat, redness, or swelling. The other subcategories (fourth characters) for myositis are "infective," "interstitial," and "foreign body granuloma;" therefore "other" is most likely to be used in a chiropractic setting. The fifth character describes the anatomic location of the involved muscles.
- The fifth and sixth characters for M62.4- "Contracture of muscle" provide detail about the anatomic location.
- The description for **M62.81** includes "generalized" in parenthesis. This is a non-essential modifier, so it is not a required part of the code.
- The sixth character for M62.83- "Muscle spasm" designates the location of the spasm.
- M79.1- "Myalgia" cannot be coded along with **M79.7** "Fibromyalgia" or M6Ø- "Myositis." It is already included in those conditions.

Pain and Stiffness

Code Options		
M25.5-	Pain in joint	*Example*: Discomfort in an extremity joint
M25.6-	Stiffness of joint, not elsewhere classified	*Example*: Stiffness in an extremity joint
M54.2	**Cervicalgia**	*Example*: Discomfort in the neck region
M54.50	**Low back pain**	*Example*: Lumbalgia or lumbago
M54.6	**Pain in thoracic spine**	*Example*: Thoracalgia
M79.6-	Pain in limb, hand, foot, fingers and toes	*Example*: Discomfort in hands or feet

Common diagnostic tests for pain and/or stiffness include: palpation and range of motion.

Sample Documentation

M54.2 "Cervicalgia"

Subjective: Patient presents today complaining of neck pain and stiffness after finals week in college. She spent many hours hunched over a desk, studying. She states that it is constant and rates 3/10 on the verbal numeric rating scale.

Objective: Palpation reveals tenderness over the paraspinal regions from C2 to C6. Pain worsens with flexion and rotation.

Coding Considerations

- The fifth and sixth characters for M25.5- describe the anatomic location of the pain, but do not include hands and fingers, feet and toes, or spinal joints. Those codes are found elsewhere.
- M25.6- "Stiffness of joint, NEC" is to be used if the documented cause of the stiffness does not include ankylosis (M24.6-), or contracture (M24.5-).
- The spinal pain codes are a restatement of the patient's subjective complaint. It does not require any clinical skill to provide these diagnoses. When using them, try to add more detail by stating "due to..." and finish the sentence. More definitive diagnoses will better communicate medical necessity to third party payers.
- Many conditions, such as strains of muscles, include pain. Signs and symptoms that are associated routinely with a condition should not be assigned as additional codes. The spinal pain codes should not be coded with certain disc disorder codes because they are included.
- Even though there are codes for "joint stiffness," there are none for "spinal stiffness." That information should still be documented and may support the selection of M99.Ø- "Segmental and somatic dysfunction" codes.
- The fifth character for M79.6- "Pain in limb, hand, foot, fingers and toes" designates the location of the pain and the sixth character designates the laterality.

Radiculopathy and Sciatica (M54-)

Code Options		
M54.1-	Radiculopathy, neuritis or radiculitis	*Example*: Pain radiating from a nerve root
M54.3-	Sciatica	*Example*: Pain or numbness following the path of the sciatic nerve
M54.4-	Lumbago with sciatica	*Example*: Low back pain accompanied by pain or numbness following the path of the sciatic nerve

Common diagnostic tests for nerve-related disorders include: pinwheel, muscle strength, deep tendon reflexes, needle EMG, nerve conduction velocity tests, and MRI. Orthopedic tests might include straight leg raiser, Bragard's, Lasegue's, and Berchterew's.

Sample Documentation

M54.17 "Lumbosacral radiculopathy"

Subjective: Patient is a 55 year old male who has worked on the docks, engaged in heavy labor, for 25 years. He reports numbness and shooting pain from the right buttock to the right posterior thigh and lateral ankle/foot which increases with sneezing or coughing.

Objective: Decreased sensation via pinwheel testing along right S1 dermatome. Lasegue's test reproduces the symptoms. Ankle plantar flexion and eversion is 4 out of 5 on the right. Achilles reflex is absent on the right.

Coding Considerations

- Definitions:
  - Neuritis or neuropathy is inflammation of a peripheral nerve. (Included in M54.1-)
  - Radiculitis is inflammation of a spinal nerve along its path of travel (dermatome). (Included in M54.1-)
  - Radiculopathy is a general term for the condition of spinal nerve root problems, including paresthesia, hyporeflexia, motor loss, and pain. (Included in M54.1-)
  - Sciatica definitions vary, but it is generally defined as numbness, tingling, weakness, and leg pain that originates in the buttock and travels down the path of the sciatic nerve in the back of the leg.
- The fifth character for M54.1- "Radiculopathy" designates the spinal level. Laterality is not an option for these codes, but it should still be documented.
- The fifth character for M54.3- "Sciatica" and M54.4- "Lumbago" with sciatica designates the laterality.
- See M5Ø.1- and M51.1- for Radiculopathy due to intervertebral disc disorders. M47.2- is for "Other spondylosis with radiculopathy."
- M54.4- "Lumbago with sciatica" is a combination code. Multiple codes should not be used when the classification provides a combination code that clearly identifies all of the elements documented in the diagnosis.

Sprain/Strain (Spinal)

Code Options		
S13.4xx_	Sprain of ligaments of cervical spine	*Example*: Stretching or tearing of ligaments
S16.1xx_	Strain of muscle, fascia, and tendon at neck level	*Example*: Stretching or tearing of muscle or tendon
S23.3xx_	Sprain of ligaments of thoracic spine	*Example*: Stretching or tearing of ligaments
S29.Ø12_	Strain of muscle, fascia, and tendon of back wall of thorax	*Example*: Stretching or tearing of muscle or tendon
S33.5xx_	Sprain of ligaments of lumbar spine	*Example*: Stretching or tearing of ligaments
S33.6xx_	Sprain of muscle, fascia, and tendon of lower back	*Example*: Stretching or tearing of ligaments
S39.Ø12_	Strain of muscle, fascia, and tendon of lower back	*Example*: Stretching or tearing of muscle or tendon
S39.Ø13_	Strain of muscle, fascia, and tendon of pelvis	*Example*: Stretching or tearing of muscle or tendon

Common diagnostic tests for *sprain* include: palpation, pain with passive assisted motion, flexion/extension or digital motion x-rays, and if necessary, MRI.

Common diagnostic tests for *strain* include: palpation, pain during muscle contraction, and if necessary, MRI.

Sample Documentation

S13.4xxA "Sprain of ligaments of cervical spine, initial encounter"

Subjective: Patient was rear-ended while at a stop light. He was facing forward and did not anticipate the impact. He did not lose consciousness or impact anything other than the headrest, which was level with the top of his head. Patient states that his neck feels "jammed" and painful throughout the posterior mid-cervical region, especially with movement.

Objective: Palpation reveals tenderness in the area of complaint, and pain increases with passive assisted flexion and rotation. Stiffness and decreased ROM is noted in all ranges. Neurological tests are negative. Flexion x-rays show 4mm of translation of C5 on C6.

Coding Considerations

- Though they commonly occur simultaneously, sprains and strains must be coded separately if both are documented.
- The seventh character "A, initial encounter" is the most likely choice for these codes, as long as the patient is undergoing "active treatment."
- Sprains and strains for extremities follow a similar pattern. They begin with the letter "S," the second character designates the anatomic location (e.g. "6" for wrist, "9" for ankle). The third character is "3" for sprains and "6" or "9" for strains.
- Many conditions, such as strains of muscles, include pain. Signs and symptoms that are associated routinely with a condition should not be assigned as additional codes. The spinal pain codes should not be coded with certain disc disorder codes because they are included.

Subluxation

Segmental and Somatic Dysfunction

Code Options	
M99.Ø-	Segmental and somatic dysfunction
M99.ØØ	**Head region**
M99.Ø1	**Cervical region**
M99.Ø2	**Thoracic region**
M99.Ø3	**Lumbar region**
M99.Ø4	**Sacral region**
M99.Ø5	**Pelvic region**
M99.Ø6	**Lower extremity**
M99.Ø7	**Upper extremity**
M99.Ø8	**Rib cage**

Common diagnostic tests for subluxations include: static and motion palpation, observation, ROM, and x-ray.

Sample Documentation

M99.Ø3 "Segmental and somatic dysfunction, lumbar region"

Subjective: Patient reports lumbar spinal pain during regular activities.

Objective:

P: Pain is reproduced when the L3/L4 region is palpated.

A: The L3 spinous process is rotated to the right, and the L4 spinous is rotated left. The right hip appears higher than the left.

R: Right lumbar lateral bending and flexion are reduced as recorded by inclinometry.

T: Hypertonicity is palpated in the lumbar paraspinal region.

Coding Considerations

- Other ICD-10-CM codes include the word "subluxation," (S13.1- Cervical, S23.1- Thoracic, S33.1- Lumbar) but it appears they are not appropriate to support chiropractic manipulative treatment. See Chapter 1 — Diagnosis Coding Essentials for more on subluxations.
- Note that the sample documentation follows the Medicare principle of P.A.R.T.

Store: See Chapter 4.2 — Evaluations & Reevaluations in the *ChiroCode DeskBook* for more details on P.A.R.T.

Notes:

4. The Alphabetic Index

Introduction

Beginning with a main term from the patient documentation, a coder can search the Alphabetic Index and locate a code that may represent the diagnosis, condition, injury, or symptom. **Do not code directly from the Alphabetic Index.** As with any other abbreviated dictionary, the Alphabetic Index does not contain enough information to allow you to code accurately. Once a code is identified in the Alphabetic Index, turn to the Tabular List for confirmation. Confirmation includes a review of the code and its components, as well as any instructional notes that may apply.

Codes appearing in the Alphabetic Index may be hyphenated (e.g., S13.4- "Sprain (joint) (ligament), spine, cervical"), which indicates additional characters are required to reach the highest specificity code or a complete code. When a code is bolded, it indicates the code is complete, or coded to the highest specificity available (e.g., **M47.22** "Spondylosis, with radiculopathy, cervical region"). While the code may be listed in the Alphabetic Index, only the Tabular List contains all the information required to properly report the code. This Alphabetic Index has been optimized to help you quickly locate Tabular List codes.

Alphabetic List Coding Conventions

The following coding conventions are used in this Alphabetic Index. See Chapter 1 — Diagnosis Coding Essentials for more commentary and examples for these conventions.

[ ]	Brackets enclose manifestation codes
See	Another term *should* be referenced
See also	Another term *can* be referenced

Disclaimer: Because of the specialty-specific nature of the Tabular List, there may be references in the Index which point to codes not found in this book's Tabular List. For the full list of ICD-10-CM codes, FindACode.com (available with subscription).

The Alphabetic List

A

- **Aftercare Z51.89** - *see also* Care
  - following surgery (for) (on)
    - amputation **Z47.81**
    - orthopedic NEC **Z47.89**
    - scoliosis **Z47.82**
    - spinal **Z47.89**
  - orthopedic NEC **Z47.89**
  - postprocedural - *see* Aftercare, following surgery
- **Age (old)** - *see* Senility
- **Agenesis**
  - coccyx **Q76.49**
  - organ
    - or site not listed - *see* Anomaly, by site
  - sacrum **Q76.49**
  - spine **Q76.49**
  - vertebra **Q76.49**
- **Agnosia (body image) (other senses) (tactile) R48.1**
  - developmental **F88**
- **AIPHI (acute idiopathic pulmonary hemorrhage in infants (over 28 days old)) RØ4.81**
- **Akathisia (drug-induced) (treatment-induced) G25.71**
  - neuroleptic induced (acute) **G25.71**
  - tardive **G25.71**
- **Akinesia R29.898**
- **Akinetic mutism R41.89**
- **Akureyri's disease G93.39**
- **Albuminuria, albuminuric (acute) (chronic) (subacute) R8Ø.9** - *see also* Proteinuria
  - complicating pregnancy - *see* Proteinuria, gestational
  - gestational - *see* Proteinuria, gestational
- **Alcohol, alcoholic, alcohol-induced**
  - counseling and surveillance **Z71.41**
    - family member **Z71.42**
- **Allergy, allergic (reaction) (to)** T78.4Ø-
  - air-borne substance NEC (rhinitis) **J3Ø.89**
  - animal (dander) (epidermal) (hair) (rhinitis) **J3Ø.81**
  - dander (animal) (rhinitis) **J3Ø.81**
  - dandruff (rhinitis) **J3Ø.81**
  - dermatitis - *see* Dermatitis, contact, allergic
  - diathesis - *see* History, allergy
  - dust (house) (stock) (rhinitis) **J3Ø.89**
    - with asthma - *see* Asthma, allergic extrinsic
  - eczema - *see* Dermatitis, contact, allergic
  - epidermal (animal) (rhinitis) **J3Ø.81**
  - feathers (rhinitis) **J3Ø.89**
  - grass (hay fever) (pollen) **J3Ø.1**
    - asthma - *see* Asthma, allergic extrinsic
  - hair (animal) (rhinitis) **J3Ø.81**
  - history (of) - *see* History, allergy
  - inhalant (rhinitis) **J3Ø.89**
  - kapok (rhinitis) **J3Ø.89**
  - pollen (any) (hay fever) **J3Ø.1**
    - asthma - *see* Asthma, allergic extrinsic
  - ragweed (hay fever) (pollen) **J3Ø.1**
    - asthma - *see* Asthma, allergic extrinsic
  - tree (any) (hay fever) (pollen) **J3Ø.1**
    - asthma - *see* Asthma, allergic extrinsic
- **ALTE (apparent life threatening event) in newborn and infant R68.13**
- **Alteration (of), Altered**
  - mental status **R41.82**
  - pattern of family relationships affecting child **Z62.898**
  - sensation
    - following
      - cerebrovascular disease **I69.998**
        - cerebral infarction **I69.398**
- **Ameba, amebic (histolytica)** - *see also* Amebiasis
- **Amebiasis AØ6.9**
  - with abscess - *see* Abscess, amebic
  - chronic (intestine) **AØ6.1**
    - with abscess - *see* Abscess, amebic
  - cystitis **AØ6.81**
  - genitourinary tract NEC **AØ6.82**
  - specified site NEC **AØ6.89**
- **Amentia** - *see* Disability, intellectual
- **AMH (asymptomatic microscopic hematuria) R31.21**
- **Amnesia R41.3**
  - postictal in epilepsy - *see* Epilepsy
- **Amnionitis** - *see* Pregnancy, complicated by
- **Amputation** - *see also* Absence, by site, acquired
- **Amyotonia M62.89**
- **Amyotrophia, amyotrophy, amyotrophic G71.8**
  - diabetic - *see* Diabetes, amyotrophy
  - lateral sclerosis **G12.21**
  - spinal progressive **G12.25**
- **Anemia (essential) (general) (hemoglobin deficiency) (infantile) (primary) (profound) D64.9**
  - complicating pregnancy, childbirth
    - or puerperium - *see* Pregnancy, complicated by (management affected by), anemia
- **Aneurysm (anastomotic) (artery) (cirsoid) (diffuse) (false) (fusiform) (multiple) (saccular) I72.9**
  - heart (wall) (chronic or with a stated duration of over 4 weeks) **I25.3**
    - valve - *see* Endocarditis
  - valve, valvular - *see* Endocarditis
- **Angiopathia, angiopathy I99.9**
  - diabetic (peripheral) - *see* Diabetes, angiopathy
  - peripheral **I73.9**
    - diabetic - *see* Diabetes, angiopathy
  - retinalis (juvenilis)
    - diabetic - *see* Diabetes, retinopathy
- **Angulation**
  - coccyx (acquired) M43.8- - *see also* subcategory
    - congenital NEC **Q76.49**
  - sacrum (acquired) M43.8- - *see also* subcategory
    - congenital NEC **Q76.49**
- **Anhedonia R45.84**
- **Ankylosis (fibrous) (osseous) (joint) M24.6Ø**
  - lumbosacral (joint) **M43.27**
  - sacro-iliac (joint) **M43.28**
  - specified site NEC **M24.69**
  - spine (joint) - *see also* Fusion, spine
- **Annular** - *see also* condition
  - organ or site, congenital NEC - *see* Distortion
- **Anoctaminopathy G71.Ø35**
- **Anomaly, anomalous (congenital) (unspecified type) Q89.9**
  - abdominal wall NEC **Q79.59**
  - coccyx **Q76.49**
  - dental
    - alveolar - *see* Anomaly, alveolar
  - dentofacial **M26.9**
    - alveolar - *see* Anomaly, alveolar
    - temporomandibular joint M26.6Ø-
      - specified type NEC **M26.69**
  - flexion (joint) NOS **Q74.9**
    - hip or thigh **Q65.89**
  - intervertebral cartilage or disc **Q76.49**
  - jaw - *see* Anomaly, dentofacial
    - alveolar - *see* Anomaly, alveolar
  - lumbosacral (joint) (region) **Q76.49**
    - kyphosis - *see* Kyphosis, congenital
    - lordosis - *see* Lordosis, congenital
  - mandible - *see* Anomaly, dentofacial
  - maxilla - *see* Anomaly, dentofacial
  - Müllerian - *see also* Anomaly, by site
  - rotation - *see* Malrotation
    - hip or thigh **Q65.89**
  - sacrum NEC **Q76.49**
    - kyphosis - *see* Kyphosis, congenital
    - lordosis - *see* Lordosis, congenital
  - spine, spinal NEC **Q76.49**
    - column NEC **Q76.49**
      - kyphosis - *see* Kyphosis, congenital
      - lordosis - *see* Lordosis, congenital
  - venous - *see* Anomaly, vein(s)
  - vertebra **Q76.49**
    - kyphosis - *see* Kyphosis, congenital
    - lordosis - *see* Lordosis, congenital
- **Anophthalmos, anophthalmus (congenital) (globe) Q11.1**
  - acquired **Z9Ø.Ø1**
- **Anorexia R63.Ø**
  - nervosa **F5Ø.ØØ**
- **Anosognosia R41.89**
- **Anoxemia RØ9.Ø2**
- **Anoxia (pathological) RØ9.Ø2**
- **Anteflexion** - *see* Anteversion
- **Antenatal**
  - care (normal pregnancy) **Z34.9Ø**
- **Anteversion**
  - femur (neck), congenital **Q65.89**
  - uterus, uterine (cervix) (postinfectional) (postpartal, old) **N85.4**
    - in pregnancy or childbirth - *see* Pregnancy, complicated by
- **Antritis J32.Ø**
  - maxilla **J32.Ø**
    - acute **JØ1.ØØ**
      - recurrent **JØ1.Ø1**
- **Anuria R34**
- **Aphasia (amnestic) (global) (nominal) (semantic) (syntactic) R47.Ø1**
  - following
    - cerebrovascular disease **I69.92Ø**
      - cerebral infarction **I69.32Ø**
- **Aplasia** - *see also* Agenesis
  - alveolar process (acquired) - *see* Anomaly, alveolar
- **Apnea, apneic (of) (spells) RØ6.81**
  - sleep **G47.3Ø**
    - central (primary) **G47.31**
      - idiopathic **G47.31**
      - in conditions classified elsewhere **G47.37**
    - obstructive (adult) (pediatric) **G47.33**
      - hypopnea **G47.33**
    - primary central **G47.31**
    - specified NEC **G47.39**
- **Apophysitis (bone)** - *see also* Osteochondropathy
- **Appearance**
  - specified NEC **R46.89**
- **Appendicitis (pneumococcal) (retrocecal) K37**
  - amebic **AØ6.89**
- **Apraxia (classic) (ideational) (ideokinetic) (ideomotor) (motor) (verbal) R48.2**
  - following
    - cerebrovascular disease **I69.99Ø**
      - cerebral infarction **I69.39Ø**
- **Arachnitis** - *see* Meningitis
- **Arachnodactyly** - *see* Syndrome, Marfan's
- **Arachnoiditis (acute) (adhesive) (basal) (brain) (cerebrospinal)** - *see* Meningitis
- **Arnold-Chiari disease, obstruction or syndrome (type II) QØ7.ØØ**
  - with
    - hydrocephalus **QØ7.Ø2**
      - with spina bifida **QØ7.Ø3**
    - spina bifida **QØ7.Ø1**
      - with hydrocephalus **QØ7.Ø3**

Arrest, arrested
cardiac **I46.9**
personal history, successfully resuscitated **Z86.74**
cardiorespiratory - *see* Arrest, cardiac
circulatory - *see* Arrest, cardiac
development or growth
child **R62.5Ø**
heart - *see* Arrest, cardiac
Arrhythmia (auricle)(cardiac)(juvenile)(nodal) (reflex)(supraventricular)(transitory) (ventricle) I49.9
vagal **R55**
Arthralgia (allergic) - *see also* Pain, joint
Arthritis, arthritic (acute) (chronic) (nonpyogenic) (subacute) M19.9Ø
allergic - *see* Arthritis, specified form NEC
ankylosing (crippling) (spine) - *see also* Spondylitis, ankylosing
sites other than spine - *see* Arthritis, specified form NEC
atrophic - *see* Osteoarthritis
back - *see* Spondylopathy, inflammatory
Charcot's - *see* Arthropathy, neuropathic
diabetic - *see* Diabetes, arthropathy, neuropathic
climacteric (any site) NEC - *see* Arthritis, specified form NEC
crystal (-induced) - *see* Arthritis, in, crystals
deformans - *see* Osteoarthritis
degenerative - *see* Osteoarthritis
due to or associated with
diabetes - *see* Diabetes, arthropathy
enteritis NEC
regional - *see* Enteritis, regional
erythema
nodosum **L52**
regional enteritis - *see* Enteritis, regional
typhoid fever **AØ1.Ø4**
facet joint **M47.819** - *see also* Spondylosis
gouty (acute) - *see* Gout
in (due to)
crystals **M11.9**
dicalcium phosphate - *see* Arthritis, in, crystals, specified type NEC
pyrophosphate - *see* Arthritis, in, crystals, specified type NEC
specified type NEC **M11.8Ø**
vertebrae **M11.88**
enteritis, infectious NEC **AØ9** - *see also* category MØ1-
erythema
nodosum **L52** (*see also* subcategory M14.8-)
gout - *see* Gout
infection - *see* Arthritis, pyogenic or pyemic
spine - *see* Spondylopathy, infective
Reiter's disease - *see* Reiter's disease
Salmonella (arizonae) (cholerae-suis) (enteritidis) (typhimurium) **AØ2.23**
typhoid fever **AØ1.Ø4**
urethritis, Reiter's - *see* Reiter's disease
infectious or infective - *see also* Arthritis, pyogenic or pyemic
spine - *see* Spondylopathy, infective
juvenile **MØ8.9Ø**
with systemic onset - *see* Still's disease
multiple site **MØ8.99**
pauciarticular **MØ8.4Ø**
specified site NEC **MØ8.4A**
vertebrae **MØ8.48**
rheumatoid - *see* Arthritis, rheumatoid, juvenile
specified site NEC **MØ8.9A**
specified type NEC **MØ8.8Ø**
multiple site **MØ8.89**
specified joint NEC **MØ8.88**
vertebrae **MØ8.88**
vertebra **MØ8.98**
meaning osteoarthritis - *see* Osteoarthritis
menopausal (any site) NEC - *see* Arthritis, specified form NEC
neuropathic (Charcot) - *see* Arthropathy, neuropathic
diabetic - *see* Diabetes, arthropathy, neuropathic
postrheumatic, chronic - *see* Arthropathy, postrheumatic, chronic
primary progressive - *see also* Arthritis, specified form NEC
purulent (any site except spine) - *see* Arthritis, pyogenic or pyemic
spine - *see* Spondylopathy, infective
pyogenic or pyemic (any site except spine) **MØØ.9**
spine - *see* Spondylopathy, infective
reactive - *see* Reiter's disease
rheumatic - *see also* Arthritis, rheumatoid
rheumatoid **MØ6.9**
with
carditis - *see* Rheumatoid, carditis
endocarditis - *see* Rheumatoid, carditis
heart involvement NEC - *see* Rheumatoid, carditis
lung involvement - *see* Rheumatoid, lung
myocarditis - *see* Rheumatoid, carditis
myopathy - *see* Rheumatoid, myopathy
pericarditis - *see* Rheumatoid, carditis
polyneuropathy - *see* Rheumatoid, polyneuropathy
rheumatoid factor - *see* Arthritis, rheumatoid, seropositive
splenoadenomegaly and leukopenia - *see* Felty's syndrome
vasculitis - *see* Rheumatoid, vasculitis
visceral involvement NEC - *see* Rheumatoid, arthritis, with involvement of organs NEC
juvenile (with or without rheumatoid factor) **MØ8.ØØ**
with systemic onset - *see* Still's disease
multiple site **MØ8.Ø9**
specified site NEC **MØ8.ØA**
vertebra **MØ8.Ø8**
seronegative **MØ6.ØØ**
multiple site **MØ6.Ø9**
specified site NEC **MØ6.ØA**
vertebra **MØ6.Ø8**
seropositive **MØ5.9**
without organ involvement **MØ5.7Ø**
multiple sites **MØ5.79**
specified site NEC **MØ5.7A**
specified NEC **MØ5.8Ø**
multiple sites **MØ5.89**
specified site NEC **MØ5.8A**
specified type NEC **MØ6.8Ø**
multiple site **MØ6.89**
specified site NEC **MØ6.8A**
vertebra **MØ6.88**
senile or senescent - *see* Osteoarthritis
septic (any site except spine) - *see* Arthritis, pyogenic or pyemic
spine - *see* Spondylopathy, infective
specified form NEC **M13.8Ø**
multiple site **M13.89**
specified joint NEC **M13.88**
spine - *see also* Spondylosis
infectious or infective NEC - *see* Spondylopathy, infective
pyogenic - *see* Spondylopathy, infective
traumatic (old) - *see* Spondylopathy, traumatic
syphilitic (late) **A52.16**
congenital **A5Ø.55 [M12.8Ø]**
toxic of menopause (any site) - *see* Arthritis, specified form NEC
transient - *see* Arthropathy, specified form NEC
traumatic (chronic) - *see* Arthropathy, traumatic
uratic - *see* Gout
urethritica (Reiter's) - *see* Reiter's disease
vertebral - *see* Spondylopathy, inflammatory
villous (any site) - *see* Arthropathy, specified form NEC
Arthrocele - *see* Effusion, joint
Arthrodynia - *see also* Pain, joint
Arthrofibrosis, joint - *see* Ankylosis
Arthropathy M12.9 - *see also* Arthritis
Charcot's - *see* Arthropathy, neuropathic
diabetic - *see* Diabetes, arthropathy, neuropathic
crystal (-induced) - *see* Arthritis, in, crystals
diabetic NEC - *see* Diabetes, arthropathy
facet joint **M47.819** - *see also* Spondylosis
gouty - *see also* Gout
in (due to)
diabetes - *see* Diabetes, arthropathy
erythema
nodosum **L52** [M14.8-]
infective endocarditis **I33.Ø [M12.8Ø]**
syphilis (late) **A52.77**
congenital **A5Ø.55 [M12.8Ø]**
ulcerative colitis **K51.9Ø [MØ7.6Ø]**
viral hepatitis (postinfectious) NEC **B19.9 [M12.8Ø]**
Jaccoud - *see* Arthropathy, postrheumatic, chronic
juvenile - *see* Arthritis, juvenile
neuropathic (Charcot) **M14.6Ø**
diabetic - *see* Diabetes, arthropathy, neuropathic
osteopulmonary - *see* Osteoarthropathy, hypertrophic, specified NEC
postinfectious NEC B99- **[M12.8Ø]**
in (due to)
enteritis due to Yersinia enterocolitica **AØ4.6 [M12.8Ø]**
viral hepatitis NEC **B19.9 [M12.8Ø]**
postrheumatic, chronic (Jaccoud) **M12.ØØ**
multiple site **M12.Ø9**
specified joint NEC **M12.Ø8**
vertebrae **M12.Ø8**
specified form NEC **M12.8Ø**
multiple site **M12.89**
specified joint NEC **M12.88**
vertebrae **M12.88**
transient - *see* Arthropathy, specified form NEC
traumatic **M12.5Ø**
multiple site **M12.59**
specified joint NEC **M12.58**
vertebrae **M12.58**
Arthrosis (deformans) (degenerative) (localized) M19.9Ø - *see also* Osteoarthritis
spine - *see* Spondylosis
Asphyxia, asphyxiation (by) RØ9.Ø1
bunny bag - *see* Asphyxia, due to, mechanical threat to breathing, trapped in bed clothes
pathological **RØ9.Ø1**

- postnatal **P84**
  - mechanical - *see* Asphyxia, due to, mechanical threat to breathing
- strangulation - *see* Asphyxia, due to, mechanical threat to breathing

Aspiration
- food or foreign body - *see* Foreign body, by site
- mucus - *see also* Foreign body, by site, causing asphyxia

Asplenia (congenital) Q89.Ø1
- postsurgical **Z9Ø.81**

Assault, sexual - *see* Maltreatment

Asthenia, asthenic R53.1
- senile **R54**

Asthma, asthmatic (bronchial) (catarrh) (spasmodic) J45.9Ø9
- with
  - hay fever - *see* Asthma, allergic extrinsic
  - rhinitis, allergic - *see* Asthma, allergic extrinsic
- allergic extrinsic **J45.9Ø9**
- atopic - *see* Asthma, allergic extrinsic
- childhood **J45.9Ø9**
- extrinsic, allergic - *see* Asthma, allergic extrinsic
- hay - *see* Asthma, allergic extrinsic
- idiosyncratic - *see* Asthma, nonallergic
- intrinsic, nonallergic - *see* Asthma, nonallergic
- late-onset **J45.9Ø9**
- mixed **J45.9Ø9**
- nervous - *see* Asthma, nonallergic
- nonallergic (intrinsic) **J45.9Ø9**
- predominantly allergic **J45.9Ø9**

Asymmetry - *see also* Distortion

Asystole (heart) - *see* Arrest, cardiac

At risk
- for
  - falling **Z91.81**

Ataxia, ataxy, ataxic R27.Ø
- following
  - cerebrovascular disease **I69.993**
    - cerebral infarction **I69.393**
- locomotor (progressive) (syphilitic) (partial) (spastic) **A52.11**
  - diabetic - *see* Diabetes, ataxia

Atheroma, atheromatous I7Ø.9Ø - *see also* Arteriosclerosis
- valve, valvular - *see* Endocarditis

Atopy - *see* History, allergy

Atrophia - *see also* Atrophy
- senilis **R54**

Atrophy, atrophic (of)
- cartilage (infectional) (joint) - *see* Disorder, cartilage, specified NEC
- disuse NEC - *see* Atrophy, muscle
- Duchenne-Aran **G12.21**
- fascioscapulohumeral (Landouzy-Déjérine) **G71.Ø2**
- Landouzy-Déjérine **G71.Ø2**
- muscle, muscular (diffuse) (general) (idiopathic) (primary) **M62.5Ø**
  - back **M62.5A9**
    - cervical **M62.5AØ**
    - lumbosacral **M62.5A2**
    - thoracic **M62.5A1**
  - Duchenne-Aran **G12.21**
  - multiple sites **M62.59**
  - myelopathic - *see* Atrophy, muscle, spinal
  - progressive (bulbar) **G12.21**
    - spinal **G12.25**
  - pseudohypertrophic **G71.Ø2**
  - specified site NEC **M62.58**
  - spinal **G12.9**
    - Aran-Duchenne **G12.21**
    - progressive **G12.25**
- myopathic NEC - *see* Atrophy, muscle
- old age **R54**
- palsy, diffuse (progressive) **G12.22**
- pseudohypertrophic (muscle) **G71.Ø2**
- senile **R54**
- spinal (acute) (cord) **G95.89**
  - muscular - *see* Atrophy, muscle, spinal
  - paralysis **G12.2Ø**
    - meaning progressive muscular atrophy **G12.25**

Attack, attacks
- benign shuddering **G25.83**
- drop NEC **R55**
- epileptic - *see* Epilepsy
- shuddering, benign **G25.83**
- syncope **R55**
- unconsciousness **R55**
- vasomotor **R55**
- vasovagal (paroxysmal) (idiopathic) **R55**

Autodigestion R68.89

Autointoxication R68.89

Autotoxemia R68.89

Avulsion (traumatic)
- cartilage - *see also* Dislocation, by site
- internal organ or site - *see* Injury, by site
- joint - *see also* Dislocation, by site
  - capsule - *see* Sprain, by site
- ligament - *see* Sprain, by site
- muscle - *see* Injury, muscle
- nerve (root) - *see* Injury, nerve
- tendon - *see* Injury, muscle

Axonotmesis - *see* Injury, nerve

B

Baastrup's disease - *see* Kissing spine

Baby
- crying constantly **R68.11**

Bacilluria R82.71

Bacillus - *see also* Infection, bacillus
- suipestifer infection - *see* Infection, salmonella

Backache (postural) M54.9
- specified NEC **M54.89**

Bacteremia R78.81
- with sepsis - *see* Sepsis

Bacterium, bacteria, bacterial
- in urine - *see* Bacteriuria

Bacteriuria, bacteruria R82.71
- asymptomatic **R82.71**

Balanitis (circinata) (erosiva) (gangrenosa) (phagedenic) (vulgaris) N48.1
- amebic **AØ6.82**

Balanorrhagia - *see* Balanitis

Bamberger-Marie disease - *see* Osteoarthropathy, hypertrophic, specified type NEC

Band (s)
- anomalous or congenital - *see also* Anomaly, by site

Bankruptcy (anxiety concerning) Z59.86

Baseball finger - *see* Dislocation, finger

Battered - *see* Maltreatment

Becker's
- dystrophy **G71.Ø1**

Bed confinement status Z74.Ø1

Bedridden Z74.Ø1

Bedwetting - *see* Enuresis

Behavior
- antisocial
  - adult **Z72.811**
  - child or adolescent **Z72.81Ø**
- obsessive-compulsive **R46.81**
- self-damaging (life-style) **Z72.89**
- sleep-incompatible **Z72.821**
- specified NEC **R46.89**

Bifurcation (congenital)
- vertebra **Q76.49**

Bilharziasis - *see also* Schistosomiasis

Birth
- complications in mother - *see* Delivery, complicated
- defect - *see* Anomaly

Black
- palm (hand) S6Ø.22-

Blackout R55

Blast (air) (hydraulic) (immersion) (underwater)
- injury
  - abdomen or thorax - *see* Injury, by site

Bleeding - *see also* Hemorrhage

Blister (nonthermal)
- beetle dermatitis **L24.89**

Blockage - *see* Obstruction

Blood
- flukes NEC - *see* Schistosomiasis
- in
  - urine - *see* Hematuria
- pressure
  - high - *see* Hypertension
- vessel rupture - *see* Hemorrhage

BMI - *see* Body, mass index

Body, bodies
- foreign - *see* Foreign body
- loose
  - joint, except knee - *see* Loose, body, joint
  - sheath, tendon - *see* Disorder, tendon, specified type NEC
- mass index (BMI)
  - adult
    - 2Ø.Ø-2Ø.9 **Z68.2Ø**
    - 21.Ø-21.9 **Z68.21**
    - 22.Ø-22.9 **Z68.22**
    - 23.Ø-23.9 **Z68.23**
    - 24.Ø-24.9 **Z68.24**
    - 25.Ø-25.9 **Z68.25**
    - 26.Ø-26.9 **Z68.26**
    - 27.Ø-27.9 **Z68.27**
    - 28.Ø-28.9 **Z68.28**
    - 29.Ø-29.9 **Z68.29**
    - 3Ø.Ø-3Ø.9 **Z68.3Ø**
    - 31.Ø-31.9 **Z68.31**
    - 32.Ø-32.9 **Z68.32**
    - 33.Ø-33.9 **Z68.33**
    - 34.Ø-34.9 **Z68.34**
    - 35.Ø-35.9 **Z68.35**
    - 36.Ø-36.9 **Z68.36**
    - 37.Ø-37.9 **Z68.37**
    - 38.Ø-38.9 **Z68.38**
    - 39.Ø-39.9 **Z68.39**
    - 4Ø.Ø-44.9 **Z68.41**
    - 45.Ø-49.9 **Z68.42**
    - 5Ø.Ø-59.9 **Z68.43**
    - 6Ø.Ø-69.9 **Z68.44**
    - 7Ø and over **Z68.45**
  - pediatric
    - less than fifth percentile for age **Z68.51**
    - 5th percentile to less than 85th percentile for age **Z68.52**
    - 85th percentile to less than 95th percentile for age **Z68.53**
    - greater than or equal to ninety-fifth percentile for age **Z68.54**
- rice - *see also* Loose, body, joint

Bony block of joint - *see* Ankylosis

Bradley's disease AØ8.19

Bradycardia (sinoatrial) (sinus) (vagal) RØØ.1
- reflex **G9Ø.Ø9**

Bradypnea RØ6.89

Brain - *see also* condition
- syndrome - *see* Syndrome, brain

Brash (water) R12

Breath
- holder, child **RØ6.89**
- holding spell **RØ6.89**
- shortness **RØ6.Ø2**

Breathing
- periodic **RØ6.3**
  - high altitude **G47.32**

Breathlessness RØ6.81

Brevicollis Q76.49

Bright's disease - *see also* Nephritis

Brion-Kayser disease - *see* Fever, parathyroid

Bronchitis (diffuse) (fibrinous) (hypostatic) (infective) (membranous) J4Ø
- with
  - tracheitis (I5 years of age and above) **J4Ø**
- allergic (acute) **J45.9Ø9**
- catarrhal (I5 years of age and above) **J4Ø**

Brown-Séquard disease, paralysis or syndrome G83.81

Bruck's disease - *see* Deformity, limb

BRUE (brief resolved unexplained event) R68.13

Bruise (skin surface intact) - *see also* Contusion
- internal organ - *see* Injury, by site

Bruit (arterial) RØ9.89

Bruxism
- sleep related **G47.63**

Bucket-handle fracture or tear (semilunar cartilage) - *see* Tear, meniscus

Bullet wound - *see also* Puncture
- internal organ - *see* Injury, by site

Bursitis M71.9
- adhesive - *see* Bursitis, specified NEC
- due to use, overuse, pressure - *see also* Disorder, soft tissue, due to use, specified type NEC
  - specified NEC - *see* Disorder, soft tissue, due to use, specified NEC
- gouty - *see* Gout
- infective NEC **M71.1Ø**
  - abscess - *see* Abscess, bursa
  - multiple sites **M71.19**
  - specified site NEC **M71.18**
- occupational NEC - *see also* Disorder, soft tissue, due to, use
- rheumatoid **MØ6.2Ø**
  - multiple site **MØ6.29**
  - vertebra **MØ6.28**
- specified NEC **M71.5Ø**
  - due to use, overuse or pressure - *see* Disorder, soft tissue, due to, use
  - specified site NEC **M71.58**

Bursopathy M71.9
- specified type NEC **M71.8Ø**
  - multiple sites **M71.89**
  - specified site NEC **M71.88**

Buschke's
- scleredema - *see* Sclerosis, systemic

C

Cachexia R64
- cancerous **R64**
- due to malnutrition **R64**
- malignant **R64**
- old age **R54**
- pulmonary **R64**
- senile **R54**

Calcification
- bursa **M71.4Ø**
  - multiple sites **M71.49**
  - specified site NEC **M71.48**
- heart - *see also* Degeneration, myocardial
  - valve - *see also* Endocarditis
- intervertebral cartilage or disc (postinfective) - *see* Disorder, disc, specified NEC
- joint - *see* Disorder, joint, specified type NEC
- massive (paraplegic) - *see* Myositis, ossificans, in, quadriplegia
- muscle **M61.9**
  - due to burns - *see* Myositis, ossificans, in, burns
  - paralytic - *see* Myositis, ossificans, in, quadriplegia
  - specified type NEC **M61.4Ø**
    - multiple sites **M61.49**
    - specified site NEC **M61.48**
- periarticular - *see* Disorder, joint, specified type NEC
- tendon (sheath) - *see also* Tenosynovitis, specified type NEC
  - with bursitis, synovitis or tenosynovitis - *see* Tendinitis, calcific

Calcified - *see* Calcification

Calcium
- deposits - *see* Calcification, by site

Callositas, callosity (infected) L84

Callus (infected) L84
- bone - *see* Osteophyte

Calpainopathy (primary) G71.Ø32
- autosomal dominant **G71.Ø31**
- autosomal recessive **G71.Ø32**

Calvé's disease - *see* Osteochondrosis, juvenile, spine

Canceled procedure (surgical) Z53.9
- because of
  - contraindication **Z53.Ø9**
    - smoking **Z53.Ø1**
  - left against medical advice (AMA) **Z53.29**
  - patient's decision **Z53.2Ø**
    - specified reason NEC **Z53.29**

Caplan's syndrome - *see* Rheumatoid, lung

Capsulitis (joint) - *see also* Enthesopathy

Cardiac - *see also* condition
- death, sudden - *see* Arrest, cardiac

Cardiomyopathy (familial) (idiopathic) I42.9
- due to
  - progressive muscular dystrophy **G71.Ø9** **[I43]** - *see also* Dystrophy, muscular, by type
- hypertensive - *see* Hypertension, heart

Carditis (acute) (bacterial) (chronic) (subacute) I51.89
- rheumatoid - *see* Rheumatoid, carditis

Care (of) (for) (following)
- improper - *see* Maltreatment

Carotid body or sinus syndrome G9Ø.Ø1

Carotidynia G9Ø.Ø1

Catabolism, senile R54

Cataract (cortical) (immature) (incipient) H26.9
- diabetic - *see* Diabetes, cataract
- in (due to)
  - diabetes - *see* Diabetes, cataract
- snowflake - *see* Diabetes, cataract

Cataracta - *see also* Cataract
- diabetic - *see* Diabetes, cataract

Catarrh, catarrhal (acute) (febrile) (infectious) (inflammation) JØØ - *see also* condition
- bronchial - *see* Bronchitis
- chest - *see* Bronchitis
- enteric - *see* Enteritis
- gastrointestinal - *see* Enteritis
- hay - *see* Fever, hay
- intestinal - *see* Enteritis
- lung - *see* Bronchitis
- nasal (chronic) - *see* Rhinitis
- nasopharyngeal (chronic) **J31.1**
  - acute **JØØ**
- pulmonary - *see* Bronchitis
- summer (hay) - *see* Fever, hay

Cephalgia, cephalalgia - *see also* Headache
- histamine **G44.ØØ9**
  - intractable **G44.ØØ1**
  - not intractable **G44.ØØ9**
- trigeminal autonomic (TAC) NEC **G44.Ø99**
  - intractable **G44.Ø91**
  - not intractable **G44.Ø99**

Cephalitis - *see* Encephalitis

Cerebellitis - *see* Encephalitis

Cerebritis - *see* Encephalitis

Cerebromalacia - *see* Softening, brain
- sequelae of cerebrovascular disease **I69.398**

Cervical - *see also* condition
- dysplasia in pregnancy - *see* Abnormal, cervix, in pregnancy or childbirth
- erosion in pregnancy - *see* Abnormal, cervix, in pregnancy or childbirth
- fibrosis in pregnancy - *see* Abnormal, cervix, in pregnancy or childbirth

Chairridden Z74.Ø9

Change (s) (in) (of) - *see also* Removal
- bone - *see also* Disorder, bone
  - diabetic - *see* Diabetes, bone change
- cognitive (mild) (organic) **R41.89**
- degenerative, spine or vertebra - *see* Spondylosis
- hip joint - *see* Derangement, joint, hip
- inflammatory - *see also* Inflammation
- joint - *see* Derangement, joint
- mental status **R41.82**
- senile **R54** - *see also* condition

Charcot's
- joint (disease) (tabetic) **A52.16**
  - diabetic - *see* Diabetes, with, arthropathy

Charley-horse (quadriceps) M62.831
- traumatic (quadriceps) S76.11-

Check-up - *see* Examination

Cheiromegaly M79.89

Childbirth - *see* Delivery

Chill (s) R68.83
- without fever **R68.83**

Choked
- on food, phlegm, or vomitus NOS - *see* Foreign body, by site
- while vomiting NOS - *see* Foreign body, by site

Choking sensation RØ9.89

Cholangiolitis (acute) (chronic) (extrahepatic) (gangrenous) (intrahepatic) K83.Ø9
- typhoidal **AØ1.Ø9**

Cholecystitis K81.9
- typhoidal **AØ1.Ø9**

Choledocholithiasis (common duct) (hepatic duct) - *see* Calculus, bile duct
- typhoidal **AØ1.Ø9**

Cholemia - *see also* Jaundice

Cholesteremia E78.ØØ

Cholesterol
- elevated (high) **E78.ØØ**
  - screening for **Z13.22Ø**

Cholesterolemia (essential) (pure) E78.ØØ
- familial **E78.Ø1**
- hereditary **E78.Ø1**

Chondritis M94.8X9

Chondrocalcinosis M11.2Ø
- familial **M11.1Ø**
  - multiple site **M11.19**
  - vertebrae **M11.18**
- multiple site **M11.29**

specified type NEC **M11.2Ø**
multiple site **M11.29**
vertebrae **M11.28**
vertebrae **M11.28**
Chondromalacia (systemic) M94.2Ø
multiple sites **M94.29**
rib **M94.28**
sacroiliac joint **M94.259**
vertebral joint **M94.28**
Chorea (chronic) (gravis) (posthemiplegic) (senile) (spasmodic) G25.5
hereditary **G1Ø**
Huntington's **G1Ø**
progressive **G25.5**
hereditary **G1Ø**
Chromoconversion R82.91
Chronic - *see* condition
fracture - *see* Fracture, pathological
Cicatricial (deformity) - *see* Cicatrix
Cicatrix (adherent) (contracted) (painful) (vicious) L9Ø.5 - *see also* Scar
muscle **M62.89**
with contracture - *see* Contraction, muscle NEC
Clavus (infected) L84
Clawfoot (congenital) Q66.89
Clawtoe (congenital) Q66.89
Climacteric (female) - *see also* Menopause
arthritis (any site) NEC - *see* Arthritis, specified form NEC
polyarthritis NEC - *see* Arthritis, specified form NEC
Closure
fistula, delayed - *see* Fistula
valve - *see* Endocarditis
Clot (blood) - *see also* Embolism
artery (obstruction) (occlusion) - *see* Embolism
vein - *see* Thrombosis
Clubfoot (congenital) Q66.89
Clutton's joints A5Ø.51 [M12.8Ø]
Coalition
calcaneo-scaphoid **Q66.89**
tarsal **Q66.89**
Cold JØØ
bronchial - *see* Bronchitis
chest - *see* Bronchitis
common (head) **JØØ**
head **JØØ**
on lung - *see* Bronchitis
symptoms **JØØ**
virus **JØØ**
Colic (bilious) (infantile) (intestinal) (recurrent) (spasmodic) R1Ø.83
abdomen **R1Ø.83**
Colicystitis - *see* Cystitis
Colitis (acute) (catarrhal) (chronic) (noninfective) (hemorrhagic) K52.9 - *see also* Enteritis
Clostridium difficile
not specified as recurrent **AØ4.72**
recurrent **AØ4.71**
infectious - *see* Enteritis, infectious
pseudomembranous
not specified as recurrent **AØ4.72**
recurrent **AØ4.71**
regional - *see* Enteritis, regional, large intestine
infectious **AØ9**
septic - *see* Enteritis, infectious
toxic NEC **K52.1**
due to Clostridium difficile
not specified as recurrent **AØ4.72**
recurrent **AØ4.71**
ulcerative (chronic) **K51.9Ø**
Collapse R55
general **R55**

valvular - *see* Endocarditis
vertebra M48.5Ø-
cervical region M48.52-
cervicothoracic region M48.53-
in (due to)
specified disease NEC M48.5Ø-
cervical region M48.52-
cervicothoracic region M48.53-
lumbar region M48.56-
lumbosacral region M48.57-
occipito-atlanto-axial region M48.51-
sacrococcygeal region M48.58-
thoracic region M48.54-
thoracolumbar region M48.55-
lumbar region M48.56-
lumbosacral region M48.57-
occipito-atlanto-axial region M48.51-
sacrococcygeal region M48.58-
thoracic region M48.54-
thoracolumbar region M48.55-
Coloenteritis - *see* Enteritis
Colpitis (acute) - *see* Vaginitis
Colpocystitis - *see* Vaginitis
Coma R4Ø.2Ø
with
motor response (none) R4Ø.231-
withdraws from pain or noxious stimuli (Ø-5 years of age) R4Ø.234-
withdraws to touch (< 2 years of age) R4Ø.235-
abnormal R4Ø.233-
abnormal extensor posturing to pain or noxious stimuli (< 2 years of age) R4Ø.232-
abnormal flexure posturing to pain or noxious stimuli (Ø-5 years of age) R4Ø.233-
extension R4Ø.232-
extensor posturing to pain or noxious stimuli (2-5 years of age) R4Ø.232-
flexion withdrawal R4Ø.234-
flexion/decorticate posturing (< 2 years of age) R4Ø.233-
localizes pain (2-5 years of age) R4Ø.235-
normal or spontaneous movement (< 2 years of age) R4Ø.236-
obeys commands (2-5 years of age) R4Ø.236-
score of
1 R4Ø.231-
2 R4Ø.232-
3 R4Ø.233-
4 R4Ø.234-
5 R4Ø.235-
6 R4Ø.236-
opening of eyes (never) R4Ø.211-
in response to
pain R4Ø.212-
sound R4Ø.213-
score of
1 R4Ø.211-
2 R4Ø.212-
3 R4Ø.213-
4 R4Ø.214-
spontaneous R4Ø.214-
verbal response (none) R4Ø.221-
confused conversation R4Ø.224-
cooing or babbling or crying appropriately (< 2 years of age) R4Ø.225-
inappropriate crying or screaming (< 2 years of age) R4Ø.223-
inappropriate words R4Ø.223-

inappropriate words (2-5 years of age) R4Ø.224-
incomprehensible sounds (2-5 years of age) R4Ø.222-
incomprehensible words R4Ø.222-
irritable cries (< 2 years of age) R4Ø.224-
oriented R4Ø.225-
score of
1 R4Ø.221-
2 R4Ø.222-
3 R4Ø.223-
4 R4Ø.224-
5 R4Ø.225-
screaming (2-5 years of age) R4Ø.223-
uses appropriate words (2- 5 years of age) R4Ø.225-
epileptic - *see* Epilepsy
hyperglycemic (diabetic) - *see* Diabetes, by type, with hyperosmolarity, with coma
hyperosmolar (diabetic) - *see* Diabetes, by type, with hyperosmolarity, with coma
hypoglycemic (diabetic) - *see* Diabetes, by type, with hypoglycemia, with coma
in diabetes - *see* Diabetes, coma
ketoacidotic (diabetic) - *see* Diabetes, by type, with ketoacidosis, with coma
Comatose - *see* Coma
Common
cold (head) **JØØ**
Commotio, commotion (current)
spinal cord - *see* Injury, spinal cord, by region
spinalis - *see* Injury, spinal cord, by region
Compartment syndrome (deep) (posterior) (traumatic) T79.AØ-
nontraumatic
abdomen **M79.A3**
specified site NEC **M79.A9**
Complaint - *see also* Disease
Complex
Costen's **M26.69**
jumped process, spine - *see* Dislocation, vertebra
subluxation (vertebral) **M99.19**
abdomen **M99.19**
acromioclavicular **M99.17**
cervical region **M99.11**
cervicothoracic **M99.11**
costochondral **M99.18**
costovertebral **M99.18**
head region **M99.1Ø**
hip **M99.15**
lower extremity **M99.16**
lumbar region **M99.13**
lumbosacral **M99.13**
occipitocervical **M99.1Ø**
pelvic region **M99.15**
pubic **M99.15**
rib cage **M99.18**
sacral region **M99.14**
sacrococcygeal **M99.14**
sacroiliac **M99.14**
specified NEC **M99.19**
sternochondral **M99.18**
sternoclavicular **M99.17**
thoracic region **M99.12**
thoracolumbar **M99.12**
upper extremity **M99.17**
Complication (s) (from) (of)
nonabsorbable (permanent) sutures - *see* Complication, sutures, permanent
orthopedic - *see also* Disorder, soft tissue
pregnancy NEC - *see* Pregnancy, complicated by
puerperium - *see* Puerperal

  transfusion (blood) (lymphocytes) (plasma) T8Ø.92-
    febrile nonhemolytic transfusion reaction **R5Ø.84**
Compression
  cord
    spinal - *see* Compression, spinal
  fracture
    nontraumatic NOS - *see* Collapse, vertebra
    pathological - *see* Fracture, pathological
    traumatic - *see* Fracture, traumatic
  nerve **G58.9** - *see also* Disorder, nerve
    root or plexus NOS (in) **G54.9**
      intervertebral disc disorder NEC - *see* Disorder, disc, with, radiculopathy
        with myelopathy - *see* Disorder, disc, with, myelopathy
      neoplastic disease **D49.9** [**G55**] - *see also* Neoplasm
      spondylosis - *see* Spondylosis, with radiculopathy
    traumatic - *see* Injury, nerve
  spinal (cord) **G95.2Ø**
    by displacement of intervertebral disc NEC - *see also* Disorder, disc, with, myelopathy
    nerve root NOS **G54.9**
      due to displacement of intervertebral disc NEC - *see* Disorder, disc, with, radiculopathy
        with myelopathy - *see* Disorder, disc, with, myelopathy
    specified NEC **G95.29**
    spondylogenic (cervical) (lumbar, lumbosacral) (thoracic) - *see* Spondylosis, with myelopathy NEC
      anterior - *see* Syndrome, anterior, spinal artery, compression
    traumatic - *see* Injury, spinal cord, by region
Concussion (brain) (cerebral) (current) SØ6.ØX9-
  with
    loss of consciousness
      3Ø minutes or less SØ6.ØX1-
      brief SØ6.ØX1-
      status unknown SØ6.ØXA-
    no loss of consciousness SØ6.ØXØ-
  without loss of consciousness SØ6.ØXØ-
  conus medullaris S34.Ø2-
  spinal (cord)
    lumbar S34.Ø1-
    sacral S34.Ø2-
  syndrome **FØ7.81**
Condition - *see also* Disease
Conditions arising in the perinatal period - *see* Newborn, affected by
Conflict (with) - *see also* Discord
  parent-child **Z62.82Ø**
    parent-adopted child **Z62.821**
    parent-biological child **Z62.82Ø**
    parent-foster child **Z62.822**
Congenital - *see also* condition
  malformation - *see* Anomaly
Congestion, congestive
  chest **RØ9.89**
  general **R68.89**
  lung **RØ9.89**
    active or acute - *see* Pneumonia
  nasal **RØ9.81**
  nose **RØ9.81**
  pulmonary - *see* Congestion, lung
  trachea - *see* Tracheitis
  viscera **R68.89**
Congestive - *see* Congestion
Consanguinity Z84.3
  counseling **Z71.89**
Constipation (atonic) (neurogenic) (simple) (spastic) K59.ØØ
  chronic **K59.Ø9**
  specified NEC **K59.Ø9**
Constriction - *see also* Stricture
  spastic - *see also* Spasm
Consultation
  without complaint or sickness **Z71.9**
    specified reason NEC **Z71.89**
  medical - *see* Counseling, medical
  religious **Z71.81**
  specified reason NEC **Z71.89**
  spiritual **Z71.81**
Contact (with) - *see also* Exposure (to)
Contamination, food - *see* Intoxication, foodborne
Contraction (s), contracture, contracted
  Achilles tendon - *see also* Short, tendon, Achilles
    congenital **Q66.89**
  burn (old) - *see* Cicatrix
  cicatricial - *see* Cicatrix
  heart valve - *see* Endocarditis
  hip - *see* Contraction, joint, hip
  joint (abduction) (acquired) (adduction) (flexion) (rotation) **M24.5Ø**
    congenital NEC **Q68.8**
      hip **Q65.89**
    hip M24.55-
      congenital **Q65.89**
    specified site NEC **M24.59**
  ligament - *see also* Disorder, ligament
  muscle (postinfective) (postural) NEC **M62.4Ø**
    with contracture of joint - *see* Contraction, joint
    multiple sites **M62.49**
    specified site NEC **M62.48**
  neck - *see* Torticollis
  paralytic
    joint - *see* Contraction, joint
    muscle - *see also* Contraction, muscle NEC
  scar - *see* Cicatrix
  tendon (sheath) **M62.4Ø**
    with contracture of joint - *see* Contraction, joint
    Achilles - *see* Short, tendon, Achilles
    ankle M62.47-
      Achilles - *see* Short, tendon, Achilles
    multiple sites **M62.49**
    neck **M62.48**
    specified site NEC **M62.48**
    thorax **M62.48**
    trunk **M62.48**
Contusion (skin surface intact) T14.8-
  alveolar process SØØ.532-
  arm (upper) S4Ø.Ø2-
  auditory canal - *see* Contusion, ear
  auricle - *see* Contusion, ear
  axilla - *see* Contusion, arm, upper
  back - *see also* Contusion, thorax, back
  brow SØØ.83-
  cheek SØØ.83-
    internal SØØ.532-
  chest (wall) - *see* Contusion, thorax
  chin SØØ.83-
  conus medullaris (spine) S34.139-
  costal region - *see* Contusion, thorax
  ear SØØ.43-
  face NEC SØØ.83-
  finger (s) S6Ø.ØØ-
    with damage to nail (matrix) S6Ø.1Ø-
    index S6Ø.Ø2-
      with damage to nail S6Ø.12-
    little S6Ø.Ø5-
      with damage to nail S6Ø.15-
    middle S6Ø.Ø3-
      with damage to nail S6Ø.13-
    ring S6Ø.Ø4-
      with damage to nail S6Ø.14-
    thumb - *see* Contusion, thumb
  foot (except toe(s) alone) S9Ø.3-
    toe - *see* Contusion, toe
  forehead SØØ.83-
  gum SØØ.532-
  hand S6Ø.22-
    finger (s) - *see* Contusion, finger
    wrist - *see* Contusion, wrist
  head SØØ.93-
    ear - *see* Contusion, ear
    lip SØØ.531-
    nose SØØ.33-
    oral cavity SØØ.532-
    scalp SØØ.Ø3-
    specified part NEC SØØ.83-
  interscapular region S2Ø.229-
  jaw SØØ.83-
  lip SØØ.531-
  malar region SØØ.83-
  mastoid region SØØ.83-
  mouth SØØ.532-
  muscle - *see* Contusion, by site
  nail
    finger - *see* Contusion, finger, with damage to nail
    toe - *see* Contusion, toe, with damage to nail
  nasal SØØ.33-
  neck S1Ø.93-
    specified site NEC S1Ø.83-
  nerve - *see* Injury, nerve
  nose SØØ.33-
  occipital
    region (scalp) SØØ.Ø3-
  palate SØØ.532-
  parietal
    region (scalp) SØØ.Ø3-
  pinna - *see* Contusion, ear
  scalp SØØ.Ø3-
  scapular region - *see* Contusion, shoulder
  shoulder S4Ø.Ø1-
  spinal cord - *see* Injury, spinal cord, by region
    conus medullaris S34.139-
  sternal region S2Ø.219-
  submaxillary region SØØ.83-
  submental region SØØ.83-
  subungual
    finger - *see* Contusion, finger, with damage to nail
    toe - *see* Contusion, toe, with damage to nail
  supraclavicular fossa S1Ø.83-
  supraorbital SØØ.83-
  temple (region) SØØ.83-
  temporal
    region SØØ.83-
  thorax (wall) S2Ø.2Ø-
    back S2Ø.22-
    front S2Ø.21-
  thumb S6Ø.Ø1-
    with damage to nail S6Ø.11-
  toe (s) (lesser) S9Ø.12-
    with damage to nail S9Ø.22-
    great S9Ø.11-
      with damage to nail S9Ø.21-

- tongue SØØ.532-
- tympanum, tympanic membrane - *see* Contusion, ear
- uvula SØØ.532-
- wrist S6Ø.21-

Conus (congenital) (any type) Q14.8
- medullaris syndrome **G95.81**

Convulsions (idiopathic) R56.9 - *see also* Seizure(s)
- epileptic - *see* Epilepsy
- epileptiform, epileptoid - *see* Seizure, epileptiform
- febrile **R56.ØØ**
  - with status epilepticus **G4Ø.9Ø1**
  - complex **R56.Ø1**
    - with status epilepticus **G4Ø.9Ø1**
  - simple **R56.ØØ**
- infantile **P9Ø**
  - epilepsy - *see* Epilepsy

Convulsive - *see also* Convulsions

Cord - *see also* condition
- bladder **G95.89**

Corn (infected) L84

Corpulence - *see* Obesity

Coryza (acute) JØØ

Costen's syndrome or complex M26.69

Costiveness - *see* Constipation

Cot death R99

Counseling (for) Z71.9
- alcohol abuser **Z71.41**
  - family **Z71.42**
- consanguinity **Z71.89**
- drug abuser **Z71.51**
  - family member **Z71.52**
- exercise **Z71.82**
- family **Z71.89**
- health (advice) (education) (instruction) - *see* Counseling, medical
- medical (for) **Z71.9**
  - consanguinity **Z71.89**
  - specified reason NEC **Z71.89**
- religious **Z71.81**
- specified reason NEC **Z71.89**
- spiritual **Z71.81**
- substance abuse **Z71.89**
  - alcohol **Z71.41**
  - drug **Z71.51**

Coxa
- valga (acquired) - *see also* Deformity, limb, specified type NEC, thigh
  - congenital **Q65.81**
- vara (acquired) - *see also* Deformity, limb, specified type NEC, thigh
  - congenital **Q65.82**

Coxsackie (virus) (infection) B34.1
- enteritis **AØ8.39**

Cramp (s) R25.2
- abdominal - *see* Pain, abdominal
- colic **R1Ø.83**
- intestinal - *see* Pain, abdominal
- leg, sleep related **G47.62**
- limb (lower) (upper) NEC **R25.2**
  - sleep related **G47.62**
- linotypist's **F48.8**
  - organic **G25.89**
- occupational (hand) **F48.8**
  - organic **G25.89**
- sleep related, leg **G47.62**
- telegrapher's **F48.8**
  - organic **G25.89**
- typist's **F48.8**
  - organic **G25.89**
- writer's **F48.8**
  - organic **G25.89**

Creaking joint - *see* Derangement, joint, specified type NEC

Creeping
- palsy or paralysis **G12.22**

Crepitus
- joint - *see* Derangement, joint, specified type NEC

Crib death R99

Crisis
- heart - *see* Failure, heart

Crohn's disease - *see* Enteritis, regional

Crush, crushed, crushing T14.8-
- nerve - *see* Injury, nerve

Crying (constant) (continuous) (excessive)
- child, adolescent, or adult **R45.83**
- infant (baby) (newborn) **R68.11**

Curse, Ondine's - *see* Apnea, sleep

Curvature
- organ or site, congenital NEC - *see* Distortion

Cut (external) - *see also* Laceration
- muscle - *see* Injury, muscle

Cyclical vomiting, in migraine, G43.AØ - *see also* Vomiting, cyclical

Cyphosis - *see* Kyphosis

Cyst (colloid) (mucous) (simple) (retention)
- bone (local) NEC **M85.6Ø**
  - aneurysmal **M85.5Ø**
    - multiple site **M85.59**
    - neck **M85.58**
    - rib **M85.58**
    - skull **M85.58**
    - specified site NEC **M85.58**
    - vertebra **M85.58**
  - solitary **M85.4Ø**
    - neck **M85.48**
    - rib **M85.48**
    - skull **M85.48**
    - specified site NEC **M85.48**
    - vertebra **M85.48**
  - specified type NEC **M85.6Ø**
    - multiple site **M85.69**
    - neck **M85.68**
    - rib **M85.68**
    - skull **M85.68**
    - specified site NEC **M85.68**
    - vertebra **M85.68**
- bursa, bursal NEC **M71.3Ø**
  - with rupture - *see* Rupture, synovium
  - multiple sites **M71.39**
  - specified site NEC **M71.38**
- cauda equina **G95.89**
- ganglion - *see* Ganglion
- intraligamentous - *see also* Disorder, ligament
  - knee - *see* Derangement, knee
- joint NEC - *see* Disorder, joint, specified type NEC
- meniscus, knee - *see* Derangement, knee, meniscus, cystic
- paralabral
  - shoulder S43.43-
- semilunar cartilage (knee) (multiple) - *see* Derangement, knee, meniscus, cystic
- solitary
  - bone - *see* Cyst, bone, solitary
- synovial - *see also* Cyst, bursa
  - ruptured - *see* Rupture, synovium
- tendon (sheath) - *see* Disorder, tendon, specified type NEC

Cystic - *see also* condition
- meniscus - *see* Derangement, knee, meniscus, cystic

Cystitis (exudative) (hemorrhagic) (septic) (suppurative) N3Ø.9Ø
- with
  - fibrosis - *see* Cystitis, chronic, interstitial
  - hematuria **N3Ø.91**
  - leukoplakia - *see* Cystitis, chronic, interstitial
  - malakoplakia - *see* Cystitis, chronic, interstitial
  - metaplasia - *see* Cystitis, chronic, interstitial
- acute **N3Ø.ØØ**
  - with hematuria **N3Ø.Ø1**
  - of trigone **N3Ø.3Ø**
    - with hematuria **N3Ø.31**
- allergic - *see* Cystitis, specified type NEC
- amebic **AØ6.81**
- bullous - *see* Cystitis, specified type NEC
- chronic **N3Ø.2Ø**
  - with hematuria **N3Ø.21**
  - interstitial **N3Ø.1Ø**
    - with hematuria **N3Ø.11**
  - of trigone **N3Ø.3Ø**
    - with hematuria **N3Ø.31**
  - specified NEC **N3Ø.2Ø**
    - with hematuria **N3Ø.21**
- cystic (a) - *see* Cystitis, specified type NEC
- emphysematous - *see* Cystitis, specified type NEC
- encysted - *see* Cystitis, specified type NEC
- eosinophilic - *see* Cystitis, specified type NEC
- follicular - *see* Cystitis, of trigone
- gangrenous - *see* Cystitis, specified type NEC
- glandularis - *see* Cystitis, specified type NEC
- incrusted - *see* Cystitis, specified type NEC
- interstitial (chronic) - *see* Cystitis, chronic, interstitial
- irradiation **N3Ø.4Ø**
  - with hematuria **N3Ø.41**
- irritation - *see* Cystitis, specified type NEC
- malignant - *see* Cystitis, specified type NEC
- of trigone **N3Ø.3Ø**
  - with hematuria **N3Ø.31**
- panmural - *see* Cystitis, chronic, interstitial
- polyposa - *see* Cystitis, specified type NEC
- radiation - *see* Cystitis, irradiation
- specified type NEC **N3Ø.8Ø**
  - with hematuria **N3Ø.81**
- subacute - *see* Cystitis, chronic
- submucous - *see* Cystitis, chronic, interstitial
- ulcerative - *see* Cystitis, chronic, interstitial

Cystopyelitis - *see* Pyelonephritis

D

Dactylitis
- bone - *see* Osteomyelitis

Death (cause unknown) (of) (unexplained) (unspecified cause) R99
- cardiac (sudden) (with successful resuscitation) - *see* Arrest, cardiac
  - family history of **Z82.41**
  - personal history of **Z86.74**

Debility (chronic) (general) (nervous) R53.81
- nervous **R53.81**
- old age **R54**
- senile **R54**

Debt, burdensome Z59.86

Decay
- senile **R54**

Decline (general) - *see* Debility
- cognitive, age-associated **R41.81**

Decrease (d)
- functional activity **R68.89**
- libido **R68.82**
- sexual desire **R68.82**

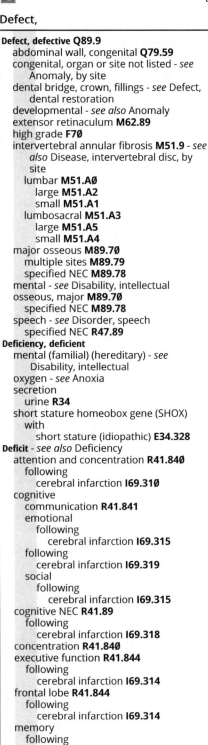

- **Defect, defective Q89.9**
  - abdominal wall, congenital **Q79.59**
  - congenital, organ or site not listed - *see* Anomaly, by site
  - dental bridge, crown, fillings - *see* Defect, dental restoration
  - developmental - *see also* Anomaly
  - extensor retinaculum **M62.89**
  - high grade **F70**
  - intervertebral annular fibrosis **M51.9** - *see also* Disease, intervertebral disc, by site
    - lumbar **M51.A0**
      - large **M51.A2**
      - small **M51.A1**
    - lumbosacral **M51.A3**
      - large **M51.A5**
      - small **M51.A4**
  - major osseous **M89.70**
    - multiple sites **M89.79**
    - specified NEC **M89.78**
  - mental - *see* Disability, intellectual
  - osseous, major **M89.70**
    - specified NEC **M89.78**
  - speech - *see* Disorder, speech
    - specified NEC **R47.89**
- **Deficiency, deficient**
  - mental (familial) (hereditary) - *see* Disability, intellectual
  - oxygen - *see* Anoxia
  - secretion
    - urine **R34**
  - short stature homeobox gene (SHOX)
    - with
      - short stature (idiopathic) **E34.328**
- **Deficit** - *see also* Deficiency
  - attention and concentration **R41.840**
    - following
      - cerebral infarction **I69.310**
  - cognitive
    - communication **R41.841**
    - emotional
      - following
        - cerebral infarction **I69.315**
    - following
      - cerebral infarction **I69.319**
    - social
      - following
        - cerebral infarction **I69.315**
  - cognitive NEC **R41.89**
    - following
      - cerebral infarction **I69.318**
  - concentration **R41.840**
  - executive function **R41.844**
    - following
      - cerebral infarction **I69.314**
  - frontal lobe **R41.844**
    - following
      - cerebral infarction **I69.314**
  - memory
    - following
      - cerebral infarction **I69.311**
  - neurologic NEC **R29.818**
  - oxygen **R09.02**
  - psychomotor **R41.843**
    - following
      - cerebral infarction **I69.313**
  - visuospatial **R41.842**
    - following
      - cerebral infarction **I69.312**
- **Deformity Q89.9**
  - abdominal wall
    - congenital **Q79.59**
  - cicatricial - *see* Cicatrix
  - clubfoot - *see* Clubfoot
  - flexion (joint) (acquired) **M21.20** - *see also* Deformity, limb, flexion
    - congenital NOS **Q74.9**
      - hip **Q65.89**
  - foot (acquired) - *see also* Deformity, limb, lower leg
    - congenital NOS Q66.9-
      - specified type NEC **Q66.89**
  - heart (congenital) **Q24.9**
    - valve (congenital) NEC **Q24.8**
      - acquired - *see* Endocarditis
  - heel (acquired) - *see* Deformity, foot
  - hip (joint) (acquired) - *see also* Deformity, limb, thigh
    - flexion - *see* Contraction, joint, hip
  - intervertebral cartilage or disc (acquired) - *see* Disorder, disc, specified NEC
  - joint (acquired) NEC **M21.90**
  - ligament (acquired) - *see* Disorder, ligament
  - limb (acquired) **M21.90**
    - flexion **M21.20**
    - specified type NEC **M21.80**
    - unequal length **M21.70**
    - valgus - *see* Deformity, valgus
    - varus - *see* Deformity, varus
  - lumbosacral (congenital) (joint) (region) **Q76.49**
    - kyphosis - *see* Kyphosis, congenital
    - lordosis - *see* Lordosis, congenital
  - metatarsus (acquired) - *see* Deformity, foot
  - muscle (acquired) **M62.89**
  - rotation (joint) (acquired) - *see* Deformity, limb, specified site NEC
    - hip - *see* Deformity, limb, specified type NEC, thigh
      - congenital **Q65.89**
  - saddle
    - back - *see* Lordosis
  - spinal - *see* Dorsopathy, deforming
    - cord (congenital) **Q06.9**
      - acquired **G95.89**
  - talipes - *see* Talipes
  - valgus NEC **M21.00**
  - valve, valvular (congenital) (heart) **Q24.8**
    - acquired - *see* Endocarditis
  - varus NEC **M21.10**
  - vertical talus (congenital) **Q66.80**
    - left foot **Q66.82**
    - right foot **Q66.81**
- **Degeneration, degenerative**
  - anterior cornua, spinal cord **G12.29**
  - anterior labral S43.49-
  - articular cartilage NEC - *see* Derangement, joint, articular cartilage, by site
  - cardiac - *see also* Degeneration, myocardial
    - valve, valvular - *see* Endocarditis
  - changes, spine or vertebra - *see* Spondylosis
  - choroid (colloid) (drusen) H31.10-
    - atrophy - *see* Atrophy, choroidal
    - hereditary - *see* Dystrophy, choroidal, hereditary
  - disc disease - *see* Degeneration, intervertebral disc, by site
  - facet joints - *see* Spondylosis
  - hyaline (diffuse) (generalized)
    - localized - *see* Degeneration, by site
  - intervertebral disc NOS
    - with
      - myelopathy - *see* Disorder, disc, with, myelopathy
      - radiculitis or radiculopathy - *see* Disorder, disc, with, radiculopathy
    - cervical, cervicothoracic - *see* Disorder, disc, cervical, degeneration
      - with
        - myelopathy - *see* Disorder, disc, cervical, with myelopathy
        - neuritis, radiculitis or radiculopathy - *see* Disorder, disc, cervical, with neuritis
    - lumbar region **M51.36**
      - with
        - myelopathy **M51.06**
        - neuritis, radiculitis, radiculopathy or sciatica **M51.16**
    - lumbosacral region **M51.37**
      - with
        - neuritis, radiculitis, radiculopathy or sciatica **M51.17**
    - thoracic region **M51.34**
      - with
        - myelopathy **M51.04**
        - neuritis, radiculitis, radiculopathy **M51.14**
    - thoracolumbar region **M51.35**
      - with
        - myelopathy **M51.05**
        - neuritis, radiculitis, radiculopathy **M51.15**
  - joint disease - *see* Osteoarthritis
  - muscle (fatty) (fibrous) (hyaline) (progressive) **M62.89**
  - myocardial, myocardium (fatty) (hyaline) (senile) **I51.5**
    - hypertensive - *see* Hypertension, heart
  - pigmentary (diffuse) (general)
    - localized - *see* Degeneration, by site
  - senile **R54**
  - sinus (cystic) - *see also* Sinusitis
  - synovial membrane (pulpy) - *see* Disorder, synovium, specified type NEC
  - vascular (senile) - *see* Arteriosclerosis
    - hypertensive - *see* Hypertension
- **Delay, delayed**
  - development **R62.50**
    - global **F88**
    - physiological **R62.50**
- **Delinquency (juvenile) (neurotic) F91.8**
  - group **Z72.810**
- **Delivery (childbirth) (labor)**
  - complicated **O75.9**
    - by
      - diabetes **O24.92**
        - gestational **O24.429**
          - diet controlled **O24.420**
          - insulin controlled **O24.424**
          - oral drug controlled (antidiabetic) (hypoglycemic) **O24.425**
        - pre-existing **O24.32**
          - specified NEC **O24.82**
          - type 1 **O24.02**
          - type 2 **O24.12**
      - gestational
        - diabetes **O24.429**
          - diet controlled **O24.420**
          - insulin (and diet) controlled **O24.424**
          - oral drug controlled (antidiabetic) (hypoglycemic) **O24.425**
        - edema **O12.04**
          - with proteinuria **O12.24**
        - proteinuria **O12.14**
      - hypertension, hypertensive (pre-existing) - *see* Hypertension, complicated by, childbirth (labor)
      - subluxation of symphysis (pubis) **O26.72**

Detachment
  cartilage - *see* Sprain
  ligament - *see* Sprain
  meniscus (knee) - *see also* Derangement, knee, meniscus, specified NEC
    current injury - *see* Tear, meniscus
Deterioration
  general physical **R53.81**
  senile (simple) **R54**
Development
  arrested **R62.5Ø**
    child **R62.5Ø**
  defective, congenital - *see also* Anomaly, by site
  delayed **R62.5Ø** - *see also* Delay, development
    mixed skills **F88**
  imperfect, congenital - *see also* Anomaly, by site
  incomplete
    organ or site not listed - *see* Hypoplasia, by site
  tardy, mental **F79** - *see also* Disability, intellectual
Developmental - *see* condition
  testing, infant or child - *see* Examination, child
Deviation (in)
  midline (jaw) (teeth) (dental arch) **M26.29**
    specified site NEC - *see* Malposition
  organ or site, congenital NEC - *see* Malposition, congenital
Diabetes, diabetic (mellitus) (sugar) E11.9
  with
    amyotrophy **E11.44**
    arthropathy NEC **E11.618**
    autonomic (poly) neuropathy **E11.43**
    cataract **E11.36**
    Charcot's joints **E11.61Ø**
    chronic kidney disease **E11.22**
    circulatory complication NEC **E11.59**
    coma due to
      hyperosmolarity **E11.Ø1**
      hypoglycemia **E11.641**
      ketoacidosis **E11.11**
    complication **E11.8**
      specified NEC **E11.69**
    dermatitis **E11.62Ø**
    foot ulcer **E11.621**
    gangrene **E11.52**
    gastroparalysis **E11.43**
    gastroparesis **E11.43**
    glomerulonephrosis, intracapillary **E11.21**
    glomerulosclerosis, intercapillary **E11.21**
    hyperglycemia **E11.65**
    hyperosmolarity **E11.ØØ**
      with coma **E11.Ø1**
    hypoglycemia **E11.649**
      with coma **E11.641**
    ketoacidosis **E11.1Ø**
      with coma **E11.11**
    kidney complications NEC **E11.29**
    Kimmelsteil-Wilson disease **E11.21**
    loss of protective sensation (LOPS) - *see* Diabetes, by type, with neuropathy
    mononeuropathy **E11.41**
    myasthenia **E11.44**
    necrobiosis lipoidica **E11.62Ø**
    nephropathy **E11.21**
    neuralgia **E11.42**
    neurologic complication NEC **E11.49**
    neuropathic arthropathy **E11.61Ø**
    neuropathy **E11.4Ø**
    ophthalmic complication NEC **E11.39**
    oral complication NEC **E11.638**
    osteomyelitis **E11.69**
    periodontal disease **E11.63Ø**
    peripheral angiopathy **E11.51**
      with gangrene **E11.52**
    polyneuropathy **E11.42**
    renal complication NEC **E11.29**
    renal tubular degeneration **E11.29**
    retinopathy **E11.319**
      with macular edema **E11.311**
        resolved following treatment E11.37-
      nonproliferative E11.329-
        with macular edema E11.321-
        mild E11.329-
          with macular edema E11.321-
        moderate E11.339-
          with macular edema E11.331-
        severe E11.349-
          with macular edema E11.341-
      proliferative E11.359-
        with
          combined traction retinal detachment and rhegmatogenous retinal detachment E11.354-
          macular edema E11.351-
          stable proliferative diabetic retinopathy E11.355-
          traction retinal detachment involving the macula E11.352-
          traction retinal detachment not involving the macula E11.353-
    skin complication NEC **E11.628**
    skin ulcer NEC **E11.622**
  brittle - *see* Diabetes, type 1
  due to
    autoimmune process - *see* Diabetes, type 1
    immune mediated pancreatic islet beta-cell destruction - *see* Diabetes, type 1
  due to drug or chemical **EØ9.9**
    with
      amyotrophy **EØ9.44**
      arthropathy NEC **EØ9.618**
      autonomic (poly) neuropathy **EØ9.43**
      cataract **EØ9.36**
      Charcot's joints **EØ9.61Ø**
      chronic kidney disease **EØ9.22**
      circulatory complication NEC **EØ9.59**
      complication **EØ9.8**
        specified NEC **EØ9.69**
      dermatitis **EØ9.62Ø**
      foot ulcer **EØ9.621**
      gangrene **EØ9.52**
      gastroparalysis **EØ9.43**
      gastroparesis **EØ9.43**
      glomerulonephrosis, intracapillary **EØ9.21**
      glomerulosclerosis, intercapillary **EØ9.21**
      hyperglycemia **EØ9.65**
      hyperosmolarity **EØ9.ØØ**
        with coma **EØ9.Ø1**
      hypoglycemia **EØ9.649**
        with coma **EØ9.641**
      ketoacidosis **EØ9.1Ø**
        with coma **EØ9.11**
      kidney complications NEC **EØ9.29**
      Kimmelstiel-Wilson disease **EØ9.21**
      mononeuropathy **EØ9.41**
      myasthenia **EØ9.44**
      necrobiosis lipoidica **EØ9.62Ø**
      nephropathy **EØ9.21**
      neuralgia **EØ9.42**
      neurologic complication NEC **EØ9.49**
      neuropathic arthropathy **EØ9.61Ø**
      neuropathy **EØ9.4Ø**
      ophthalmic complication NEC **EØ9.39**
      oral complication NEC **EØ9.638**
      periodontal disease **EØ9.63Ø**
      peripheral angiopathy **EØ9.51**
        with gangrene **EØ9.52**
      polyneuropathy **EØ9.42**
      renal complication NEC **EØ9.29**
      renal tubular degeneration **EØ9.29**
      retinopathy **EØ9.319**
        with macular edema **EØ9.311**
        nonproliferative EØ9.329-
          with macular edema EØ9.321-
          mild EØ9.329-
            with macular edema EØ9.321-
          moderate EØ9.339-
            with macular edema EØ9.331-
          severe EØ9.349-
            with macular edema EØ9.341-
        proliferative EØ9.359-
          with
            combined traction retinal detachment and rhegmatogenous retinal detachment EØ9.354-
            macular edema EØ9.351-
            stable proliferative diabetic retinopathy EØ9.355-
            traction retinal detachment involving the macula EØ9.352-
            traction retinal detachment not involving the macula EØ9.353-
        resolved following treatment EØ9.37-
      skin complication NEC **EØ9.628**
      skin ulcer NEC **EØ9.622**
  due to underlying condition **EØ8.9**
    with
      amyotrophy **EØ8.44**
      arthropathy NEC **EØ8.618**
      autonomic (poly) neuropathy **EØ8.43**
      cataract **EØ8.36**
      Charcot's joints **EØ8.61Ø**
      chronic kidney disease **EØ8.22**
      circulatory complication NEC **EØ8.59**
      complication **EØ8.8**
        specified NEC **EØ8.69**
      dermatitis **EØ8.62Ø**
      foot ulcer **EØ8.621**
      gangrene **EØ8.52**
      gastroparalysis **EØ8.43**
      gastroparesis **EØ8.43**
      glomerulonephrosis, intracapillary **EØ8.21**
      glomerulosclerosis, intercapillary **EØ8.21**
      hyperglycemia **EØ8.65**
      hyperosmolarity **EØ8.ØØ**
        with coma **EØ8.Ø1**
      hypoglycemia **EØ8.649**
        with coma **EØ8.641**
      ketoacidosis **EØ8.1Ø**
        with coma **EØ8.11**
      kidney complications NEC **EØ8.29**
      Kimmelsteil-WIlson disease **EØ8.21**
      mononeuropathy **EØ8.41**
      myasthenia **EØ8.44**
      necrobiosis lipoidica **EØ8.62Ø**
      nephropathy **EØ8.21**
      neuralgia **EØ8.42**
      neurologic complication NEC **EØ8.49**
      neuropathic arthropathy **EØ8.61Ø**
      neuropathy **EØ8.4Ø**
      ophthalmic complication NEC **EØ8.39**

- - coma due to
    - hyperosmolarity **E11.Ø1**
    - hypoglycemia **E11.641**
  - complication **E11.8**
    - specified NEC **E11.69**
  - dermatitis **E11.62Ø**
  - foot ulcer **E11.621**
  - gangrene **E11.52**
  - gastroparalysis **E11.43**
  - gastroparesis **E11.43**
  - glomerulonephrosis, intracapillary **E11.21**
  - glomerulosclerosis, intercapillary **E11.21**
  - hyperglycemia **E11.65**
  - hyperosmolarity **E11.ØØ**
    - with coma **E11.Ø1**
  - hypoglycemia **E11.649**
    - with coma **E11.641**
  - ketoacidosis **E11.1Ø**
    - with coma **E11.11**
  - kidney complications NEC **E11.29**
  - Kimmelsteil-Wilson disease **E11.21**
  - mononeuropathy **E11.41**
  - myasthenia **E11.44**
  - necrobiosis lipoidica **E11.62Ø**
  - nephropathy **E11.21**
  - neuralgia **E11.42**
  - neurologic complication NEC **E11.49**
  - neuropathic arthropathy **E11.61Ø**
  - neuropathy **E11.4Ø**
  - ophthalmic complication NEC **E11.39**
  - oral complication NEC **E11.638**
  - osteomyelitis **E11.69**
  - periodontal disease **E11.63Ø**
  - peripheral angiopathy **E11.51**
    - with gangrene **E11.52**
  - polyneuropathy **E11.42**
  - renal complication NEC **E11.29**
  - renal tubular degeneration **E11.29**
  - retinopathy **E11.319**
    - with macular edema **E11.311**
    - nonproliferative E11.329-
      - with macular edema E11.321-
      - mild E11.329-
        - with macular edema E11.321-
      - moderate E11.339-
        - with macular edema E11.331-
      - severe E11.349-
        - with macular edema E11.341-
    - proliferative E11.359-
      - with
        - combined traction retinal detachment and rhegmatogenous retinal detachment E11.354-
        - macular edema E11.351-
        - stable proliferative diabetic retinopathy E11.355-
        - traction retinal detachment involving the macula E11.352-
        - traction retinal detachment not involving the macula E11.353-
    - resolved following treatment E11.37-
  - skin complication NEC **E11.628**
  - skin ulcer NEC **E11.622**
- uncontrolled
  - meaning
    - hyperglycemia - *see* Diabetes, by type, with, hyperglycemia
    - hypoglycemia - *see* Diabetes, by type, with, hypoglycemia

Diagnosis deferred R69

Dialysis (intermittent) (treatment)
- noncompliance (with) **Z91.15**

Diaper rash L22

Diaphoresis (excessive) R61

Diarrhea, diarrheal (disease) (infantile) (inflammatory) R19.7
- amebic **AØ6.Ø** - *see also* Amebiasis
  - with abscess - *see* Abscess, amebic
- due to
  - Clostridium difficile
    - not specified as recurrent **AØ4.72**
    - recurrent **AØ4.71**
  - specified organism NEC **AØ8.8**
    - viral **AØ8.39**
  - virus - *see* Enteritis, viral
- dysenteric **AØ9**
- endemic **AØ9**
- epidemic **AØ9**
- infectious **AØ9**
- specified
  - virus NEC **AØ8.39**
- viral - *see* Enteritis, viral

Diastasis
- joint (traumatic) - *see* Dislocation
- muscle **M62.ØØ**
  - specified site NEC **M62.Ø8**
- recti (abdomen)
  - congenital **Q79.59**

Diathesis
- allergic - *see* History, allergy
- gouty - *see* Gout

Difficult, difficulty (in)
- micturition
  - need to immediately re-void **R39.191**
  - position dependent **R39.192**
  - specified NEC **R39.198**
- swallowing - *see* Dysphagia

Dilatation
- cardiac (acute) (chronic) - *see also* Hypertrophy, cardiac
  - valve - *see* Endocarditis
- heart (acute) (chronic) - *see also* Hypertrophy, cardiac
  - valve - *see* Endocarditis
- organ or site, congenital NEC - *see* Distortion

Diplegia (upper limbs) G83.Ø
- lower limbs **G82.2Ø**

Disability, disabilities
- intellectual **F79**
  - mild (I.Q.5Ø-69) **F7Ø**
  - moderate (I.Q.35-49) **F71**
  - profound (I.Q. under 2Ø) **F73**
  - severe (I.Q.2Ø-34) **F72**

Discharge (from)
- postnasal **RØ9.82**

Discitis, diskitis M46.4Ø
- cervical region **M46.42**
- cervicothoracic region **M46.43**
- lumbar region **M46.46**
- lumbosacral region **M46.47**
- multiple sites **M46.49**
- occipito-atlanto-axial region **M46.41**
- pyogenic - *see* Infection, intervertebral disc, pyogenic
- sacrococcygeal region **M46.48**
- thoracic region **M46.44**
- thoracolumbar region **M46.45**

Discomfort
- chest **RØ7.89**

Discrepancy
- leg length (acquired) - *see* Deformity, limb, unequal length

Disease, diseased - *see also* Syndrome
- airway
  - reactive - *see* Asthma
- anterior
  - horn cell **G12.29**
- antral - *see* Sinusitis, maxillary
- aponeuroses - *see* Enthesopathy
- Arnold-Chiari - *see* Arnold-Chiari disease
- atticoantral, chronic **H66.2Ø**
  - left **H66.22**
    - with right **H66.23**
  - right **H66.21**
    - with left **H66.23**
- basal ganglia **G25.9**
  - specified NEC **G25.89**
- bone - *see also* Disorder, bone
- brain **G93.9**
  - inflammatory - *see* Encephalitis
- Bright's - *see* Nephritis
- bursa - *see* Bursopathy
- cardiovascular (atherosclerotic) **I25.1Ø**
  - hypertensive - *see* Hypertension, heart
- cartilage - *see* Disorder, cartilage
- Crohn's - *see* Enteritis, regional
- demyelinating, demyelinizating (nervous system) **G37.9**
  - multiple sclerosis **G35**
- deposition, hydroxyapatite - *see* Disease, hydroxyapatite deposition
- diarrheal, infectious NEC **AØ9**
- disc, degenerative - *see* Degeneration, intervertebral disc
- discogenic - *see also* Displacement, intervertebral disc NEC
  - with myelopathy - *see* Disorder, disc, with, myelopathy
- Duchenne-Griesinger **G71.Ø1**
- Duchenne's
  - muscular dystrophy **G71.Ø1**
  - pseudohypertrophy, muscles **G71.Ø1**
- Eberth's - *see* Fever, typhoid
- Erb (-Landouzy) **G71.Ø2**
- extrapyramidal **G25.9**
  - specified NEC **G25.89**
- fascia NEC - *see also* Disorder, muscle
  - inflammatory - *see* Myositis
  - specified NEC **M62.89**
- Forestier's (rhizomelic pseudopolyarthritis) **M35.3**
  - meaning ankylosing hyperostosis - *see* Hyperostosis, ankylosing
- Fothergill's
  - neuralgia - *see* Neuralgia, trigeminal
- frontal sinus - *see* Sinusitis, frontal
- gallbladder **K82.9**
  - cholecystitis - *see* Cholecystitis
- glomerular - *see also* Glomerulonephritis
- Hansen's - *see* Leprosy
- heart (organic) **I51.9**
  - fibroid - *see* Myocarditis
  - hypertensive - *see* Hypertension, heart
  - senile - *see* Myocarditis
  - valve, valvular (obstructive) (regurgitant) - *see also* Endocarditis
- heredodegenerative NEC
  - spinal cord **G95.89**
- hip (joint) **M25.9**
  - congenital **Q65.89**
- Huntington's **G1Ø**
  - with dementia **G1Ø** [**FØ2.8Ø**] - *see also* Dementia, in, diseases specified elsewhere
- hydroxyapatite deposition **M11.ØØ**
  - multiple site **M11.Ø9**
  - vertebra **M11.Ø8**
- hypertensive - *see* Hypertension
- Iceland **G93.39**
- intervertebral disc - *see also* Disorder, disc
  - with myelopathy - *see* Disorder, disc, with, myelopathy

- cervical, cervicothoracic - *see* Disorder, disc, cervical
  - with
    - myelopathy - *see* Disorder, disc, cervical, with myelopathy
    - neuritis, radiculitis or radiculopathy - *see* Disorder, disc, cervical, with neuritis
    - specified NEC - *see* Disorder, disc, cervical, specified type NEC
- lumbar (with)
  - myelopathy **M51.Ø6**
  - neuritis, radiculitis, radiculopathy or sciatica **M51.16**
  - specified NEC **M51.86**
- lumbosacral (with)
  - neuritis, radiculitis, radiculopathy or sciatica **M51.17**
  - specified NEC **M51.87**
- specified NEC - *see* Disorder, disc, specified NEC
- thoracic (with)
  - myelopathy **M51.Ø4**
  - neuritis, radiculitis or radiculopathy **M51.14**
  - specified NEC **M51.84**
- thoracolumbar (with)
  - myelopathy **M51.Ø5**
  - neuritis, radiculitis or radiculopathy **M51.15**
  - specified NEC **M51.85**

joint - *see also* Disorder, joint
- degenerative - *see* Osteoarthritis
  - spine - *see* Spondylosis
- facet joint **M47.819** - *see also* Spondylosis
- hypertrophic - *see* Osteoarthritis
- specified NEC - *see* Disorder, joint, specified type NEC
- spine NEC - *see* Dorsopathy

König's (osteochondritis dissecans) - *see* Osteochondritis, dissecans

liver (chronic) (organic) **K76.9**
- end stage K72.1-
  - due to hepatitis - *see* Hepatitis

lumbosacral region **M53.87**

lung **J98.4**
- in
  - Sjögren's syndrome **M35.Ø2**
  - systemic
    - sclerosis **M34.81**
- rheumatoid (diffuse) (interstitial) - *see* Rheumatoid, lung

mental **F99**

motor neuron (bulbar) (mixed type) (spinal) **G12.2Ø**
- amyotrophic lateral sclerosis **G12.21**
- familial **G12.24**
- progressive bulbar palsy **G12.22**
- specified NEC **G12.29**

muscle - *see also* Disorder, muscle
- inflammatory - *see* Myositis

musculoskeletal system, soft tissue - *see also* Disorder, soft tissue
- specified NEC - *see* Disorder, soft tissue, specified type NEC

nucleus pulposus - *see* Disorder, disc

Parkinson's **G2Ø**

peripheral
- nerves - *see* Polyneuropathy

persistent mucosal (middle ear) **H66.2Ø**
- left **H66.22**
  - with right **H66.23**
- right **H66.21**
  - with left **H66.23**

psychiatric **F99**

pulmonary - *see also* Disease, lung

reactive airway - *see* Asthma

renal (functional) (pelvis) **N28.9** - *see also* Disease, kidney
- with
  - glomerular lesion - *see* Glomerulonephritis

rheumatoid - *see* Arthritis, rheumatoid

Rotes Quérol - *see* Hyperostosis, ankylosing

Schmorl's - *see* Schmorl's disease or nodes

semilunar cartilage, cystic - *see also* Derangement, knee, meniscus, cystic

sinus - *see* Sinusitis

spinal (cord) **G95.9**
- specified NEC **G95.89**

spine - *see also* Spondylopathy
- joint - *see* Dorsopathy

striatopallidal system NEC **G25.89**

synovium - *see* Disorder, synovium

tendon, tendinous - *see also* Disorder, tendon
- nodular - *see* Trigger finger

thromboembolic - *see* Embolism

vascular **I99.9**
- hypertensive - *see* Hypertension

vertebra, vertebral - *see also* Spondylopathy
- disc - *see* Disorder, disc

wasting NEC **R64**

Willis' - *see* Diabetes

DISH (diffuse idiopathic skeletal hyperostosis) - *see* Hyperostosis, ankylosing

Dislocation (articular)
- acromioclavicular (joint) S43.1Ø-
  - with displacement
    - 1ØØ%-2ØØ% S43.12-
    - more than 2ØØ% S43.13-
  - inferior S43.14-
  - posterior S43.15-
- atlantoaxial S13.121-
- atlantooccipital S13.111-
- atloidooccipital S13.111-
- breast bone S23.29-
- carpal (bone) - *see* Dislocation, wrist
- carpometacarpal (joint) NEC S63.Ø5-
  - thumb S63.Ø4-
- cervical spine (vertebra) - *see* Dislocation, vertebra, cervical
- chronic - *see* Dislocation, recurrent
- clavicle - *see* Dislocation, acromioclavicular joint
- coracoid - *see* Dislocation, shoulder
- costal cartilage S23.29-
- costochondral S23.29-
- cricoarytenoid articulation S13.29-
- cricothyroid articulation S13.29-
- dorsal vertebra - *see* Dislocation, vertebra, thoracic
- elbow S53.1Ø-
  - radial head alone - *see* Dislocation, radial head
  - traumatic S53.1Ø-
    - anterior S53.11-
    - lateral S53.14-
    - medial S53.13-
    - posterior S53.12-
    - specified type NEC S53.19-
- femur
  - distal end - *see* Dislocation, knee
  - proximal end - *see* Dislocation, hip
- fibula
  - proximal end - *see* Dislocation, knee
- finger S63.25-
  - index S63.25-
  - interphalangeal S63.27-
    - distal S63.29-
      - index S63.29-
      - little S63.29-
      - middle S63.29-
      - ring S63.29-
    - index S63.27-
    - little S63.27-
    - middle S63.27-
    - proximal S63.28-
      - index S63.28-
      - little S63.28-
      - middle S63.28-
      - ring S63.28-
    - ring S63.27-
  - little S63.25-
  - metacarpophalangeal S63.26-
    - index S63.26-
    - little S63.26-
    - middle S63.26-
    - ring S63.26-
  - middle S63.25-
  - ring S63.25-
  - thumb - *see* Dislocation, thumb
- foot S93.3Ø-
  - specified site NEC S93.33-
  - tarsal joint S93.31-
  - tarsometatarsal joint S93.32-
  - toe - *see* Dislocation, toe
- glenohumeral (joint) - *see* Dislocation, shoulder
- glenoid - *see* Dislocation, shoulder
- habitual - *see* Dislocation, recurrent
- hip S73.ØØ-
  - anterior S73.Ø3-
    - obturator S73.Ø2-
  - central S73.Ø4-
  - posterior S73.Ø1-
- humerus, proximal end - *see* Dislocation, shoulder
- incomplete - *see* Subluxation, by site
- infracoracoid - *see* Dislocation, shoulder
- innominate (pubic junction) (sacral junction) S33.39-
  - acetabulum - *see* Dislocation, hip
- interphalangeal (joint(s))
  - finger S63.279-
    - distal S63.29-
      - index S63.29-
      - little S63.29-
      - middle S63.29-
      - ring S63.29-
    - index S63.27-
    - little S63.27-
    - middle S63.27-
    - proximal S63.28-
      - index S63.28-
      - little S63.28-
      - middle S63.28-
      - ring S63.28-
    - ring S63.27-
  - foot or toe - *see* Dislocation, toe
  - thumb S63.12-
- knee S83.1Ø6-
  - cap - *see* Dislocation, patella
  - patella - *see* Dislocation, patella
  - proximal tibia
    - anteriorly S83.11-
    - laterally S83.14-
    - medially S83.13-
    - posteriorly S83.12-
  - specified type NEC S83.19-
- lumbar (vertebra) - *see* Dislocation, vertebra, lumbar

- disc (intervertebral) **M51.9**
  - with
    - myelopathy
      - cervical region **M50.00**
      - cervicothoracic region **M50.03**
      - high cervical region **M50.01**
      - lumbar region **M51.06**
      - mid-cervical region **M50.020**
      - thoracic region **M51.04**
      - thoracolumbar region **M51.05**
    - radiculopathy
      - cervical region **M50.10**
      - cervicothoracic region **M50.13**
      - high cervical region **M50.11**
      - lumbar region **M51.16**
      - lumbosacral region **M51.17**
      - mid-cervical region **M50.120**
      - thoracic region **M51.14**
      - thoracolumbar region **M51.15**
  - cervical **M50.90**
    - with
      - myelopathy **M50.00**
        - C2-C3 **M50.01**
        - C3-C4 **M50.01**
        - C4-C5 **M50.021**
        - C5-C6 **M50.022**
        - C6-C7 **M50.023**
        - C7-T1 **M50.03**
        - cervicothoracic region **M50.03**
        - high cervical region **M50.01**
        - mid-cervical region **M50.020**
      - neuritis, radiculitis or radiculopathy **M50.10**
        - C2-C3 **M50.11**
        - C3-C4 **M50.11**
        - C4-C5 **M50.121**
        - C5-C6 **M50.122**
        - C6-C7 **M50.123**
        - C7-T1 **M50.13**
        - cervicothoracic region **M50.13**
        - high cervical region **M50.11**
        - mid-cervical region **M50.120**
    - C2-C3 **M50.91**
    - C3-C4 **M50.91**
    - C4-C5 **M50.921**
    - C5-C6 **M50.922**
    - C6-C7 **M50.923**
    - C7-T1 **M50.93**
    - cervicothoracic region **M50.93**
    - degeneration **M50.30**
      - C2-C3 **M50.31**
      - C3-C4 **M50.31**
      - C4-C5 **M50.321**
      - C5-C6 **M50.322**
      - C6-C7 **M50.323**
      - C7-T1 **M50.33**
      - cervicothoracic region **M50.33**
      - high cervical region **M50.31**
      - mid-cervical region **M50.320**
    - displacement **M50.20**
      - C2-C3 **M50.21**
      - C3-C4 **M50.21**
      - C4-C5 **M50.221**
      - C5-C6 **M50.222**
      - C6-C7 **M50.223**
      - C7-T1 **M50.23**
      - cervicothoracic region **M50.23**
      - high cervical region **M50.21**
      - mid-cervical region **M50.220**
    - high cervical region **M50.91**
    - mid-cervical region **M50.920**
    - specified type NEC **M50.80**
      - C2-C3 **M50.81**
      - C3-C4 **M50.81**
      - C4-C5 **M50.821**
      - C5-C6 **M50.822**
      - C6-C7 **M50.823**
      - C7-T1 **M50.83**
      - cervicothoracic region **M50.83**
      - high cervical region **M50.81**
      - mid-cervical region **M50.820**
  - specified NEC
    - lumbar region **M51.86**
    - lumbosacral region **M51.87**
    - thoracic region **M51.84**
    - thoracolumbar region **M51.85**
- drug related **F19.99**
  - abuse - *see* Abuse, drug
  - dependence - *see* Dependence, drug
- eating (adult) (psychogenic) **F50.9**
  - anorexia - *see* Anorexia
- erythematous - *see* Erythema
- extrapyramidal **G25.9**
  - specified type NEC **G25.89**
- fluency
  - following
    - cerebral infarction **I69.323**
  - in conditions classified elsewhere **R47.82**
- joint **M25.9**
  - derangement - *see* Derangement, joint
  - effusion - *see* Effusion, joint
  - fistula - *see* Fistula, joint
  - hemarthrosis - *see* Hemarthrosis
  - instability - *see* Instability, joint
  - osteophyte - *see* Osteophyte
  - pain - *see* Pain, joint
  - specified type NEC **M25.80**
  - stiffness - *see* Stiffness, joint
- ligament **M24.20**
  - attachment, spine - *see* Enthesopathy, spinal
  - specified site NEC **M24.29**
  - vertebra **M24.28**
- ligamentous attachments - *see also* Enthesopathy
  - spine - *see* Enthesopathy, spinal
- low back - *see also* Dorsopathy, specified NEC
- meniscus - *see* Derangement, knee, meniscus
- mental (or behavioral) (nonpsychotic) **F99**
  - due to (secondary to)
    - cannabis use
      - due to drug abuse - *see* Abuse, drug, cannabis
    - tobacco (nicotine) use - *see* Dependence, drug, nicotine
  - following organic brain damage **F07.9**
    - postconcussional syndrome **F07.81**
- micturition NEC **R39.198** - *see also* Difficulty, micturition
  - feeling of incomplete emptying **R39.14**
  - hesitancy **R39.11**
  - poor stream **R39.12**
  - split stream **R39.13**
  - straining **R39.16**
  - urgency **R39.15**
- movement **G25.9**
  - drug-induced **G25.70**
    - akathisia **G25.71**
    - specified NEC **G25.79**
  - periodic limb **G47.61**
    - sleep related **G47.61**
  - sleep related NEC **G47.69**
  - specified NEC **G25.89**
- muscle **M62.9**
  - attachment, spine - *see* Enthesopathy, spinal
  - in trichinellosis - *see* Trichinellosis, with muscle disorder
  - specified type NEC **M62.89**
- muscular
  - attachments - *see also* Enthesopathy
    - spine - *see* Enthesopathy, spinal
- musculoskeletal system, soft tissue - *see* Disorder, soft tissue
- myoneural **G70.9**
  - specified NEC **G70.89**
- neck region NEC - *see* Dorsopathy, specified NEC
- neurodevelopmental **F89**
  - specified NEC **F88**
- neurological NEC **R29.818**
- neuromuscular **G70.9**
  - specified NEC **G70.89**
- nicotine use - *see* Dependence, drug, nicotine
- opioid use
  - due to drug abuse - *see* Abuse, drug, opioid
  - mild **F11.10**
- pain
  - with related psychological factors **F45.42**
  - exclusively related to psychological factors **F45.41**
- persistent
  - (somatoform) pain **F45.41**
- postconcussional **F07.81**
- psychological **F99**
- psychophysiologic - *see* Disorder, somatoform
- psychosomatic NOS - *see* Disorder, somatoform
- seizure **G40.909** - *see also* Epilepsy
  - intractable **G40.919**
    - with status epilepticus **G40.911**
- sleep **G47.9**
  - breathing-related - *see* Apnea, sleep
  - circadian rhythm **G47.20**
  - excessive somnolence - *see* Hypersomnia
  - hypersomnia type - *see* Hypersomnia
  - initiating or maintaining - *see* Insomnia
- soft tissue **M79.9**
  - due to use, overuse and pressure **M70.90**
    - bursitis - *see* Bursitis
    - multiple sites **M70.99**
    - specified site NEC **M70.98**
    - specified type NEC **M70.80**
      - multiple sites **M70.89**
      - specified site NEC **M70.88**
  - occupational - *see* Disorder, soft tissue, due to use, overuse and pressure
  - specified type NEC **M79.89**
- somatoform **F45.9**
  - pain (persistent) **F45.41**
- somnolence, excessive - *see* Hypersomnia
- speech **R47.9**
  - specified NEC **R47.89**
- spine - *see also* Dorsopathy
  - ligamentous or muscular attachments, peripheral - *see* Enthesopathy, spinal
  - specified NEC - *see* Dorsopathy, specified NEC
- synovium **M67.90**
  - multiple sites **M67.99**
  - rupture - *see* Rupture, synovium
  - specified type NEC **M67.80**
    - multiple sites **M67.89**
  - synovitis - *see* Synovitis

- tendon **M67.90**
  - multiple sites **M67.99**
  - rupture - *see* Rupture, tendon
  - specified type NEC **M67.80**
    - multiple sites **M67.89**
    - trunk **M67.88**
  - synovitis - *see* Synovitis
  - tendinitis - *see* Tendinitis
  - tenosynovitis - *see* Tenosynovitis
  - trunk **M67.98**
- tic - *see* Tic
- tobacco use
  - mild **F17.200**
  - moderate **F17.200**
  - severe **F17.200**
- tubulo-interstitial (in)
  - Salmonella infection **A02.25**
- vestibular function H81.9-
  - vertigo - *see* Vertigo

Displacement, displaced
- acquired traumatic of bone, cartilage, joint, tendon NEC - *see* Dislocation
- intervertebral disc NEC
  - with myelopathy - *see* Disorder, disc, with, myelopathy
  - cervical, cervicothoracic (with) **M50.20**
    - myelopathy - *see* Disorder, disc, cervical, with myelopathy
    - neuritis, radiculitis or radiculopathy - *see* Disorder, disc, cervical, with neuritis
  - due to trauma - *see* Dislocation, vertebra
  - lumbar region **M51.26**
    - with
      - myelopathy **M51.06**
      - neuritis, radiculitis, radiculopathy or sciatica **M51.16**
  - lumbosacral region **M51.27**
    - with
      - neuritis, radiculitis, radiculopathy or sciatica **M51.17**
  - thoracic region **M51.24**
    - with
      - myelopathy **M51.04**
      - neuritis, radiculitis, radiculopathy **M51.14**
  - thoracolumbar region **M51.25**
    - with
      - myelopathy **M51.05**
      - neuritis, radiculitis, radiculopathy **M51.15**
- organ or site, congenital NEC - *see* Malposition, congenital

Disruption (of)
- family **Z63.8**
  - due to
    - absence of family member due to military deployment **Z63.31**
    - absence of family member NEC **Z63.32**
    - alcoholism and drug addiction in family **Z63.72**
    - drug addiction in family **Z63.72**
    - return of family member from military deployment (current or past conflict) **Z63.71**
    - stressful life events NEC **Z63.79**
- ligament (s) - *see also* Sprain
  - knee
    - current injury - *see* Dislocation, knee
    - spontaneous NEC - *see* Derangement, knee, disruption ligament
- pelvic ring (stable) S32.810-
  - unstable S32.811-

Distortion (s) (congenital)
- coccyx **Q76.49**
- lumbar spine **Q76.49**
- lumbosacral (joint) (region) **Q76.49**
  - kyphosis - *see* Kyphosis, congenital
  - lordosis - *see* Lordosis, congenital
- organ
  - or site not listed - *see* Anomaly, by site
- sacrum **Q76.49**
- spine **Q76.49**
  - kyphosis - *see* Kyphosis, congenital
  - lordosis - *see* Lordosis, congenital
- vertebra **Q76.49**
  - kyphosis - *see* Kyphosis, congenital
  - lordosis - *see* Lordosis, congenital
- visual - *see also* Disturbance, vision

Distress
- abdomen - *see* Pain, abdominal
- epigastric **R10.13**
- respiratory (adult) (child) **R06.03**
  - orthopnea **R06.01**
  - shortness of breath **R06.02**
  - specified type NEC **R06.09**

Disturbance (s) - *see also* Disease
- equilibrium **R42**
- gait - *see* Gait
- hearing, except deafness and tinnitus - *see* Abnormal, auditory perception
- mental **F99**
- speech **R47.9**
  - specified NEC **R47.89**
- vision, visual **H53.9**
  - following
    - cerebral infarction **I69.398**

Diverticulitis (acute) K57.92
- bladder - *see* Cystitis

Diverticulum, diverticula (multiple) K57.90
- organ or site, congenital NEC - *see* Distortion

Division
- ligament (partial or complete) (current) - *see also* Sprain
- muscle (partial or complete) (current) - *see also* Injury, muscle
- nerve (traumatic) - *see* Injury, nerve
- spinal cord - *see* Injury, spinal cord, by region

Dizziness R42

Dolichostenomelia - *see* Syndrome, Marfan's

Dorsalgia M54.9
- psychogenic **F45.41**
- specified NEC **M54.89**

Dorsopathy M53.9
- specified NEC **M53.80**
  - cervical region **M53.82**
  - cervicothoracic region **M53.83**
  - lumbar region **M53.86**
  - lumbosacral region **M53.87**
  - occipito-atlanto-axial region **M53.81**
  - sacrococcygeal region **M53.88**
  - thoracic region **M53.84**
  - thoracolumbar region **M53.85**

Drinking (alcohol)
- excessive, to excess NEC (without dependence) **F10.10**

Drip, postnasal (chronic) R09.82
- due to
  - allergic rhinitis - *see* Rhinitis, allergic
  - common cold **J00**
  - nasopharyngitis - *see* Nasopharyngitis
  - sinusitis - *see* Sinusitis

Droop
- facial **R29.810**
  - cerebrovascular disease **I69.992**
    - cerebral infarction **I69.392**

Drop (in)
- attack NEC **R55**

Drug
- abuse counseling and surveillance **Z71.51**
- addiction - *see* Dependence
- dependence - *see* Dependence
- habit - *see* Dependence
- harmful use - *see* Abuse, drug
- therapy
  - long term (current) (prophylactic) - *see* Therapy, drug long-term (current) (prophylactic)

Duchenne-Aran muscular atrophy G12.21

Duchenne-Griesinger disease G71.01

Duchenne's
- disease or syndrome
  - motor neuron disease **G12.22**
  - muscular dystrophy **G71.01**
- paralysis
  - due to or associated with
    - motor neuron disease **G12.22**
    - muscular dystrophy **G71.01**

Dumbness - *see* Aphasia

Duplication, duplex - *see also* Accessory

Dwarfism E34.328 - *see also* Stature, short
- congenital **E34.328** - *see also* Stature, short
- constitutional **E34.31**
- infantile **E34.328** - *see also* Stature, short
- Laron-type **E34.321** - *see also* Stature, short

Dysacusis - *see* Abnormal, auditory perception

Dysarthria R47.1
- following
  - cerebral infarction **I69.322**

Dyschezia K59.00

Dysentery, dysenteric (catarrhal) (diarrhea) (epidemic) (hemorrhagic) (infectious) (sporadic) (tropical) A09
- amebic **A06.0** - *see also* Amebiasis
  - with abscess - *see* Abscess, amebic
- arthritis **A09** - *see also* category M01-

Dysequilibrium R42

Dysferlinopathy G71.033

Dysfunction
- physiological NEC **R68.89**
- reflex (sympathetic) - *see* Syndrome, pain, complex regional I
- segmental - *see* Dysfunction, somatic
- senile **R54**
- sexual (due to) **R37**
- somatic **M99.09**
  - abdomen **M99.09**
  - acromioclavicular **M99.07**
  - cervical region **M99.01**
  - cervicothoracic **M99.01**
  - costochondral **M99.08**
  - costovertebral **M99.08**
  - head region **M99.00**
  - hip **M99.05**
  - lower extremity **M99.06**
  - lumbar region **M99.03**
  - lumbosacral **M99.03**
  - occipitocervical **M99.00**
  - pelvic region **M99.05**
  - pubic **M99.05**
  - rib cage **M99.08**
  - sacral region **M99.04**
  - sacrococcygeal **M99.04**
  - sacroiliac **M99.04**
  - specified NEC **M99.09**
  - sternochondral **M99.08**
  - sternoclavicular **M99.07**
  - thoracic region **M99.02**
  - thoracolumbar **M99.02**
  - upper extremity **M99.07**
- temporomandibular (joint) **M26.69**

Dysnomia R47.01

- **Dyspepsia R10.13**
- **Dysphagia R13.10**
  - cervical **R13.19**
  - following
    - cerebral infarction **I69.391**
  - neurogenic **R13.19**
  - oral phase **R13.11**
  - oropharyngeal phase **R13.12**
  - pharyngeal phase **R13.13**
  - pharyngoesophageal phase **R13.14**
  - specified NEC **R13.19**
- **Dysphasia R47.02**
  - following
    - cerebrovascular disease **I69.921**
      - cerebral infarction **I69.321**
- **Dysplasia** - *see also* Anomaly
  - acetabular, congenital **Q65.89**
  - fibrous
    - bone NEC (monostotic) **M85.00**
  - hip, congenital **Q65.89**
- **Dyspnea (nocturnal) (paroxysmal) R06.00**
  - asthmatic (bronchial) **J45.909**
    - with
      - bronchitis **J45.909**
  - orthopnea **R06.01**
  - shortness of breath **R06.02**
  - specified type NEC **R06.09**
- **Dysrhythmia**
  - cerebral or cortical - *see* Epilepsy
- **Dyssomnia** - *see* Disorder, sleep
- **Dystonia G24.9**
  - drug induced NEC **G24.09**
    - specified NEC **G24.09**
- **Dystrophy, dystrophia**
  - autosomal recessive, childhood type, muscular dystrophy resembling Duchenne or Becker **G71.01**
  - Becker's type **G71.01**
  - Duchenne's type **G71.01**
  - Erb's **G71.02**
  - Gower's muscular **G71.01**
  - Landouzy-Déjérine **G71.02**
  - Leyden-Möbius **G71.039** - *see also* Dystrophy, muscular, limb-girdle, by type
    - meaning Limb girdle muscular dystrophy NOS **G71.039**
    - meaning Limb girdle muscular dystrophy type 2A (autosomal recessive) **G71.032**
    - meaning Limb girdle muscular dystrophy, specified type NEC **G71.038**
  - muscular **G71.00**
    - autosomal recessive, childhood type, muscular dystrophy resembling Duchenne or Becker **G71.01**
    - benign (Becker type) **G71.01**
      - scapuloperoneal with early contractures [Emery-Dreifuss] **G71.09**
    - congenital (hereditary) (progressive) (with specific morphological abnormalities of the muscle fiber) **G71.09**
    - distal **G71.09**
    - Duchenne type **G71.01**
    - Emery-Dreifuss **G71.09**
    - Erb type **G71.02**
    - facioscapulohumeral **G71.02**
    - Gower's **G71.01**
    - hereditary (progressive) **G71.09** - *see also* Dystrophy, muscular, by type
    - Landouzy-Déjérine type **G71.02**
    - limb-girdle **G71.039**
      - R10- (autosomal recessive) **G71.038**
      - R11- (autosomal recessive) **G71.038**
      - **R12** (autosomal recessive) **G71.035**
      - R13- (autosomal recessive) **G71.038**
      - R14- (autosomal recessive) **G71.038**
      - R15- (autosomal recessive) **G71.038**
      - R16- (autosomal recessive) **G71.038**
      - **R17** (autosomal recessive) **G71.038**
      - R18- (autosomal recessive) **G71.038**
      - R19- (autosomal recessive) **G71.038**
      - R20- (autosomal recessive) **G71.038**
      - **R21** (autosomal recessive) **G71.038**
      - R22- (autosomal recessive) **G71.038**
      - R23- (autosomal recessive) **G71.038**
      - anoctamin-5-related autosomal recessive (**R12**) **G71.035**
      - autosomal recessive NEC **G71.038**
      - calpain-3-related **G71.032**
        - autosomal dominant **G71.031**
        - autosomal recessive **G71.032**
      - collagen VI related
        - autosomal dominant **G71.031**
        - autosomal recessive **G71.038**
      - D1 (autosomal dominant) **G71.031**
      - D2 (autosomal dominant) **G71.031**
      - D3 (autosomal dominant) **G71.031**
      - D4 (autosomal dominant) **G71.031**
      - D5 (autosomal dominant) **G71.031**
      - due to
        - anoctamin-5 dysfunction **G71.035**
        - fukutin related protein dysfunction **G71.038**
      - FKRP-related autosomal recessive **G71.038**
      - R1 (autosomal recessive) **G71.032**
      - R2 (autosomal recessive) **G71.033**
      - R24 (autosomal recessive) **G71.038**
      - R7 (autosomal recessive) **G71.038**
      - R8 (autosomal recessive) **G71.038**
      - R9 (autosomal recessive) **G71.038**
      - type 1 (autosomal dominant) **G71.031**
      - type 1A (autosomal dominant) **G71.031**
      - type 1B (autosomal dominant) **G71.031**
      - type 1C (autosomal dominant) **G71.031**
      - type 1E (autosomal dominant) **G71.031**
      - type 1H (autosomal dominant) **G71.031**
      - type 1I (autosomal dominant) **G71.031**
      - type 2 (autosomal recessive) **G71.038**
        - specified NEC **G71.038**
      - type 2A (autosomal recessive) **G71.032**
      - type 2B (autosomal recessive) **G71.033**
      - type 2I (autosomal recessive) **G71.038**
      - type 2L (autosomal recessive) **G71.035**
    - progressive (hereditary) **G71.09** - *see also* Dystrophy, muscular, by type
    - pseudohypertrophic (infantile) **G71.01**
    - scapulohumeral **G71.02**
    - scapuloperoneal **G71.09**
    - severe (Duchenne type) **G71.01**
    - specified type NEC **G71.09**
  - ocular **G71.09**
  - oculopharyngeal **G71.09**
  - reflex (neuromuscular) (sympathetic) - *see* Syndrome, pain, complex regional I
  - scapuloperoneal **G71.09**
  - sympathetic (reflex) - *see* Syndrome, pain, complex regional I

E

- **Ear** - *see also* condition
  - wax (impacted) **H61.20**
    - left **H61.22**
      - with right **H61.23**
    - right **H61.21**
      - with left **H61.23**
- **Early satiety R68.81**
- **Eaton-Lambert syndrome** - *see* Syndrome, Lambert-Eaton
- **Eberth's disease (typhoid fever) A01.00**
- **Ecchymosis R58**
  - traumatic - *see* Contusion
- **Ectopic, ectopia (congenital)**
  - abdominal viscera **Q45.8**
    - due to defect in anterior abdominal wall **Q79.59**
  - gestation - *see* Pregnancy, by site
  - mole - *see* Pregnancy, by site
  - organ or site NEC - *see* Malposition, congenital
- **Eczema (acute) (chronic) (erythematous) (fissum) (rubrum) (squamous) L30.9** - *see also* Dermatitis
  - contact - *see* Dermatitis, contact
  - hypostatic - *see* Varix, leg, with, inflammation
  - stasis **I87.2**
    - with varicose veins - *see* Varix, leg, with, inflammation
  - varicose - *see* Varix, leg, with, inflammation
- **Edema, edematous (infectious) (pitting) (toxic) R60.9**
  - joint - *see* Effusion, joint
  - macula **H35.81**
    - diabetic - *see* Diabetes, by type, with, retinopathy, with macular edema
  - retina **H35.81**
    - diabetic - *see* Diabetes, by type, with, retinopathy, with macular edema
- **Effect, adverse**
  - abuse - *see* Maltreatment
  - exposure - *see* Exposure
- **Effects, late** - *see* Sequelae
- **Effusion**
  - bronchial - *see* Bronchitis
  - cerebrospinal - *see also* Meningitis
  - joint **M25.40**
    - specified joint NEC **M25.48**
  - meninges - *see* Meningitis
  - spinal - *see* Meningitis
- **Ekbom's syndrome (restless legs) G25.81**
- **Elevated, elevation**
  - blood pressure - *see also* Hypertension
  - cholesterol **E78.00**
  - finding on laboratory examination - *see* Findings, abnormal, inconclusive, without diagnosis, by type of exam
  - GFR (glomerular filtration rate) - *see* Findings, abnormal, inconclusive, without diagnosis, by type of exam
  - liver function
    - test **R79.89**
      - bilirubin **R17**
- **Elongated, elongation (congenital)** - *see also* Distortion
- **Emaciation R64**

- **Embolism (multiple) (paradoxical) I74.9**
  - artery **I74.9**
    - pulmonary - *see* Embolism, pulmonary
  - lung (massive) - *see* Embolism, pulmonary
  - pulmonary (acute) (artery) (vein) **I26.99**
    - healed or old **Z86.711**
    - personal history of **Z86.711**
- **Embolus** - *see* Embolism
- **Emesis** - *see* Vomiting
- **Emotional lability R45.86**
- **Empyema (acute) (chest) (double) (pleura) (supradiaphragmatic) (thorax) J86.9**
  - accessory sinus (chronic) - *see* Sinusitis
  - antrum (chronic) - *see* Sinusitis, maxillary
  - ethmoidal (chronic) (sinus) - *see* Sinusitis, ethmoidal
  - frontal (chronic) (sinus) - *see* Sinusitis, frontal
  - maxilla, maxillary **M27.2**
    - sinus (chronic) - *see* Sinusitis, maxillary
  - nasal sinus (chronic) - *see* Sinusitis
  - sinus (accessory) (chronic) (nasal) - *see* Sinusitis
  - sphenoidal (sinus) (chronic) - *see* Sinusitis, sphenoidal
- **Encephalitis (chronic) (hemorrhagic) (idiopathic) (nonepidemic) (spurious) (subacute) GØ4.9Ø**
  - otitic NEC **H66.4Ø** [GØ5.3]
- **Encephalomyelitis GØ4.9Ø** - *see also* Encephalitis
  - myalgic **G93.32**
    - chronic fatigue syndrome [ME/CFS] **G93.32**
- **Encephalopathy (acute) G93.4Ø**
  - in (due to) (with)
    - trauma (postconcussional) **FØ7.81**
  - postcontusional **FØ7.81**
  - traumatic (postconcussional) **FØ7.81**
- **Encephalosis, posttraumatic FØ7.81**
- **Encounter (with health service) (for) Z76.89**
  - administrative purpose only **ZØ2.9**
    - examination for
      - disability determination **ZØ2.71**
      - medical certificate NEC **ZØ2.79**
    - specified reason NEC **ZØ2.89**
  - aftercare - *see* Aftercare
  - check-up - *see* Examination
  - counseling - *see* Counseling
  - examination - *see* Examination
  - laboratory (as part of a general medical examination) **ZØØ.ØØ**
    - with abnormal findings **ZØØ.Ø1**
  - radiological (as part of a general medical examination) **ZØØ.ØØ**
    - with abnormal findings **ZØØ.Ø1**
  - removal (of) - *see also* Removal
  - respirator [ventilator] use during power failure **Z99.12**
  - screening - *see* Screening
  - specified NEC **Z76.89**
  - testing - *see* Test
  - X-ray of chest (as part of a general medical examination) **ZØØ.ØØ**
    - with abnormal findings **ZØØ.Ø1**
- **Encystment** - *see* Cyst
- **Endarteritis (bacterial, subacute) (infective) I77.6**
  - embolic - *see* Embolism
- **Endocarditis (chronic) (marantic) (nonbacterial) (thrombotic) (valvular) I38**
  - due to
    - typhoid (fever) **AØ1.Ø2**
  - rheumatoid - *see* Rheumatoid, carditis
  - typhoid **AØ1.Ø2**
- **Endomyocarditis** - *see* Endocarditis
- **Endopericarditis** - *see* Endocarditis
- **Endosteitis** - *see* Osteomyelitis
- **Enlargement, enlarged** - *see also* Hypertrophy
  - alveolar ridge **KØ8.89**
    - congenital - *see* Anomaly, alveolar
  - organ or site, congenital NEC - *see* Anomaly, by site
- **Entamebic, entamebiasis** - *see* Amebiasis
- **Enteralgia** - *see* Pain, abdominal
- **Enteritis (acute) (diarrheal) (hemorrhagic) (noninfective) K52.9**
  - amebic (acute) **AØ6.Ø**
    - with abscess - *see* Abscess, amebic
    - chronic **AØ6.1**
      - with abscess - *see* Abscess, amebic
  - astrovirus **AØ8.32**
  - calicivirus **AØ8.31**
  - chronic (noninfectious) **K52.9**
    - ulcerative - *see* Colitis, ulcerative
  - Clostridium
    - difficile
      - not specified as recurrent **AØ4.72**
      - recurrent **AØ4.71**
  - coxsackie virus **AØ8.39**
  - due to
    - astrovirus **AØ8.32**
    - calicivirus **AØ8.31**
    - coxsackie virus **AØ8.39**
    - echovirus **AØ8.39**
    - enterovirus NEC **AØ8.39**
    - infectious organism (bacterial) (viral) - *see* Enteritis, infectious
    - torovirus **AØ8.39**
  - echovirus **AØ8.39**
  - enterovirus NEC **AØ8.39**
  - epidemic (infectious) **AØ9**
  - gangrenous - *see* Enteritis, infectious
  - infectious NOS **AØ9**
    - due to
      - Clostridium difficile
        - not specified as recurrent **AØ4.72**
        - recurrent **AØ4.71**
      - enterovirus **AØ8.39**
      - specified
        - virus NEC **AØ8.39**
      - virus NEC **AØ8.4**
        - specified type NEC **AØ8.39**
  - norovirus **AØ8.11**
  - regional (of) **K5Ø.9Ø**
  - segmental - *see* Enteritis, regional
  - septic **AØ9**
  - small round structured NEC **AØ8.19**
  - torovirus **AØ8.39**
  - toxic NEC **K52.1**
    - due to Clostridium difficile
      - not specified as recurrent **AØ4.72**
      - recurrent **AØ4.71**
  - typhosa **AØ1.ØØ**
  - ulcerative (chronic) - *see* Colitis, ulcerative
  - viral **AØ8.4**
    - enterovirus **AØ8.39**
    - small round structured NEC **AØ8.19**
    - specified NEC **AØ8.39**
    - virus specified NEC **AØ8.39**
- **Enterocolitis K52.9** - *see also* Enteritis
  - due to Clostridium difficile
    - not specified as recurrent **AØ4.72**
    - recurrent **AØ4.71**
  - granulomatous - *see* Enteritis, regional
  - infectious NEC **AØ9**
  - necrotizing **K55.3Ø**
    - due to Clostridium difficile
      - not specified as recurrent **AØ4.72**
      - recurrent **AØ4.71**
  - pseudomembranous (newborn)
    - not specified as recurrent **AØ4.72**
    - recurrent **AØ4.71**
- **Enterogastritis** - *see* Enteritis
- **Enthesopathy (peripheral) M77.9**
  - spinal **M46.ØØ**
    - cervical region **M46.Ø2**
    - cervicothoracic region **M46.Ø3**
    - lumbar region **M46.Ø6**
    - lumbosacral region **M46.Ø7**
    - multiple sites **M46.Ø9**
    - occipito-atlanto-axial region **M46.Ø1**
    - sacrococcygeal region **M46.Ø8**
    - thoracic region **M46.Ø4**
    - thoracolumbar region **M46.Ø5**
- **Enuresis R32**
- **Ependymitis (acute) (cerebral) (chronic) (granular)** - *see* Encephalomyelitis
- **Epicystitis** - *see* Cystitis
- **Epilepsy, epileptic, epilepsia (attack) (cerebral) (convulsion) (fit) (seizure) G4Ø.9Ø9**
  - intractable **G4Ø.919**
    - with status epilepticus **G4Ø.911**
    - without status epilepticus **G4Ø.919**
  - not intractable **G4Ø.9Ø9**
    - with status epilepticus **G4Ø.9Ø1**
    - without status epilepticus **G4Ø.9Ø9**
- **Epipharyngitis** - *see* Nasopharyngitis
- **Epiphyseolysis, epiphysiolysis** - *see* Osteochondropathy
- **Epiphysitis** - *see also* Osteochondropathy
- **Erb-Goldflam disease or syndrome G7Ø.ØØ**
  - with exacerbation (acute) **G7Ø.Ø1**
  - in crisis **G7Ø.Ø1**
- **Erb's**
  - disease **G71.Ø2**
  - pseudohypertrophic muscular dystrophy **G71.Ø2**
- **Erosion**
  - bone - *see* Disorder, bone, density and structure, specified NEC
  - cartilage (joint) - *see* Disorder, cartilage, specified type NEC
- **Eruption**
  - napkin **L22**
  - skin (nonspecific) **R21**
    - meaning dermatitis - *see* Dermatitis
- **Erythema, erythematous (infectional) (inflammation) L53.9**
  - diaper **L22**
  - gluteal **L22**
  - induratum (nontuberculous) **L52**
  - napkin **L22**
  - nodosum **L52**
- **Estrangement (marital) Z63.5**
  - parent-child NEC **Z62.89Ø**
- **Ethmoiditis (chronic) (nonpurulent) (purulent)** - *see also* Sinusitis, ethmoidal
- **Event**
  - apparent life threatening in newborn and infant (ALTE) **R68.13**
  - brief resolved unexplained event (BRUE) **R68.13**
- **Examination (for) (following) (general) (of) (routine) ZØØ.ØØ**
  - with abnormal findings **ZØØ.Ø1**
  - annual (adult) (periodic) (physical) **ZØØ.ØØ**
    - with abnormal findings **ZØØ.Ø1**
  - blood - *see* Examination, laboratory
  - child (over 28 days old) **ZØØ.129**
    - with abnormal findings **ZØØ.121**
    - under 28 days old - *see* Newborn, examination
  - developmental - *see* Examination, child
  - health - *see* Examination, medical
  - hearing **ZØ1.1Ø**
    - infant or child (over 28 days old) **ZØØ.129**
      - with abnormal findings **ZØØ.121**

F

- **Flatback syndrome M4Ø.3Ø**
  - lumbar region **M4Ø.36**
  - lumbosacral region **M4Ø.37**
  - thoracolumbar region **M4Ø.35**
- **Flea bite** - *see* Injury, bite, by site, superficial, insect
- **Flexion**
  - contracture, joint - *see* Contraction, joint
  - deformity, joint **M21.2Ø** - *see also* Deformity, limb, flexion
    - hip, congenital **Q65.89**
- **Flexure** - *see* Flexion
- **Floating**
  - cartilage (joint) - *see also* Loose, body, joint
- **Fluid**
  - joint - *see* Effusion, joint
- **Flukes NEC** - *see also* Infestation, fluke
  - blood NEC - *see* Schistosomiasis
- **Fluorosis**
  - skeletal **M85.1Ø**
- **FNHTR (febrile nonhemolytic transfusion reaction) R5Ø.84**
- **Fold, folds (anomalous)** - *see also* Anomaly, by site
- **Food**
  - asphyxia (from aspiration or inhalation) - *see* Foreign body, by site
  - choked on - *see* Foreign body, by site
  - strangulation or suffocation - *see* Foreign body, by site
- **Foreign body**
  - with
    - laceration - *see* Laceration, by site, with foreign body
  - entering through orifice
    - suffocation by - *see* Foreign body, by site
  - feeling of, in throat **RØ9.89**
  - granuloma (old) (soft tissue) - *see also* Granuloma, foreign body
  - in
    - laceration - *see* Laceration, by site, with foreign body
  - inhalation or inspiration - *see* Foreign body, by site
- **Forestier's disease (rhizomelic pseudopolyarthritis) M35.3**
  - meaning ankylosing hyperostosis - *see* Hyperostosis, ankylosing
- **Fothergill's**
  - disease (trigeminal neuralgia) - *see also* Neuralgia, trigeminal
- **Fracture, pathological (pathologic)** - *see also* Fracture, traumatic M84.4Ø-
  - compression (not due to trauma) M48.5Ø- - *see also* Collapse, vertebra
- **Fracture, traumatic (abduction) (adduction) (separation)** T14.8- - *see also* Fracture, pathological
  - acetabulum S32.4Ø-
    - column
      - anterior (displaced) (iliopubic) S32.43-
        - nondisplaced S32.436-
      - posterior (displaced) (ilioischial) S32.443-
        - nondisplaced S32.44-
    - dome (displaced) S32.48-
      - nondisplaced S32.48-
    - specified NEC S32.49-
    - transverse (displaced) S32.45-
      - with associated posterior wall fracture (displaced) S32.46-
        - nondisplaced S32.46-
      - nondisplaced S32.45-
    - wall
      - anterior (displaced) S32.41-
        - nondisplaced S32.41-
      - medial (displaced) S32.47-
        - nondisplaced S32.47-
      - posterior (displaced) S32.42-
        - with associated transverse fracture (displaced) S32.46-
          - nondisplaced S32.46-
        - nondisplaced S32.42-
  - atlas - *see* Fracture, neck, cervical vertebra, first
  - axis - *see* Fracture, neck, cervical vertebra, second
  - base of skull - *see* Fracture, skull, base
  - bone NEC T14.8-
    - pathological (cause unknown) - *see* Fracture, pathological
  - breast bone - *see* Fracture, sternum
  - bucket handle (semilunar cartilage) - *see* Tear, meniscus
  - burst - *see* Fracture, traumatic, by site
  - collapsed - *see* Collapse, vertebra
  - costochondral cartilage S23.41-
  - ethmoid (bone) (sinus) - *see* Fracture, skull, base
  - face bone SØ2.92-
  - fatigue - *see also* Fracture, stress
    - vertebra M48.4Ø-
      - cervical region M48.42-
      - cervicothoracic region M48.43-
      - lumbar region M48.46-
      - lumbosacral region M48.47-
      - occipito-atlanto-axial region M48.41-
      - sacrococcygeal region M48.48-
      - thoracic region M48.44-
      - thoracolumbar region M48.45-
  - fossa (anterior) (middle) (posterior) SØ2.19-
  - frontal (bone) (skull) SØ2.Ø-
    - sinus SØ2.19-
  - ilium S32.3Ø-
    - with disruption of pelvic ring - *see* Disruption, pelvic ring
    - avulsion (displaced) S32.31-
      - nondisplaced S32.31-
    - specified NEC S32.39-
  - ischium S32.6Ø-
    - with disruption of pelvic ring - *see* Disruption, pelvic ring
    - avulsion (displaced) S32.61-
      - nondisplaced S32.61-
    - specified NEC S32.69-
  - jaw (bone) (lower) - *see* Fracture, mandible
    - upper - *see* Fracture, maxilla
  - lumbar spine - *see* Fracture, vertebra, lumbar
  - malar bone SØ2.4ØØ- - *see also* Fracture, maxilla
    - left side SØ2.4ØB-
    - right side SØ2.4ØA-
  - mandible (lower jaw (bone)) SØ2.6Ø9-
    - alveolus SØ2.67-
    - angle (of jaw) SØ2.65-
    - body, unspecified SØ2.6ØØ-
      - left side SØ2.6Ø2-
      - right side SØ2.6Ø1-
    - condylar process SØ2.61-
    - coronoid process SØ2.63-
    - ramus, unspecified SØ2.64-
    - specified site NEC SØ2.69-
    - subcondylar process SØ2.62-
    - symphysis SØ2.66-
  - manubrium (sterni) S22.21-
    - dissociation from sternum S22.23-
  - march - *see* Fracture, traumatic, stress, by site
  - maxilla, maxillary (bone) (sinus) (superior) (upper jaw) SØ2.4Ø1-
    - alveolus SØ2.42-
    - inferior - *see* Fracture, mandible
    - LeFort I SØ2.411-
    - LeFort II SØ2.412-
    - LeFort III SØ2.413-
    - left side SØ2.4ØD-
    - right side SØ2.4ØC-
  - metaphyseal - *see* Fracture, traumatic, by site, shaft
  - neck S12.9-
    - cervical vertebra S12.9-
      - fifth (displaced) S12.4ØØ-
        - nondisplaced S12.4Ø1-
        - specified type NEC (displaced) S12.49Ø-
          - nondisplaced S12.491-
      - first (displaced) S12.ØØØ-
        - burst (stable) S12.Ø1-
          - unstable S12.Ø2-
        - lateral mass (displaced) S12.Ø4Ø-
          - nondisplaced S12.Ø41-
        - nondisplaced S12.ØØ1-
        - posterior arch (displaced) S12.Ø3Ø-
          - nondisplaced S12.Ø31-
        - specified type NEC (displaced) S12.Ø9Ø-
          - nondisplaced S12.Ø91-
      - fourth (displaced) S12.3ØØ-
        - nondisplaced S12.3Ø1-
        - specified type NEC (displaced) S12.39Ø-
          - nondisplaced S12.391-
      - second (displaced) S12.1ØØ-
        - dens (anterior) (displaced) (type II) S12.11Ø-
          - nondisplaced S12.112-
          - posterior S12.111-
          - specified type NEC (displaced) S12.12Ø-
            - nondisplaced S12.121-
        - nondisplaced S12.1Ø1-
        - specified type NEC (displaced) S12.19Ø-
          - nondisplaced S12.191-
      - seventh (displaced) S12.6ØØ-
        - nondisplaced S12.6Ø1-
        - specified type NEC (displaced) S12.69Ø-
          - nondisplaced S12.691-
      - sixth (displaced) S12.5ØØ-
        - nondisplaced S12.5Ø1-
        - specified type NEC (displaced) S12.59Ø-
          - nondisplaced S12.591-
      - third (displaced) S12.2ØØ-
        - nondisplaced S12.2Ø1-
        - specified type NEC (displaced) S12.29Ø-
          - nondisplaced S12.291-
  - nontraumatic - *see* Fracture, pathological
  - occiput - *see* Fracture, skull, base, occiput
  - odontoid process - *see* Fracture, neck, cervical vertebra, second
  - orbit, orbital (bone) (region) SØ2.85-
    - roof SØ2.12-
    - wall SØ2.85-
      - lateral SØ2.84-
      - medial SØ2.83-
  - os
    - pubis - *see* Fracture, pubis

- pelvis, pelvic (bone) S32.9-
  - acetabulum - *see* Fracture, acetabulum
  - circle - *see* Disruption, pelvic ring
  - multiple
    - with disruption of pelvic ring (circle) - *see* Disruption, pelvic ring
    - without disruption of pelvic ring (circle) S32.82-
  - pubis - *see* Fracture, pubis
  - sacrum - *see* Fracture, sacrum
  - specified site NEC S32.89-
- pubis S32.5Ø-
  - with disruption of pelvic ring - *see* Disruption, pelvic ring
  - specified site NEC S32.59-
  - superior rim S32.51-
- ramus
  - inferior or superior, pubis - *see* Fracture, pubis
  - mandible - *see* Fracture, mandible
- sacrum S32.1Ø-
  - specified NEC S32.19-
  - Type
    - 1 S32.14-
    - 2 S32.15-
    - 3 S32.16-
    - 4 S32.17-
  - Zone
    - I S32.119-
      - displaced (minimally) S32.111-
        - severely S32.112-
      - nondisplaced S32.11Ø-
    - II S32.129-
      - displaced (minimally) S32.121-
        - severely S32.122-
      - nondisplaced S32.12Ø-
    - III S32.139-
      - displaced (minimally) S32.131-
        - severely S32.132-
      - nondisplaced S32.13Ø-
- sesamoid bone
  - other - *see* Fracture, traumatic, by site
- sinus (ethmoid) (frontal) SØ2.19-
- skull SØ2.91-
  - base SØ2.1Ø-
    - occiput SØ2.119-
      - condyle SØ2.113-
        - specified NEC SØ2.118-
          - left side SØ2.11H-
          - right side SØ2.11G-
        - type I SØ2.11Ø-
          - left side SØ2.11B-
          - right side SØ2.11A-
        - type II SØ2.111-
          - left side SØ2.11D-
          - right side SØ2.11C-
        - type III SØ2.112-
          - left side SØ2.11F-
          - right side SØ2.11E-
    - specified NEC SØ2.19-
  - temporal bone SØ2.19-
- sphenoid (bone) (sinus) SØ2.19-
- spontaneous (cause unknown) - *see* Fracture, pathological
- sternum S22.2Ø-
  - body S22.22-
  - manubrium S22.21-
  - xiphoid (process) S22.24-
- stress M84.3Ø-
  - femoral neck M84.359-
  - hip M84.359-
  - ilium M84.35Ø-
  - ischium M84.35Ø-
  - neck - *see* Fracture, fatigue, vertebra
  - pelvis M84.35Ø-
  - rib M84.38-
  - skull M84.38-
  - vertebra - *see* Fracture, fatigue, vertebra
- symphysis pubis - *see* Fracture, pubis
- temporal bone (styloid) SØ2.19-
- thorax (bony) S22.9-
  - sternum S22.2Ø-
    - body S22.22-
    - manubrium S22.21-
    - xiphoid process S22.24-
  - vertebra (displaced) S22.ØØ9-
    - burst (stable) S22.ØØ1-
      - unstable S22.ØØ2-
    - eighth S22.Ø69-
      - burst (stable) S22.Ø61-
        - unstable S22.Ø62-
      - specified type NEC S22.Ø68-
      - wedge compression S22.Ø6Ø-
    - eleventh S22.Ø89-
      - burst (stable) S22.Ø81-
        - unstable S22.Ø82-
      - specified type NEC S22.Ø88-
      - wedge compression S22.Ø8Ø-
    - fifth S22.Ø59-
      - burst (stable) S22.Ø51-
        - unstable S22.Ø52-
      - specified type NEC S22.Ø58-
      - wedge compression S22.Ø5Ø-
    - first S22.Ø19-
      - burst (stable) S22.Ø11-
        - unstable S22.Ø12-
      - specified type NEC S22.Ø18-
      - wedge compression S22.Ø1Ø-
    - fourth S22.Ø49-
      - burst (stable) S22.Ø41-
        - unstable S22.Ø42-
      - specified type NEC S22.Ø48-
      - wedge compression S22.Ø4Ø-
    - ninth S22.Ø79-
      - burst (stable) S22.Ø71-
        - unstable S22.Ø72-
      - specified type NEC S22.Ø78-
      - wedge compression S22.Ø7Ø-
    - nondisplaced S22.ØØ1-
    - second S22.Ø29-
      - burst (stable) S22.Ø21-
        - unstable S22.Ø22-
      - specified type NEC S22.Ø28-
      - wedge compression S22.Ø2Ø-
    - seventh S22.Ø69-
      - burst (stable) S22.Ø61-
        - unstable S22.Ø62-
      - specified type NEC S22.Ø68-
      - wedge compression S22.Ø6Ø-
    - sixth S22.Ø59-
      - burst (stable) S22.Ø51-
        - unstable S22.Ø52-
      - specified type NEC S22.Ø58-
      - wedge compression S22.Ø5Ø-
    - specified type NEC S22.ØØ8-
    - tenth S22.Ø79-
      - burst (stable) S22.Ø71-
        - unstable S22.Ø72-
      - specified type NEC S22.Ø78-
      - wedge compression S22.Ø7Ø-
    - third S22.Ø39-
      - burst (stable) S22.Ø31-
        - unstable S22.Ø32-
      - specified type NEC S22.Ø38-
      - wedge compression S22.Ø3Ø-
    - twelfth S22.Ø89-
      - burst (stable) S22.Ø81-
        - unstable S22.Ø82-
      - specified type NEC S22.Ø88-
      - wedge compression S22.Ø8Ø-
    - wedge compression S22.ØØØ-
- tuberosity (external) - *see* Fracture, traumatic, by site
- vertebra, vertebral (arch) (body) (column) (neural arch) (pedicle) (spinous process) (transverse process)
  - atlas - *see* Fracture, neck, cervical vertebra, first
  - axis - *see* Fracture, neck, cervical vertebra, second
  - cervical (teardrop) S12.9-
    - axis - *see* Fracture, neck, cervical vertebra, second
    - first (atlas) - *see* Fracture, neck, cervical vertebra, first
    - second (axis) - *see* Fracture, neck, cervical vertebra, second
  - dorsal - *see* Fracture, thorax, vertebra
  - lumbar S32.ØØ9-
    - burst (stable) S32.ØØ1-
      - unstable S32.ØØ2-
    - fifth S32.Ø59-
      - burst (stable) S32.Ø51-
        - unstable S32.Ø52-
      - specified type NEC S32.Ø58-
      - wedge compression S32.Ø5Ø-
    - first S32.Ø19-
      - burst (stable) S32.Ø11-
        - unstable S32.Ø12-
      - specified type NEC S32.Ø18-
      - wedge compression S32.Ø1Ø-
    - fourth S32.Ø49-
      - burst (stable) S32.Ø41-
        - unstable S32.Ø42-
      - specified type NEC S32.Ø48-
      - wedge compression S32.Ø4Ø-
    - second S32.Ø29-
      - burst (stable) S32.Ø21-
        - unstable S32.Ø22-
      - specified type NEC S32.Ø28-
      - wedge compression S32.Ø2Ø-
    - specified type NEC S32.ØØ8-
    - third S32.Ø39-
      - burst (stable) S32.Ø31-
        - unstable S32.Ø32-
      - specified type NEC S32.Ø38-
      - wedge compression S32.Ø3Ø-
    - wedge compression S32.ØØØ-
  - sacrum S32.1Ø-
    - specified NEC S32.19-
    - Type
      - 1 S32.14-
      - 2 S32.15-
      - 3 S32.16-
      - 4 S32.17-
    - Zone
      - I S32.119-
        - displaced (minimally) S32.111-
          - severely S32.112-
        - nondisplaced S32.11Ø-
      - II S32.129-
        - displaced (minimally) S32.121-
          - severely S32.122-
        - nondisplaced S32.12Ø-
      - III S32.139-
        - displaced (minimally) S32.131-
          - severely S32.132-
        - nondisplaced S32.13Ø-
  - thoracic - *see* Fracture, thorax, vertebra
- xiphisternum, xiphoid (process) S22.24-
- zygoma SØ2.4Ø2-
  - left side SØ2.4ØF-
  - right side SØ2.4ØE-

Fracture, burst - *see* Fracture, traumatic, by site

Fracture, chronic - *see* Fracture, pathological, by site

- **Fracture, insufficiency** - *see* Fracture, pathological, by site
- **Frailty (frail) R54**
  - mental **R41.81**
- **Frederickson's hyperlipoproteinemia, type** IIA **E78.ØØ**
- **Friction**
  - sounds, chest **RØ9.89**
- **Fugue R68.89**
  - postictal in epilepsy - *see* Epilepsy
- **Functioning, intellectual, borderline R41.83**
- **Fused** - *see* Fusion, fused
- **Fusion, fused (congenital)**
  - cervical spine **M43.22**
  - joint (acquired) - *see also* Ankylosis
  - lumbosacral (acquired) **M43.27**
    - congenital **Q76.49**
  - organ or site not listed - *see* Anomaly, by site
  - sacroiliac (joint) (acquired) **M43.28**
  - spine (acquired) NEC **M43.2Ø**
    - cervical region **M43.22**
    - cervicothoracic region **M43.23**
    - congenital **Q76.49**
    - lumbar **M43.26**
    - lumbosacral region **M43.27**
    - occipito-atlanto-axial region **M43.21**
    - sacrococcygeal region **M43.28**
    - thoracic region **M43.24**
    - thoracolumbar region **M43.25**
  - vertebra (arch) - *see* Fusion, spine
- **Fussy baby R68.12**

G

- **Gait abnormality R26.9**
  - specified type NEC **R26.89**
  - unsteadiness **R26.81**
- **Gang**
  - membership offenses **Z72.81Ø**
- **Ganglion (compound) (diffuse) (joint) (tendon (sheath)) M67.4Ø**
  - multiple sites **M67.49**
  - specified site NEC **M67.48**
- **Ganglionitis**
  - fifth nerve - *see* Neuralgia, trigeminal
  - gasserian (postherpetic) (postzoster) **BØ2.21**
  - geniculate **G51.1**
    - postherpetic, postzoster **BØ2.21**
  - herpes zoster **BØ2.21**
  - postherpetic geniculate **BØ2.21**
- **Gangrene, gangrenous (connective tissue) (dropsical) (dry) (moist) (skin) (ulcer) I96** - *see also* Necrosis
  - with diabetes (mellitus) - *see* Diabetes, with, gangrene
  - bladder (infectious) - *see* Cystitis, specified type NEC
  - diabetic (any site) - *see* Diabetes, with, gangrene
  - hernia - *see* Hernia, by site, with gangrene
- **Gastralgia** - *see also* Pain, abdominal
- **Gastroduodenitis K29.9Ø**
  - virus, viral **AØ8.4**
    - specified type NEC **AØ8.39**
- **Gastrodynia** - *see* Pain, abdominal
- **Gastroenteritis (acute) (chronic) (noninfectious) K52.9** - *see also* Enteritis
  - due to
    - food poisoning - *see* Intoxication, foodborne
  - epidemic (infectious) **AØ9**
  - infectious - *see* Enteritis, infectious
  - viral NEC **AØ8.4**
    - acute infectious **AØ8.39**
      - type Norwalk **AØ8.11**
    - infantile (acute) **AØ8.39**
    - Norwalk agent **AØ8.11**
    - severe of infants **AØ8.39**
    - specified type NEC **AØ8.39**
- **Gastroenteropathy K52.9** - *see also* Gastroenteritis
  - acute, due to Norovirus **AØ8.11**
  - acute, due to Norwalk agent **AØ8.11**
  - infectious **AØ9**
- **Gastroparalysis K31.84**
  - diabetic - *see* Diabetes, gastroparalysis
- **Gastroparesis K31.84**
  - diabetic - *see* Diabetes, by type, with gastroparesis
- **Gestation (period)** - *see also* Pregnancy
  - ectopic - *see* Pregnancy, by site
- **Giddiness R42**
- **Gliosis (cerebral) G93.89**
  - spinal **G95.89**
- **Glomerular**
  - nephritis - *see* Glomerulonephritis
- **Glomerulitis** - *see* Glomerulonephritis
- **Glomerulonephritis NØ5.9** - *see also* Nephritis
  - in (due to)
    - diabetes mellitus - *see* Diabetes, glomerulosclerosis
    - typhoid fever **AØ1.Ø9**
- **Glomerulopathy** - *see* Glomerulonephritis
- **Glomerulosclerosis** - *see also* Sclerosis, renal
  - intercapillary (nodular) (with diabetes) - *see* Diabetes, glomerulosclerosis
  - intracapillary - *see* Diabetes, glomerulosclerosis
- **Glycogenosis (diffuse) (generalized)** - *see also* Disease, glycogen storage
  - diabetic, secondary - *see* Diabetes, glycogenosis, secondary
- **Glycosuria R81**
- **Goldflam-Erb disease or syndrome G7Ø.ØØ**
  - with exacerbation (acute) **G7Ø.Ø1**
  - in crisis **G7Ø.Ø1**
- **Gonecystitis** - *see* Vesiculitis
- **Goodall's disease AØ8.19**
- **Gout, gouty (acute) (attack) (flare) M1Ø.9** - *see also* Gout, chronic
  - drug-induced **M1Ø.2Ø**
    - multiple site **M1Ø.29**
    - vertebrae **M1Ø.28**
  - idiopathic **M1Ø.ØØ**
    - multiple site **M1Ø.Ø9**
    - vertebrae **M1Ø.Ø8**
  - in (due to) renal impairment **M1Ø.3Ø**
    - multiple site **M1Ø.39**
    - vertebrae **M1Ø.38**
  - lead-induced **M1Ø.1Ø**
    - multiple site **M1Ø.19**
    - vertebrae **M1Ø.18**
  - primary - *see* Gout, idiopathic
  - saturnine - *see* Gout, lead-induced
  - secondary NEC **M1Ø.4Ø**
    - multiple site **M1Ø.49**
    - vertebrae **M1Ø.48**
  - tophi - *see* Gout, chronic
- **Gout, chronic** M1A.9- - *see also* Gout, gouty
  - drug-induced M1A.2Ø-
    - multiple site M1A.29-
    - vertebrae M1A.28-
  - idiopathic M1A.ØØ-
    - multiple site M1A.Ø9-
    - vertebrae M1A.Ø8-
  - in (due to) renal impairment M1A.3Ø-
    - multiple site M1A.39-
    - vertebrae M1A.38-
  - lead-induced M1A.1Ø-
    - multiple site M1A.19-
    - vertebrae M1A.18-
  - primary - *see* Gout, chronic, idiopathic
  - saturnine - *see* Gout, chronic, lead-induced
  - secondary NEC M1A.4Ø-
    - multiple site M1A.49-
    - vertebrae M1A.48-
- **Gower's**
  - muscular dystrophy **G71.Ø1**
  - syndrome (vasovagal attack) **R55**
- **Granuloma L92.9**
  - foreign body (in soft tissue) NEC **M6Ø.2Ø**
    - specified site NEC **M6Ø.28**
  - nasal sinus - *see* Sinusitis
  - Schistosoma - *see* Schistosomiasis
  - sinus (accessory) (infective) (nasal) - *see* Sinusitis
  - talc - *see also* Granuloma, foreign body
- **Graphospasm F48.8**
  - organic **G25.89**
- **Grinding, teeth**
  - sleep related **G47.63**
- **Growing pains, children R29.898**
- **Gunshot wound** - *see also* Puncture, open
  - internal organs - *see* Injury, by site

H

- **Habit, habituation**
  - bad sleep **Z72.821**
  - drug - *see* Dependence, drug
  - irregular sleep **Z72.821**
  - spasm - *see* Tic
  - tic - *see* Tic
- **Half vertebra Q76.49**
- **Hammer toe (acquired) NEC** - *see also* Deformity, toe, hammer toe
  - congenital **Q66.89**
- **Hansen's disease** - *see* Leprosy
- **Harmful use (of)**
  - alcohol **F1Ø.1Ø**
  - cannabinoids - *see* Abuse, drug, cannabis
  - drug - *see* Abuse, drug
  - opioids - *see* Abuse, drug, opioid
- **Headache R51.9**
  - allergic NEC **G44.89**
  - associated with sexual activity **G44.82**
  - cervicogenic **G44.86**
  - cluster **G44.ØØ9**
    - chronic **G44.Ø29**
      - intractable **G44.Ø21**
      - not intractable **G44.Ø29**
    - episodic **G44.Ø19**
      - intractable **G44.Ø11**
      - not intractable **G44.Ø19**
    - intractable **G44.ØØ1**
    - not intractable **G44.ØØ9**
  - cough (primary) **G44.83**
  - drug-induced NEC **G44.4Ø**
    - intractable **G44.41**
    - not intractable **G44.4Ø**
  - exertional (primary) **G44.84**
  - histamine **G44.ØØ9**
    - intractable **G44.ØØ1**
    - not intractable **G44.ØØ9**
  - hypnic **G44.81**
  - medication overuse **G44.4Ø**
    - intractable **G44.41**
    - not intractable **G44.4Ø**
  - menstrual - *see* Migraine, menstrual

- migraine (type) **G43.9Ø9** - *see also* Migraine
- neuralgiform, short lasting unilateral, with conjunctival injection and tearing (SUNCT) **G44.Ø59**
  - intractable **G44.Ø51**
  - not intractable **G44.Ø59**
- new daily persistent (NDPH) **G44.52**
- orgasmic **G44.82**
- periodic syndromes in adults and children **G43.CØ**
  - with refractory migraine **G43.C1**
  - without refractory migraine **G43.CØ**
  - intractable **G43.C1**
  - not intractable **G43.CØ**
- post-traumatic **G44.3Ø9**
  - acute **G44.319**
    - intractable **G44.311**
    - not intractable **G44.319**
  - chronic **G44.329**
    - intractable **G44.321**
    - not intractable **G44.329**
  - intractable **G44.3Ø1**
  - not intractable **G44.3Ø9**
- pre-menstrual - *see* Migraine, menstrual
- preorgasmic **G44.82**
- primary
  - cough **G44.83**
  - exertional **G44.84**
  - stabbing **G44.85**
  - thunderclap **G44.53**
- rebound **G44.4Ø**
  - intractable **G44.41**
  - not intractable **G44.4Ø**
- short lasting unilateral neuralgiform, with conjunctival injection and tearing (SUNCT) **G44.Ø59**
  - intractable **G44.Ø51**
  - not intractable **G44.Ø59**
- specified syndrome NEC **G44.89**
- stabbing (primary) **G44.85**
- tension (-type) **G44.2Ø9**
  - chronic **G44.229**
    - intractable **G44.221**
    - not intractable **G44.229**
  - episodic **G44.219**
    - intractable **G44.211**
    - not intractable **G44.219**
  - intractable **G44.2Ø1**
  - not intractable **G44.2Ø9**
- thunderclap (primary) **G44.53**

Hearing examination ZØ1.1Ø
- infant or child (over 28 days old) **ZØØ.129**
  - with abnormal findings **ZØØ.121**

Heartburn R12

Hebra's
- pityriasis **L26**

Heloma L84

Hemarthrosis (nontraumatic) M25.ØØ
- specified joint NEC **M25.Ø8**
- traumatic - *see* Sprain, by site
- vertebrae **M25.Ø8**

Hematoma (traumatic) (skin surface intact) - *see also* Contusion
- with
  - injury of internal organs - *see* Injury, by site
- auricle - *see* Contusion, ear
- epidural (traumatic) - *see* Injury, intracranial, epidural hemorrhage
  - spinal - *see* Injury, spinal cord, by region
- internal organs - *see* Injury, by site
- nontraumatic
  - muscle **M79.81**
  - soft tissue **M79.81**
- pelvis (female) (nontraumatic) (nonobstetric) **N94.89**
  - traumatic - *see* Injury, by site
- pinna - *see* Contusion, ear
- spinal (cord) (meninges) - *see also* Injury, spinal cord, by region

Hematuria R31.9
- microscopic NEC (with symptoms) **R31.29**
  - asymptomatic **R31.21**

Hemiatrophy R68.89

Hemicrania
- continua **G44.51**
- meaning migraine **G43.9Ø9** - *see also* Migraine
- paroxysmal **G44.Ø39**
  - chronic **G44.Ø49**
    - intractable **G44.Ø41**
    - not intractable **G44.Ø49**
  - episodic **G44.Ø39**
    - intractable **G44.Ø31**
    - not intractable **G44.Ø39**
  - intractable **G44.Ø31**
  - not intractable **G44.Ø39**

Hemidystrophy - *see* Hemiatrophy

Hemiparalysis - *see* Hemiplegia

Hemiparesis - *see* Hemiplegia

Hemiparkinsonism G2Ø

Hemiplegia G81.9-
- alternans facialis **G83.89**
- ascending NEC **G81.9Ø**
  - spinal **G95.89**

Hemisection, spinal cord - *see* Injury, spinal cord, by region

Hemivertebra Q76.49

Hemorrhage, hemorrhagic (concealed) R58
- abdomen **R58**
- acute idiopathic pulmonary, in infants **RØ4.81**
- artery **R58**
- bronchial tube - *see* Hemorrhage, lung
- bronchopulmonary - *see* Hemorrhage, lung
- bronchus - *see* Hemorrhage, lung
- endotracheal - *see* Hemorrhage, lung
- internal (organs) NEC **R58**
- intra-abdominal **R58**
- joint (nontraumatic) - *see* Hemarthrosis
- lung **RØ4.89**
- mediastinum - *see* Hemorrhage, lung
- mucous membrane NEC **R58**
- muscle **M62.89**
- pleura - *see* Hemorrhage, lung
- polymyositis - *see* Polymyositis
- pulmonary **RØ4.89**
- respiratory passage or tract **RØ4.9**
  - specified NEC **RØ4.89**
- retroperitoneal **R58**
- scalp **R58**
- secondary (nontraumatic) **R58**
- subdiaphragmatic **R58**
- thorax - *see* Hemorrhage, lung
- trachea - *see* Hemorrhage, lung
- tracheobronchial **RØ4.89**
- viscera NEC **R58**

Hepatitis K75.9
- history of
  - B **Z86.19**
  - C **Z86.19**

Hernia, hernial (acquired) (recurrent) K46.9
- with
  - gangrene - *see* Hernia, by site, with, gangrene
  - incarceration - *see* Hernia, by site, with, obstruction
  - irreducible - *see* Hernia, by site, with, obstruction
  - obstruction - *see* Hernia, by site, with, obstruction
  - strangulation - *see* Hernia, by site, with, obstruction
- bladder (mucosa) (sphincter)
  - congenital (female) (male) **Q79.51**
- cartilage, vertebra - *see* Displacement, intervertebral disc
- fascia **M62.89**
- incarcerated - *see also* Hernia, by site, with obstruction
  - with gangrene - *see* Hernia, by site, with gangrene
- intervertebral cartilage or disc - *see* Displacement, intervertebral disc
- intestine, intestinal - *see* Hernia, by site
- irreducible - *see also* Hernia, by site, with obstruction
  - with gangrene - *see* Hernia, by site, with gangrene
- muscle (sheath) **M62.89**
- nucleus pulposus - *see* Displacement, intervertebral disc
- obstructive - *see also* Hernia, by site, with obstruction
  - with gangrene - *see* Hernia, by site, with gangrene
- pregnant uterus - *see* Abnormal, uterus in pregnancy or childbirth
- strangulated - *see also* Hernia, by site, with obstruction
  - with gangrene - *see* Hernia, by site, with gangrene
- tendon - *see* Disorder, tendon, specified type NEC
- uterus **N81.4**
  - pregnant - *see* Abnormal, uterus in pregnancy or childbirth
- vesical
  - congenital (female) (male) **Q79.51**

Herniation - *see also* Hernia
- nucleus pulposus - *see* Displacement, intervertebral disc

Herpes, herpesvirus, herpetic BØØ.9
- geniculate ganglionitis **BØ2.21**
- zoster **BØ2.9** - *see also* condition
  - auricularis **BØ2.21**
  - geniculate ganglionitis **BØ2.21**
  - myelitis **BØ2.24**
  - neuritis, neuralgia **BØ2.29**
  - oticus **BØ2.21**
  - polyneuropathy **BØ2.23**
  - trigeminal neuralgia **BØ2.22**

Herpesvirus (human) - *see* Herpes

Herxheimer's reaction R68.89

Hesitancy
- of micturition **R39.11**
- urinary **R39.11**

Heterotopia, heterotopic - *see also* Malposition, congenital

High
- arterial tension - *see* Hypertension
- blood pressure - *see also* Hypertension
- cholesterol **E78.ØØ**
- risk
  - sexual behavior (heterosexual) **Z72.51**
    - bisexual **Z72.53**
    - homosexual **Z72.52**

History
- family (of) - *see also* History, personal (of)
  - arthritis **Z82.61**
  - cardiac death (sudden) **Z82.41**
  - chromosomal anomaly **Z82.79**
  - colonic polyps **Z83.71**

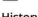

- congenital malformations and deformations **Z82.79**
  - polycystic kidney **Z82.71**
- disease or disorder (of)
  - cardiovascular NEC **Z82.49**
  - digestive **Z83.79**
  - ear NEC **Z83.52**
  - endocrine NEC **Z83.49**
  - eye NEC **Z83.518**
    - glaucoma **Z83.511**
  - glaucoma **Z83.511**
  - ischemic heart **Z82.49**
  - metabolic **Z83.49**
  - musculoskeletal NEC **Z82.69**
  - nutritional **Z83.49**
- glaucoma **Z83.511**
- malignant neoplasm (of) NOS **Z8Ø.9**
  - bladder **Z8Ø.52**
  - genital organ **Z8Ø.49**
    - ovary **Z8Ø.41**
    - prostate **Z8Ø.42**
    - specified organ NEC **Z8Ø.49**
    - testis **Z8Ø.43**
  - kidney **Z8Ø.51**
  - ovary **Z8Ø.41**
  - prostate **Z8Ø.42**
  - testis **Z8Ø.43**
  - urinary organ or tract **Z8Ø.59**
    - bladder **Z8Ø.52**
    - kidney **Z8Ø.51**
- multiple endocrine neoplasia (MEN) syndrome **Z83.41**
- osteoporosis **Z82.62**
- polycystic kidney **Z82.71**
- polyps (colon) **Z83.71**
- sudden
  - cardiac death **Z82.41**

personal (of) - *see also* History, family (of)
- abuse
  - childhood **Z62.819**
    - physical **Z62.81Ø**
    - psychological **Z62.811**
    - sexual **Z62.81Ø**
- anaphylactic shock **Z87.892**
- anaphylaxis **Z87.892**
- behavioral disorders **Z86.59**
- benign carcinoid tumor **Z86.Ø12**
- benign neoplasm **Z86.Ø18**
  - brain **Z86.Ø11**
  - carcinoid **Z86.Ø12**
  - colonic polyps **Z86.Ø1Ø**
- brain injury (traumatic) **Z87.82Ø**
- calculi, renal **Z87.442**
- cancer - *see* History, personal (of), malignant neoplasm (of)
- cardiac arrest (death), successfully resuscitated **Z86.74**
- cerebral infarction without residual deficit **Z86.73**
- cervical dysplasia **Z87.41Ø**
- childhood abuse - *see* History, personal (of), abuse
- cleft lip (corrected) **Z87.73Ø**
- cleft palate (corrected) **Z87.73Ø**
- collapsed vertebra (healed) **Z87.311**
  - due to osteoporosis **Z87.31Ø**
- combat and operational stress reaction **Z86.51**
- congenital malformation (corrected) **Z87.798**
  - circulatory system (corrected) **Z87.74**
  - digestive system (corrected) NEC **Z87.738**
  - ear (corrected) **Z87.721**
  - eye (corrected) **Z87.72Ø**
  - face and neck (corrected) **Z87.79Ø**
  - genitourinary system (corrected) NEC **Z87.718**
  - heart (corrected) **Z87.74**
  - neck (corrected) **Z87.79Ø**
  - nervous system (corrected) NEC **Z87.728**
  - respiratory system (corrected) **Z87.75**
  - sense organs (corrected) NEC **Z87.728**
  - specified NEC **Z87.798**
- deployment (military) **Z91.82**
- diabetic foot ulcer **Z86.31**
- disease or disorder (of) **Z87.898**
  - circulatory system **Z86.79**
    - specified condition NEC **Z86.79**
  - connective tissue NEC **Z87.39**
  - digestive system **Z87.19**
    - colonic polyp **Z86.Ø1Ø**
    - peptic ulcer disease **Z87.11**
    - specified condition NEC **Z87.19**
  - ear **Z86.69**
  - endocrine **Z86.39**
    - diabetic foot ulcer **Z86.31**
    - gestational diabetes **Z86.32**
    - specified type NEC **Z86.39**
  - eye **Z86.69**
  - genital (track) system NEC
    - female **Z87.42**
    - male **Z87.438**
  - Hodgkin **Z85.71**
  - infectious **Z86.19**
    - malaria **Z86.13**
    - Methicillin resistant Staphylococcus aureus (MRSA) **Z86.14**
    - poliomyelitis **Z86.12**
    - specified NEC **Z86.19**
    - tuberculosis **Z86.11**
  - mental NEC **Z86.59**
  - metabolic **Z86.39**
    - diabetic foot ulcer **Z86.31**
    - gestational diabetes **Z86.32**
    - specified type NEC **Z86.39**
  - musculoskeletal NEC **Z87.39**
  - nervous system **Z86.69**
  - nutritional **Z86.39**
  - parasitic **Z86.19**
  - respiratory system NEC **Z87.Ø9**
  - sense organs **Z86.69**
  - specified site or type NEC **Z87.898**
  - trophoblastic **Z87.59**
  - urinary system NEC **Z87.448**
- drug dependence - *see* Dependence, drug, by type, in remission
- dysplasia
  - cervical (mild) (moderate) **Z87.41Ø**
    - severe (grade III) **Z86.ØØ1**
  - prostatic **Z87.43Ø**
  - vaginal (mild) (moderate) **Z87.411**
  - vulvar (mild) (moderate) **Z87.412**
- embolism (venous) **Z86.718**
  - pulmonary **Z86.711**
- encephalitis **Z86.61**
- fall, falling **Z91.81**
- fracture (healed)
  - fatigue **Z87.312**
  - fragility **Z87.31Ø**
  - osteoporosis **Z87.31Ø**
  - pathological NEC **Z87.311**
  - stress **Z87.312**
  - traumatic **Z87.81**
- gestational diabetes **Z86.32**
- hepatitis
  - B **Z86.19**
  - C **Z86.19**
- Hodgkin disease **Z85.71**
- hypospadias (corrected) **Z87.71Ø**
- hysterectomy **Z9Ø.71Ø**
- in situ neoplasm
  - breast **Z86.ØØØ**
  - cervix uteri **Z86.ØØ1**
  - specified NEC **Z86.ØØ8**
- infection NEC **Z86.19**
  - central nervous system **Z86.61**
  - Methicillin resistant Staphylococcus aureus (MRSA) **Z86.14**
  - urinary (recurrent) (tract) **Z87.44Ø**
- injury NEC **Z87.828**
- kidney stones **Z87.442**
- lymphoma (non-Hodgkin) **Z85.72**
- malignant melanoma (skin) **Z85.82Ø**
- malignant neoplasm (of) **Z85.9**
  - accessory sinuses **Z85.22**
  - anus NEC **Z85.Ø48**
    - carcinoid **Z85.Ø4Ø**
  - bladder **Z85.51**
  - bone **Z85.83Ø**
  - brain **Z85.841**
  - bronchus NEC **Z85.118**
    - carcinoid **Z85.11Ø**
  - carcinoid - *see* History, personal (of), malignant neoplasm, by site, carcinioid
  - cervix **Z85.41**
  - colon NEC **Z85.Ø38**
    - carcinoid **Z85.Ø3Ø**
  - digestive organ **Z85.ØØ**
    - specified NEC **Z85.Ø9**
  - endocrine gland NEC **Z85.858**
  - epididymis **Z85.48**
  - esophagus **Z85.Ø1**
  - eye **Z85.84Ø**
  - gastrointestinal tract - *see* History, malignant neoplasm, digestive organ
  - genital organ
    - female **Z85.4Ø**
      - specified NEC **Z85.44**
    - male **Z85.45**
      - specified NEC **Z85.49**
  - hematopoietic NEC **Z85.79**
  - intrathoracic organ **Z85.2Ø**
  - kidney NEC **Z85.528**
    - carcinoid **Z85.52Ø**
  - large intestine NEC **Z85.Ø38**
    - carcinoid **Z85.Ø3Ø**
  - larynx **Z85.21**
  - liver **Z85.Ø5**
  - lung NEC **Z85.118**
    - carcinoid **Z85.11Ø**
  - mediastinum **Z85.29**
  - Merkel cell **Z85.821**
  - middle ear **Z85.22**
  - nasal cavities **Z85.22**
  - nervous system NEC **Z85.848**
  - oral cavity **Z85.819**
    - specified site NEC **Z85.818**
  - ovary **Z85.43**
  - pancreas **Z85.Ø7**
  - pelvis **Z85.53**
  - pharynx **Z85.819**
    - specified site NEC **Z85.818**
  - pleura **Z85.29**
  - prostate **Z85.46**
  - rectosigmoid junction NEC **Z85.Ø48**
    - carcinoid **Z85.Ø4Ø**
  - rectum NEC **Z85.Ø48**
    - carcinoid **Z85.Ø4Ø**
  - respiratory organ **Z85.2Ø**
  - sinuses, accessory **Z85.22**
  - skin NEC **Z85.828**
    - melanoma **Z85.82Ø**
    - Merkel cell **Z85.821**

small intestine NEC **Z85.Ø68**
carcinoid **Z85.Ø6Ø**
soft tissue **Z85.831**
specified site NEC **Z85.89**
stomach NEC **Z85.Ø28**
carcinoid **Z85.Ø2Ø**
testis **Z85.47**
thymus NEC **Z85.238**
carcinoid **Z85.23Ø**
thyroid **Z85.85Ø**
tongue **Z85.81Ø**
trachea **Z85.12**
ureter **Z85.54**
urinary organ or tract **Z85.5Ø**
specified NEC **Z85.59**
uterus **Z85.42**
maltreatment **Z91.89**
medical treatment NEC **Z92.89**
melanoma **Z85.82Ø**
malignant (skin) **Z85.82Ø**
meningitis **Z86.61**
mental disorder **Z86.59**
Merkel cell carcinoma (skin) **Z85.821**
Methicillin resistant Staphylococcus aureus (MRSA) **Z86.14**
military deployment **Z91.82**
military war, peacekeeping and humanitarian deployment (current or past conflict) **Z91.82**
neglect (in)
childhood **Z62.812**
neoplasm
benign **Z86.Ø18**
brain **Z86.Ø11**
colon polyp **Z86.Ø1Ø**
in situ
breast **Z86.ØØØ**
cervix uteri **Z86.ØØ1**
specified NEC **Z86.ØØ8**
malignant - *see* History of, malignant neoplasm
uncertain behavior **Z86.Ø3**
nephrotic syndrome **Z87.441**
nicotine dependence **Z87.891**
noncompliance with medical treatment or regimen - *see* Noncompliance
nutritional deficiency **Z86.39**
obstetric complications **Z87.59**
childbirth **Z87.59**
pregnancy **Z87.59**
pre-term labor **Z87.51**
puerperium **Z87.59**
physical trauma NEC **Z87.828**
pneumonia (recurrent) **Z87.Ø1**
poisoning NEC **Z91.89**
poor personal hygiene **Z91.89**
preterm labor **Z87.51**
prolonged reversible ischemic neurologic deficit (PRIND) **Z86.73**
prostatic dysplasia **Z87.43Ø**
psychological
abuse
child **Z62.811**
renal calculi **Z87.442**
respiratory condition NEC **Z87.Ø9**
retained foreign body fully removed **Z87.821**
risk factors NEC **Z91.89**
sex reassignment **Z87.89Ø**
sleep-wake cycle problem **Z72.821**
specified NEC **Z87.898**
stroke without residual deficits **Z86.73**
sudden cardiac arrest **Z86.74**
sudden cardiac death successfully resuscitated **Z86.74**
surgery NEC **Z98.89Ø**
sex reassignment **Z87.89Ø**
thrombophlebitis **Z86.72**
thrombosis (venous) **Z86.718**
pulmonary **Z86.711**
tobacco dependence **Z87.891**
transient ischemic attack (TIA) without residual deficits **Z86.73**
trauma (physical) NEC **Z87.828**
traumatic brain injury **Z87.82Ø**
unhealthy sleep-wake cycle **Z72.821**
urinary calculi **Z87.442**
urinary (recurrent) (tract) infection(s) **Z87.44Ø**
vaginal dysplasia **Z87.411**
venous thrombosis or embolism **Z86.718**
pulmonary **Z86.711**
vulvar dysplasia **Z87.412**

Horton's headache or neuralgia G44.Ø99
intractable **G44.Ø91**
not intractable **G44.Ø99**

Human
herpesvirus - *see* Herpes

Humiliation (experience) in childhood Z62.898

Humpback (acquired) - *see* Kyphosis

Hunchback (acquired) - *see* Kyphosis

Hunner's ulcer - *see* Cystitis, chronic, interstitial

Huntington's disease or chorea G1Ø
with dementia **G1Ø** [**FØ2.8Ø**] - *see also* Dementia, in, diseases specified elsewhere
with behavioral disturbance **G1Ø** [FØ2.81-] - *see also* Dementia, in, diseases specified elsewhere

Hunt's
disease or syndrome (herpetic geniculate ganglionitis) **BØ2.21**
neuralgia **BØ2.21**

Hydrarthrosis - *see also* Effusion, joint
syphilitic (late) **A52.77**
congenital **A5Ø.55** [**M12.8Ø**]

Hydromeningitis - *see* Meningitis

Hydrops R6Ø.9
joint - *see* Effusion, joint

Hygiene, sleep
abuse **Z72.821**
inadequate **Z72.821**
poor **Z72.821**

Hyperactive, hyperactivity F9Ø.9
bowel sounds **R19.12**

Hyperbetalipoproteinemia (familial) E78.ØØ

Hypercapnia RØ6.89

Hypercholesterinemia - *see* Hypercholesterolemia

Hypercholesterolemia (essential) (primary) (pure) E78.ØØ
familial **E78.Ø1**
hereditary **E78.Ø1**

Hyperemesis R11.1Ø
projectile **R11.12**

Hyperemia (acute) (passive) R68.89

Hyperglycemia, hyperglycemic (transient) R73.9
coma - *see* Diabetes, by type, with coma

Hyperhidrosis, hyperidrosis R61
generalized **R61**
secondary **R61**

Hyperlipemia, hyperlipidemia E78.5
group
A **E78.ØØ**

Hyperlipoproteinemia E78.5
Fredrickson's type
IIa **E78.ØØ**
low-density-lipoprotein-type (LDL) **E78.ØØ**

Hypermobility, hypermotility
meniscus (knee) - *see* Derangement, knee, meniscus

Hypernasality R49.21

Hyperostosis (monomelic) - *see also* Disorder, bone, density and structure, specified NEC
ankylosing (spine) **M48.1Ø**
cervical region **M48.12**
cervicothoracic region **M48.13**
lumbar region **M48.16**
lumbosacral region **M48.17**
multiple sites **M48.19**
occipito-atlanto-axial region **M48.11**
sacrococcygeal region **M48.18**
thoracic region **M48.14**
thoracolumbar region **M48.15**
skeletal, diffuse idiopathic - *see* Hyperostosis, ankylosing
vertebral, ankylosing - *see* Hyperostosis, ankylosing

Hyperpiesis, hyperpiesia - *see* Hypertension

Hyperplasia, hyperplastic
bone - *see also* Hypertrophy, bone
organ or site, congenital NEC - *see* Anomaly, by site

Hypersensitive, hypersensitiveness, hypersensitivity - *see also* Allergy
carotid sinus **G9Ø.Ø1**

Hypersomnia (organic) G47.1Ø

Hypersusceptibility - *see* Allergy

Hypertension, hypertensive (accelerated) (benign) (essential) (idiopathic) (malignant) (systemic) I1Ø
cardiovascular
disease (arteriosclerotic) (sclerotic) - *see* Hypertension, heart
complicating
puerperium, pre-existing **O16.5**
pre-existing
essential **O1Ø.Ø3**

Hypertensive urgency - *see* Hypertension

Hypertrophy, hypertrophic
alveolar process or ridge - *see* Anomaly, alveolar
bone **M89.3Ø**
ilium **M89.359**
ischium **M89.359**
multiple sites **M89.39**
neck **M89.38**
rib **M89.38**
skull **M89.38**
vertebra **M89.38**
cardiac (chronic) (idiopathic) **I51.7**
hypertensive - *see* Hypertension, heart
valve - *see* Endocarditis
cartilage - *see* Disorder, cartilage, specified type NEC
cecum - *see* Megacolon
colon - *see also* Megacolon
facet joint **M47.819** - *see also* Spondylosis
ligament - *see* Disorder, ligament
muscle **M62.89**
organ or site, congenital NEC - *see* Anomaly, by site
pseudomuscular **G71.Ø9** - *see also* Dystrophy, muscular, by type, if applicable
sigmoid - *see* Megacolon
spondylitis - *see* Spondylosis
synovial NEC **M67.2Ø**
multiple sites **M67.29**
specified site NEC **M67.28**
tendon - *see* Disorder, tendon, specified type NEC

- **Hypofunction**
  - cerebral **R29.818**
- **Hypoglycemia (spontaneous) E16.2**
  - coma **E15**
    - diabetic - *see* Diabetes, by type, with hypoglycemia, with coma
  - diabetic - *see* Diabetes, hypoglycemia
- **Hyponasality R49.22**
- **Hypoplasia, hypoplastic**
  - coccyx **Q76.49**
  - sacrum **Q76.49**
  - spine **Q76.49**
  - vertebra **Q76.49**
- **Hypopnea, obstructive sleep apnea G47.33**
- **Hypoventilation RØ6.89**
  - congenital central alveolar **G47.35**
  - sleep related
    - idiopathic nonobstructive alveolar **G47.34**
    - in conditions classified elsewhere **G47.36**
- **Hypoxemia RØ9.Ø2**
  - sleep related, in conditions classified elsewhere **G47.36**
- **Hypoxia RØ9.Ø2** - *see also* Anoxia
  - sleep-related **G47.34**

I

- **Ichthyotoxism** - *see* Poisoning, fish
  - bacterial - *see* Intoxication, foodborne
- **Icterus** - *see also* Jaundice
  - conjunctiva **R17**
- **Ideation**
  - homicidal **R45.85Ø**
  - suicidal **R45.851**
- **Idiot, idiocy (congenital) F73**
- **IgE asthma J45.9Ø9**
- **Ileitis (chronic) (noninfectious) K52.9** - *see also* Enteritis
  - infectious **AØ9**
  - segmental - *see* Enteritis, regional
- **Ileocolitis K52.9** - *see also* Enteritis
  - infectious **AØ9**
  - regional - *see* Enteritis, regional
- **Ileotyphus** - *see* Typhoid
- **Illness R69** - *see also* Disease
- **Imbalance R26.89**
- **Imbecile, imbecility (I.Q.35-49) F71**
- **Immaturity (less than 37 completed weeks)** - *see also* Preterm, newborn
  - organ or site NEC - *see* Hypoplasia
- **Immunization** - *see also* Vaccination
  - appropriate for age
    - child (over 28 days old) **ZØØ.129**
      - with abnormal findings **ZØØ.121**
- **Impaired, impairment (function)**
  - auditory discrimination - *see* Abnormal, auditory perception
  - mobility
    - requiring care provider **Z74.Ø9**
- **Impediment, speech R47.9** - *see also* Disorder, speech
  - slurring **R47.81**
  - specified NEC **R47.89**
- **Imperfect**
  - closure (congenital)
    - organ or site not listed - *see* Anomaly, by site
- **Impingement (on teeth)**
  - joint - *see* Disorder, joint, specified type NEC
- **Implantation**
  - anomalous - *see* Anomaly, by site
- **Improper care (child) (newborn)** - *see* Maltreatment
- **Impulsiveness (impulsive) R45.87**
- **Inability to swallow** - *see* Aphagia
  - comply with dietary regimen **Z91.118**
- **Inadequate, inadequacy**
  - development
    - child **R62.5Ø**
    - organ or site not listed - *see* Anomaly, by site
  - mental - *see* Disability, intellectual
  - pulmonary
    - function **RØ6.89**
- **Inanition R64**
- **Inattention at or after birth** - *see* Neglect
- **Incarceration, incarcerated**
  - hernia - *see also* Hernia, by site, with obstruction
    - with gangrene - *see* Hernia, by site, with gangrene
  - rupture - *see* Hernia, by site
- **Incised wound**
  - external - *see* Laceration
  - internal organs - *see* Injury, by site
- **Incision, incisional**
  - traumatic
    - external - *see* Laceration
    - internal organs - *see* Injury, by site
- **Incompetency, incompetent, incompetence**
  - cardiac valve - *see* Endocarditis
  - valvular - *see* Endocarditis
  - vein, venous (saphenous) (varicose) - *see* Varix, leg
- **Incontinence R32**
  - urethral sphincter **R32**
  - urine (urinary) **R32**
    - due to cognitive impairment, or severe physical disability or immobility **R39.81**
    - functional **R39.81**
- **Incoordinate, incoordination**
  - esophageal-pharyngeal (newborn) - *see* Dysphagia
- **Inequality, leg (length) (acquired)** - *see also* Deformity, limb, unequal length
  - lower leg - *see* Deformity, limb, unequal length
- **Infant (s)** - *see also* Infancy
  - excessive crying **R68.11**
  - irritable child **R68.12**
  - lack of care - *see* Neglect
- **Infarct, infarction**
  - embolic - *see* Embolism
  - lung (embolic) (thrombotic) - *see* Embolism, pulmonary
  - muscle (ischemic) **M62.2Ø**
    - specified site NEC **M62.28**
  - pulmonary (artery) (vein) (hemorrhagic) - *see* Embolism, pulmonary
  - thrombotic - *see also* Thrombosis
    - artery, arterial - *see* Embolism
- **Infection, infected, infective (opportunistic) B99.9**
  - with
    - organ dysfunction (acute) **R65.2Ø**
      - with septic shock **R65.21**
  - accessory sinus (chronic) - *see* Sinusitis
  - aertrycke - *see* Infection, salmonella
  - alimentary canal NOS - *see* Enteritis, infectious
  - Ameba, amebic (histolytica) - *see* Amebiasis
  - antrum (chronic) - *see* Sinusitis, maxillary
  - Bacillus **A49.9**
    - suipestifer - *see* Infection, salmonella
    - typhosa **AØ1.ØØ**
  - Bacterium
    - typhosum **AØ1.ØØ**
  - bladder - *see* Cystitis
  - bone - *see* Osteomyelitis
  - brain **GØ4.9Ø** - *see also* Encephalitis
    - membranes - *see* Meningitis
  - bronchus - *see* Bronchitis
  - bursa - *see* Bursitis, infective
  - cartilage - *see* Disorder, cartilage, specified type NEC
  - cerebrospinal - *see* Meningitis
  - chest **J22**
  - Clostridium NEC
    - difficile
      - foodborne (disease)
        - not specified as recurrent **AØ4.72**
        - recurrent **AØ4.71**
      - necrotizing enterocolitis
        - not specified as recurrent **AØ4.72**
        - recurrent **AØ4.71**
  - colon - *see* Enteritis, infectious
  - coxsackie - *see* Coxsackie
  - cyst - *see* Cyst
  - ear (middle) - *see also* Otitis media
  - Eberthella typhosa **AØ1.ØØ**
  - Entamoeba - *see* Amebiasis
  - enteric - *see* Enteritis, infectious
  - ethmoidal (chronic) (sinus) - *see* Sinusitis, ethmoidal
  - food - *see* Intoxication, foodborne
  - frontal (sinus) (chronic) - *see* Sinusitis, frontal
  - gallbladder - *see* Cholecystitis
  - gastrointestinal - *see* Enteritis, infectious
  - generalized NEC - *see* Sepsis
  - herpes (simplex) - *see also* Herpes
  - herpesvirus, herpesviral - *see* Herpes
  - intervertebral disc, pyogenic **M46.3Ø**
    - cervical region **M46.32**
    - cervicothoracic region **M46.33**
    - lumbar region **M46.36**
    - lumbosacral region **M46.37**
    - multiple sites **M46.39**
    - occipito-atlanto-axial region **M46.31**
    - sacrococcygeal region **M46.38**
    - thoracic region **M46.34**
    - thoracolumbar region **M46.35**
  - intestine, intestinal - *see* Enteritis, infectious
  - maxilla, maxillary **M27.2**
    - sinus (chronic) - *see* Sinusitis, maxillary
  - muscle NEC - *see* Myositis, infective
  - nasal sinus (chronic) - *see* Sinusitis
  - nasopharynx - *see* Nasopharyngitis
  - purulent - *see* Abscess
  - respiratory (tract) NEC **J98.8**
    - acute **J22**
    - lower (acute) **J22**
    - rhinovirus **JØØ**
  - Salmonella (aertrycke) (arizonae) (callinarum) (cholerae-suis) (enteritidis) (suipestifer) (typhimurium) **AØ2.9**
    - localized **AØ2.2Ø**
      - arthritis **AØ2.23**
      - meningitis **AØ2.21**
      - osteomyelitis **AØ2.24**
      - pneumonia **AØ2.22**
      - pyelonephritis **AØ2.25**
      - specified NEC **AØ2.29**
    - typhi, typhosa - *see* Typhoid
  - seminal vesicle - *see* Vesiculitis
  - septic
    - localized, skin - *see* Abscess
  - sinus (accessory) (chronic) (nasal) - *see also* Sinusitis

- sphenoidal (sinus) - *see* Sinusitis, sphenoidal
- spinal cord NOS **GØ4.91** - *see also* Myelitis
  - meninges - *see* Meningitis
- suipestifer - *see* Infection, salmonella
- tendon (sheath) - *see* Tenosynovitis, infective NEC
- typhoid (abortive) (ambulant) (bacillus) - *see* Typhoid
- urinary (tract) **N39.Ø**
  - bladder - *see* Cystitis
- vagina (acute) - *see* Vaginitis
- varicose veins - *see* Varix
- vesical - *see* Cystitis
- virus, viral NOS **B34.9**
  - intestine - *see* Enteritis, viral

Infestation B88.9
- fluke **B66.9**
  - blood NOS - *see* Schistosomiasis

Infiltrate, infiltration
- calcareous NEC **R89.7**
  - localized - *see* Degeneration, by site
- muscle, fatty **M62.89**

Infirmity R68.89
- senile **R54**

Inflammation, inflamed, inflammatory (with exudation)
- accessory sinus (chronic) - *see* Sinusitis
- antrum (chronic) - *see* Sinusitis, maxillary
- appendix - *see* Appendicitis
- arachnoid - *see* Meningitis
- bladder - *see* Cystitis
- bone - *see* Osteomyelitis
- brain - *see also* Encephalitis
  - membrane - *see* Meningitis
- bronchi - *see* Bronchitis
- catarrhal **JØØ**
- cecum - *see* Appendicitis
- cerebral - *see also* Encephalitis
  - membrane - *see* Meningitis
- colon - *see* Enteritis
- connective tissue (diffuse) NEC - *see* Disorder, soft tissue, specified type NEC
- dura mater - *see* Meningitis
- ear (middle) - *see also* Otitis, media
- ethmoidal (sinus) (chronic) - *see* Sinusitis, ethmoidal
- fascia - *see* Myositis
- frontal (sinus) (chronic) - *see* Sinusitis, frontal
- gallbladder - *see* Cholecystitis
- gastrointestinal - *see* Enteritis
- gland (lymph) - *see* Lymphadenitis
- ileum - *see also* Enteritis
  - regional or terminal - *see* Enteritis, regional
- intestine (any part) - *see* Enteritis
- joint NEC - *see* Arthritis
- kidney - *see* Nephritis
- knee (joint) **M13.169**
- liver (capsule) - *see also* Hepatitis
- lung (acute) - *see also* Pneumonia
- lymph gland or node - *see* Lymphadenitis
- maxilla, maxillary **M27.2**
  - sinus (chronic) - *see* Sinusitis, maxillary
- membranes of brain or spinal cord - *see* Meningitis
- meninges - *see* Meningitis
- muscle - *see* Myositis
- myocardium - *see* Myocarditis
- nasal sinus (chronic) - *see* Sinusitis
- nasopharynx - *see* Nasopharyngitis
- nerve NEC - *see* Neuritis
- nose - *see* Rhinitis
- perivesical - *see* Cystitis
- pia mater - *see* Meningitis
- retrocecal - *see* Appendicitis
- seminal vesicle - *see* Vesiculitis
- sigmoid - *see* Enteritis
- sinus - *see* Sinusitis
- sphenoidal (sinus) - *see* Sinusitis, sphenoidal
- spinal
  - cord - *see* Encephalitis
  - membrane - *see* Meningitis
- spine - *see* Spondylopathy, inflammatory
- synovial - *see* Tenosynovitis
- tendon (sheath) NEC - *see* Tenosynovitis
- trachea - *see* Tracheitis
- vagina - *see* Vaginitis

Inhalation
- food or foreign body - *see* Foreign body, by site
- liquid or vomitus - *see* Asphyxia
- oil or gasoline (causing suffocation) - *see* Foreign body, by site
- stomach contents or secretions - *see* Foreign body, by site

Injury T14.9Ø- - *see also* specified injury type
- abdomen, abdominal S39.91-
  - specified NEC S39.81-
- Achilles tendon S86.ØØ-
  - laceration S86.Ø2-
  - specified type NEC S86.Ø9-
  - strain S86.Ø1-
- ankle S99.91-
  - specified type NEC S99.81-
  - sprain - *see* Sprain, ankle
- anus - *see* Injury, abdomen
- arm (upper) S49.9-
  - contusion - *see* Contusion, arm, upper
  - lower - *see* Injury, forearm
  - muscle - *see* Injury, muscle, shoulder
- blast (air) (hydraulic) (immersion) (underwater) NEC T14.8-
  - brain - *see* Concussion
- broad ligament - *see* Injury, pelvic organ, specified site NEC
- conus medullaris - *see* Injury, spinal, sacral cord
  - spinal - *see* Injury, spinal cord, by region
- cortex (cerebral) - *see also* Injury, intracranial
  - visual - *see* Injury, nerve, optic
- cranial
  - nerve - *see* Injury, nerve, cranial
- deep tissue - *see* Contusion, by site
- ear (auricle) (external) (canal) SØ9.91-
  - bruise - *see* Contusion, ear
  - contusion - *see* Contusion, ear
  - hematoma - *see* Hematoma, ear
- elbow S59.9Ø-
  - dislocation - *see* Dislocation, elbow
  - specified NEC S59.8Ø-
  - sprain - *see* Sprain, elbow
- fascia - *see* Injury, muscle
- finger (nail) S69.9-
  - contusion - *see* Contusion, finger
  - dislocation - *see* Dislocation, finger
  - muscle - *see* Injury, muscle, finger
  - nerve - *see* Injury, nerve, digital, finger
  - sprain - *see* Sprain, finger
- first cranial nerve (olfactory) - *see* Injury, nerve, olfactory
- flank - *see* Injury, abdomen
- foot S99.92-
  - dislocation - *see* Dislocation, foot
  - muscle - *see* Injury, muscle, foot
  - specified type NEC S99.82-
  - sprain - *see* Sprain, foot
- forearm S59.91-
  - muscle - *see* Injury, muscle, forearm
  - specified NEC S59.81-
- groin - *see* Injury, abdomen
- hand S69.9-
  - contusion - *see* Contusion, hand
  - muscle - *see* Injury, muscle, hand
- heel - *see* Injury, foot
- hip S79.91-
  - dislocation - *see* Dislocation, hip
  - muscle - *see* Injury, muscle, hip
  - specified NEC S79.81-
  - sprain - *see* Sprain, hip
- instrumental (during surgery) - *see* Laceration, accidental complicating surgery
  - nonsurgical - *see* Injury, by site
- internal T14.8-
  - pelvis, pelvic (organ) S37.9Ø-
    - specified NEC S39.83-
- joint NOS T14.8-
  - old or residual - *see* Disorder, joint, specified type NEC
- knee S89.9-
  - dislocation - *see* Dislocation, knee
  - meniscus (lateral) (medial) - *see* Sprain, knee, specified site NEC
  - sprain - *see* Sprain, knee
- leg (lower) S89.9-
  - muscle - *see* Injury, muscle, leg
- lower back S39.92-
  - specified NEC S39.82-
- mesosalpinx - *see* Injury, pelvic organ, specified site NEC
- muscle (and fascia) (and tendon)
  - abdomen S39.ØØ1-
    - specified type NEC S39.Ø91-
    - strain S39.Ø11-
  - abductor
    - thumb, forearm level - *see* Injury, muscle, thumb, abductor
  - adductor
    - thigh S76.2Ø-
      - laceration S76.22-
      - specified type NEC S76.29-
      - strain S76.21-
  - ankle - *see* Injury, muscle, foot
  - anterior muscle group, at leg level (lower) S86.2Ø-
    - laceration S86.22-
    - specified type NEC S86.29-
    - strain S86.21-
  - arm (upper) - *see* Injury, muscle, shoulder
  - biceps (parts NEC) S46.2Ø-
    - laceration S46.22-
    - long head S46.1Ø-
      - laceration S46.12-
      - specified type NEC S46.19-
      - strain S46.11-
    - specified type NEC S46.29-
    - strain S46.21-
  - extensor
    - finger (s) (other than thumb) - *see* Injury, muscle, finger by site, extensor
    - forearm level, specified NEC - *see* Injury, muscle, forearm, extensor
    - thumb - *see* Injury, muscle, thumb, extensor
    - toe (large) (ankle level) (foot level) - *see* Injury, muscle, toe, extensor

    - flexor (forearm level) S56.ØØ-
      - hand level S66.ØØ-
        - specified type NEC S66.Ø9-
        - strain S66.Ø1-
      - specified type NEC S56.Ø9-
      - strain S56.Ø1-
      - wrist level - *see* Injury, muscle, thumb, flexor, hand level
    - intrinsic S66.4Ø-
      - specified type NEC S66.49-
      - strain S66.41-
  - toe - *see also* Injury, muscle, foot
    - extensor, long S96.1Ø-
      - laceration S96.12-
      - specified type NEC S96.19-
      - strain S96.11-
    - flexor, long S96.ØØ-
      - laceration S96.Ø2-
      - specified type NEC S96.Ø9-
      - strain S96.Ø1-
  - triceps S46.3Ø-
    - laceration S46.32-
    - specified type NEC S46.39-
    - strain S46.31-
  - wrist (and hand) level - *see* Injury, muscle, hand
- nerve NEC T14.8-
  - cranial SØ4.9-
    - first (olfactory) - *see* Injury, nerve, olfactory
    - ninth (glossopharyngeal) - *see* Injury, nerve, glossopharyngeal
    - second (optic) - *see* Injury, nerve, optic
    - specified
      - nerve NEC SØ4.89-
        - contusion SØ4.89-
        - laceration SØ4.89-
        - specified type NEC SØ4.89-
    - tenth (pneumogastric or vagus) - *see* Injury, nerve, vagus
    - twelfth (hypoglossal) - *see* Injury, nerve, hypoglossal
  - digital
    - finger S64.4-
      - index S64.49-
      - little S64.49-
      - middle S64.49-
      - ring S64.49-
  - finger (digital) - *see* Injury, nerve, digital, finger
  - first cranial (olfactory) - *see* Injury, nerve, olfactory
  - glossopharyngeal SØ4.89-
    - specified type NEC SØ4.89-
  - hypoglossal SØ4.89-
    - specified type NEC SØ4.89-
  - lumbar spinal - *see* Injury, spinal, lumbar
    - root S34.21-
  - ninth cranial (glossopharyngeal) - *see* Injury, nerve, glossopharyngeal
  - olfactory SØ4.81-
    - specified type NEC SØ4.81-
  - optic SØ4.Ø1-
    - contusion SØ4.Ø1-
    - laceration SØ4.Ø1-
    - specified type NEC SØ4.Ø1-
  - pneumogastric - *see* Injury, nerve, vagus
  - root - *see* Injury, nerve, spinal, root
  - sacral spinal - *see* Injury, spinal, sacral
    - root S34.22-
  - second cranial (optic) - *see* Injury, nerve, optic
  - spinal
    - root
      - lumbar S34.21-
      - sacral S34.22-
  - tenth cranial (pneumogastric or vagus) - *see* Injury, nerve, vagus
  - twelfth cranial (hypoglossal) - *see* Injury, nerve, hypoglossal
  - vagus SØ4.89-
    - specified type NEC SØ4.89-
- ninth cranial nerve (glossopharyngeal) - *see* Injury, nerve, glossopharyngeal
- optic chiasm SØ4.Ø2-
- optic radiation SØ4.Ø3-
- optic tract and pathways SØ4.Ø3-
- patellar ligament (tendon) S76.1Ø-
  - laceration S76.12-
  - specified NEC S76.19-
  - strain S76.11-
- pelvis, pelvic (floor) S39.93-
  - specified NEC S39.83-
- phalanges
  - foot - *see* Injury, foot
- rectovaginal septum NEC S39.83-
- rotator cuff (muscle(s)) (tendon(s)) S46.ØØ-
  - laceration S46.Ø2-
  - specified type NEC S46.Ø9-
  - strain S46.Ø1-
- round ligament - *see* Injury, pelvic organ, specified site NEC
- second cranial nerve (optic) - *see* Injury, nerve, optic
- seminal vesicle - *see* Injury, pelvic organ, specified site NEC
- shoulder S49.9-
  - contusion - *see* Contusion, shoulder
  - dislocation - *see* Dislocation, shoulder
  - muscle - *see* Injury, muscle, shoulder
- spinal (cord)
  - cervical (neck) S14.1Ø9-
    - anterior cord syndrome S14.139-
      - C1 level S14.131-
      - C2 level S14.132-
      - C3 level S14.133-
      - C4 level S14.134-
      - C5 level S14.135-
      - C6 level S14.136-
      - C7 level S14.137-
      - C8 level S14.138-
    - Brown-Séquard syndrome S14.149-
      - C1 level S14.141-
      - C2 level S14.142-
      - C3 level S14.143-
      - C4 level S14.144-
      - C5 level S14.145-
      - C6 level S14.146-
      - C7 level S14.147-
      - C8 level S14.148-
    - C1 level S14.1Ø1-
    - C2 level S14.1Ø2-
    - C3 level S14.1Ø3-
    - C4 level S14.1Ø4-
    - C5 level S14.1Ø5-
    - C6 level S14.1Ø6-
    - C7 level S14.1Ø7-
    - C8 level S14.1Ø8-
    - central cord syndrome S14.129-
      - C1 level S14.121-
      - C2 level S14.122-
      - C3 level S14.123-
      - C4 level S14.124-
      - C5 level S14.125-
      - C6 level S14.126-
      - C7 level S14.127-
      - C8 level S14.128-
    - complete lesion S14.119-
      - C1 level S14.111-
      - C2 level S14.112-
      - C3 level S14.113-
      - C4 level S14.114-
      - C5 level S14.115-
      - C6 level S14.116-
      - C7 level S14.117-
      - C8 level S14.118-
    - incomplete lesion specified NEC S14.159-
      - C1 level S14.151-
      - C2 level S14.152-
      - C3 level S14.153-
      - C4 level S14.154-
      - C5 level S14.155-
      - C6 level S14.156-
      - C7 level S14.157-
      - C8 level S14.158-
    - posterior cord syndrome S14.159-
      - C1 level S14.151-
      - C2 level S14.152-
      - C3 level S14.153-
      - C4 level S14.154-
      - C5 level S14.155-
      - C6 level S14.156-
      - C7 level S14.157-
      - C8 level S14.158-
  - dorsal - *see* Injury, spinal, thoracic
  - lumbar S34.1Ø9-
    - complete lesion S34.119-
      - L1 level S34.111-
      - L2 level S34.112-
      - L3 level S34.113-
      - L4 level S34.114-
      - L5 level S34.115-
    - concussion S34.Ø1-
    - edema S34.Ø1-
    - incomplete lesion S34.129-
      - L1 level S34.121-
      - L2 level S34.122-
      - L3 level S34.123-
      - L4 level S34.124-
      - L5 level S34.125-
    - L1 level S34.1Ø1-
    - L2 level S34.1Ø2-
    - L3 level S34.1Ø3-
    - L4 level S34.1Ø4-
    - L5 level S34.1Ø5-
  - nerve root NEC
    - lumbar S34.21-
    - sacral S34.22-
  - sacral S34.139-
    - complete lesion S34.131-
    - incomplete lesion S34.132-
  - thoracic S24.1Ø9-
    - anterior cord syndrome S24.139-
    - Brown-Séquard syndrome S24.149-
    - complete lesion S24.119-
    - incomplete lesion specified NEC S24.159-
    - posterior cord syndrome S24.159-
    - T1 level S24.1Ø1-
    - T11-T12 level S24.1Ø4-
    - T2-T6 level S24.1Ø2-
    - T7-T1Ø level S24.1Ø3-
- subungual
  - toes - *see* Injury, foot
- superficial NEC T14.8-
  - arm (upper) S4Ø.92-
    - contusion - *see* Contusion, arm
  - blister - *see* Blister, by site
  - contusion - *see* Contusion, by site
  - ear (auricle) (canal) (external) SØØ.4Ø-
    - contusion - *see* Contusion, ear

finger (s) S6Ø.949-
contusion - *see* Contusion, finger
hand S6Ø.92-
contusion - *see* Contusion, hand
shoulder S4Ø.91-
contusion - *see* Contusion, shoulder
thorax, thoracic (wall) S2Ø.9Ø-
contusion - *see* Contusion, thorax
thumb S6Ø.93-
contusion - *see* Contusion, thumb
toe (s) S9Ø.93-
contusion - *see* Contusion, toe
tendon - *see also* Injury, muscle, by site
abdomen - *see* Injury, muscle, abdomen
Achilles - *see* Injury, Achilles tendon
lower back - *see* Injury, muscle, lower back
pelvic organs - *see* Injury, muscle, pelvis
tenth cranial nerve (pneumogastric or vagus) - *see* Injury, nerve, vagus
thigh S79.92-
muscle - *see* Injury, muscle, thigh
specified NEC S79.82-
thorax, thoracic S29.9-
dislocation - *see* Dislocation, thorax
external (wall) S29.9-
contusion - *see* Contusion, thorax
sprain - *see* Sprain, thorax
fracture - *see* Fracture, thorax
thumb S69.9-
contusion - *see* Contusion, thumb
dislocation - *see* Dislocation, thumb
muscle - *see* Injury, muscle, thumb
sprain - *see* Sprain, thumb
toe S99.92-
contusion - *see* Contusion, toe
dislocation - *see* Dislocation, toe
muscle - *see* Injury, muscle, toe
specified type NEC S99.82-
sprain - *see* Sprain, toe
twelfth cranial nerve (hypoglossal) - *see* Injury, nerve, hypoglossal
vas deferens - *see* Injury, pelvic organ, specified site NEC
visual cortex SØ4.Ø4-
wrist S69.9-
contusion - *see* Contusion, wrist
dislocation - *see* Dislocation, wrist
muscle - *see* Injury, muscle, hand
sprain - *see* Sprain, wrist

Insecurity
financial **Z59.86**

Insomnia (organic) G47.ØØ
due to
medical condition **G47.Ø1**
specified NEC **G47.Ø9**

Inspiration
food or foreign body - *see* Foreign body, by site

Instability
joint (post-traumatic) **M25.3Ø**
due to old ligament injury - *see* Disorder, ligament
flail - *see* Flail, joint
secondary to
old ligament injury - *see* Disorder, ligament
specified site NEC **M25.39**
vasomotor **R55**

Institutionalization, affecting child Z62.22

Insufficiency, insufficient
heart - *see also* Insufficiency, myocardial
valve - *see* Endocarditis
idiopathic autonomic **G9Ø.Ø9**
mental (congenital) - *see* Disability, intellectual
myocardial, myocardium (with arteriosclerosis) **I5Ø.9** - *see also* Failure, heart
hypertensive - *see* Hypertension, heart
respiratory **RØ6.89**
urethral sphincter **R32**

Interruption
phase-shift, sleep cycle - *see* Disorder, sleep, circadian rhythm
sleep phase-shift, or 24 hour sleep-wake cycle - *see* Disorder, sleep, circadian rhythm

Intoxication
drug
acute (without dependence) - *see* Abuse, drug, by type with intoxication
with dependence - *see* Dependence, drug, by type with intoxication
foodborne **AØ5.9**
due to
Salmonella **AØ2.9**
with
localized infection (s) **AØ2.2Ø**
arthritis **AØ2.23**
meningitis **AØ2.21**
osteomyelitis **AØ2.24**
pneumonia **AØ2.22**
pyelonephritis **AØ2.25**
specified NEC **AØ2.29**

Intrinsic deformity - *see* Deformity

Inversion
circadian rhythm - *see* Disorder, sleep, circadian rhythm
nyctohemeral rhythm - *see* Disorder, sleep, circadian rhythm
organ or site, congenital NEC - *see* Anomaly, by site
sleep rhythm - *see* Disorder, sleep, circadian rhythm

I.Q.
2Ø-34 **F72**
35-49 **F71**
5Ø-69 **F7Ø**
under 2Ø **F73**

Irregular, irregularity
breathing **RØ6.89**
respiratory **RØ6.89**
shape, organ or site, congenital NEC - *see* Distortion

Irritable, irritability R45.4
bronchial - *see* Bronchitis
infant **R68.12**

Irritation
bronchial - *see* Bronchitis
spinal (cord) (traumatic) - *see also* Injury, spinal cord, by region
nerve **G58.9**
root NEC - *see* Radiculopathy
nontraumatic - *see* Myelopathy

Ischemia, ischemic I99.8
infarction, muscle - *see* Infarct, muscle

Ischuria R34

Isolation, isolated
family **Z63.79**

Issue of
medical certificate **ZØ2.79**
for disability determination **ZØ2.71**

J

Jaccoud's syndrome - *see* Arthropathy, postrheumatic, chronic

Jackson's
paralysis or syndrome **G83.89**

Jacquet's dermatitis (diaper dermatitis) L22

Jaffe-Lichtenstein (-Uehlinger) syndrome - *see* Dysplasia, fibrous, bone NEC

Jaundice (yellow) R17
cholestatic (benign) **R17**
symptomatic **R17**

Jejunitis - *see* Enteritis

Joint - *see also* condition
mice - *see* Loose, body, joint

K

Keratoderma, keratodermia (congenital) (palmaris et plantaris) (symmetrical) Q82.8
Reiter's - *see* Reiter's disease

Ketoacidosis E87.29
diabetic - *see* Diabetes, by type, with ketoacidosis

Ketosis NEC E88.89
diabetic - *see* Diabetes, by type, with ketoacidosis

Kimmelstiel (-Wilson) disease - *see* Diabetes, Kimmelstiel (-Wilson) disease

Kink, kinking
organ or site, congenital NEC - *see* Anomaly, by site

Kissing spine M48.2Ø
cervical region **M48.22**
cervicothoracic region **M48.23**
lumbar region **M48.26**
lumbosacral region **M48.27**
occipito-atlanto-axial region **M48.21**
thoracic region **M48.24**
thoracolumbar region **M48.25**

Köenig's disease (osteochondritis dissecans) - *see* Osteochondritis, dissecans

Korsakoff's (Wernicke) disease, psychosis or syndrome (alcoholic) F1Ø.96
drug-induced
due to drug abuse - *see* Abuse, drug, by type, with amnestic disorder
due to drug dependence - *see* Dependence, drug, by type, with amnestic disorder

Kümmell's disease or spondylitis - *see* Spondylopathy, traumatic

Kussmaul's
respiration **E87.29**
in diabetic acidosis - *see* Diabetes, by type, with ketoacidosis

Kyphosis, kyphotic (acquired) M4Ø.2Ø9
cervical region **M4Ø.2Ø2**
cervicothoracic region **M4Ø.2Ø3**
congenital **Q76.419**
cervical region **Q76.412**
cervicothoracic region **Q76.413**
occipito-atlanto-axial region **Q76.411**
thoracic region **Q76.414**
thoracolumbar region **Q76.415**
postural (adolescent) **M4Ø.ØØ**
cervicothoracic region **M4Ø.Ø3**
thoracic region **M4Ø.Ø4**
thoracolumbar region **M4Ø.Ø5**
secondary NEC **M4Ø.1Ø**
cervical region **M4Ø.12**
cervicothoracic region **M4Ø.13**
thoracic region **M4Ø.14**
thoracolumbar region **M4Ø.15**
specified type NEC **M4Ø.299**
cervical region **M4Ø.292**
cervicothoracic region **M4Ø.293**
thoracic region **M4Ø.294**
thoracolumbar region **M4Ø.295**
thoracic region **M4Ø.2Ø4**
thoracolumbar region **M4Ø.2Ø5**

L

M

Maladaptation - *see* Maladjustment
Maladjustment
- occupational NEC **Z56.89**

Malaise R53.81
Maldevelopment - *see also* Anomaly
- spine **Q76.49**

Malformation (congenital) - *see also* Anomaly
- auricle
  - ear (congenital) **Q17.3**
    - acquired **H61.119**
      - left **H61.112**
        - with right **H61.113**
      - right **H61.111**
        - with left **H61.113**
- Chiari
  - Type II **QØ7.Ø1**
- joint **Q74.9**
  - lumbosacral **Q76.49**
- spine **Q76.49**
  - kyphosis - *see* Kyphosis, congenital
  - lordosis - *see* Lordosis, congenital
- venous - *see* Anomaly, vein(s)

Malfunction - *see also* Dysfunction
Malocclusion (teeth) M26.4
- temporomandibular (joint) **M26.69**

Malposition
- congenital
  - hip (joint) **Q65.89**
  - organ or site not listed - *see* Anomaly, by site
- fetus - *see* Pregnancy, complicated by (management affected by), presentation, fetal

Maltreatment
- child
  - history of - *see* History, personal (of), abuse
  - neglect
    - history of - *see* History, personal (of), abuse
  - physical abuse
    - history of - *see* History, personal (of), abuse
  - psychological abuse
    - history of - *see* History, personal (of), abuse
  - sexual abuse
    - history of - *see* History, personal (of), abuse
- personal history of **Z91.89**

Marasmus E41
- senile **R54**

March
- fracture - *see* Fracture, traumatic, stress, by site

Marfan's syndrome - *see* Syndrome, Marfan's
Marie-Bamberger disease - *see* Osteoarthropathy, hypertrophic, specified NEC
Mass
- abdominal **R19.ØØ**
  - epigastric **R19.Ø6**
  - generalized **R19.Ø7**
  - left lower quadrant **R19.Ø4**
  - left upper quadrant **R19.Ø2**
  - periumbilic **R19.Ø5**
  - right lower quadrant **R19.Ø3**
  - right upper quadrant **R19.Ø1**
  - specified site NEC **R19.Ø9**
- cystic - *see* Cyst
- intra-abdominal (diffuse) (generalized) - *see* Mass, abdominal
- pelvic (diffuse) (generalized) - *see* Mass, abdominal
- specified organ NEC - *see* Disease, by site
- umbilical (diffuse) (generalized) **R19.Ø9**

Maternal care (for) - *see* Pregnancy (complicated by) (management affected by)
ME/CFS (myalgic encephalomyelitis/chronic fatigue syndrome) G93.32
Megacolon (acquired) (functional) (not Hirschsprung's disease) (in) K59.39
- toxic NEC **K59.31**
  - due to Clostridium difficile
    - not specified as recurrent **AØ4.72**
    - recurrent **AØ4.71**

Megrim - *see* Migraine
Mellitus, diabetes - *see* Diabetes
Melorheostosis (bone) - *see* Disorder, bone, density and structure, specified NEC
Meningitis (basal) (basic) (brain) (cerebral) (cervical) (congestive) (diffuse) (hemorrhagic) (infantile) (membranous) (metastatic) (nonspecific) (pontine) (progressive) (simple) (spinal) (subacute) (sympathetic) (toxic) GØ3.9
- in (due to)
  - Salmonella infection **AØ2.21**
  - typhoid fever **AØ1.Ø1**
- Salmonella (arizonae) (Cholerae-Suis) (enteritidis) (typhimurium) **AØ2.21**
- typhoid **AØ1.Ø1**

Meningoradiculitis - *see* Meningitis
Menopause, menopausal (asymptomatic) (state) Z78.Ø
- arthritis (any site) NEC - *see* Arthritis, specified form NEC
- toxic polyarthritis NEC - *see* Arthritis, specified form NEC

Mental - *see also* condition
- deficiency - *see* Disability, intellectual
- disorder - *see* Disorder, mental
- insufficiency (congenital) - *see* Disability, intellectual
- retardation - *see* Disability, intellectual
- subnormality - *see* Disability, intellectuall
- upset - *see* Disorder, mental

Mesencephalitis - *see* Encephalitis
Metastasis, metastatic
- abscess - *see* Abscess

Methadone use - *see* Use, opioid
Mice, joint - *see* Loose, body, joint
Micturition
- disorder NEC **R39.198** - *see also* Difficulty, micturition
- hesitancy **R39.11**
- incomplete emptying **R39.14**
- poor stream **R39.12**
- position dependent **R39.192**
- split stream **R39.13**
- straining **R39.16**
- urgency **R39.15**

Migraine (idiopathic) G43.9Ø9
- with aura (acute-onset) (prolonged) (typical) (without headache) **G43.1Ø9**
  - with refractory migraine **G43.119**
    - with status migrainosus **G43.111**
    - without status migrainosus **G43.119**
  - without mention of refractory migraine **G43.1Ø9**
    - with status migrainosus **G43.1Ø1**
    - without status migrainosus **G43.1Ø9**
  - intractable **G43.119**
    - with status migrainosus **G43.111**
    - without status migrainosus **G43.119**
  - not intractable **G43.1Ø9**
    - with status migrainosus **G43.1Ø1**
    - without status migrainosus **G43.1Ø9**
  - persistent **G43.5Ø9**
    - with cerebral infarction **G43.6Ø9**
      - with refractory migraine **G43.619**
        - with status migrainosus **G43.611**
        - without status migrainosus **G43.619**
      - without refractory migraine **G43.6Ø9**
        - with status migrainosus **G43.6Ø1**
        - without status migrainosus **G43.6Ø9**
      - intractable **G43.619**
        - with status migrainosus **G43.611**
        - without status migrainosus **G43.619**
      - not intractable **G43.6Ø9**
        - with status migrainosus **G43.6Ø1**
        - without status migrainosus **G43.6Ø9**
    - without cerebral infarction **G43.5Ø9**
      - with refractory migraine **G43.519**
        - with status migrainosus **G43.511**
        - without status migrainosus **G43.519**
      - without refractory migraine **G43.5Ø9**
        - with status migrainosus **G43.5Ø1**
        - without status migrainosus **G43.5Ø9**
      - intractable **G43.519**
        - with status migrainosus **G43.511**
        - without status migrainosus **G43.519**
      - not intractable **G43.5Ø9**
        - with status migrainosus **G43.5Ø1**
        - without status migrainosus **G43.5Ø9**
- with refractory migraine **G43.919**
  - with status migrainosus **G43.911**
  - without status migrainosus **G43.919**
- without aura **G43.ØØ9**
  - with refractory migraine **G43.Ø19**
    - with status migrainosus **G43.Ø11**
    - without status migrainosus **G43.Ø19**
  - without mention of refractory migraine **G43.ØØ9**
    - with status migrainosus **G43.ØØ1**
    - without status migrainosus **G43.ØØ9**
  - chronic **G43.7Ø9**
    - with refractory migraine **G43.719**
      - with status migrainosus **G43.711**
      - without status migrainosus **G43.719**
    - without refractory migraine **G43.7Ø9**
      - with status migrainosus **G43.7Ø1**
      - without status migrainosus **G43.7Ø9**
    - intractable
      - with status migrainosus **G43.711**
      - without status migrainosus **G43.719**
    - not intractable
      - with status migrainosus **G43.7Ø1**
      - without status migrainosus **G43.7Ø9**
  - intractable
    - with status migrainosus **G43.Ø11**
    - without status migrainosus **G43.Ø19**
  - not intractable
    - with status migrainosus **G43.ØØ1**
    - without status migrainosus **G43.ØØ9**
- without refractory migraine **G43.9Ø9**
  - with status migrainosus **G43.9Ø1**
  - without status migrainosus **G43.9Ø9**
- abdominal **G43.DØ**
  - with refractory migraine **G43.D1**
  - without refractory migraine **G43.DØ**
  - intractable **G43.D1**
  - not intractable **G43.DØ**
- basilar - *see* Migraine, with aura
- classical - *see* Migraine, with aura
- common - *see* Migraine, without aura
- complicated **G43.1Ø9**
- equivalents - *see* Migraine, with aura
- familiar - *see* Migraine, hemiplegic

- hemiplegic **G43.4Ø9**
  - with refractory migraine **G43.419**
    - with status migrainosus **G43.411**
    - without status migrainosus **G43.419**
  - without refractory migraine **G43.4Ø9**
    - with status migrainosus **G43.4Ø1**
    - without status migrainosus **G43.4Ø9**
  - intractable **G43.419**
    - with status migrainosus **G43.411**
    - without status migrainosus **G43.419**
  - not intractable **G43.4Ø9**
    - with status migrainosus **G43.4Ø1**
    - without status migrainosus **G43.4Ø9**
- intractable **G43.919**
  - with status migrainosus **G43.911**
  - without status migrainosus **G43.919**
- menstrual **G43.829**
  - with refractory migraine **G43.839**
    - with status migrainosus **G43.831**
    - without status migrainosus **G43.839**
  - without refractory migraine **G43.829**
    - with status migrainosus **G43.821**
    - without status migrainosus **G43.829**
  - intractable **G43.839**
    - with status migrainosus **G43.831**
    - without status migrainosus **G43.839**
  - not intractable **G43.829**
    - with status migrainosus **G43.821**
    - without status migrainosus **G43.829**
- menstrually related - *see* Migraine, menstrual
- not intractable **G43.9Ø9**
  - with status migrainosus **G43.9Ø1**
  - without status migrainosus **G43.919**
- ophthalmoplegic **G43.BØ**
  - with refractory migraine **G43.B1**
  - without refractory migraine **G43.BØ**
  - intractable **G43.B1**
  - not intractable **G43.BØ**
- persistent aura (with, without) cerebral infarction - *see* Migraine, with aura, persistent
- preceded or accompanied by transient focal neurological phenomena - *see* Migraine, with aura
- pre-menstrual - *see* Migraine, menstrual
- pure menstrual - *see* Migraine, menstrual
- retinal - *see* Migraine, with aura
- specified NEC **G43.8Ø9**
  - intractable **G43.819**
    - with status migrainosus **G43.811**
    - without status migrainosus **G43.819**
  - not intractable **G43.8Ø9**
    - with status migrainosus **G43.8Ø1**
    - without status migrainosus **G43.8Ø9**
- sporadic - *see* Migraine, hemiplegic
- transformed - *see* Migraine, without aura, chronic
- triggered seizures - *see* Migraine, with aura

Mills' disease - *see* Hemiplegia

Misplaced, misplacement
- organ or site, congenital NEC - *see* Malposition, congenital

Missing - *see also* Absence

Mobile, mobility
- organ or site, congenital NEC - *see* Malposition, congenital

Moebius, Möbius
- disease (ophthalmoplegic migraine) - *see* Migraine, ophthalmoplegic
- syndrome **Q87.Ø**
  - ophthalmoplegic migraine - *see* Migraine, ophthalmoplegic

Monoarthritis M13.1Ø

Mononeuropathy G58.9
- in diseases classified elsewhere - *see* **G59**

Monoplegia G83.3-
- transient **R29.818**

Morbidity not stated or unknown R69

Morbus - *see also* Disease
- caducus - *see* Epilepsy
- comitialis - *see* Epilepsy
- cordis **I51.9** - *see also* Disease, heart
  - valvulorum - *see* Endocarditis

Moron (I.Q.5Ø-69) F7Ø

Mouse, joint - *see* Loose, body, joint

Münchmeyer's syndrome - *see* Myositis, ossificans, progressiva

Murmur (cardiac) (heart) (organic) RØ1.1
- abdominal **R19.15**
- diastolic - *see* Endocarditis
- valvular - *see* Endocarditis

Musculoneuralgia - *see* Neuralgia

Mushrooming hip - *see* Derangement, joint, specified NEC, hip

Mutism - *see also* Aphasia

Myalgia M79.1Ø
- auxiliary muscles, head and neck **M79.12**
- mastication muscle **M79.11**
- site specified NEC **M79.18**

Myasthenia G7Ø.9
- cordis - *see* Failure, heart
- gravis **G7Ø.ØØ**
  - with exacerbation (acute) **G7Ø.Ø1**
  - in crisis **G7Ø.Ø1**
  - pseudoparalytica **G7Ø.ØØ**
    - with exacerbation (acute) **G7Ø.Ø1**
    - in crisis **G7Ø.Ø1**

Myasthenic M62.81

Myelitis (acute) (ascending) (childhood) (chronic) (descending) (diffuse) (disseminated) (idiopathic) (pressure) (progressive) (spinal cord) (subacute) GØ4.91 - *see also* Encephalitis
- herpes zoster **BØ2.24**
- postherpetic **BØ2.24**

Myeloencephalitis - *see* Encephalitis

Myelomalacia G95.89

Myelopathic
- muscle atrophy - *see* Atrophy, muscle, spinal

Myelopathy (spinal cord) G95.9
- drug-induced **G95.89**
- in (due to)
  - degeneration or displacement, intervertebral disc NEC - *see* Disorder, disc, with, myelopathy
  - infection - *see* Encephalitis
  - intervertebral disc disorder - *see also* Disorder, disc, with, myelopathy
  - spondylosis - *see* Spondylosis, with myelopathy NEC
- radiation-induced **G95.89**
- spondylogenic NEC - *see* Spondylosis, with myelopathy NEC
- toxic **G95.89**

Myelosclerosis D75.89
- disseminated, of nervous system **G35**

Myocardiopathy (congestive) (constrictive) (familial) (hypertrophic nonobstructive) (idiopathic) (infiltrative) (obstructive) (primary) (restrictive) (sporadic) I42.9 - *see also* Cardiomyopathy
- in (due to)
  - progressive muscular dystrophy **G71.Ø9** [**I43**] - *see also* Dystrophy, muscular, by type

Myocarditis (with arteriosclerosis)(chronic) (fibroid) (interstitial) (old) (progressive) (senile) I51.4
- hypertensive - *see* Hypertension, heart
- in (due to)
  - typhoid **AØ1.Ø2**
- rheumatoid - *see* Rheumatoid, carditis
- typhoid **AØ1.Ø2**
- valvular - *see* Endocarditis

Myocardosis - *see* Cardiomyopathy

Myodiastasis - *see* Diastasis, muscle

Myoendocarditis - *see* Endocarditis

Myofasciitis (acute) - *see* Myositis

Myofibrosis M62.89
- heart - *see* Myocarditis

Myomalacia M62.89

Myopathy G72.9
- distal **G71.Ø9**
- facioscapulohumeral **G71.Ø2**
- in (due to)
  - rheumatoid arthritis - *see* Rheumatoid, myopathy
  - scleroderma **M34.82**
  - sicca syndrome **M35.Ø3**
  - Sjögren's syndrome **M35.Ø3**
- limb-girdle - *see* Dystrophy, muscular, limb-girdle
- Miyoshi, type 3 **G71.Ø35**
- ocular **G71.Ø9**
- oculopharyngeal **G71.Ø9**
- scapulohumeral **G71.Ø2**

Myositis M6Ø.9
- due to posture - *see* Myositis, specified type NEC
- foreign body granuloma - *see* Granuloma, foreign body
- infective **M6Ø.ØØ9**
- interstitial **M6Ø.1Ø**
- ossificans or ossifying (circumscripta) - *see also* Ossification, muscle, specified NEC
  - in (due to)
    - burns **M61.3Ø**
      - multiple sites **M61.39**
      - specified site NEC **M61.38**
    - quadriplegia or paraplegia **M61.2Ø**
      - multiple sites **M61.29**
      - specified site NEC **M61.28**
  - progressiva **M61.1Ø**
    - multiple sites **M61.19**
    - specified site NEC **M61.18**
  - traumatica **M61.ØØ**
    - multiple sites **M61.Ø9**
    - specified site NEC **M61.Ø8**
- purulent - *see* Myositis, infective
- specified type NEC **M6Ø.8Ø**
  - multiple sites **M6Ø.89**
  - specified site NEC **M6Ø.88**
- suppurative - *see* Myositis, infective
- traumatic (old) - *see* Myositis, specified type NEC

Myotonia (acquisita) (intermittens) M62.89

Myringitis H73.2-
- with otitis media - *see* Otitis, media

N

Nanism, nanosomia - *see* Dwarfism

Napkin rash L22

Narcosis RØ6.89

Narcotism - *see* Dependence

Narrowing - *see also* Stenosis

Nasopharyngitis (acute) (infective) (streptococcal) (subacute) JØØ

Near-syncope R55

O

- fecal **K56.41**
  - with hernia - *see* Hernia, by site, with obstruction
- foreign body - *see* Foreign body
- labor - *see* Delivery
- thrombotic - *see* Thrombosis
- valvular - *see* Endocarditis
- vein, venous **I87.1**
  - thrombotic - *see* Thrombosis

Occlusion, occluded
- embolic - *see* Embolism
- vein - *see* Thrombosis

Occupational
- problems NEC **Z56.89**

Old age (without mention of debility) R54

Oligophrenia - *see also* Disability, intellectual

Oliguria R34

Ondine's curse - *see* Apnea, sleep

Ophthalmia H1Ø.9 - *see also* Conjunctivitis
- migraine - *see* Migraine, ophthalmoplegic

Ophthalmoplegia - *see also* Strabismus, paralytic
- migraine - *see* Migraine, ophthalmoplegic

Opioid (s)
- abuse - *see* Abuse, drug, opioids
- dependence - *see* Dependence, drug, opioids

Orthopnea RØ6.Ø1

Ossification
- cartilage (senile) - *see* Disorder, cartilage, specified type NEC
- heart - *see also* Degeneration, myocardial
  - valve - *see* Endocarditis
- ligament - *see* Disorder, tendon, specified type NEC
- muscle - *see also* Calcification, muscle
  - due to burns - *see* Myositis, ossificans, in, burns
  - paralytic - *see* Myositis, ossificans, in, quadriplegia
  - progressive - *see* Myositis, ossificans, progressiva
  - specified NEC **M61.5Ø**
    - multiple sites **M61.59**
    - specified site NEC **M61.58**
  - traumatic - *see* Myositis, ossificans, traumatica
- periarticular - *see* Disorder, joint, specified type NEC
- rider's bone - *see* Ossification, muscle, specified NEC
- tendon - *see* Disorder, tendon, specified type NEC

Osteitis - *see also* Osteomyelitis
- condensans **M85.3Ø**
- deformans **M88.9**
  - specified NEC - *see* Paget's disease, bone, by site
- fibrosa NEC - *see* Cyst, bone, by site
  - circumscripta - *see* Dysplasia, fibrous, bone NEC

Osteoarthritis M19.9Ø
- post-traumatic NEC **M19.92**
  - specified site NEC **M19.19**
- primary **M19.91**
  - specified site NEC **M19.Ø9**
  - spine - *see* Spondylosis
- secondary **M19.93**
  - specified site NEC **M19.29**
  - spine - *see* Spondylosis
- specified site NEC **M19.Ø9**
- spine - *see* Spondylosis

Osteoarthropathy (hypertrophic) M19.9Ø
- pulmonary - *see also* Osteoarthropathy, specified type NEC
  - hypertrophic - *see* Osteoarthropathy, hypertrophic, specified type NEC
- specified joint NEC - *see* Osteoarthritis, primary, specified joint NEC
- spine - *see* Spondylosis

Osteoarthrosis (degenerative) (hypertrophic) (joint) - *see also* Osteoarthritis
- spine - *see* Spondylosis

Osteochondritis - *see also* Osteochondropathy, by site
- dissecans **M93.2Ø**
  - multiple sites **M93.29**
  - specified site NEC **M93.28**

Osteochondrolysis - *see* Osteochondritis, dissecans

Osteochondropathy M93.9Ø
- multiple joints **M93.99**
- osteochondritis dissecans - *see* Osteochondritis, dissecans
- osteochondrosis - *see* Osteochondrosis
- specified joint NEC **M93.98**
- specified type NEC **M93.8Ø**
  - multiple joints **M93.89**
  - specified joint NEC **M93.88**

Osteochondrosis - *see also* Osteochondropathy, by site
- adult - *see* Osteochondropathy, specified type NEC, by site
- dissecans (knee) (shoulder) - *see* Osteochondritis, dissecans
- juvenile, juvenilis **M92.9**
  - spine **M42.ØØ**
    - cervical region **M42.Ø2**
    - cervicothoracic region **M42.Ø3**
    - lumbar region **M42.Ø6**
    - lumbosacral region **M42.Ø7**
    - multiple sites **M42.Ø9**
    - occipito-atlanto-axial region **M42.Ø1**
    - sacrococcygeal region **M42.Ø8**
    - thoracic region **M42.Ø4**
    - thoracolumbar region **M42.Ø5**
  - vertebra (body) (epiphyseal plates) (Calvé's) (Scheuermann's) - *see* Osteochondrosis, juvenile, spine
- Scheuermann's - *see* Osteochondrosis, juvenile, spine
- spine **M42.9**
  - adult **M42.1Ø**
    - cervical region **M42.12**
    - cervicothoracic region **M42.13**
    - lumbar region **M42.16**
    - lumbosacral region **M42.17**
    - multiple sites **M42.19**
    - occipito-atlanto-axial region **M42.11**
    - sacrococcygeal region **M42.18**
    - thoracic region **M42.14**
    - thoracolumbar region **M42.15**
  - juvenile - *see* Osteochondrosis, juvenile, spine
- vertebral - *see* Osteochondrosis, spine

Osteolysis M89.5Ø
- ilium **M89.559**
- ischium **M89.559**
- multiple sites **M89.59**
- neck **M89.58**
- rib **M89.58**
- skull **M89.58**
- vertebra **M89.58**

Osteomyelitis (general) (infective) (localized) (neonatal) (purulent) (septic) (staphylococcal) (streptococcal) (suppurative) (with periostitis) M86.9
- acute **M86.1Ø**
  - hematogenous **M86.ØØ**
    - vertebra - *see* Osteomyelitis, vertebra
  - vertebra - *see* Osteomyelitis, vertebra
- chronic (or old) **M86.6Ø**
  - with draining sinus **M86.4Ø**
    - vertebra - *see* Osteomyelitis, vertebra
  - hematogenous NEC **M86.5Ø**
    - multifocal **M86.3Ø**
      - vertebra - *see* Osteomyelitis, vertebra
    - vertebra - *see* Osteomyelitis, vertebra
  - vertebra - *see* Osteomyelitis, vertebra
- Salmonella (arizonae) (cholerae-suis) (enteritidis) (typhimurium) **AØ2.24**
- specified type NEC M86.8X- - *see also* subcategory
  - vertebra - *see* Osteomyelitis, vertebra
- subacute **M86.2Ø**
  - vertebra - *see* Osteomyelitis, vertebra
- typhoid **AØ1.Ø5**
- vertebra **M46.2Ø**
  - cervical region **M46.22**
  - cervicothoracic region **M46.23**
  - lumbar region **M46.26**
  - lumbosacral region **M46.27**
  - occipito-atlanto-axial region **M46.21**
  - sacrococcygeal region **M46.28**
  - thoracic region **M46.24**
  - thoracolumbar region **M46.25**

Osteonecrosis M87.9
- due to
  - trauma - *see* Osteonecrosis, secondary, due to, trauma
- secondary NEC **M87.3Ø**
  - due to
    - trauma (previous) **M87.2Ø**
      - multiple sites **M87.29**
      - neck **M87.28**
      - rib **M87.28**
      - skull **M87.28**
      - vertebra **M87.28**

Osteopathy - *see also* Osteomyelitis, Osteonecrosis, Osteoporosis

Osteophyte M25.7Ø
- spine **M25.78**
- vertebrae **M25.78**

Otitis (acute) H66.9Ø
- chronic - *see also* Otitis, media, chronic
- media (hemorrhagic) (staphylococcal) (streptococcal) H66.9-
  - acute, subacute **H66.9Ø**
  - chronic **H66.9Ø**

Overdevelopment - *see* Hypertrophy

Overgrowth, bone - *see* Hypertrophy, bone

Overlapping toe (acquired) - *see also* Deformity, toe, specified NEC
- congenital (fifth toe) **Q66.89**

Overriding
- toe (acquired) - *see also* Deformity, toe, specified NEC
  - congenital **Q66.89**

Overstrained R53.83

Overworked R53.83

P

Pachydermoperiostosis - *see also* Osteoarthropathy, hypertrophic, specified type NEC

Pachymeningitis (adhesive) (basal) (brain) (cervical) (chronic)(circumscribed) (external) (fibrous) (hemorrhagic) (hypertrophic) (internal) (purulent) (spinal) (suppurative) - *see* Meningitis

Paget's disease
- bone **M88.9**
  - multiple sites **M88.89**
- osteitis deformans - *see* Paget's disease, bone

- **Pain (s) R52** - *see also* Painful
  - abdominal **R1Ø.9**
    - colic **R1Ø.83**
    - generalized **R1Ø.84**
    - lower **R1Ø.3Ø**
      - left quadrant **R1Ø.32**
      - periumbilical **R1Ø.33**
      - right quadrant **R1Ø.31**
    - rebound - *see* Tenderness, abdominal, rebound
    - tenderness - *see* Tenderness, abdominal
    - upper **R1Ø.1Ø**
      - epigastric **R1Ø.13**
      - left quadrant **R1Ø.12**
      - right quadrant **R1Ø.11**
  - acute **R52**
    - due to trauma **G89.11**
    - postprocedural NEC **G89.18**
    - post-thoracotomy **G89.12**
  - bladder **R39.89**
    - chronic **R39.82**
  - cecum - *see* Pain, abdominal
  - chest (central) **RØ7.9**
    - anterior wall **RØ7.89**
    - atypical **RØ7.89**
    - musculoskeletal **RØ7.89**
    - non-cardiac **RØ7.89**
    - pleurodynia **RØ7.81**
    - wall (anterior) **RØ7.89**
  - chronic **G89.29**
    - due to trauma **G89.21**
    - postoperative NEC **G89.28**
    - postprocedural NEC **G89.28**
    - post-thoracotomy **G89.22**
    - specified NEC **G89.29**
  - colon - *see* Pain, abdominal
  - epigastric, epigastrium **R1Ø.13**
  - flank - *see* Pain, abdominal
  - gastric - *see* Pain, abdominal
  - generalized NOS **R52**
  - groin - *see* Pain, abdominal, lower
  - head - *see* Headache
  - infra-orbital - *see* Neuralgia, trigeminal
  - intercostal **RØ7.82**
  - jaw **R68.84**
  - joint **M25.5Ø**
    - specified site NEC **M25.59**
  - limb **M79.6Ø9**
  - loin **M54.5Ø**
  - low back **M54.5Ø**
    - specified NEC **M54.59**
    - vertebral end plate **M54.51**
    - vertebrogenic **M54.51**
  - lumbar region **M54.5Ø**
    - vertebral end plate **M54.51**
    - vertebrogenic **M54.51**
  - mandibular **R68.84**
  - maxilla **R68.84**
  - muscle - *see* Myalgia
  - musculoskeletal **M79.18** - *see also* Pain, by site
  - myofascial **M79.18**
  - nerve NEC - *see* Neuralgia
  - neuromuscular - *see* Neuralgia
  - pleura, pleural, pleuritic **RØ7.81**
  - postoperative NOS **G89.18**
  - postprocedural NOS **G89.18**
  - post-thoracotomy **G89.12**
  - psychogenic (persistent) (any site) **F45.41**
  - radicular (spinal) - *see* Radiculopathy
  - rheumatoid, muscular - *see* Myalgia
  - rib **RØ7.81**
  - root (spinal) - *see* Radiculopathy
  - spinal root - *see* Radiculopathy
  - spine **M54.9**
    - low back **M54.5Ø**
  - stomach - *see* Pain, abdominal
  - thoracic spine **M54.6**
    - with radicular and visceral pain **M54.14**
  - trigeminal - *see* Neuralgia, trigeminal
  - vertebral end plate - *see* Pain, vertebrogenic
  - vertebrogenic **M54.89**
    - low back **M54.51**
    - lumbar **M54.51**
    - syndrome **M54.89**
  - vesical **R39.89**
- **Painful** - *see also* Pain
- **Palsy G83.9** - *see also* Paralysis
  - atrophic diffuse (progressive) **G12.22**
  - bulbar (progressive) (chronic) **G12.22**
    - pseudo NEC **G12.29**
  - cranial nerve - *see also* Disorder, nerve, cranial
    - multiple **G52.7**
      - in
        - infectious disease B99- [**G53**]
        - neoplastic disease **D49.9** [**G53**] - *see also* Neoplasm
        - parasitic disease **B89** [**G53**]
  - creeping **G12.22**
  - pseudobulbar NEC **G12.29**
  - shaking - *see* Parkinsonism
  - wasting **G12.29**
- **Panniculitis (nodular) (nonsuppurative) M79.3**
  - back **M54.ØØ**
    - cervical region **M54.Ø2**
    - cervicothoracic region **M54.Ø3**
    - lumbar region **M54.Ø6**
    - lumbosacral region **M54.Ø7**
    - multiple sites **M54.Ø9**
    - occipito-atlanto-axial region **M54.Ø1**
    - sacrococcygeal region **M54.Ø8**
    - thoracic region **M54.Ø4**
    - thoracolumbar region **M54.Ø5**
  - neck **M54.Ø2**
    - cervicothoracic region **M54.Ø3**
    - occipito-atlanto-axial region **M54.Ø1**
- **Pansinusitis (chronic) (hyperplastic) (nonpurulent) (purulent) J32.4**
  - acute **JØ1.4Ø**
    - recurrent **JØ1.41**
- **Paralysis, paralytic (complete) (incomplete) G83.9**
  - agitans **G2Ø** - *see also* Parkinsonism
  - alternating (oculomotor) **G83.89**
  - amyotrophic **G12.21**
  - association **G12.29**
  - asthenic bulbar **G7Ø.ØØ**
    - with exacerbation (acute) **G7Ø.Ø1**
    - in crisis **G7Ø.Ø1**
  - atrophic **G58.9**
    - progressive **G12.22**
  - Babinski-Nageotte's **G83.89**
  - brain **G83.9**
    - triplegia **G83.89**
  - Brown-Séquard **G83.81**
  - bulbar (chronic) (progressive) **G12.22**
    - pseudo **G12.29**
  - bulbospinal **G7Ø.ØØ**
    - with exacerbation (acute) **G7Ø.Ø1**
    - in crisis **G7Ø.Ø1**
  - cervical
    - sympathetic **G9Ø.Ø9**
  - cordis - *see* Failure, heart
  - creeping **G12.22**
  - crossed leg **G83.89**
  - descending (spinal) NEC **G12.29**
  - diplegic - *see* Diplegia
  - Duchenne's
    - due to or associated with
      - motor neuron disease **G12.22**
      - muscular dystrophy **G71.Ø1**
  - heart - *see* Arrest, cardiac
  - hemiplegic - *see* Hemiplegia
  - Jackson's **G83.89**
  - labioglossal (laryngeal) (pharyngeal) **G12.29**
  - lateral **G12.23**
  - left side - *see* Hemiplegia
  - leg G83.1-
    - both - *see* Paraplegia
    - crossed **G83.89**
    - transient or transitory **R29.818**
  - limb - *see* Monoplegia
  - lower limb - *see* Monoplegia, lower limb
    - both - *see* Paraplegia
  - medullary (tegmental) **G83.89**
  - mesencephalic NEC **G83.89**
    - tegmental **G83.89**
  - middle alternating **G83.89**
  - monoplegic - *see* Monoplegia
  - muscle, muscular NEC **G72.89**
    - progressive **G12.21**
    - progressive, spinal **G12.25**
    - pseudohypertrophic **G71.Ø2**
    - spinal progressive **G12.25**
  - ocular **H49.9**
    - alternating **G83.89**
  - peripheral autonomic nervous system - *see* Neuropathy, peripheral, autonomic
  - postepileptic transitory **G83.84**
  - progressive (atrophic) (bulbar) (spinal) **G12.22**
  - pseudobulbar **G12.29**
  - pseudohypertrophic (muscle) **G71.Ø9** - *see also* Dystrophy, muscular, by type, if applicable
  - quadriplegic - *see* Tetraplegia
  - respiratory (muscle) (system) (tract) **RØ6.81**
  - right side - *see* Hemiplegia
  - shaking - *see* Parkinsonism
  - spinal (cord) **G83.9**
    - hereditary **G95.89**
    - progressive **G12.21**
      - muscle **G12.25**
    - sequelae NEC **G83.89**
  - stomach **K31.84**
    - diabetic - *see* Diabetes, by type, with gastroparesis
    - nerve **G52.2**
      - diabetic - *see* Diabetes, by type, with gastroparesis
  - sympathetic **G9Ø.8**
    - cervical **G9Ø.Ø9**
    - nervous system - *see* Neuropathy, peripheral, autonomic
  - syndrome **G83.9**
    - specified NEC **G83.89**
  - Todd's (postepileptic transitory paralysis) **G83.84**
  - transient **R29.5**
    - arm or leg NEC **R29.818**
    - traumatic NEC - *see* Injury, nerve
  - traumatic, transient NEC - *see* Injury, nerve
  - trembling - *see* Parkinsonism
  - wasting **G12.29**
- **Paraparesis** - *see* Paraplegia
- **Paraphasia R47.Ø2**
- **Paraplegia (lower) G82.2Ø**
  - complete **G82.21**
  - incomplete **G82.22**

Paratyphilitis - *see* Appendicitis
Paravaginitis - *see* Vaginitis
Parencephalitis - *see also* Encephalitis
Parent-child conflict - *see* Conflict, parent-child
  estrangement NEC **Z62.89Ø**
Paresis - *see also* Paralysis
  heart - *see* Failure, heart
  pseudohypertrophic **G71.Ø9** - *see also* Dystrophy, muscular, by type, if applicable
Parkinsonism (idiopathic) (primary) G2Ø
  dementia **G2Ø** [**FØ2.8Ø**] - *see also* Dementia, in, diseases specified elsewhere
    with behavioral disturbance **G2Ø** [FØ2.81-] - *see also* Dementia, in, diseases specified elsewhere
Parkinson's disease, syndrome or tremor - *see* Parkinsonism
Parturition - *see* Delivery
Pathologic, pathological - *see also* condition
  asphyxia **RØ9.Ø1**
Pathology (of) - *see* Disease
Penetrating wound - *see also* Puncture
  with internal injury - *see* Injury, by site
Perforation, perforated (nontraumatic) (of)
  antrum - *see* Sinusitis, maxillary
  ethmoidal sinus - *see* Sinusitis, ethmoidal
  frontal sinus - *see* Sinusitis, frontal
  heart valve - *see* Endocarditis
  maxillary sinus - *see* Sinusitis, maxillary
  nasal
    sinus **J34.89**
      due to sinusitis - *see* Sinusitis
  sphenoidal sinus - *see* Sinusitis, sphenoidal
  traumatic
    internal organ - *see* Injury, by site
  typhoid, gastrointestinal - *see* Typhoid
  ulcer - *see* Ulcer, by site, with perforation
Periappendicitis (acute) - *see* Appendicitis
Periarthritis (joint) - *see also* Enthesopathy
Periarthrosis (angioneural) - *see* Enthesopathy
Pericarditis (with decompensation) (with effusion) I31.9
  rheumatoid - *see* Rheumatoid, carditis
Perichondritis
  larynx **J38.7**
    typhoid **AØ1.Ø9**
Pericystitis N3Ø.9Ø
  with hematuria **N3Ø.91**
Periendocarditis - *see* Endocarditis
Perimeningitis - *see* Meningitis
Perineuritis NEC - *see* Neuralgia
Periostitis (albuminosa) (circumscribed) (diffuse) (infective) (monomelic) - *see also* Osteomyelitis
Peritendinitis - *see* Enthesopathy
Perivaginitis - *see* Vaginitis
Perivesiculitis (seminal) - *see* Vesiculitis
Persistence, persistent (congenital)
  organ or site not listed - *see* Anomaly, by site
Pes (congenital) - *see also* Talipes
  adductus **Q66.89**
Phenomenon
  vasomotor **R55**
  vasovagal **R55**
Phlebectasia - *see also* Varix
Phlebitis (infective) (pyemic) (septic) (suppurative) I8Ø.9
  varicose (leg) (lower limb) - *see* Varix, leg, with, inflammation
Phlebothrombosis - *see also* Thrombosis
Phlegmon - *see* Abscess
Phrenitis - *see* Encephalitis
Pill roller hand (intrinsic) - *see* Parkinsonism
Pityriasis (capitis) L21.Ø
  Hebra's **L26**
Placenta, placental - *see* Pregnancy, complicated by (care of) (management affected by), specified condition
Plaque (s)
  calcareous - *see* Calcification
Platyspondylisis Q76.49
Pleuralgia RØ7.81
Pleurodynia RØ7.81
Pneumaturia R39.89
Pneumoconiosis (due to) (inhalation of) J64
  rheumatoid - *see* Rheumatoid, lung
Pneumonia (acute) (double) (migratory) (purulent) (septic) (unresolved) J18.9
  with
    lung abscess **J85.1**
      due to specified organism - *see* Pneumonia, in (due to)
  basal, basic, basilar - *see* Pneumonia, by type
  embolic, embolism - *see* Embolism, pulmonary
  in (due to)
    Salmonella (infection) **AØ2.22**
      typhi **AØ1.Ø3**
    typhoid (fever) **AØ1.Ø3**
  multilobar - *see* Pneumonia, by type
  Salmonella (arizonae) (cholerae-suis) (enteritidis) (typhimurium) **AØ2.22**
    typhi **AØ1.Ø3**
    typhoid fever **AØ1.Ø3**
Pneumonitis (acute) (primary) - *see also* Pneumonia
Pneumorrhagia - *see also* Hemorrhage, lung
Poikilodermatomyositis M33.1Ø
  with
    myopathy **M33.12**
    respiratory involvement **M33.11**
    specified organ involvement NEC **M33.19**
Poisoning (acute) - *see also* Table of Drugs and Chemicals
  fish (noxious) T61.9-
    bacterial - *see* Intoxication, foodborne, by agent
  food NEC **AØ5.9**
    bacterial - *see* Intoxication, foodborne, by agent
  mussels - *see also* Poisoning, shellfish
    bacterial - *see* Intoxication, foodborne, by agent
  seafood (noxious) T61.9-
    bacterial - *see* Intoxication, foodborne, by agent
  shellfish (amnesic) (azaspiracid) (diarrheic) (neurotoxic) (noxious) (paralytic) T61.78-
    bacterial - *see* Intoxication, foodborne, by agent
Polioencephalitis (acute) (bulbar) A8Ø.9
  inferior **G12.22**
Polyadenitis - *see also* Lymphadenitis
Polyalgia M79.89
Polyarthralgia - *see* Pain, joint
Polyarthritis, polyarthropathy M13.Ø - *see also* Arthritis
  due to or associated with other specified conditions - *see* Arthritis
Polychondritis (atrophic) (chronic) - *see also* Disorder, cartilage, specified type NEC
Polymyositis (acute) (chronic) (hemorrhagic) M33.2Ø
  with
    myopathy **M33.22**
    respiratory involvement **M33.21**
    skin involvement - *see* Dermatopolymyositis
    specified organ involvement NEC **M33.29**
  ossificans (generalisata) (progressiva) - *see* Myositis, ossificans, progressiva
Polyneuritis, polyneuritic - *see also* Polyneuropathy
  diabetic - *see* Diabetes, polyneuropathy
Polyneuropathy (peripheral) G62.9
  diabetic - *see* Diabetes, polyneuropathy
  in (due to)
    diabetes - *see* Diabetes, polyneuropathy
    herpes zoster **BØ2.23**
    rheumatoid arthritis - *see* Rheumatoid, polyneuropathy
    zoster **BØ2.23**
  postherpetic (zoster) **BØ2.23**
Polyradiculitis - *see* Polyneuropathy
Poor
  urinary stream **R39.12**
Positive
  culture (nonspecific)
    urine **R82.79**
Postconcussional syndrome FØ7.81
Postcontusional syndrome FØ7.81
Posthemiplegic chorea - *see* Monoplegia
Postherpetic neuralgia (zoster) BØ2.29
  trigeminal **BØ2.22**
Postnasal drip RØ9.82
  due to
    allergic rhinitis - *see* Rhinitis, allergic
    common cold **JØØ**
    nasopharyngitis - *see* Nasopharyngitis
    sinusitis - *see* Sinusitis
Postpartum - *see* Puerperal
Postpolio (myelitic) syndrome G14
Postsurgery status - *see also* Status (post)
Post-traumatic brain syndrome, nonpsychotic FØ7.81
Post-typhoid abscess AØ1.Ø9
Pregnancy (single) (uterine) Z33.1 - *see also* Delivery and Puerperal
  complicated by (care of) (management affected by)
    diabetes (mellitus) O24.91-
      gestational (pregnancy induced) - *see* Diabetes, gestational
    mental disorders (conditions in FØ1-FØ9, F2Ø-F52 and F54-F99) O99.34-
    respiratory condition (conditions in JØØ-J99) O99.51-
  weeks of gestation
    less than 8 weeks **Z3A.Ø1**
    8 weeks **Z3A.Ø8**
    9 weeks **Z3A.Ø9**
    1Ø weeks **Z3A.1Ø**
    11 weeks **Z3A.11**
    12 weeks **Z3A.12**
    13 weeks **Z3A.13**
    14 weeks **Z3A.14**
    15 weeks **Z3A.15**
    16 weeks **Z3A.16**
    17 weeks **Z3A.17**
    18 weeks **Z3A.18**
    19 weeks **Z3A.19**
    2Ø weeks **Z3A.2Ø**
    21 weeks **Z3A.21**
    22 weeks **Z3A.22**
    23 weeks **Z3A.23**
    24 weeks **Z3A.24**
    25 weeks **Z3A.25**

- 26 weeks **Z3A.26**
- 27 weeks **Z3A.27**
- 28 weeks **Z3A.28**
- 29 weeks **Z3A.29**
- 3Ø weeks **Z3A.3Ø**
- 31 weeks **Z3A.31**
- 32 weeks **Z3A.32**
- 33 weeks **Z3A.33**
- 34 weeks **Z3A.34**
- 35 weeks **Z3A.35**
- 36 weeks **Z3A.36**
- 37 weeks **Z3A.37**
- 38 weeks **Z3A.38**
- 39 weeks **Z3A.39**
- 4Ø weeks **Z3A.4Ø**
- 41 weeks **Z3A.41**
- 42 weeks **Z3A.42**
- greater than 42 weeks **Z3A.49**
- not specified **Z3A.ØØ**

Presbycardia R54

Presence (of)
- artificial
  - limb (complete) (partial) Z97.1-
    - arm Z97.1-
      - bilateral **Z97.15**
    - leg Z97.1-
      - bilateral **Z97.16**
- bone
  - joint (prosthesis) - *see* Presence, joint implant
- device (external) NEC **Z97.8**
  - implanted (functional) **Z96.9**
    - specified NEC **Z96.89**
- functional implant **Z96.9**
  - specified NEC **Z96.89**
- implanted device (artificial) (functional) (prosthetic) **Z96.9**
  - joint **Z96.6Ø**
    - specified NEC **Z96.698**
  - skin **Z96.81**
  - specified NEC **Z96.89**
- joint implant (prosthetic) (any) **Z96.6Ø**
  - specified joint NEC **Z96.698**
- neurostimulator (brain) (gastric) (peripheral nerve) (sacral nerve) (spinal cord) (vagus nerve) **Z96.82**
- orthopedic-joint implant (prosthetic) (any) - *see* Presence, joint implant

Pressure
- chest **RØ7.89**
- spinal cord **G95.2Ø**

Pre-syncope R55

Problem (with) (related to)
- adopted child **Z62.821**
- alcoholism in family **Z63.72**
- birth of sibling affecting child **Z62.898**
- child
  - in care of non-parental family member **Z62.21**
  - in foster care **Z62.21**
  - in welfare custody **Z62.21**
  - living in orphanage or group home **Z62.22**
- child-rearing **Z62.9**
  - specified NEC **Z62.898**
- drug addict in family **Z63.72**
- economic **Z59.9**
  - strain **Z59.86**
- employment **Z56.9**
  - sexual harassment **Z56.81**
  - specified NEC **Z56.89**
- falling **Z91.81**
- foster child **Z62.822**
- frightening experience (s) in childhood **Z62.898**
- impaired mobility **Z74.Ø9**
- institutionalization, affecting child **Z62.22**
- life-style **Z72.9**
  - high-risk sexual behavior (heterosexual) **Z72.51**
    - bisexual **Z72.53**
    - homosexual **Z72.52**
  - self-damaging behavior NEC **Z72.89**
  - specified NEC **Z72.89**
- loss of love relationship in childhood **Z62.898**
- money **Z59.86**
- negative life events in childhood **Z62.9**
  - altered pattern of family relationships **Z62.898**
  - frightening experience **Z62.898**
  - loss of
    - love relationship **Z62.898**
    - self-esteem **Z62.898**
  - removal from home **Z62.29**
  - specified event NEC **Z62.898**
- neurological NEC **R29.818**
- new step-parent affecting child **Z62.898**
- occupational NEC **Z56.89**
- parent-child - *see* Conflict, parent-child
- personal hygiene **Z91.89**
- presence of sick or disabled person in family or household **Z63.79**
- psychiatric **F99**
- removal from home affecting child **Z62.29**
- speech **R47.9**
  - specified NEC **R47.89**
- swallowing - *see* Dysphagia
- upbringing **Z62.9**
  - specified NEC **Z62.898**
- voice production **R47.89**

Procedure (surgical)
- not done **Z53.9**
  - because of
    - contraindication **Z53.Ø9**
      - smoking **Z53.Ø1**
    - patient's decision **Z53.2Ø**
      - left against medical advice (AMA) **Z53.29**
      - left without being seen **Z53.21**
      - specified reason NEC **Z53.29**

Profichet's disease - *see* Disorder, soft tissue, specified type NEC

Prolapse, prolapsed
- ciliary body (traumatic) - *see* Laceration, eye(ball), with prolapse or loss of interocular tissue
- disc (intervertebral) - *see* Displacement, intervertebral disc
- intervertebral disc - *see* Displacement, intervertebral disc
- iris (traumatic) - *see* Laceration, eye(ball), with prolapse or loss of interocular tissue
- organ or site, congenital NEC - *see* Malposition, congenital
- uveal (traumatic) - *see* Laceration, eye(ball), with prolapse or loss of interocular tissue
- vitreous (humor) H43.Ø-
  - in wound - *see* Laceration, eye(ball), with prolapse or loss of interocular tissue

Prolonged, prolongation (of)
- QT interval **R94.31**

Promiscuity - *see* High, risk, sexual behavior

Prophylactic
- administration of
  - drug **Z79.899** - *see also* Long-term (current) drug therapy (use of)
- medication **Z79.899**

Prostration R53.83
- senile **R54**

Protection (against) (from) - *see* Prophylactic

Proteinuria R8Ø.9
- complicating pregnancy - *see* Proteinuria, gestational
- gestational
  - complicating
    - childbirth **O12.14**
    - puerperium **O12.15**
- puerperal **O12.15**

Protrusion, protrusio
- intervertebral disc - *see* Displacement, intervertebral disc
- nucleus pulposus - *see* Displacement, intervertebral disc

Pseudohypertrophic muscular dystrophy (Erb's) G71.Ø2

Pseudohypertrophy, muscle G71.Ø9 - *see also* Dystrophy, muscular, by type, if applicable

Pseudoparalysis
- arm or leg **R29.818**

Pseudotetanus - *see* Convulsions

Psoitis M6Ø.88

Psychiatric disorder or problem F99

Psychopathy, psychopathic
- constitution, post-traumatic **FØ7.81**

Ptosis - *see also* Blepharoptosis
- congenital (eyelid) **Q1Ø.Ø**
  - specified site NEC - *see* Anomaly, by site

Puerperal, puerperium (complicated by, complications)
- albuminuria (acute) (subacute) - *see* Proteinuria, gestational
- diabetes **O24.93**
  - gestational - *see* Puerperal, gestational diabetes
  - pre-existing **O24.33**
    - specified NEC **O24.83**
    - type 1 **O24.Ø3**
    - type 2 **O24.13**
- endophlebitis - *see* Puerperal, phlebitis
- gestational
  - diabetes **O24.439**
    - diet controlled **O24.43Ø**
    - insulin (and diet) controlled **O24.434**
    - oral drug controlled (antidiabetic) (hypoglycemic) **O24.435**
  - edema **O12.Ø5**
    - with proteinuria **O12.25**
  - proteinuria **O12.15**
- hypertension - *see* Hypertension, complicating, puerperium
- infection **O86.4**
  - vein - *see* Puerperal, phlebitis
- subluxation of symphysis (pubis) **O26.73**

Puerperium - *see* Puerperal

Pulse
- weak **RØ9.89**

Punch drunk FØ7.81

Puncture
- internal organs - *see* Injury, by site

Pyelitis (congenital) (uremic) - *see also* Pyelonephritis

Pyelocystitis - *see* Pyelonephritis

Pyelonephritis - *see also* Nephritis, tubulo-interstitial
- in (due to)
  - Salmonella infection **AØ2.25**
  - Sjögren's disease **M35.Ø4**

Pyemia, pyemic (fever) (infection) (purulent) - *see also* Sepsis

Pyocele
- sinus (accessory) - *see* Sinusitis

Pyocolpos - *see* Vaginitis

Q

R

- **Rotes Quérol disease or syndrome** - *see* Hyperostosis, ankylosing
- **Round**
  - back (with wedging of vertebrae) - *see* Kyphosis
- **Rudimentary (congenital)** - *see also* Agenesis
- **Rumination R11.1Ø**
- **Running out of money Z59.86**
- **Runny nose RØ9.89**
- **Rupture, ruptured**
  - blood vessel - *see also* Hemorrhage
  - cartilage (articular) (current) - *see also* Sprain
    - semilunar - *see* Tear, meniscus
  - cyst - *see* Cyst
  - internal organ, traumatic - *see* Injury, by site
  - intervertebral disc - *see* Displacement, intervertebral disc
  - joint capsule, traumatic - *see* Sprain
  - ligament, traumatic - *see* Rupture, traumatic, ligament, by site
  - meniscus (knee) - *see also* Tear, meniscus
  - muscle (traumatic) - *see also* Strain
    - diastasis - *see* Diastasis, muscle
    - nontraumatic **M62.1Ø**
      - specified site NEC **M62.18**
    - traumatic - *see* Strain, by site
  - musculotendinous junction NEC, nontraumatic - *see* Rupture, tendon, spontaneous
  - nontraumatic, meaning hernia - *see* Hernia
  - obstructed - *see* Hernia, by site, obstructed
  - spinal cord - *see also* Injury, spinal cord, by region
  - splenic vein **R58**
  - supraspinatus (complete) (incomplete) (nontraumatic) - *see* Tear, rotator cuff
  - synovium (cyst) **M66.1Ø**
    - specified site NEC **M66.18**
  - tendon (traumatic) - *see* Strain
    - nontraumatic (spontaneous) **M66.9**
      - extensor **M66.2Ø**
        - multiple sites **M66.29**
        - specified site NEC **M66.28**
      - flexor **M66.3Ø**
        - multiple sites **M66.39**
        - specified site NEC **M66.38**
      - multiple sites **M66.89**
      - specified
        - site NEC **M66.88**
        - tendon **M66.8Ø**
  - traumatic
    - internal organ - *see* Injury, by site
    - ligament - *see also* Sprain
      - ankle - *see* Sprain, ankle
      - carpus - *see* Rupture, traumatic, ligament, wrist
      - collateral (hand) - *see* Rupture, traumatic, ligament, finger, collateral
      - finger (metacarpophalangeal) (interphalangeal) S63.4Ø-
        - collateral S63.41-
          - index S63.41-
          - little S63.41-
          - middle S63.41-
          - ring S63.41-
        - index S63.4Ø-
        - little S63.4Ø-
        - middle S63.4Ø-
        - palmar S63.42-
          - index S63.42-
          - little S63.42-
          - middle S63.42-
          - ring S63.42-
        - ring S63.4Ø-
        - specified site NEC S63.499-
          - index S63.49-
          - little S63.49-
          - middle S63.49-
          - ring S63.49-
        - volar plate S63.43-
          - index S63.43-
          - little S63.43-
          - middle S63.43-
          - ring S63.43-
      - foot - *see* Sprain, foot
      - radiocarpal - *see* Rupture, traumatic, ligament, wrist, radiocarpal
      - ulnocarpal - *see* Rupture, traumatic, ligament, wrist, ulnocarpal
      - wrist S63.3Ø-
        - collateral S63.31-
        - radiocarpal S63.32-
        - specified site NEC S63.39-
        - ulnocarpal (palmar) S63.33-
    - muscle or tendon - *see* Strain
  - valve, valvular (heart) - *see* Endocarditis
  - varicose vein - *see* Varix
  - varix - *see* Varix
  - vena cava **R58**
  - vessel (blood) **R58**

S

- **Sacculation**
  - organ or site, congenital - *see* Distortion
- **Sacralization Q76.49**
- **Saddle**
  - back - *see* Lordosis
- **Salmonella** - *see* Infection, Salmonella
- **Sarcoepiplocele** - *see* Hernia
- **Sarcopenia (age-related) M62.84**
- **Satiety, early R68.81**
- **Scapulohumeral myopathy G71.Ø2**
- **Scar, scarring L9Ø.5** - *see also* Cicatrix
  - muscle **M62.89**
- **Scarlatina (anginosa) (maligna) A38.9**
  - myocarditis (acute) **A38.1**
    - old - *see* Myocarditis
- **Scheuermann's disease or osteochondrosis** - *see* Osteochondrosis, juvenile, spine
- **Schistosomiasis B65.9**
  - with muscle disorder **B65.9** [**M63.8Ø**]
    - multiple sites **B65.9** [**M63.89**]
    - specified site NEC **B65.9** [**M63.88**]
- **Schmorl's disease or nodes**
  - lumbar region **M51.46**
  - lumbosacral region **M51.47**
  - thoracic region **M51.44**
  - thoracolumbar region **M51.45**
- **Sciatica (infective)** M54.3-
  - with lumbago M54.4-
    - due to intervertebral disc disorder - *see* Disorder, disc, with, radiculopathy
  - due to displacement of intervertebral disc (with lumbago) - *see* Disorder, disc, with, radiculopathy
- **Scleredema**
  - adultorum - *see* Sclerosis, systemic
  - Buschke's - *see* Sclerosis, systemic
- **Sclerema (adiposum) (edematosum) (neonatorum) (newborn) P83.Ø**
  - adultorum - *see* Sclerosis, systemic
- **Sclérose en plaques G35**
- **Sclerosis, sclerotic**
  - amyotrophic (lateral) **G12.21**
  - ascending multiple **G35**
  - brain (generalized) (lobular) **G37.9**
    - disseminated **G35**
    - insular **G35**
    - miliary **G35**
    - multiple **G35**
    - stem, multiple **G35**
  - bulbar, multiple **G35**
  - cerebellar - *see* Sclerosis, brain
  - cerebral - *see* Sclerosis, brain
  - cerebrospinal (disseminated) (multiple) **G35**
  - combined (spinal cord) - *see also* Degeneration, combined
    - multiple **G35**
  - disseminated **G35**
  - dorsal **G35**
  - insular **G35**
  - lateral (amyotrophic) (descending) (spinal) **G12.21**
    - primary **G12.23**
  - multiple (brain stem) (cerebral) (generalized) (spinal cord) **G35**
  - plaques **G35**
  - primary, lateral **G12.23**
  - spinal (cord) (progressive) **G95.89**
    - combined - *see also* Degeneration, combined
      - multiple **G35**
    - disseminated **G35**
    - lateral (amyotrophic) **G12.21**
      - progressive **G12.23**
    - multiple **G35**
  - systemic **M34.9**
    - with
      - lung involvement **M34.81**
      - myopathy **M34.82**
      - polyneuropathy **M34.83**
    - specified NEC **M34.89**
  - valve, valvular (heart) - *see* Endocarditis
- **Scoliosis (acquired) (postural) M41.9**
  - adolescent (idiopathic) - *see* Scoliosis, idiopathic, adolescent
  - idiopathic **M41.2Ø**
    - adolescent **M41.129**
      - cervical region **M41.122**
      - cervicothoracic region **M41.123**
      - lumbar region **M41.126**
      - lumbosacral region **M41.127**
      - thoracic region **M41.124**
      - thoracolumbar region **M41.125**
    - cervical region **M41.22**
    - cervicothoracic region **M41.23**
    - infantile **M41.ØØ**
      - cervical region **M41.Ø2**
      - cervicothoracic region **M41.Ø3**
      - lumbar region **M41.Ø6**
      - lumbosacral region **M41.Ø7**
      - sacrococcygeal region **M41.Ø8**
      - thoracic region **M41.Ø4**
      - thoracolumbar region **M41.Ø5**
    - juvenile **M41.119**
      - cervical region **M41.112**
      - cervicothoracic region **M41.113**
      - lumbar region **M41.116**
      - lumbosacral region **M41.117**
      - thoracic region **M41.114**
      - thoracolumbar region **M41.115**
    - lumbar region **M41.26**
    - lumbosacral region **M41.27**
    - thoracic region **M41.24**
    - thoracolumbar region **M41.25**
  - infantile - *see* Scoliosis, idiopathic, infantile

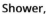

- organ or site, congenital NEC - *see* Distortion
- radius (acquired) - *see also* Deformity, limb, unequal length
- stature (child) (hereditary) (idiopathic) NEC **R62.52**
  - constitutional **E34.31**
  - due to
    - endocrine disorder **E34.3Ø**
      - specified type NEC, due to endocrine disorder **E34.39**
    - genetic causes **E34.329**
      - acid-labile subunit gene (IGFALS) defect **E34.321**
      - genetic syndrome with resistance to insulin-like growth factor-1 **E34.322**
      - growth hormone gene 1 (GH1) defect with growth hormone neutralizing antibodies **E34.321**
      - growth hormone insensitivity syndrome (GHIS) **E34.321**
      - insulin-like growth factor 1 gene (IGF1) defect **E34.321**
      - insulin-like growth factor-1 (IGF1) resistance **E34.322**
      - insulin-like growth factor-1 receptor (IGF1R) defect **E34.322**
      - post-insulin-like growth factor-1 receptor signaling defect **E34.322**
      - primary insulin-like growth factor-1 (IGF1) deficiency **E34.321**
      - severe primary insulin-like growth factor-1 deficiency (SPIGFD) **E34.321**
      - signal transducer and activator of transcription 5B gene (STAT5b) defect **E34.321**
  - Laron-type **E34.321**
- tendon - *see also* Contraction, tendon
  - with contracture of joint - *see* Contraction, joint
  - Achilles (acquired) M67.Ø-
    - congenital **Q66.89**
- thigh (acquired) - *see also* Deformity, limb, unequal length, femur
- tibialis anterior (tendon) - *see* Contraction, tendon

Shower, thromboembolic - *see* Embolism

Sibling rivalry Z62.891

Sicca syndrome - *see* Syndrome, Sjögren

Sick R69
- or handicapped person in family **Z63.79**

Sighing RØ6.89

Sigmoiditis K52.9 - *see also* Enteritis
- infectious **AØ9**

Sinus - *see also* Fistula
- tract (postinfective) - *see* Fistula

Sinusitis (accessory) (chronic) (hyperplastic) (nasal) (nonpurulent) (purulent) J32.9
- acute **JØ1.9Ø**
  - ethmoidal **JØ1.2Ø**
    - recurrent **JØ1.21**
  - frontal **JØ1.1Ø**
    - recurrent **JØ1.11**
  - involving more than one sinus, other than pansinusitis **JØ1.8Ø**
    - recurrent **JØ1.81**
  - maxillary **JØ1.ØØ**
    - recurrent **JØ1.Ø1**
  - pansinusitis **JØ1.4Ø**
    - recurrent **JØ1.41**
  - recurrent **JØ1.91**
  - specified NEC **JØ1.8Ø**
    - recurrent **JØ1.81**
  - sphenoidal **JØ1.3Ø**
    - recurrent **JØ1.31**
- allergic - *see* Rhinitis, allergic
- ethmoidal **J32.2**
  - acute **JØ1.2Ø**
    - recurrent **JØ1.21**
- frontal **J32.1**
  - acute **JØ1.1Ø**
    - recurrent **JØ1.11**
- involving more than one sinus but not pansinusitis **J32.8**
  - acute **JØ1.8Ø**
    - recurrent **JØ1.81**
- maxillary **J32.Ø**
  - acute **JØ1.ØØ**
    - recurrent **JØ1.Ø1**
- sphenoidal **J32.3**
  - acute **JØ1.3Ø**
    - recurrent **JØ1.31**

Situation, psychiatric F99

Sjögren's syndrome or disease - *see* Syndrome, Sjögren

Sleep
- apnea - *see* Apnea, sleep
- deprivation **Z72.82Ø**

Sleep hygiene
- abuse **Z72.821**
- inadequate **Z72.821**
- poor **Z72.821**

Sleeplessness - *see* Insomnia

Sleep-wake schedule disorder G47.2Ø

Slipped, slipping
- epiphysis (traumatic) - *see also* Osteochondropathy, specified type NEC
- intervertebral disc - *see* Displacement, intervertebral disc
- tendon - *see* Disorder, tendon
- vertebra NEC - *see* Spondylolisthesis

Sloughing (multiple) (phagedena) (skin) - *see also* Gangrene
- abscess - *see* Abscess
- fascia - *see* Disorder, soft tissue, specified type NEC
- tendon - *see* Disorder, tendon

Slowing, urinary stream R39.198

Sluder's neuralgia (syndrome) G44.89

Slurred, slurring speech R47.81

Smoker - *see* Dependence, drug, nicotine

Smothering spells RØ6.81

Snapping
- finger - *see* Trigger finger
- knee - *see* Derangement, knee

Snoring RØ6.83

Softening
- spinal cord **G95.89**

Somatization reaction, somatic reaction - *see* Disorder, somatoform

Sore
- muscle **M79.1Ø**

Spasm (s), spastic, spasticity R25.2 - *see also* condition
- compulsive - *see* Tic
- habit - *see* Tic
- muscle NEC **M62.838**
  - back **M62.83Ø**
- trigeminal nerve - *see* Neuralgia, trigeminal
- viscera - *see* Pain, abdominal

Spastic, spasticity - *see also* Spasm

Speech
- defect, disorder, disturbance, impediment **R47.9** - *see* Disorder, speech
  - slurring **R47.81**
  - specified NEC **R47.89**

Spencer's disease AØ8.19

Sphenoiditis (chronic) - *see* Sinusitis, sphenoidal

Sphenopalatine ganglion neuralgia G9Ø.Ø9

Spider
- fingers - *see* Syndrome, Marfan's
- toes - *see* Syndrome, Marfan's

Split, splitting
- urinary stream **R39.13**

Spondylarthrosis - *see* Spondylosis

Spondylitis (chronic) - *see also* Spondylopathy, inflammatory
- deformans (chronic) - *see* Spondylosis
- gouty **M1Ø.Ø8** - *see also* Gout, by type, vertebrae
- in (due to)
  - brucellosis **A23.9** [**M49.8Ø**]
    - cervical region **A23.9** [**M49.82**]
    - cervicothoracic region **A23.9** [**M49.83**]
    - lumbar region **A23.9** [**M49.86**]
    - lumbosacral region **A23.9** [**M49.87**]
    - multiple sites **A23.9** [**M49.89**]
    - occipito-atlanto-axial region **A23.9** [**M49.81**]
    - sacrococcygeal region **A23.9** [**M49.88**]
    - thoracic region **A23.9** [**M49.84**]
    - thoracolumbar region **A23.9** [**M49.85**]
- infectious NEC - *see* Spondylopathy, infective
- Kümmell's - *see* Spondylopathy, traumatic
- senescent, senile - *see* Spondylosis
- traumatic (chronic) or post-traumatic - *see* Spondylopathy, traumatic
- typhosa **AØ1.Ø5**

Spondyloarthritis
- axial - *see also* Spondlyitis, ankylosing
  - non-radiographic **M45.AØ**
    - cervical **M45.A2**
    - cervicothoracic **M45.A3**
    - lumbar **M45.A6**
    - lumbosacral **M45.A7**
    - multiple sites **M45.AB**
    - occipito-atlanto-axial region **M45.A1**
    - sacral and sacrococcygeal **M45.A8**
    - thoracic **M45.A4**
    - thoracolumbar **M45.A5**

Spondylolisthesis (acquired) (degenerative) M43.1Ø
- cervical region **M43.12**
- cervicothoracic region **M43.13**
- lumbar region **M43.16**
- lumbosacral region **M43.17**
- multiple sites **M43.19**
- occipito-atlanto-axial region **M43.11**
- sacrococcygeal region **M43.18**
- thoracic region **M43.14**
- thoracolumbar region **M43.15**
- traumatic (old) **M43.1Ø**
  - acute
    - fifth cervical (displaced) S12.43Ø-
      - nondisplaced S12.431-
      - specified type NEC (displaced) S12.45Ø-
        - nondisplaced S12.451-
      - type III S12.44-

meniscus
jaw SØ3.4-
old **M26.69**
knee - *see* Sprain, knee, specified site NEC
with current tear - *see* Tear, meniscus
mandible SØ3.4-
old **M26.69**
metacarpophalangeal - *see* Sprain, finger, metacarpophalangeal (joint)
metatarsophalangeal - *see* Sprain, toe, metatarsophalangeal joint
midtarsal - *see* Sprain, foot, specified site NEC
orbicular, hip - *see* Sprain, hip
patella - *see* Sprain, knee, specified site NEC
patellar ligament S76.11-
phalanx
finger - *see* Sprain, finger
toe - *see* Sprain, toe
pubofemoral - *see* Sprain, hip
radiocarpal - *see* Sprain, wrist
radiohumeral - *see* Sprain, elbow
rib (cage) S23.41-
rotator cuff (capsule) S43.42-
semilunar cartilage (knee) - *see* Sprain, knee, specified site NEC
with current tear - *see* Tear, meniscus
shoulder joint S43.4Ø-
coracohumeral ligament - *see* Sprain, coracohumeral joint
rotator cuff - *see* Sprain, rotator cuff
specified site NEC S43.49-
sternum S23.429-
chondrosternal joint S23.421-
specified site NEC S23.428-
sternoclavicular (joint) (ligament) S23.42Ø-
symphysis
jaw SØ3.4-
old **M26.69**
mandibular SØ3.4-
old **M26.69**
talofibular - *see* Sprain, ankle
tarsal - *see* Sprain, foot, specified site NEC
tarsometatarsal - *see* Sprain, foot, specified site NEC
temporomandibular SØ3.4-
old **M26.69**
thorax S23.9-
ribs S23.41-
sternum - *see* Sprain, sternum
thumb S63.6Ø-
interphalangeal (joint) S63.62-
metacarpophalangeal (joint) S63.64-
specified site NEC S63.68-
tibia (proximal end) - *see* Sprain, knee, specified site NEC
tibial collateral, knee - *see* Sprain, knee, collateral
tibiofibular
distal - *see* Sprain, ankle
superior - *see* Sprain, knee, specified site NEC
toe (s) S93.5Ø-
great S93.5Ø-
interphalangeal joint S93.51-
great S93.51-
lesser S93.51-
lesser S93.5Ø-
metatarsophalangeal joint S93.52-
great S93.52-
lesser S93.52-
ulnohumeral - *see* Sprain, elbow
wrist S63.5Ø-
carpal S63.51-
radiocarpal S63.52-
specified site NEC S63.59-
xiphoid cartilage - *see* Sprain, sternum

Spur, bone - *see also* Enthesopathy

Stab - *see also* Laceration
internal organs - *see* Injury, by site

Standstill
cardiac - *see* Arrest, cardiac
ventricular - *see* Arrest, cardiac

Stasis
bronchus **J98.Ø9**
with infection - *see* Bronchitis
dermatitis **I87.2**
with
varicose veins - *see* Varix, leg, with, inflammation
eczema - *see* Varix, leg, with, inflammation
ulcer - *see* Varix, leg, with, ulcer

State (of)
convulsive - *see* Convulsions

Status (post) - *see also* Presence (of)
absence, epileptic - *see* Epilepsy, by type, with status epilepticus
asthmaticus - *see* Asthma, by type, with status asthmaticus
bed confinement **Z74.Ø1**
cholecystectomy **Z9Ø.49**
colectomy (complete) (partial) **Z9Ø.49**
convulsivus idiopathicus - *see* Epilepsy, by type, with status epilepticus
deployment (current) (military) **Z56.82**
epileptic, epilepticus **G4Ø.9Ø1** - *see also* Epilepsy, by type, with status epilepticus
hysterectomy (complete) (total) **Z9Ø.71Ø**
partial (with remaining cervial stump) **Z9Ø.711**
laryngectomy **Z9Ø.Ø2**
military deployment status (current) **Z56.82**
in theater or in support of military war, peacekeeping and humanitarian operations **Z56.82**
oophorectomy
bilateral **Z9Ø.722**
unilateral **Z9Ø.721**
organ replacement
by artificial or mechanical device or prosthesis of
joint **Z96.6Ø**
specified site NEC **Z96.698**
limbs - *see* Presence, artificial, limb
pacemaker
brain **Z96.89**
specified NEC **Z96.89**
pancreatectomy **Z9Ø.41Ø**
complete **Z9Ø.41Ø**
partial **Z9Ø.411**
total **Z9Ø.41Ø**
postcommotio cerebri **FØ7.81**
salpingo-oophorectomy
bilateral **Z9Ø.722**
unilateral **Z9Ø.721**
sex reassignment surgery status **Z87.89Ø**
splenectomy **Z9Ø.81**

Stealing
child problem **F91.8**
in company with others **Z72.81Ø**

Stenosis, stenotic (cicatricial) - *see also* Stricture
caudal **M48.Ø8**
intervertebral foramina - *see also* Lesion, biomechanical, specified NEC
connective tissue **M99.79**
abdomen **M99.79**
cervical region **M99.71**
cervicothoracic **M99.71**
head region **M99.7Ø**
lumbar region **M99.73**
lumbosacral **M99.73**
occipitocervical **M99.7Ø**
sacral region **M99.74**
sacrococcygeal **M99.74**
sacroiliac **M99.74**
specified NEC **M99.79**
thoracic region **M99.72**
thoracolumbar **M99.72**
disc **M99.79**
abdomen **M99.79**
cervical region **M99.71**
cervicothoracic **M99.71**
head region **M99.7Ø**
lower extremity **M99.76**
lumbar region **M99.73**
lumbosacral **M99.73**
occipitocervical **M99.7Ø**
pelvic **M99.75**
rib cage **M99.78**
sacral region **M99.74**
sacrococcygeal **M99.74**
sacroiliac **M99.74**
specified NEC **M99.79**
thoracic region **M99.72**
thoracolumbar **M99.72**
upper extremity **M99.77**
osseous **M99.69**
abdomen **M99.69**
cervical region **M99.61**
cervicothoracic **M99.61**
head region **M99.6Ø**
lower extremity **M99.66**
lumbar region **M99.63**
lumbosacral **M99.63**
occipitocervical **M99.6Ø**
pelvic **M99.65**
rib cage **M99.68**
sacral region **M99.64**
sacrococcygeal **M99.64**
sacroiliac **M99.64**
specified NEC **M99.69**
thoracic region **M99.62**
thoracolumbar **M99.62**
upper extremity **M99.67**
subluxation - *see* Stenosis, intervertebral foramina, osseous
neural canal - *see also* Lesion, biomechanical, specified NEC
connective tissue **M99.49**
abdomen **M99.49**
cervical region **M99.41**
cervicothoracic **M99.41**
head region **M99.4Ø**
lower extremity **M99.46**
lumbar region **M99.43**
lumbosacral **M99.43**
occipitocervical **M99.4Ø**
pelvic **M99.45**
rib cage **M99.48**
sacral region **M99.44**
sacrococcygeal **M99.44**
sacroiliac **M99.44**
specified NEC **M99.49**
thoracic region **M99.42**
thoracolumbar **M99.42**
upper extremity **M99.47**

- traumatic S43.ØØ-
  - anterior S43.Ø1-
  - inferior S43.Ø3-
  - posterior S43.Ø2-
  - specified type NEC S43.Ø8-
- sternoclavicular (joint) S43.2Ø-
  - anterior S43.21-
  - posterior S43.22-
- thumb S63.1Ø3-
  - interphalangeal joint - *see* Subluxation, interphalangeal (joint), thumb
  - metacarpophalangeal joint - *see* Subluxation, metacarpophalangeal (joint), thumb
- toe (s) S93.1Ø-
  - great S93.1Ø-
    - interphalangeal joint S93.13-
    - metatarsophalangeal joint S93.14-
  - interphalangeal joint S93.13-
  - lesser S93.1Ø-
    - interphalangeal joint S93.13-
    - metatarsophalangeal joint S93.14-
  - metatarsophalangeal joint S93.149-
- ulna
  - distal end S63.Ø7-
  - proximal end - *see* Subluxation, elbow
- ulnohumeral joint - *see* Subluxation, elbow
- vertebral
  - traumatic
    - cervical S13.1ØØ-
      - atlantoaxial joint S13.12Ø-
      - atlantooccipital joint S13.11Ø-
      - atloidooccipital joint S13.11Ø-
      - joint between
        - CØ and C1 S13.11Ø-
        - C1 and C2 S13.12Ø-
        - C2 and C3 S13.13Ø-
        - C3 and C4 S13.14Ø-
        - C4 and C5 S13.15Ø-
        - C5and C6 S13.16Ø-
        - C6and C7 S13.17Ø-
        - C7and T1 S13.18Ø-
      - occipitoatloid joint S13.11Ø-
    - lumbar S33.1ØØ-
      - joint between
        - L1and L2 S33.11Ø-
        - L2and L3 S33.12Ø-
        - L3 and L4 S33.13Ø-
        - L4and L5 S33.14Ø-
    - thoracic S23.1ØØ-
      - joint between
        - T1Ø and T11 S23.16Ø-
        - T11 and T12 S23.162-
        - T12 and L1 S23.17Ø-
        - T1and T2 S23.11Ø-
        - T2and T3 S23.12Ø-
        - T3 and T4 S23.122-
        - T4 and T5 S23.13Ø-
        - T5 and T6 S23.132-
        - T6 and T7 S23.14Ø-
        - T7 and T8 S23.142-
        - T8 and T9 S23.15Ø-
        - T9 and T1Ø S23.152-
- wrist (carpal bone) S63.ØØ-
  - carpometacarpal joint - *see* Subluxation, carpometacarpal (joint)
  - distal radioulnar joint - *see* Subluxation, radioulnar (joint), distal
  - metacarpal bone, proximal - *see* Subluxation, metacarpal (bone), proximal end
  - midcarpal - *see* Subluxation, midcarpal (joint)
  - radiocarpal joint - *see* Subluxation, radiocarpal (joint)
  - specified site NEC S63.Ø9-
  - ulna - *see* Subluxation, ulna, distal end

Subnormal, subnormality
- mental - *see* Disability, intellectual

Sudden
- heart failure - *see* Failure, heart

Sugar
- in urine **R81**

Suicide, suicidal (attempted) T14.91-
- ideation - *see* Ideation, suicidal
- risk
  - meaning suicidal ideation - *see* Ideation, suicidal
- tendencies
  - meaning suicidal ideation - *see* Ideation, suicidal

Suipestifer infection - *see* Infection, salmonella

SUNCT (short lasting unilateral neuralgiform headache with conjunctival injection and tearing) G44.Ø59
- intractable **G44.Ø51**
- not intractable **G44.Ø59**

Supernumerary (congenital)
- organ or site not listed - *see* Accessory
- vertebra **Q76.49**

Suppression
- urine, urinary secretion **R34**

Suppuration, suppurative - *see also* condition
- accessory sinus (chronic) - *see* Sinusitis
- antrum (chronic) - *see* Sinusitis, maxillary
- bladder - *see* Cystitis
- ear (middle) - *see also* Otitis, media
- ethmoidal (chronic) (sinus) - *see* Sinusitis, ethmoidal
- frontal (chronic) (sinus) - *see* Sinusitis, frontal
- maxilla, maxillary **M27.2**
  - sinus (chronic) - *see* Sinusitis, maxillary
- muscle - *see* Myositis, infective
- nasal sinus (chronic) - *see* Sinusitis
- pericranial - *see* Osteomyelitis
- sinus (accessory) (chronic) (nasal) - *see* Sinusitis
- sphenoidal sinus (chronic) - *see* Sinusitis, sphenoidal

Surveillance (of) (for) - *see also* Observation
- alcohol abuse **Z71.41**
- drug abuse **Z71.51**

Swallowed, swallowing
- difficulty - *see* Dysphagia

Sweat, sweats
- night **R61**

Sweating, excessive R61

Swelling (of) RGØ.9
- abdomen, abdominal (not referable to any particular organ) - *see* Mass, abdominal
- arm **M79.89**
  - forearm **M79.89**
- extremity (lower) (upper) - *see* Disorder, soft tissue, specified type NEC
- finger **M79.89**
- foot **M79.89**
- hand **M79.89**
- inflammatory - *see* Inflammation
- intra-abdominal - *see* Mass, abdominal
- joint - *see* Effusion, joint
- leg **M79.89**
  - lower **M79.89**
- limb - *see* Disorder, soft tissue, specified type NEC
- pelvic - *see* Mass, abdominal
- toe **M79.89**
- umbilical **R19.Ø9**

Swimming in the head R42

Swollen - *see* Swelling

Symptoms NEC R68.89
- cold **JØØ**
- involving
  - appearance NEC **R46.89**
  - awareness **R41.9**
    - altered mental status **R41.82**
    - borderline intellectual functioning **R41.83**
    - coma - *see* Coma
    - senile cognitive decline **R41.81**
    - specified symptom NEC **R41.89**
  - behavior NEC **R46.89**
  - cardiovascular system NEC **RØ9.89**
  - chest NEC **RØ9.89**
  - circulatory system NEC **RØ9.89**
  - cognitive functions **R41.9**
    - altered mental status **R41.82**
    - borderline intellectual functioning **R41.83**
    - coma - *see* Coma
    - senile cognitive decline **R41.81**
    - specified symptom NEC **R41.89**
  - development NEC **R62.5Ø**
  - emotional state NEC **R45.89**
    - emotional lability **R45.86**
  - musculoskeletal system **R29.91**
    - specified NEC **R29.898**
  - nervous system **R29.9Ø**
    - specified NEC **R29.818**
  - respiratory system NEC **RØ9.89**
- of infancy **R68.19**
- viral cold **JØØ**

Syncope (near) (pre-) R55
- cardiac **R55**
- carotid sinus **G9Ø.Ø1**
- heart **R55**
- vasoconstriction **R55**
- vasodepressor **R55**
- vasomotor **R55**
- vasovagal **R55**

Syndrome - *see also* Disease
- anterior
  - chest wall **RØ7.89**
  - cord **G83.82**
  - spinal artery **G95.19**
    - compression **M47.Ø19**
      - cervical region **M47.Ø12**
      - cervicothoracic region **M47.Ø13**
      - lumbar region **M47.Ø16**
      - occipito-atlanto-axial region **M47.Ø11**
      - thoracic region **M47.Ø14**
      - thoracolumbar region **M47.Ø15**
- Arnold-Chiari - *see* Arnold-Chiari disease
- autosomal - *see* Abnormal, autosomes
- Babinski-Nageotte **G83.89**
- Beals **Q87.4Ø**
- Bing-Horton's - *see* Horton's headache
- brain (nonpsychotic) **FØ9**
  - congenital - *see* Disability, intellectual
  - organic **FØ9**
    - post-traumatic (nonpsychotic) **FØ7.81**
  - postcontusional **FØ7.81**
  - post-traumatic, nonpsychotic **FØ7.81**
- Brown-Sequard **G83.81**
- bulbar (progressive) **G12.22**
- carotid
  - body **G9Ø.Ø1**
  - sinus **G9Ø.Ø1**
- cervical (root) **M53.1**
  - disc - *see* Disorder, disc, cervical, with neuritis
- Charcot-Weiss-Baker **G9Ø.Ø9**
- cluster headache **G44.ØØ9**
  - intractable **G44.ØØ1**
  - not intractable **G44.ØØ9**

- compartment (deep) (posterior) (traumatic) T79.AØ-
  - nontraumatic
    - abdomen **M79.A3**
    - specified site NEC **M79.A9**
  - postprocedural - *see* Syndrome, compartment, nontraumatic
- complex regional pain - *see* Syndrome, pain, complex regional
- compression T79.5-
  - anterior spinal - *see* Syndrome, anterior, spinal artery, compression
  - vertebral artery **M47.Ø29**
    - cervical region **M47.Ø22**
    - occipito-atlanto-axial region **M47.Ø21**
- concussion **FØ7.81**
- congenital
  - central alveolar hypoventilation **G47.35**
- conus medullaris **G95.81**
- cord
  - anterior **G83.82**
  - posterior **G83.83**
- Costen's (complex) **M26.69**
- crib death **R99**
- cricopharyngeal - *see* Dysphagia
- CRPS I - *see* Syndrome, pain, complex regional I
- Dandy-Walker **QØ3.1**
  - with spina bifida **QØ7.Ø1**
- diabetes mellitus-hypertension-nephrosis - *see* Diabetes, nephrosis
- diabetes-nephrosis - *see* Diabetes, nephrosis
- diabetic amyotrophy - *see* Diabetes, amyotrophy
- Eaton-Lambert - *see* Syndrome, Lambert-Eaton
- epileptic - *see also* Epilepsy, by type
- extrapyramidal **G25.9**
  - specified NEC **G25.89**
- facet joint **M47.819** - *see also* Spondylosis
- fatigue
  - chronic **G93.32**
  - postviral **G93.31**
- Felty's - *see* Felty's syndrome
- flatback - *see* Flatback syndrome
- Froin's **G95.89**
- Gower's **R55**
- headache NEC **G44.89**
  - complicated NEC **G44.59**
- Hilger's **G9Ø.Ø9**
- Hoppe-Goldflam **G7Ø.ØØ**
  - with exacerbation (acute) **G7Ø.Ø1**
  - in crisis **G7Ø.Ø1**
- Jaccoud's - *see* Arthropathy, postrheumatic, chronic
- Jackson's **G83.89**
- Kimmelsteil-Wilson - *see* Diabetes, specified type, with Kimmelsteil-Wilson disease
- Lambert-Eaton **G7Ø.8Ø**
  - in
    - specified disease NEC **G7Ø.81**
- low
  - back **M54.5Ø**
- Mal de Debarquement **R42**
- Marfan's **Q87.4Ø**
- migraine **G43.9Ø9** - *see also* Migraine
- Möbius, ophthalmoplegic migraine - *see* Migraine, ophthalmoplegic
- myasthenic **G7Ø.9**
  - in
    - diabetes mellitus - *see* Diabetes, amyotrophy
- myofascial pain **M79.18**
- nephritic - *see also* Nephritis
- nephrotic (congenital) **NØ4.9** - *see also* Nephrosis
  - diabetic - *see* Diabetes, nephrosis
- pain - *see also* Pain
  - complex regional I **G9Ø.5Ø**
    - specified site NEC **G9Ø.59**
- paralysis agitans - *see* Parkinsonism
- paralytic **G83.9**
  - specified NEC **G83.89**
- parkinsonian - *see* Parkinsonism
- Parkinson's - *see* Parkinsonism
- periodic headache, in adults and children - *see* Headache, periodic syndromes in adults and children
- postbacterial fatigue **G93.39**
- postconcussional **FØ7.81**
- postcontusional **FØ7.81**
- posterior
  - cord **G83.83**
- postinfectious fatigue **G93.39**
- postpolio (myelitic) **G14**
- postviral NEC **G93.31**
  - fatigue **G93.31**
- pseudoparalytica **G7Ø.ØØ**
  - with exacerbation (acute) **G7Ø.Ø1**
  - in crisis **G7Ø.Ø1**
- pyramidopallidonigral **G2Ø**
- radicular NEC - *see* Radiculopathy
- renal glomerulohyalinosis-diabetic - *see* Diabetes, nephrosis
- restless legs **G25.81**
- Rotes Quérol - *see* Hyperostosis, ankylosing
- scapuloperoneal **G71.Ø9**
- sicca - *see* Syndrome, Sjögren
- Sjögren **M35.ØØ**
  - with
    - keratoconjunctivitis **M35.Ø1**
    - lung involvement **M35.Ø2**
    - myopathy **M35.Ø3**
    - renal tubular acidosis **M35.Ø4**
    - specified organ involvement, NEC **M35.Ø9**
    - tubulo-interstitial nephropathy **M35.Ø4**
- Sluder's **G44.89**
- stiff man **G25.82**
- Still-Felty - *see* Felty's syndrome
- straight back, congenital **Q76.49**
- systemic inflammatory response (SIRS), of non-infectious origin (without organ dysfunction) **R65.1Ø**
  - with acute organ dysfunction **R65.11**
- urethro-oculo-articular - *see* Reiter's disease
- vasovagal **R55**
- vertebral
  - artery **G45.Ø**
    - compression - *see* Syndrome, anterior, spinal artery, compression
- vertebrogenic (pain) **M54.89** - *see also* Pain, vertebrogenic
- Weiss-Baker **G9Ø.Ø9**

Synovitis M65.9 - *see also* Tenosynovitis
- gouty - *see* Gout
- in (due to)
  - use, overuse, pressure - *see* Disorder, soft tissue, due to use
- infective NEC - *see* Tenosynovitis, infective NEC
- specified NEC - *see* Tenosynovitis, specified type NEC
- toxic - *see* Synovitis, transient
- transient M67.3-
  - multiple site **M67.39**
  - specified joint NEC **M67.38**
- traumatic, current - *see* Sprain

Syringomyelitis - *see* Encephalitis

System, systemic - *see also* condition
- inflammatory response syndrome (SIRS)
  - of non-infectious origin (without organ dysfunction) **R65.1Ø**
  - with acute organ dysfunction **R65.11**

Systemic exertion intolerance disease [SEID] G93.32

T

Tabacism, tabacosis, tabagism - *see also* Poisoning, tobacco
- meaning dependence (without remission) **F17.2ØØ**

TAC (trigeminal autonomic cephalgia) NEC G44.Ø99
- intractable **G44.Ø91**
- not intractable **G44.Ø99**

Tache noir S6Ø.22-

Tachypnea RØ6.82

Talipes (congenital) Q66.89
- asymmetric **Q66.89**
- calcaneus **Q66.89**
- equinus **Q66.89**

Talma's disease M62.89

Talon noir S9Ø.3-
- hand S6Ø.22-

Tear, torn (traumatic) - *see also* Laceration
- annular fibrosis **M51.35**
- articular cartilage, old - *see* Derangement, joint, articular cartilage, by site
- bucket handle (knee) (meniscus) - *see* Tear, meniscus
- capsule, joint - *see* Sprain
- cartilage - *see also* Sprain
  - articular, old - *see* Derangement, joint, articular cartilage, by site
- internal organ - *see* Injury, by site
- ligament - *see* Sprain
- meniscus (knee) (current injury) S83.2Ø9-
  - bucket-handle S83.2Ø-
  - lateral
    - bucket-handle S83.25-
    - complex S83.27-
    - peripheral S83.26-
    - specified type NEC S83.28-
  - medial
    - bucket-handle S83.21-
    - complex S83.23-
    - peripheral S83.22-
    - specified type NEC S83.24-
  - specified type NEC S83.2Ø-
- muscle - *see* Strain
- rotator cuff (nontraumatic) M75.1Ø-
  - traumatic S46.Ø1-
    - capsule S43.42-
- semilunar cartilage, knee - *see* Tear, meniscus
- tendon - *see* Strain

Teeth - *see also* condition
- grinding
  - sleep related **G47.63**

Tendency
- suicide
  - meaning suicidal ideation - *see* Ideation, suicidal

Tenderness, abdominal R1Ø.819
- epigastric **R1Ø.816**
- generalized **R1Ø.817**
- left lower quadrant **R1Ø.814**
- left upper quadrant **R1Ø.812**
- periumbilic **R1Ø.815**

- rebound **R1Ø.829**
  - epigastric **R1Ø.826**
  - generalized **R1Ø.827**
  - left lower quadrant **R1Ø.824**
  - left upper quadrant **R1Ø.822**
  - periumbilic **R1Ø.825**
  - right lower quadrant **R1Ø.823**
  - right upper quadrant **R1Ø.821**
- right lower quadrant **R1Ø.813**
- right upper quadrant **R1Ø.811**

Tendinitis, tendonitis - *see also* Enthesopathy
- adhesive - *see* Tenosynovitis, specified type NEC
- calcific M65.2-
  - multiple sites **M65.29**
  - specified site NEC **M65.28**
- due to use, overuse, pressure - *see also* Disorder, soft tissue, due to use
  - specified NEC - *see* Disorder, soft tissue, due to use, specified NEC

Tendosynovitis - *see* Tenosynovitis

Tenonitis - *see also* Tenosynovitis

Tenontosynovitis - *see* Tenosynovitis

Tenontothecitis - *see* Tenosynovitis

Tenophyte - *see* Disorder, synovium, specified type NEC

Tenosynovitis M65.9 - *see also* Synovitis
- adhesive - *see* Tenosynovitis, specified type NEC
- in (due to)
  - use, overuse, pressure - *see also* Disorder, soft tissue, due to use
    - specified NEC - *see* Disorder, soft tissue, due to use, specified NEC
- infective NEC M65.1-
  - multiple sites **M65.19**
  - specified site NEC **M65.18**
- specified type NEC **M65.88**
  - multiple sites **M65.89**
  - specified site NEC **M65.88**

Tenovaginitis - *see* Tenosynovitis

Tension
- arterial, high - *see also* Hypertension
- headache **G44.2Ø9**
  - intractable **G44.2Ø1**
  - not intractable **G44.2Ø9**

Termination
- anomalous - *see also* Malposition, congenital

Test, tests, testing (for)
- blood-alcohol **ZØ2.83**
- blood-drug **ZØ2.83**
- hearing **ZØ1.1Ø**
  - infant or child (over 28 days old) **ZØØ.129**
    - with abnormal findings **ZØØ.121**
- laboratory (as part of a general medical examination) **ZØØ.ØØ**
  - with abnormal finding **ZØØ.Ø1**
- skin, diagnostic
  - allergy **ZØ1.82**
    - special screening examination - *see* Screening, by name of disease
- vision **ZØ1.ØØ**
  - infant or child (over 28 days old) **ZØØ.129**
    - with abnormal findings **ZØØ.121**

Tetraplegia (chronic) G82.5Ø - *see also* Quadriplegia

Therapy
- drug, long-term (current) (prophylactic)
  - aspirin **Z79.82**
  - drug, specified NEC **Z79.899**
  - hormone replacement **Z79.89Ø**

Thibierge-Weissenbach syndrome - *see* Sclerosis, systemic

Thickening
- bone - *see* Hypertrophy, bone
- periosteal - *see* Hypertrophy, bone
- valve, heart - *see* Endocarditis

Thromboembolism - *see* Embolism

Thrombosis, thrombotic (bland) (multiple) (progressive) (silent) (vessel) I82.9Ø
- artery, arteries (postinfectional) **I74.9**
  - pulmonary (iatrogenic) - *see* Embolism, pulmonary
- cardiac - *see also* Infarct, myocardium
  - valve - *see* Endocarditis
- history (of) **Z86.718**
- lung (iatrogenic) (postoperative) - *see* Embolism, pulmonary
- personal history (of) **Z86.718**
- pulmonary (artery) (iatrogenic) (postoperative) (vein) - *see* Embolism, pulmonary

Thrombus - *see* Thrombosis

Tic (disorder) F95.9
- degenerative (generalized) (localized) **G25.69**
  - facial **G25.69**
- douloureux **G5Ø.Ø**
  - postherpetic, postzoster **BØ2.22**
- drug-induced **G25.61**
- organic origin **G25.69**
- postchoreic **G25.69**

Tight, tightness
- chest **RØ7.89**
- fascia (lata) **M62.89**
- tendon - *see* Short, tendon

Tiredness R53.83

Tobacco (nicotine)
- abuse - *see* Tobacco, use
- dependence - *see* Dependence, drug, nicotine
- use **Z72.Ø**
  - history **Z87.891**

Todd's
- paralysis (postepileptic) (transitory) **G83.84**

Tophi - *see* Gout, chronic

Torn - *see* Tear

Torsion
- organ or site, congenital NEC - *see* Anomaly, by site

Torticollis (intermittent) (spastic) M43.6
- ocular **R29.891**
- rheumatoid **MØ6.88**

Tortuous
- organ or site, congenital NEC - *see* Distortion
- vein - *see* Varix

Toxemia R68.89
- bacterial - *see* Sepsis
- fatigue **R68.89**
- stasis **R68.89**

Toxicemia - *see* Toxemia

Toxicosis - *see also* Toxemia

Tracheitis (catarrhal) (infantile) (membranous) (plastic) (septal) (suppurative) (viral) JØ4.1Ø
- with
  - bronchitis (15 years of age and above) **J4Ø**

Tracheobronchitis (15 years of age and above) - *see also* Bronchitis

Trance R41.89

Transposition (congenital) - *see also* Malposition, congenital

Trauma, traumatism - *see also* Injury

Trembling paralysis - *see* Parkinsonism

Tremor (s) R25.1
- Parkinson's - *see* Parkinsonism
- senilis **R54**

Trichinellosis, trichiniasis, trichinelliasis, trichinosis B75
- with muscle disorder **B75** [**M63.8Ø**]
  - multiple sites **B75** [**M63.89**]
  - specified site NEC **B75** [**M63.88**]

Trifid - *see also* Accessory

Trigeminal neuralgia - *see* Neuralgia, trigeminal

Trigger finger (acquired) M65.3Ø

Trigonitis (bladder) (chronic) (pseudomembranous) N3Ø.3Ø
- with hematuria **N3Ø.31**

Triple - *see also* Accessory

Triplegia G83.89

Triplication - *see* Accessory

Trouble - *see also* Disease
- sinus - *see* Sinusitis

Truancy, childhood
- from school **Z72.81Ø**

Tumefaction - *see also* Swelling

Tumor - *see also* Neoplasm, unspecified behavior, by site
- ovary, in pregnancy - *see* Pregnancy, complicated by
- pelvic, in pregnancy or childbirth - *see* Pregnancy, complicated by
- vagina, in pregnancy or childbirth - *see* Pregnancy, complicated by
- varicose - *see* Varix
- vulva or perineum, in pregnancy or childbirth - *see* Pregnancy, complicated by

Twist, twisted
- organ or site, congenital NEC - *see* Anomaly, by site

Tylosis (acquired) L84

Tympany
- chest **RØ9.89**

Typhoenteritis - *see* Typhoid

Typhoid (abortive) (ambulant) (any site) (clinical) (fever) (hemorrhagic) (infection) (intermittent) (malignant) (rheumatic) (Widal negative) AØ1.ØØ
- with pneumonia **AØ1.Ø3**
- abdominal **AØ1.Ø9**
- arthritis **AØ1.Ø4**
- cholecystitis (current) **AØ1.Ø9**
- endocarditis **AØ1.Ø2**
- heart involvement **AØ1.Ø2**
- meningitis **AØ1.Ø1**
- mesenteric lymph nodes **AØ1.Ø9**
- myocarditis **AØ1.Ø2**
- osteomyelitis **AØ1.Ø5**
- perichondritis, larynx **AØ1.Ø9**
- pneumonia **AØ1.Ø3**
- specified NEC **AØ1.Ø9**
- spine **AØ1.Ø5**
- ulcer (perforating) **AØ1.Ø9**

Typhomania AØ1.ØØ

Typhoperitonitis AØ1.Ø9

Typhus (fever) A75.9
- abdominal, abdominalis - *see* Typhoid

U

Ulcer, ulcerated, ulcerating, ulceration, ulcerative
- diabetes, diabetic - *see* Diabetes, ulcer
- dysenteric **AØ9**
- intestine, intestinal **K63.3**
  - typhoid (fever) - *see* Typhoid
- lower limb (atrophic) (chronic) (neurogenic) (perforating) (pyogenic) (trophic) (tropical) **L97.9Ø9**
  - varicose - *see* Varix, leg, with, ulcer
- stasis (venous) - *see* Varix, leg, with, ulcer
- typhoid (perforating) - *see* Typhoid

- varicose (lower limb, any part) - *see also* Varix, leg, with, ulcer

Ulcus - *see also* Ulcer

Unable to
- make ends meet **Z59.86**

Unconscious (ness) - *see* Coma

Underdosing Z91.14 - *see also* Table of Drugs and Chemicals, categories T36-T5Ø, with final character 6
- intentional NEC **Z91.128**
  - due to financial hardship of patient **Z91.12Ø**
- unintentional NEC **Z91.138**
  - due to patient's age related debility **Z91.13Ø**

Undescended - *see also* Malposition, congenital

Undeveloped, undevelopment - *see also* Hypoplasia

Undiagnosed (disease) R69

Unequal length (acquired) (limb) - *see also* Deformity, limb, unequal length
- leg - *see also* Deformity, limb, unequal length

Unilateral - *see also* condition
- organ or site, congenital NEC - *see* Agenesis, by site

Union, abnormal - *see also* Fusion

Unstable
- joint - *see* Instability, joint

Unsteadiness on feet R26.81

Upbringing, institutional Z62.22
- away from parents NEC **Z62.29**
- in care of non-parental family member **Z62.21**
- in foster care **Z62.21**
- in orphanage or group home **Z62.22**
- in welfare custody **Z62.21**

Urethralgia R39.89

Urethritis (anterior) (posterior) N34.2
- nongonococcal **N34.1**
  - Reiter's - *see* Reiter's disease
- Reiter's - *see* Reiter's disease

Urethrotrigonitis - *see* Trigonitis

Urgency
- hypertensive - *see* Hypertension
- urinary **R39.15**

Urine
- blood in - *see* Hematuria
- incontinence **R32**
- intermittent stream **R39.198**
- secretion
  - deficient **R34**
- stream
  - intermittent **R39.198**
  - slowing **R39.198**
  - splitting **R39.13**
  - weak **R39.12**

Uroarthritis, infectious (Reiter's) - *see* Reiter's disease

Urodialysis R34

Use (of)
- alcohol **F1Ø.9Ø**
  - harmful - *see* Abuse, alcohol
  - in remission **F1Ø.91**
- amphetamines - *see* Use, stimulant NEC
- caffeine - *see* Use, stimulant NEC
- cannabis **F12.9Ø**
  - with
    - unspecified disorder **F12.99**
  - in remission **F12.91**
- cocaine **F14.9Ø**
  - in remission **F14.91**
- drug (s) NEC **F19.9Ø**
  - harmful - *see* Abuse, drug, by type
- hallucinogen NEC **F16.9Ø**
  - in remission **F16.91**
- inhalants **F18.9Ø**
  - in remission **F18.91**
- methadone - *see* Use, opioid
- opioid **F11.9Ø**
  - with
    - disorder **F11.99**
  - harmful - *see* Abuse, drug, opioid
  - in remission **F11.91**
- psychoactive drug NEC **F19.9Ø**
  - in remission **F19.91**
- sedative, hypnotic, or anxiolytic **F13.9Ø**
  - in remission **F13.91**
- stimulant NEC **F15.9Ø**
  - in remission **F15.91**
- tobacco **Z72.Ø**
  - with dependence - *see* Dependence, drug, nicotine

V

Vaginitis (acute) (circumscribed) (diffuse) (emphysematous) (nonvenereal) (ulcerative) N76.Ø
- amebic **AØ6.82**

Vaginosis - *see* Vaginitis

Valvulitis (chronic) - *see* Endocarditis

Valvulopathy - *see* Endocarditis

Varices - *see* Varix

Varicose
- dermatitis - *see* Varix, leg, with, inflammation
- eczema - *see* Varix, leg, with, inflammation
- phlebitis - *see* Varix, with, inflammation
- tumor - *see* Varix
- ulcer (lower limb, any part) - *see also* Varix, leg, with, ulcer
- vein - *see* Varix
- vessel - *see* Varix, leg

Varicosis, varicosities, varicosity - *see* Varix

Varix (lower limb) I83.9Ø
- with
  - bleeding **I83.899**
  - edema **I83.899**
  - inflammation **I83.1Ø**
    - with ulcer (venous) **I83.2Ø9**
  - pain **I83.819**
  - rupture **I83.899**
  - specified complication NEC **I83.899**
  - stasis dermatitis **I83.1Ø**
    - with ulcer (venous) **I83.2Ø9**
  - swelling **I83.899**
  - ulcer **I83.ØØ9**
    - with inflammation **I83.2Ø9**
- inflamed or infected **I83.1Ø**
  - ulcerated **I83.2Ø9**
- leg (asymptomatic) I83.9-
  - with
    - edema **I83.899**
    - inflammation **I83.1Ø**
    - pain **I83.819**
    - specified complication NEC **I83.899**
    - swelling **I83.899**
    - ulcer I83.Ø-
      - ankle **I83.ØØ3**
        - with inflammation **I83.2Ø3**
      - calf **I83.ØØ2**
        - with inflammation **I83.2Ø2**
      - foot NEC **I83.ØØ5**
        - with inflammation **I83.2Ø5**
      - heel **I83.ØØ4**
        - with inflammation **I83.2Ø4**
      - lower leg NEC **I83.ØØ8**
        - with inflammation **I83.2Ø8**
      - midfoot **I83.ØØ4**
        - with inflammation **I83.2Ø4**
      - thigh **I83.ØØ1**
        - with inflammation **I83.2Ø1**
  - bilateral (asymptomatic) **I83.93**
    - with
      - edema **I83.893**
      - pain **I83.813**
      - specified complication NEC **I83.893**
      - swelling **I83.893**
      - ulcer I83.Ø-
        - with inflammation **I83.2Ø9**
  - left (asymptomatic) **I83.92**
    - with
      - edema **I83.892**
      - inflammation **I83.12**
      - pain **I83.812**
      - specified complication NEC **I83.892**
      - swelling **I83.892**
      - ulcer **I83.Ø29**
        - with inflammation **I83.229**
        - ankle **I83.Ø23**
          - with inflammation **I83.223**
        - calf **I83.Ø22**
          - with inflammation **I83.222**
        - foot NEC **I83.Ø25**
          - with inflammation **I83.225**
        - heel **I83.Ø24**
          - with inflammation **I83.224**
        - lower leg NEC **I83.Ø28**
          - with inflammation **I83.228**
        - midfoot **I83.Ø24**
          - with inflammation **I83.224**
        - thigh **I83.Ø21**
          - with inflammation **I83.221**
  - right (asymptomatic) **I83.91**
    - with
      - edema **I83.891**
      - inflammation **I83.11**
      - pain **I83.811**
      - specified complication NEC **I83.891**
      - swelling **I83.891**
      - ulcer **I83.Ø19**
        - with inflammation **I83.219**
        - ankle **I83.Ø13**
          - with inflammation **I83.213**
        - calf **I83.Ø12**
          - with inflammation **I83.212**
        - foot NEC **I83.Ø15**
          - with inflammation **I83.215**
        - heel **I83.Ø14**
          - with inflammation **I83.214**
        - lower leg NEC **I83.Ø18**
          - with inflammation **I83.218**
        - midfoot **I83.Ø14**
          - with inflammation **I83.214**
        - thigh **I83.Ø11**
          - with inflammation **I83.211**
- ulcerated **I83.ØØ9**
  - inflamed or infected **I83.2Ø9**

Vasculitis I77.6
- rheumatoid - *see* Rheumatoid, vasculitis

Vasovagal attack (paroxysmal) R55

Vertical talus (congenital) Q66.8Ø
- left foot **Q66.82**
- right foot **Q66.81**

Vertigo R42

Vesiculitis (seminal) N49.Ø
- amebic **AØ6.82**

Vitality, lack or want of R53.83

Vomiting R11.1Ø
- without nausea **R11.11**
- asphyxia - *see* Foreign body, by site, causing asphyxia, gastric contents

Notes:

Notes:

5. The Tabular List

Introduction

Always code from this list! After identifying a potential code from the Alphabetic Index, turn to the Tabular List to see the full description and rules associated with the code. First, identify whether you have arrived at the correct code by verifying that it accurately describes the diagnosis documented in the patient's medical record. Second, review the instructions specific to the code and follow them precisely.

The format of this Tabular List is designed to be as functional and useful as possible. Highest specificity codes, which may be anywhere from three to seven characters, will be **bold** (e.g., **F33.41**). Incomplete codes are not bold and end with a hyphen (e.g., F33.4-). When encountering a hyphen, continue looking at the codes beneath that code (moving from top to bottom and left to right), until you reach a final, bolded code. Codes requiring a seventh character will be bolded but end with an underscore (e.g., **S42.351_**), signifying the code is only complete once the final 7th character is added to the code. To find the appropriate seventh character, look for the gray shaded box at the preceding subcategory or category level. Reporting an incomplete code will result in claim denial. Always code to the highest specificity.

To avoid needless repetition of the same code description, many of the descriptions have been shortened when the words are repeated at a higher level. This is a favorite feature of the book for many coders, making it easy to identify the unique descriptors added to the code with each new character. The example below shows how easy it is to identify the final code selection with the shortened code descriptions, as compared to the regular descriptions on the left column for the same code.

Example:

ChiroCode Shortened Descriptions	Full Length Description
M99.0- Segmental and somatic dysfunction	M99.0- Segmental and somatic dysfunction
M99.00 Head region	**M99.00** Segmental and somatic dysfunction of head region
M99.01 Cervical region	**M99.01** Segmental and somatic dysfunction of cervical region
M99.02 Thoracic region	**M99.02** Segmental and somatic dysfunction of thoracic region
M99.03 Lumbar region	**M99.03** Segmental and somatic dysfunction of lumbar region
M99.04 Sacral region	**M99.04** Segmental and somatic dysfunction of sacral region
M99.05 Pelvic region	**M99.05** Segmental and somatic dysfunction of pelvic region
M99.06 Lower extremity	**M99.06** Segmental and somatic dysfunction of lower extremity
M99.07 Upper extremity	**M99.07** Segmental and somatic dysfunction of upper extremity
M99.08 Rib cage	**M99.08** Segmental and somatic dysfunction of rib cage
M99.09 Abdomen and other regions	**M99.09** Segmental and somatic dysfunction of abdomen and other regions

The user should move backwards through each character and read the descriptions for each subcategory, category, block, and chapter so all the proper descriptions are seen, including the relevant instructional notes, guideline references, and special indicators to assist with accurate code selection.

Codes that require additional characters must be fully reported or risk denial. This means provider documentation needs to be more detailed to allow for higher specificity code selection. When the documentation doesn't contain the necessary details, it often results in selection of an unspecified code, which can also lead to claim denial. Coding to the highest specificity demonstrates to claims reviewers that details were provided in the documentation and the coder is aware of how they should be reported.

An emerging trend, for which auditors are on the lookout, is "code cloning," cutting and pasting the same diagnosis from visit to visit and patient to patient. When viewed from a payer's perspective, this may indicate a possible attempt at fraud (filing claims for patient visits that did not occur or were incorrect). Coding to the highest specificity is a simple way for ethical practitioners to indicate they have indeed spent time with a patient and are rendering their clinical judgment as part of patient care.

Book: See Chapter 1 — Diagnosis Coding Essentials for a thorough discussion on how to correctly code using ICD-10-CM.

This Tabular List only contains HIPAA approved diagnosis codes (ICD-10-CM).

Store: See the *ChiroCode DeskBook* for CPT and HCPCS codes.

You will you see these icons below throughout The Tabular List.

N Signifies a code added this year.

R Signifies a code revised this year. Revised codes may have had a change to their description, inclusion terms, and/or instructional notes.

Tabular List Coding Conventions

Here is a list of the conventions you will need to know when coding from the ICD-10-CM Tabular List.

Coding Conventions	
Inclusion Terms	When these terms appear under the code description, they are included in the same category/subcategory/code as the main term listed.
Includes	This instructional note further defines the content of the category/subcategory/code.
Excludes1	This instructional note conveys which codes cannot be coded with the codes this note applies to.
Excludes2	This instructional note coveys which codes can be coded with the codes this note applies to, but must be coded separately.
Code First	This instructional note points to a code which must be sequenced first.
Use additional code	This instructional note points to a code which, if applicable, must be sequenced after the code this note applies to.
Code Also	This instructional note indicates that another code may be required to fully explain a condition, but the order they are sequenced in depends on whichever is the primary reason for the encounter.
Notes	This instructional note provides information necessary to properly understand how to code the conditions in the chapter or block this note applies to.
See Guidelines	This ChiroCode enhanced instructional note directs to guidelines applicable to the chapter/block/category/etc. it falls under.
Indicators	This ChiroCode enhanced instructional note provides additional information regarding the correct use of a code. See the next page for a list of the indicators you may see.
Placeholder "x"	This is used for codes with fewer than six characters that require a seventh character extension. The placeholder may be used in the fourth, fifth, and/or sixth character positions. The seventh character extension must always appear as the seventh character.
NEC	"Not Elsewhere Classifiable" means the diagnosis is specified in the documentation, but there is no code that accurately represents it.
NOS	"Not Otherwise Specified" represents the unspecified option.
[ ]	Brackets enclose words that are synonyms, alternative wordings, or explanatory phrases.
( )	Parentheses enclose supplementary words, which are nonessential modifiers.
And	When the word "and" appears, it should be read as "and/or."
With	When the word "with" appears, it should be read as "associated with" or "due to."

 See Appendix A — Coding Reference Tables for lists of the ICD-10-CM Tabular indicators, HAC categories, and HCC codes.

Notes

Book: See Chapter 1 — Diagnosis Coding Essentials for more detail on these conventions.

Alert: — The instructional notes above can appear at the chapter, block, category, subcategory, and code levels. When reporting codes, it is essential to be aware of the instructions at each level (block, category, subcategory, and code). Instructional notes appearing at any level within the block pertain to all codes beneath them, unless otherwise specified. To make sure all the pertinent information is gathered, work backward. Find the instructions at the code level, then subcategory, category, and so on to ensure compliance at all levels.

Book: See Appendix A — Coding Reference Tables for lists of the ICD-10-CM Tabular indicators.

Content — The Tabular List

 See Appendix A — Coding Reference Tables for lists of the ICD-10-CM Tabular indicators, HAC categories, and HCC codes.

The Tabular List

1. Certain infectious and parasitic diseases (AØØ-B99)

Includes:
diseases generally recognized as communicable or transmissible
Use additional *code to identify resistance to antimicrobial drugs (Z16.-)*
Excludes1:
certain localized infections - see body system-related chapters
Excludes2:
carrier or suspected carrier of infectious disease (Z22.-)
infectious and parasitic diseases complicating pregnancy, childbirth and the puerperium (O98.-)
infectious and parasitic diseases specific to the perinatal period (P35-P39)
influenza and other acute respiratory infections (JØØ-J22)
See Guidelines: *1;C.2Ø.a.1*

INTESTINAL INFECTIOUS DISEASES (AØØ-AØ9)

AØØ- CHOLERA
Indicator(s): *CC*

AØØ.Ø **Due to Vibrio cholerae Ø1, biovar cholerae**
Including: Classical cholera

AØØ.1 **Due to Vibrio cholerae Ø1, biovar eltor**
Including: Cholera eltor

AØØ.9 **Unspecified**

AØ1- TYPHOID AND PARATYPHOID FEVERS
Indicator(s): *CC*

AØ1.Ø- **Typhoid fever**
Including: Infection due to Salmonella typhi

AØ1.ØØ **Unspecified**

AØ1.Ø1 **Meningitis**
Indicator(s): *HHSØ5: 3 | HHSØ7: 3*

AØ1.Ø2 **With heart involvement**
Including: Typhoid endocarditis; Typhoid myocarditis
Indicator(s): *HHSØ5: 135 | HHSØ7: 135*

AØ1.Ø3 **Pneumonia**
Indicator(s): *CMS22: 115 | CMS24: 115 | ESRD21: 115*

AØ1.Ø4 **Arthritis**
Indicator(s): *CMS22: 39 | CMS24: 39 | ESRD21: 39 | HHSØ5: 55 | HHSØ7: 55*

AØ1.Ø5 **Osteomyelitis**
Indicator(s): *CMS22: 39 | CMS24: 39 | ESRD21: 39 | HHSØ5: 55 | HHSØ7: 55*

AØ1.Ø9 **With other complications**

AØ1.1 **Paratyphoid fever A**

AØ1.2 **Paratyphoid fever B**

AØ1.3 **Paratyphoid fever C**

AØ1.4 **Paratyphoid fever, unspecified**
Including: Infection due to Salmonella paratyphi NOS

AØ2- OTHER SALMONELLA INFECTIONS
Includes:
infection or foodborne intoxication due to any Salmonella species other than S. typhi and S. paratyphi

AØ2.Ø **Salmonella enteritis**
Including: Salmonellosis
Indicator(s): *CC*

AØ2.1 **Salmonella sepsis**
Indicator(s): *MCC | CMS22: 2 | CMS24: 2 | ESRD21: 2 | HHSØ5: 2 | HHSØ7: 2*

AØ2.2- **Localized salmonella infections**

AØ2.2Ø **Unspecified**

AØ2.21 **Meningitis**
Indicator(s): *MCC | HHSØ5: 3 | HHSØ7: 3*

AØ2.22 **Pneumonia**
Indicator(s): *MCC | CMS22: 115 | CMS24: 115 | ESRD21: 115*

AØ2.23 **Arthritis**
Indicator(s): *CC | CMS22: 39 | CMS24: 39 | ESRD21: 39 | HHSØ5: 55 | HHSØ7: 55*

AØ2.24 **Osteomyelitis**
Indicator(s): *CC | CMS22: 39 | CMS24: 39 | ESRD21: 39 | HHSØ5: 55 | HHSØ7: 55*

AØ2.25 **Pyelonephritis**
Including: Tubulo-interstitial nephropathy
Indicator(s): *CC*

AØ2.29 **Other localized infection**
Indicator(s): *CC*

AØ2.8 **Other specified salmonella infections**
Indicator(s): *CC*

AØ2.9 **Salmonella infection, unspecified**
Indicator(s): *CC*

AØ3- SHIGELLOSIS

AØ3.Ø **Due to Shigella dysenteriae**
Including: Group A [Shiga-Kruse dysentery]
Indicator(s): *CC*

AØ3.1 **Due to Shigella flexneri**
Including: Group B shigellosis

AØ3.2 **Due to Shigella boydii**
Including: Group C shigellosis

AØ3.3 **Due to Shigella sonnei**
Including: Group D shigellosis

AØ3.8 **Other**

AØ3.9 **Unspecified**
Including: Bacillary dysentery NOS

AØ4- OTHER BACTERIAL INTESTINAL INFECTIONS
Excludes1:
bacterial foodborne intoxications, NEC (AØ5.-)
tuberculous enteritis (A18.32)
Indicator(s): *CC*

AØ4.Ø **Enteropathogenic Escherichia coli**

AØ4.1 **Enterotoxigenic Escherichia coli**

AØ4.2 **Enteroinvasive Escherichia coli**

AØ4.3 **Enterohemorrhagic Escherichia coli**

AØ4.4 **Other Escherichia coli**
Including: Escherichia coli enteritis NOS

AØ4.5 **Campylobacter enteritis**

AØ4.6 **Enteritis due to Yersinia enterocolitica**
Excludes1:
extraintestinal yersiniosis (A28.2)

AØ4.7- **Enterocolitis due to Clostridium difficile**
Including: Foodborne intoxication by C. diff, Pseudomembraneous colitis

AØ4.71 **Recurrent**

AØ4.72 **Not specified as recurrent**

AØ4.8 **Other specified**

AØ4.9 **Unspecified**
Including: enteritis NOS

See Appendix A — Coding Reference Tables for lists of the ICD-10-CM Tabular indicators, HAC categories, and HCC codes.

AØ5- OTHER BACTERIAL FOODBORNE INTOXICATIONS, NOT ELSEWHERE CLASSIFIED

Excludes1:
Clostridium difficile foodborne intoxication and infection (AØ4.7-)
Escherichia coli infection (AØ4.Ø-AØ4.4)
listeriosis (A32.-)
salmonella foodborne intoxication and infection (AØ2.-)
toxic effect of noxious foodstuffs (T61-T62)

AØ5.Ø **Staphylococcal intoxication**
Indicator(s): CC

AØ5.1 **Botulism food poisoning**
Including: Botulism NOS, Classical foodborne intoxication due to Clostridium botulinum
Excludes1:
infant botulism (A48.51)
wound botulism (A48.52)
Indicator(s): CC

AØ5.2 **Clostridium perfringens [Clostridium welchii]**
Including: Enteritis necroticans, Pig-bel
Indicator(s): CC

AØ5.3 **Vibrio parahaemolyticus**
Indicator(s): CC

AØ5.4 **Bacillus cereus**
Indicator(s): CC

AØ5.5 **Vibrio vulnificus**
Indicator(s): CC

AØ5.8 **Other specified**
Indicator(s): CC

AØ5.9 **Unspecified**

AØ6- AMEBIASIS

Includes:
infection due to Entamoeba histolytica
Excludes1:
other protozoal intestinal diseases (AØ7.-)
Excludes2:
acanthamebiasis (B6Ø.1-)
Naegleriasis (B6Ø.2)

AØ6.Ø **Acute amebic dysentery**
Including: Acute amebiasis; Intestinal amebiasis NOS
Indicator(s): CC

AØ6.1 **Chronic intestinal amebiasis**
Indicator(s): CC

AØ6.2 **Amebic nondysenteric colitis**
Indicator(s): CC

AØ6.3 **Ameboma of intestine**
Including: Ameboma NOS
Indicator(s): CC

AØ6.4 **Amebic liver abscess**
Including: Hepatic amebiasis
Indicator(s): MCC | HHSØ5: 38 | HHSØ7: 35.1

AØ6.5 **Amebic lung abscess**
Including: Amebic abscess of lung (and liver)
Indicator(s): MCC | CMS22: 115 | CMS24: 115 | ESRD21: 115 | HHSØ5: 163 | HHSØ7: 163

AØ6.6 **Amebic brain abscess**
Including: Amebic abscess of brain (and liver) (and lung)
Indicator(s): MCC | HHSØ5: 3 | HHSØ7: 3

AØ6.7 **Cutaneous amebiasis**

AØ6.8- **Amebic infection of other sites**
Indicator(s): CC

AØ6.81 **Cystitis**

AØ6.82 **Other genitourinary**
Including: Amebic balanitis, vesiculitis, and vulvovaginitis

AØ6.89 **Other**
Including: Amebic appendicitis; Amebic splenic abscess

AØ6.9 **Amebiasis, unspecified**

AØ7- OTHER PROTOZOAL INTESTINAL DISEASES

AØ7.Ø **Balantidiasis**
Including: Balantidial dysentery

AØ7.1 **Giardiasis [lambliasis]**
Indicator(s): CC

AØ7.2 **Cryptosporidiosis**
Indicator(s): CC | CMS22: 6 | CMS24: 6 | RxØ5: 5 | ESRD21: 6 | HHSØ5: 6 | HHSØ7: 6

AØ7.3 **Isosporiasis**
Including: Infection due to Isospora belli and Isospora hominis; Intestinal coccidiosis; Isosporosis
Indicator(s): CC

AØ7.4 **Cyclosporiasis**
Indicator(s): CC

AØ7.8 **Other specified**
Including: Intestinal microsporidiosis; Intestinal trichomoniasis; Sarcocystosis; Sarcosporidiosis
Indicator(s): CC

AØ7.9 **Unspecified**
Including: Flagellate diarrhea; Protozoal colitis, diarrhea and dysentery
Indicator(s): CC

AØ8- VIRAL AND OTHER SPECIFIED INTESTINAL INFECTIONS

Excludes1:
influenza with involvement of gastrointestinal tract (JØ9.X3, J1Ø.2, J11.2)

AØ8.Ø **Rotaviral enteritis**
Indicator(s): CC

AØ8.1- **Acute gastroenteropathy due to Norwalk agent and other small round viruses**
Indicator(s): CC

AØ8.11 **Due to Norwalk agent**
Including: Norovirus or Norwalk-like agent

AØ8.19 **Due to other small round viruses**
Including: Small round virus [SRV] NOS

AØ8.2 **Adenoviral enteritis**
Indicator(s): CC

AØ8.3- **Other viral enteritis**
Indicator(s): CC

AØ8.31 **Calicivirus enteritis**

AØ8.32 **Astrovirus enteritis**

AØ8.39 **Other viral enteritis**
Including: Coxsackie virus; Echovirus; Enterovirus NEC; Torovirus

AØ8.4 **Viral intestinal infection, unspecified**
Including: Enteritis NOS, gastroenteritis NOS, gastroenteropathy NOS

AØ8.8 **Other specified intestinal infections**

See Appendix A — Coding Reference Tables for lists of the ICD-10-CM Tabular indicators, HAC categories, and HCC codes.

AØ9 **Infectious gastroenteritis and colitis, unspecified**
Including: Infectious colitis NOS; enteritis NOS; gastroenteritis NOS
Excludes1:
colitis NOS (K52.9)
diarrhea NOS (R19.7)
enteritis NOS (K52.9)
gastroenteritis NOS (K52.9)
noninfective gastroenteritis and colitis, unspecified (K52.9)
Indicator(s): *CC*

VIRAL INFECTIONS CHARACTERIZED BY SKIN AND MUCOUS MEMBRANE LESIONS (BØØ-BØ9)

BØ2- ZOSTER [HERPES ZOSTER]
Includes:
shingles
zona

BØ2.2- **Zoster with other nervous system involvement**

BØ2.21 **Postherpetic geniculate ganglionitis**
Indicator(s): *CC | RxØ5: 168*

BØ2.22 **Postherpetic trigeminal neuralgia**
Indicator(s): *CC | RxØ5: 168*

BØ2.23 **Postherpetic polyneuropathy**
Indicator(s): *CC | RxØ5: 168*

BØ2.24 **Postherpetic myelitis**
Including: Herpes zoster myelitis
Indicator(s): *MCC | CMS22: 72 | CMS24: 72 | RxØ5: 157 | ESRD21: 72 | HHSØ5: 11Ø | HHSØ7: 11Ø*

BØ2.29 **Other postherpetic involvement**
Including: radiculopathy
Indicator(s): *CC | RxØ5: 168*

BØ2.9 **Without complications**
Including: zoster NOS

SEQUELAE OF INFECTIOUS AND PARASITIC DISEASES (B9Ø-B94)

Notes:
Categories B9Ø-B94 are to be used to indicate conditions in categories AØØ-B89 as the cause of sequelae, which are themselves classified elsewhere. The 'sequelae' include conditions specified as such; they also include residuals of diseases classifiable to the above categories if there is evidence that the disease itself is no longer present. Codes from these categories are not to be used for chronic infections. Code chronic current infections to active infectious disease as appropriate.
Code First:
condition resulting from (sequela) the infectious or parasitic disease
Indicator(s): *POAEx*

B91 **Sequelae of poliomyelitis**
Excludes1:
postpolio syndrome (G14)

2. Neoplasms (CØØ-D49)

This Chapter was not included in this common codes list. For a complete listing of ICD-10-CM codes see FindACode.com

3. Diseases of the blood and blood-forming organs and certain disorders involving the immune mechanism (D5Ø-D89)

Excludes2:
autoimmune disease (systemic) NOS (M35.9)
certain conditions originating in the perinatal period (PØØ-P96)
complications of pregnancy, childbirth and the puerperium (OØØ-O9A)
congenital malformations, deformations and chromosomal abnormalities (QØØ-Q99)
endocrine, nutritional and metabolic diseases (EØØ-E88)
human immunodeficiency virus [HIV] disease (B2Ø)
injury, poisoning and certain other consequences of external causes (SØØ-T88)
neoplasms (CØØ-D49)
symptoms, signs and abnormal clinical and laboratory findings, not elsewhere classified (RØØ-R94)
See Guidelines: *1;C.2Ø.a.1*

NUTRITIONAL ANEMIAS (D5Ø-D53)

See Guidelines: *1;C.2.c.1-2*

D5Ø- IRON DEFICIENCY ANEMIA
Includes:
asiderotic anemia
hypochromic anemia

D5Ø.Ø **Secondary to blood loss (chronic)**
Including: Posthemorrhagic anemia
Excludes1:
acute posthemorrhagic anemia (D62)
congenital anemia from fetal blood loss (P61.3)

D5Ø.1 **Sideropenic dysphagia**
Including: Kelly-Paterson syndrome, Plummer-Vinson syndrome

D5Ø.8 **Other**
Including: anemia due to inadequate dietary iron intake

D5Ø.9 **Unspecified**

4. Endocrine, nutritional and metabolic diseases (EØØ-E89)

Notes:
All neoplasms, whether functionally active or not, are classified in Chapter 2. Appropriate codes in this chapter (i.e. EØ5.8, EØ7.Ø, E16-E31, E34.-) may be used as additional codes to indicate either functional activity by neoplasms and ectopic endocrine tissue or hyperfunction and hypofunction of endocrine glands associated with neoplasms and other conditions classified elsewhere.

Excludes1:
transitory endocrine and metabolic disorders specific to newborn (P7Ø-P74)

See Guidelines: *1;C.4 | 1;C.2Ø.a.1*

DISORDERS OF THYROID GLAND (EØØ-EØ7)

EØ3- OTHER HYPOTHYROIDISM

Excludes1:
iodine-deficiency related hypothyroidism (EØØ-EØ2)
postprocedural hypothyroidism (E89.Ø)

Indicator(s): *RxØ5: 42*

EØ3.9 **Unspecified**
Including: Myxedema NOS

DIABETES MELLITUS (EØ8-E13)

See Guidelines: *1;C.15.g | 1;C.15.g-i*

EØ8- DIABETES MELLITUS DUE TO UNDERLYING CONDITION

Code First:
the underlying condition, such as:
congenital rubella (P35.Ø)
Cushing's syndrome (E24.-)
cystic fibrosis (E84.-)
malignant neoplasm (CØØ-C96)
malnutrition (E4Ø-E46)
pancreatitis and other diseases of the pancreas (K85-K86.-)

Use additional *code to identify control using:*
insulin (Z79.4)
oral antidiabetic drugs (Z79.84)
oral hypoglycemic drugs (Z79.84)

Excludes1:
drug or chemical induced diabetes mellitus (EØ9.-)
gestational diabetes (O24.4-)
neonatal diabetes mellitus (P7Ø.2)
postpancreatectomy diabetes mellitus (E13.-)
postprocedural diabetes mellitus (E13.-)
secondary diabetes mellitus NEC (E13.-)
type 1 diabetes mellitus (E1Ø.-)
type 2 diabetes mellitus (E11.-)

See Guidelines: *1;C.4.a.6*

EØ8.Ø- **Diabetes mellitus due to underlying condition with hyperosmolarity**
Indicator(s): *MCC | HAC: Ø9 | CMS22: 17 | CMS24: 17 | RxØ5: 3Ø | ESRD21: 17 | HHSØ5: 19 | HHSØ7: 19*

EØ8.ØØ **Without nonketotic hyperglycemic-hyperosmolar coma (NKHHC)**

EØ8.Ø1 **With coma**

EØ8.1- **Diabetes mellitus due to underlying condition with ketoacidosis**
Indicator(s): *MCC | HAC: Ø9 | CMS22: 17 | CMS24: 17 | RxØ5: 3Ø | ESRD21: 17 | HHSØ5: 19 | HHSØ7: 19*

EØ8.1Ø **Without coma**

EØ8.11 **With coma**

EØ8.2- **Diabetes mellitus due to underlying condition with kidney complications**
Indicator(s): *CMS22: 18 | CMS24: 18 | RxØ5: 3Ø | ESRD21: 18 | HHSØ5: 2Ø | HHSØ7: 2Ø*

EØ8.21 **Diabetic nephropathy**
Including: intercapillary glomerulosclerosis, intracapillary glomerulonephrosis, Kimmelstiel-Wilson disease

EØ8.22 **Diabetic chronic kidney disease**
Use additional *code to identify stage of chronic kidney disease (N18.1-N18.6)*

EØ8.29 **Other complication**
Including: Renal tubular degeneration

EØ8.3- **Diabetes mellitus due to underlying condition with ophthalmic complications**
Indicator(s): *CMS22: 18 | CMS24: 18 | RxØ5: 3Ø | HHSØ5: 2Ø | HHSØ7: 2Ø*

EØ8.31- **Diabetes mellitus due to underlying condition with unspecified diabetic retinopathy**

EØ8.311 **With macular edema**

EØ8.319 **Without macular edema**

EØ8.32- **Diabetes mellitus due to underlying condition with mild nonproliferative diabetic retinopathy**
Including: Diabetes mellitus due to underlying condition with nonproliferative diabetic retinopathy NOS

One of the following 7th characters is to be assigned to codes in subcategory EØ8.32 to designate laterality of the disease:
1 - right eye
2 - left eye
3 - bilateral
9 - unspecified eye

EØ8.321_ **With macular edema**

EØ8.329_ **Without macular edema**

EØ8.33- **Diabetes mellitus due to underlying condition with moderate nonproliferative diabetic retinopathy**

One of the following 7th characters is to be assigned to codes in subcategory EØ8.33 to designate laterality of the disease:
1 - right eye
2 - left eye
3 - bilateral
9 - unspecified eye

EØ8.331_ **With macular edema**

EØ8.339_ **Without macular edema**

EØ8.34- **Diabetes mellitus due to underlying condition with severe nonproliferative diabetic retinopathy**

One of the following 7th characters is to be assigned to codes in subcategory EØ8.34 to designate laterality of the disease:
1 - right eye
2 - left eye
3 - bilateral
9 - unspecified eye

EØ8.341_ **With macular edema**

EØ8.349_ **Without macular edema**

E08.35- **Diabetes mellitus due to underlying condition with proliferative diabetic retinopathy**

One of the following 7th characters is to be assigned to codes in subcategory E08.35 to designate laterality of the disease:

1 - right eye
2 - left eye
3 - bilateral
9 - unspecified eye

E08.351_ With macular edema

E08.352_ With traction retinal detachment involving the macula

E08.353_ With traction retinal detachment not involving the macula

E08.354_ With combined traction retinal detachment and rhegmatogenous retinal detachment

E08.355_ With stable proliferative diabetic retinopathy

E08.359_ Without macular edema

E08.36 Diabetic cataract

E08.37x_ Diabetic macular edema, resolved following treatment

One of the following 7th characters is to be assigned to code E08.37 to designate laterality of the disease:

1 - right eye
2 - left eye
3 - bilateral
9 - unspecified eye

E08.39 Other complication

Use additional code to identify manifestation, such as:
diabetic glaucoma (H40-H42)

E08.4- **Diabetes mellitus due to underlying condition with neurological complications**

Indicator(s): CMS22: 18 | CMS24: 18 | Rx05: 30 | HHS05: 20 | HHS07: 20

E08.40 Diabetic neuropathy, unspecified

E08.41 Diabetic mononeuropathy

E08.42 Diabetic polyneuropathy

Including: neuralgia

E08.43 Diabetic autonomic (poly)neuropathy

Including: gastroparesis

E08.44 Diabetic amyotrophy

E08.49 Other complication

E08.5- **Diabetes mellitus due to underlying condition with circulatory complications**

Indicator(s): CMS22: 18 | CMS24: 18 | Rx05: 30 | ESRD21: 18 | HHS05: 20 | HHS07: 20

E08.51 Diabetic peripheral angiopathy without gangrene

E08.52 Diabetic peripheral angiopathy with gangrene

Including: Diabetic gangrene

Indicator(s): CC

E08.59 Other complication

E08.6- **Diabetes mellitus due to underlying condition with other specified complications**

Indicator(s): Rx05: 30

E08.61- **Diabetes mellitus due to underlying condition with diabetic arthropathy**

E08.610 Neuropathic

Including: Charcôt's joints

E08.618 Other arthropathy

E08.62- **Diabetes mellitus due to underlying condition with skin complications**

E08.620 Diabetic dermatitis

Including: necrobiosis lipoidica

E08.621 Foot ulcer

Use additional code to identify site of ulcer (L97.4-, L97.5-)

E08.622 Other skin ulcer

Use additional code to identify site of ulcer (L97.1-L97.9, L98.41-L98.49)

E08.628 Other complication

E08.63- **Diabetes mellitus due to underlying condition with oral complications**

E08.630 Periodontal disease

E08.638 Other complication

E08.64- **Diabetes mellitus due to underlying condition with hypoglycemia**

E08.641 With coma

Indicator(s): MCC

E08.649 Without coma

E08.65 Hyperglycemia

E08.69 Other complication

Use additional code to identify complication

E08.8 Diabetes mellitus due to underlying condition with unspecified complications

Indicator(s): CMS22: 18 | CMS24: 18 | Rx05: 30 | ESRD21: 18 | HHS05: 20 | HHS07: 21

E08.9 Diabetes mellitus due to underlying condition without complications

Indicator(s): CMS22: 19 | CMS24: 19 | Rx05: 31 | ESRD21: 19 | HHS05: 21 | HHS07: 21

E09- DRUG OR CHEMICAL INDUCED DIABETES MELLITUS

Code First:
poisoning due to drug or toxin, if applicable (T36-T65 with fifth or sixth character 1-4 or 6)
Use additional code for adverse effect, if applicable, to identify drug (T36-T50 with fifth or sixth character 5)
Use additional code to identify control using:
insulin (Z79.4)
oral antidiabetic drugs (Z79.84)
oral hypoglycemic drugs (Z79.84)
Excludes1:
diabetes mellitus due to underlying condition (E08.-)
gestational diabetes (O24.4-)
neonatal diabetes mellitus (P70.2)
postpancreatectomy diabetes mellitus (E13.-)
postprocedural diabetes mellitus (E13.-)
secondary diabetes mellitus NEC (E13.-)
type 1 diabetes mellitus (E10.-)
type 2 diabetes mellitus (E11.-)
See Guidelines: 1;C.4.a.6

E09.0- **Drug or chemical induced diabetes mellitus with hyperosmolarity**

Indicator(s): MCC | HAC: 09 | CMS22: 17 | CMS24: 17 | Rx05: 30 | ESRD21: 17 | HHS05: 19 | HHS07: 19

E09.00 Without nonketotic hyperglycemic-hyperosmolar coma (NKHHC)

E09.01 With coma

E09.1- **Drug or chemical induced diabetes mellitus with ketoacidosis**
Indicator(s): MCC | HAC: 09 | CMS22: 17 | CMS24: 17 | Rx05: 30 | ESRD21: 17 | HHS05: 19 | HHS07: 19

E09.10 **Without coma**

E09.11 **With coma**

E09.2- **Drug or chemical induced diabetes mellitus with kidney complications**
Indicator(s): CMS22: 18 | CMS24: 18 | Rx05: 30 | ESRD21: 18 | HHS05: 20 | HHS07: 20

E09.21 **Diabetic nephropathy**
Including: intercapillary glomerulosclerosis, intracapillary glomerulonephrosis, Kimmelstiel-Wilson disease

E09.22 **Diabetic chronic kidney disease**
Use additional code to identify stage of chronic kidney disease (N18.1-N18.6)

E09.29 **Other complication**
Including: renal tubular degeneration

E09.3- **Drug or chemical induced diabetes mellitus with ophthalmic complications**
Indicator(s): CMS22: 18 | CMS24: 18 | Rx05: 30 | HHS05: 20 | HHS07: 20

E09.31- **Drug or chemical induced diabetes mellitus with unspecified diabetic retinopathy**

E09.311 **With macular edema**

E09.319 **Without macular edema**

E09.32- **Drug or chemical induced diabetes mellitus with mild nonproliferative diabetic retinopathy**
Including: Drug or chemical induced diabetes mellitus with nonproliferative diabetic retinopathy NOS

One of the following 7th characters is to be assigned to codes in subcategory E09.32 to designate laterality of the disease:
- *1 - right eye*
- *2 - left eye*
- *3 - bilateral*
- *9 - unspecified eye*

E09.321_ **With macular edema**

E09.329_ **Without macular edema**

E09.33- **Drug or chemical induced diabetes mellitus with moderate nonproliferative diabetic retinopathy**

One of the following 7th characters is to be assigned to codes in subcategory E09.33 to designate laterality of the disease:
- *1 - right eye*
- *2 - left eye*
- *3 - bilateral*
- *9 - unspecified eye*

E09.331_ **With macular edema**

E09.339_ **Without macular edema**

E09.34- **Drug or chemical induced diabetes mellitus with severe nonproliferative diabetic retinopathy**

One of the following 7th characters is to be assigned to codes in subcategory E09.34 to designate laterality of the disease:
- *1 - right eye*
- *2 - left eye*
- *3 - bilateral*
- *9 - unspecified eye*

E09.341_ **With macular edema**

E09.349_ **Without macular edema**

E09.35- **Drug or chemical induced diabetes mellitus with proliferative diabetic retinopathy**

One of the following 7th characters is to be assigned to codes in subcategory E09.35 to designate laterality of the disease:
- *1 - right eye*
- *2 - left eye*
- *3 - bilateral*
- *9 - unspecified eye*

E09.351_ **With macular edema**

E09.352_ **With traction retinal detachment involving the macula**

E09.353_ **With traction retinal detachment not involving the macula**

E09.354_ **With combined traction retinal detachment and rhegmatogenous retinal detachment**

E09.355_ **With stable proliferative diabetic retinopathy**

E09.359_ **Without macular edema**

E09.36 **Diabetic cataract**

E09.37x_ **Diabetic macular edema, resolved following treatment**

One of the following 7th characters is to be assigned to code E09.37 to designate laterality of the disease:
- *1 - right eye*
- *2 - left eye*
- *3 - bilateral*
- *9 - unspecified eye*

E09.39 **Other complication**
Use additional code to identify manifestation, such as:
diabetic glaucoma (H40-H42)

E09.4- **Drug or chemical induced diabetes mellitus with neurological complications**
Indicator(s): CMS22: 18 | CMS24: 18 | Rx05: 30 | HHS05: 20 | HHS07: 20

E09.40 **Diabetic neuropathy, unspecified**

E09.41 **Diabetic mononeuropathy**

E09.42 **Diabetic polyneuropathy**
Including: neuralgia

E09.43 **Diabetic autonomic (poly)neuropathy**
Including: gastroparesis

E09.44 **Diabetic amyotrophy**

E09.49 **Other complication**

See Appendix A — Coding Reference Tables for lists of the ICD-10-CM Tabular indicators, HAC categories, and HCC codes.

E09.5- **Drug or chemical induced diabetes mellitus with circulatory complications**
Indicator(s): CMS22: 18 | CMS24: 18 | Rx05: 30 | ESRD21: 18 | HHS05: 20 | HHS07: 20

E09.51 Diabetic peripheral angiopathy without gangrene

E09.52 Diabetic peripheral angiopathy with gangrene
Including: gangrene
Indicator(s): CC

E09.59 Other complication

E09.6- **Drug or chemical induced diabetes mellitus with other specified complications**
Indicator(s): Rx05: 30

E09.61- **Drug or chemical induced diabetes mellitus with diabetic arthropathy**

E09.610 Neuropathic
Including: Charcôt's joints

E09.618 Other arthropathy

E09.62- **Drug or chemical induced diabetes mellitus with skin complications**

E09.620 Diabetic dermatitis
Including: necrobiosis lipoidica

E09.621 Foot ulcer
Use additional code to identify site of ulcer (L97.4-, L97.5-)

E09.622 Other skin ulcer
Use additional code to identify site of ulcer (L97.1-L97.9, L98.41-L98.49)

E09.628 Other complication

E09.63- **Drug or chemical induced diabetes mellitus with oral complications**

E09.630 Periodontal disease

E09.638 Other complication

E09.64- **Drug or chemical induced diabetes mellitus with hypoglycemia**

E09.641 With coma
Indicator(s): MCC

E09.649 Without coma

E09.65 Hyperglycemia

E09.69 Other complication
Use additional code to identify complication

E09.8 Drug or chemical induced diabetes mellitus with unspecified complications
Indicator(s): CMS22: 18 | CMS24: 18 | Rx05: 30 | ESRD21: 18 | HHS05: 20 | HHS07: 21

E09.9 Drug or chemical induced diabetes mellitus without complications
Indicator(s): CMS22: 19 | CMS24: 19 | Rx05: 31 | ESRD21: 19 | HHS05: 21 | HHS07: 21

E10- TYPE 1 DIABETES MELLITUS

Includes:
- *brittle diabetes (mellitus)*
- *diabetes (mellitus) due to autoimmune process*
- *diabetes (mellitus) due to immune mediated pancreatic islet beta-cell destruction*
- *idiopathic diabetes (mellitus)*
- *juvenile onset diabetes (mellitus)*
- *ketosis-prone diabetes (mellitus)*

Excludes1:
- *diabetes mellitus due to underlying condition (E08.-)*
- *drug or chemical induced diabetes mellitus (E09.-)*
- *gestational diabetes (O24.4-)*
- *hyperglycemia NOS (R73.9)*
- *neonatal diabetes mellitus (P70.2)*
- *postpancreatectomy diabetes mellitus (E13.-)*
- *postprocedural diabetes mellitus (E13.-)*
- *secondary diabetes mellitus NEC (E13.-)*
- *type 2 diabetes mellitus (E11.-)*

E10.1- **Type 1 diabetes mellitus with ketoacidosis**
Indicator(s): MCC | HAC: 09 | CMS22: 17 | CMS24: 17 | Rx05: 30 | ESRD21: 17 | HHS05: 19 | HHS07: 19

E10.10 Without coma

E10.11 With coma

E10.2- **Type 1 diabetes mellitus with kidney complications**
Indicator(s): CMS22: 18 | CMS24: 18 | Rx05: 30 | ESRD21: 18 | HHS05: 20 | HHS07: 20

E10.21 Diabetic nephropathy
Including: intercapillary glomerulosclerosis, intracapillary glomerulonephrosis, Kimmelstiel-Wilson disease

E10.22 Diabetic chronic kidney disease
Use additional code to identify stage of chronic kidney disease (N18.1-N18.6)

E10.29 Other diabetic kidney complication
Including: renal tubular degeneration

E10.3- **Type 1 diabetes mellitus with ophthalmic complications**
Indicator(s): CMS22: 18 | CMS24: 18 | Rx05: 30 | HHS05: 20 | HHS07: 20

E10.31- **Type 1 diabetes mellitus with unspecified diabetic retinopathy**

E10.311 With macular edema

E10.319 Without macular edema

E10.32- **Type 1 diabetes mellitus with mild nonproliferative diabetic retinopathy**
Including: nonproliferative diabetic retinopathy NOS

One of the following 7th characters is to be assigned to codes in subcategory E10.32 to designate laterality of the disease:
- *1 - right eye*
- *2 - left eye*
- *3 - bilateral*
- *9 - unspecified eye*

E10.321_ With macular edema

E10.329_ Without macular edema

Ch5

5. The Tabular List

E1Ø.33- **Type 1 diabetes mellitus with moderate nonproliferative diabetic retinopathy**

One of the following 7th characters is to be assigned to codes in subcategory E1Ø.33 to designate laterality of the disease:
1 - right eye
2 - left eye
3 - bilateral
9 - unspecified eye

E1Ø.331_ With macular edema

E1Ø.339_ Without macular edema

E1Ø.34- **Type 1 diabetes mellitus with severe nonproliferative diabetic retinopathy**

One of the following 7th characters is to be assigned to codes in subcategory E1Ø.34 to designate laterality of the disease:
1 - right eye
2 - left eye
3 - bilateral
9 - unspecified eye

E1Ø.341_ With macular edema

E1Ø.349_ Without macular edema

E1Ø.35- **Type 1 diabetes mellitus with proliferative diabetic retinopathy**

One of the following 7th characters is to be assigned to codes in subcategory E1Ø.35 to designate laterality of the disease:
1 - right eye
2 - left eye
3 - bilateral
9 - unspecified eye

E1Ø.351_ With macular edema

E1Ø.352_ With traction retinal detachment involving the macula

E1Ø.353_ With traction retinal detachment not involving the macula

E1Ø.354_ With combined traction retinal detachment and rhegmatogenous retinal detachment

E1Ø.355_ With stable proliferative diabetic retinopathy

E1Ø.359_ Without macular edema

E1Ø.36 With diabetic cataract

E1Ø.37x_ Diabetic macular edema, resolved following treatment

One of the following 7th characters is to be assigned to code E1Ø.37 to designate laterality of the disease:
1 - right eye
2 - left eye
3 - bilateral
9 - unspecified eye

E1Ø.39 Other complication

Use additional code to identify manifestation, such as:
diabetic glaucoma (H4Ø-H42)

E1Ø.4- **Type 1 diabetes mellitus with neurological complications**

Indicator(s): CMS22: 18 | CMS24: 18 | RxØ5: 3Ø | HHSØ5: 2Ø | HHSØ7: 2Ø

E1Ø.4Ø Diabetic neuropathy, unspecified

E1Ø.41 Diabetic mononeuropathy

E1Ø.42 Diabetic polyneuropathy

Including: neuralgia

E1Ø.43 Diabetic autonomic (poly)neuropathy

Including: gastroparesis

E1Ø.44 Diabetic amyotrophy

E1Ø.49 Other complication

E1Ø.5- **With circulatory complications**

Indicator(s): CMS22: 18 | CMS24: 18 | RxØ5: 3Ø | ESRD21: 18 | HHSØ5: 2Ø | HHSØ7: 2Ø

E1Ø.51 Diabetic peripheral angiopathy without gangrene

E1Ø.52 Diabetic peripheral angiopathy with gangrene

Including: gangrene

Indicator(s): CC

E1Ø.59 Other complication

E1Ø.6- **Type 1 diabetes mellitus with other specified complications**

Indicator(s): RxØ5: 3Ø

E1Ø.61- **Type 1 diabetes mellitus with diabetic arthropathy**

E1Ø.61Ø Neuropathic

Including: Charcôt's joints

E1Ø.618 Other arthropathy

E1Ø.62- **Type 1 diabetes mellitus with skin complications**

E1Ø.62Ø Diabetic dermatitis

Including: necrobiosis lipoidica

E1Ø.621 Foot ulcer

Use additional code to identify site of ulcer (L97.4-, L97.5-)

E1Ø.622 Other skin ulcer

Use additional code to identify site of ulcer (L97.1-L97.9, L98.41-L98.49)

E1Ø.628 Other complication

E1Ø.63- **Type 1 diabetes mellitus with oral complications**

E1Ø.63Ø Periodontal disease

E1Ø.638 Other complication

E1Ø.64- **Type 1 diabetes mellitus with hypoglycemia**

E1Ø.641 With coma

Indicator(s): MCC

E1Ø.649 Without coma

E1Ø.65 Hyperglycemia

E1Ø.69 Other complication

Use additional code to identify complication

E1Ø.8 Type 1 diabetes mellitus with unspecified complications

Indicator(s): CMS22: 18 | CMS24: 18 | RxØ5: 3Ø | ESRD21: 18 | HHSØ5: 2Ø | HHSØ7: 21

E1Ø.9 Type 1 diabetes mellitus without complications

Indicator(s): CMS22: 19 | CMS24: 19 | RxØ5: 31 | ESRD21: 19 | HHSØ5: 21 | HHSØ7: 21

Ch5

5. The Tabular List

E11- TYPE 2 DIABETES MELLITUS

Includes:
diabetes (mellitus) due to insulin secretory defect
diabetes NOS
insulin resistant diabetes (mellitus)
Use additional code to identify control using:
insulin (Z79.4)
oral antidiabetic drugs (Z79.84)
oral hypoglycemic drugs (Z79.84)
Excludes1:
diabetes mellitus due to underlying condition (EØ8.-)
drug or chemical induced diabetes mellitus (EØ9.-)
gestational diabetes (O24.4-)
neonatal diabetes mellitus (P7Ø.2)
postpancreatectomy diabetes mellitus (E13.-)
postprocedural diabetes mellitus (E13.-)
secondary diabetes mellitus NEC (E13.-)
type 1 diabetes mellitus (E1Ø.-)
See Guidelines: 1;C.4.a.2

E11.Ø- **Type 2 diabetes mellitus with hyperosmolarity**
Indicator(s): MCC | HAC: Ø9 | CMS22: 17 | CMS24: 17 | RxØ5: 3Ø | ESRD21: 17 | HHSØ5: 19 | HHSØ7: 19

E11.ØØ Without nonketotic hyperglycemic-hyperosmolar coma (NKHHC)

E11.Ø1 With coma

E11.1- **Type 2 diabetes mellitus with ketoacidosis**
Indicator(s): MCC | HAC: Ø9 | CMS22: 17 | CMS24: 17 | RxØ5: 3Ø | ESRD21: 17 | HHSØ5: 19 | HHSØ7: 19

E11.1Ø Without coma

E11.11 With coma

E11.2- **Type 2 diabetes mellitus with kidney complications**
Indicator(s): CMS22: 18 | CMS24: 18 | RxØ5: 3Ø | ESRD21: 18 | HHSØ5: 2Ø | HHSØ7: 2Ø

E11.21 Diabetic nephropathy
Including: intercapillary glomerulosclerosis, intracapillary glomerulonephrosis, Kimmelstiel-Wilson disease

E11.22 Diabetic chronic kidney disease
Use additional code to identify stage of chronic kidney disease (N18.1-N18.6)

E11.29 Other complication
Including: renal tubular degeneration

E11.3- **Type 2 diabetes mellitus with ophthalmic complications**
Indicator(s): CMS22: 18 | CMS24: 18 | RxØ5: 3Ø | HHSØ5: 2Ø | HHSØ7: 2Ø

E11.31- **Type 2 diabetes mellitus with unspecified diabetic retinopathy**

E11.311 With macular edema

E11.319 Without macular edema

E11.32- **Type 2 diabetes mellitus with mild nonproliferative diabetic retinopathy**
Including: with nonproliferative diabetic retinopathy NOS

One of the following 7th characters is to be assigned to codes in subcategory E11.32 to designate laterality of the disease:
1 - right eye
2 - left eye
3 - bilateral
9 - unspecified eye

E11.321_ With macular edema

E11.329_ Without macular edema

E11.33- **Type 2 diabetes mellitus with moderate nonproliferative diabetic retinopathy**

One of the following 7th characters is to be assigned to codes in subcategory E11.33 to designate laterality of the disease:
1 - right eye
2 - left eye
3 - bilateral
9 - unspecified eye

E11.331_ With macular edema

E11.339_ Without macular edema

E11.34- **Type 2 diabetes mellitus with severe nonproliferative diabetic retinopathy**

One of the following 7th characters is to be assigned to codes in subcategory E11.34 to designate laterality of the disease:
1 - right eye
2 - left eye
3 - bilateral
9 - unspecified eye

E11.341_ With macular edema

E11.349_ Without macular edema

E11.35- **Type 2 diabetes mellitus with proliferative diabetic retinopathy**

One of the following 7th characters is to be assigned to codes in subcategory E11.35 to designate laterality of the disease:
1 - right eye
2 - left eye
3 - bilateral
9 - unspecified eye

E11.351_ With macular edema

E11.352_ With traction retinal detachment involving the macula

E11.353_ With traction retinal detachment not involving the macula

E11.354_ With combined traction retinal detachment and rhegmatogenous retinal detachment

E11.355_ With stable proliferative diabetic retinopathy

E11.359_ Without macular edema

E11.36 Diabetic cataract

E11.37x_ Diabetic macular edema, resolved following treatment

One of the following 7th characters is to be assigned to code E11.37 to designate laterality of the disease:
1 - right eye
2 - left eye
3 - bilateral
9 - unspecified eye

E11.39 Other complication
Use additional code to identify manifestation, such as:
diabetic glaucoma (H4Ø-H42)

E11.4- **Type 2 diabetes mellitus with neurological complications**
Indicator(s): CMS22: 18 | CMS24: 18 | RxØ5: 3Ø | HHSØ5: 2Ø | HHSØ7: 2Ø

E11.4Ø Diabetic neuropathy, unspecified

E11.41 Diabetic mononeuropathy

E11.42 Diabetic polyneuropathy
Including: neuralgia

E11.43 Diabetic autonomic (poly)neuropathy
Including: gastroparesis

E11.44 Diabetic amyotrophy

E11.49 Other complication

E11.5- **Type 2 diabetes mellitus with circulatory complications**
Indicator(s): CMS22: 18 | CMS24: 18 | RxØ5: 3Ø | ESRD21: 18 | HHSØ5: 2Ø | HHSØ7: 2Ø

E11.51 Diabetic peripheral angiopathy without gangrene

E11.52 Diabetic peripheral angiopathy with gangrene
Including: gangrene
Indicator(s): CC

E11.59 Other complication

E11.6- **Type 2 diabetes mellitus with other specified complications**
Indicator(s): RxØ5: 3Ø

E11.61- **Type 2 diabetes mellitus with diabetic arthropathy**

E11.61Ø Neuropathic
Including: Charcôt's joints

E11.618 Other arthropathy

E11.62- **Type 2 diabetes mellitus with skin complications**

E11.62Ø Diabetic dermatitis
Including: necrobiosis lipoidica

E11.621 Foot ulcer
Use additional code to identify site of ulcer (L97.4-, L97.5-)

E11.622 Other skin ulcer
Use additional code to identify site of ulcer (L97.1-L97.9, L98.41-L98.49)

E11.628 Other complication

E11.63- **Type 2 diabetes mellitus with oral complications**

E11.63Ø Periodontal disease

E11.638 Other complication

E11.64- **Type 2 diabetes mellitus with hypoglycemia**

E11.641 With coma
Indicator(s): MCC

E11.649 Without coma

E11.65 Hyperglycemia

E11.69 Other complication
Use additional code to identify complication

E11.8 Type 2 diabetes mellitus with unspecified complications
Indicator(s): CMS22: 18 | CMS24: 18 | RxØ5: 3Ø | ESRD21: 18 | HHSØ5: 2Ø | HHSØ7: 21

E11.9 Type 2 diabetes mellitus without complications
Indicator(s): QAdmit | CMS22: 19 | CMS24: 19 | RxØ5: 31 | ESRD21: 19 | HHSØ5: 21 | HHSØ7: 21

E13- OTHER SPECIFIED DIABETES MELLITUS

Includes:
diabetes mellitus due to genetic defects of beta-cell function
diabetes mellitus due to genetic defects in insulin action
postpancreatectomy diabetes mellitus
postprocedural diabetes mellitus
secondary diabetes mellitus NEC

Use additional code to identify control using:
insulin (Z79.4)
oral antidiabetic drugs (Z79.84)
oral hypoglycemic drugs (Z79.84)

Excludes1:
diabetes (mellitus) due to autoimmune process (E1Ø.-)
diabetes (mellitus) due to immune mediated pancreatic islet beta-cell destruction (E1Ø.-)
diabetes mellitus due to underlying condition (EØ8.-)
drug or chemical induced diabetes mellitus (EØ9.-)
gestational diabetes (O24.4-)
neonatal diabetes mellitus (P7Ø.2)
type 1 diabetes mellitus (E1Ø.-)

See Guidelines: 1;C.4.a.6

E13.Ø- **Other specified diabetes mellitus with hyperosmolarity**
Indicator(s): MCC | HAC: Ø9 | CMS22: 17 | CMS24: 17 | RxØ5: 3Ø | ESRD21: 17 | HHSØ5: 19 | HHSØ7: 19

E13.ØØ Without nonketotic hyperglycemic-hyperosmolar coma (NKHHC)
Excludes2:
type 2 diabetes mellitus (E11.-)

E13.Ø1 With coma

E13.1- **Other specified diabetes mellitus with ketoacidosis**
Indicator(s): MCC | HAC: Ø9 | CMS22: 17 | CMS24: 17 | RxØ5: 3Ø | ESRD21: 17 | HHSØ5: 19 | HHSØ7: 19

E13.1Ø Without coma

E13.11 With coma

E13.2- **Other specified diabetes mellitus with kidney complications**
Indicator(s): CMS22: 18 | CMS24: 18 | RxØ5: 3Ø | ESRD21: 18 | HHSØ5: 2Ø | HHSØ7: 2Ø

E13.21 Diabetic nephropathy
Including: intercapillary glomerulosclerosis, intracapillary glomerulonephrosis, Kimmelstiel-Wilson disease

E13.22 Diabetic chronic kidney disease
Use additional code to identify stage of chronic kidney disease (N18.1-N18.6)

E13.29 Other complication
Including: renal tubular degeneration

E13.3- **Other specified diabetes mellitus with ophthalmic complications**
Indicator(s): CMS22: 18 | CMS24: 18 | RxØ5: 3Ø | HHSØ5: 2Ø | HHSØ7: 2Ø

E13.31- **Other specified diabetes mellitus with unspecified diabetic retinopathy**

E13.311 With macular edema

E13.319 Without macular edema

E13.32- **Other specified diabetes mellitus with mild nonproliferative diabetic retinopathy**
Including: with nonproliferative diabetic retinopathy NOS
One of the following 7th characters is to be assigned to codes in subcategory E13.32 to designate laterality of the disease:
1 - right eye
2 - left eye
3 - bilateral
9 - unspecified eye

E13.321_ With macular edema

E13.329_ Without macular edema

E13.33- **Other specified diabetes mellitus with moderate nonproliferative diabetic retinopathy**
One of the following 7th characters is to be assigned to codes in subcategory E13.33 to designate laterality of the disease:
1 - right eye
2 - left eye
3 - bilateral
9 - unspecified eye

E13.331_ With macular edema

E13.339_ Without macular edema

E13.34- **Other specified diabetes mellitus with severe nonproliferative diabetic retinopathy**
One of the following 7th characters is to be assigned to codes in subcategory E13.34 to designate laterality of the disease:
1 - right eye
2 - left eye
3 - bilateral
9 - unspecified eye

E13.341_ With macular edema

E13.349_ Without macular edema

E13.35- **Other specified diabetes mellitus with proliferative diabetic retinopathy**
One of the following 7th characters is to be assigned to codes in subcategory E13.35 to designate laterality of the disease:
1 - right eye
2 - left eye
3 - bilateral
9 - unspecified eye

E13.351_ With macular edema

E13.352_ With traction retinal detachment involving the macula

E13.353_ With traction retinal detachment not involving the macula

E13.354_ With combined traction retinal detachment and rhegmatogenous retinal detachment

E13.355_ With stable proliferative diabetic retinopathy

E13.359_ Without macular edema

E13.36 Diabetic cataract

E13.37x_ Diabetic macular edema, resolved following treatment
One of the following 7th characters is to be assigned to code E13.37 to designate laterality of the disease:
1 - right eye
2 - left eye
3 - bilateral
9 - unspecified eye

E13.39 Other complication
Use additional code to identify manifestation, such as:
diabetic glaucoma (H40-H42)

E13.4- **Other specified diabetes mellitus with neurological complications**
Indicator(s): CMS22: 18 | CMS24: 18 | Rx05: 30 | HHS05: 20 | HHS07: 20

E13.40 Diabetic neuropathy, unspecified

E13.41 Diabetic mononeuropathy

E13.42 Diabetic polyneuropathy
Including: neuralgia

E13.43 Diabetic autonomic (poly)neuropathy
Including: gastroparesis

E13.44 Diabetic amyotrophy

E13.49 Other complication

E13.5- **Other specified diabetes mellitus with circulatory complications**
Indicator(s): CMS22: 18 | CMS24: 18 | Rx05: 30 | ESRD21: 18 | HHS05: 20 | HHS07: 20

E13.51 Diabetic peripheral angiopathy without gangrene

E13.52 Diabetic peripheral angiopathy with gangrene
Including: gangrene
Indicator(s): CC

E13.59 Other complication

E13.6- **Other specified diabetes mellitus with other specified complications**
Indicator(s): Rx05: 30

E13.61- **Other specified diabetes mellitus with diabetic arthropathy**

E13.610 Neuropathic
Including: Charcôt's joints

E13.618 Other arthropathy

E13.62- **Other specified diabetes mellitus with skin complications**

E13.620 Diabetic dermatitis
Including: necrobiosis lipoidica

E13.621 Foot ulcer
Use additional code to identify site of ulcer (L97.4-, L97.5-)

E13.622 Other skin ulcer
Use additional code to identify site of ulcer (L97.1-L97.9, L98.41-L98.49)

E13.628 Other complication

E13.63- **Other specified diabetes mellitus with oral complications**

E13.630 Periodontal disease

E13.638 Other complication

Ch5

5. The Tabular List

E13.64- **Other specified diabetes mellitus with hypoglycemia**

E13.641 **With coma**
Indicator(s): MCC

E13.649 **Without coma**

E13.65 **Hyperglycemia**

E13.69 **Other complication**
Use additional code to identify complication

E13.8 **Other specified diabetes mellitus with unspecified complications**
Indicator(s): CMS22: 18 | CMS24: 18 | RxØ5: 3Ø | ESRD21: 18 | HHSØ5: 2Ø | HHSØ7: 21

E13.9 **Other specified diabetes mellitus without complications**
Indicator(s): QAdmit | CMS22: 19 | CMS24: 19 | RxØ5: 31 | ESRD21: 19 | HHSØ5: 21 | HHSØ7: 21

OTHER DISORDERS OF GLUCOSE REGULATION AND PANCREATIC INTERNAL SECRETION (E15-E16)

E16- OTHER DISORDERS OF PANCREATIC INTERNAL SECRETION

E16.2 **Hypoglycemia, unspecified**
Excludes1:
diabetes with hypoglycemia (EØ8.649, E1Ø.649, E11.649, E13.649)

DISORDERS OF OTHER ENDOCRINE GLANDS (E2Ø-E35)

Excludes1:
galactorrhea (N64.3)
gynecomastia (N62)

E2Ø- HYPOPARATHYROIDISM
Excludes1:
Di George's syndrome (D82.1)
postprocedural hypoparathyroidism (E89.2)
tetany NOS (R29.Ø)
transitory neonatal hypoparathyroidism (P71.4)

E2Ø.Ø **Idiopathic**
Indicator(s): CMS22: 23 | CMS24: 23 | RxØ5: 41 | ESRD21: 23 | HHSØ5: 3Ø | HHSØ7: 3Ø

E2Ø.1 **Pseudohypoparathyroidism**

E2Ø.8 **Other**
Indicator(s): CMS22: 23 | CMS24: 23 | RxØ5: 41 | ESRD21: 23 | HHSØ5: 3Ø | HHSØ7: 3Ø

E2Ø.9 **Unspecified**
Including: Parathyroid tetany
Indicator(s): CMS22: 23 | CMS24: 23 | RxØ5: 41 | ESRD21: 23 | HHSØ5: 3Ø | HHSØ7: 3Ø

E21- HYPERPARATHYROIDISM AND OTHER DISORDERS OF PARATHYROID GLAND
Excludes1:
adult osteomalacia (M83.-)
ectopic hyperparathyroidism (E34.2)
hungry bone syndrome (E83.81)
infantile and juvenile osteomalacia (E55.Ø)
Excludes2:
familial hypocalciuric hypercalcemia (E83.52)
Indicator(s): CMS22: 23 | CMS24: 23 | RxØ5: 41 | ESRD21: 23 | HHSØ5: 3Ø | HHSØ7: 3Ø

E21.Ø **Primary hyperparathyroidism**
Including: Hyperplasia of parathyroid, Osteitis fibrosa cystica generalisata [von Recklinghausen's disease of bone]

E21.1 **Secondary hyperparathyroidism, NEC**
Excludes1:
secondary hyperparathyroidism of renal origin (N25.81)

E21.2 **Other hyperparathyroidism**
Including: Tertiary
Excludes1:
familial hypocalciuric hypercalcemia (E83.52)

E21.3 **Hyperparathyroidism, unspecified**

E34- OTHER ENDOCRINE DISORDERS
Excludes1:
pseudohypoparathyroidism (E2Ø.1)

E34.3- **Short stature due to endocrine disorder**
Including: Constitutional, Laron-type
Excludes1:
achondroplastic short stature (Q77.4)
hypochondroplastic short stature (Q77.4)
nutritional short stature (E45)
pituitary short stature (E23.Ø)
progeria (E34.8)
renal short stature (N25.Ø)
Russell-Silver syndrome (Q87.19)
short-limbed stature with immunodeficiency (D82.2)
short stature in specific dysmorphic syndromes - code to syndrome - see Alphabetical Index
short stature NOS (R62.52)

N **E34.3Ø** **Unspecified**

N **E34.31** **Constitutional short stature**
Including: delay of growth, puberty, or maturation

E34.32- **Genetic causes**

N **E34.321** **Primary insulin-like growth factor-1 (IGF-1) deficiency**
Including: Acid-labile subunit gene (IGFALS) defect, Growth hormone gene 1 (GH1) defect with growth hormone neutralizing antibodies, Growth hormone insensitivity syndrome (GHIS), Insulin-like growth factor 1 gene (IGF1) defect, Laron type short stature, Severe primary insulin-like growth factor-1 deficiency (SPIGFD), Signal transducer and activator of transcription 5B gene (STAT5b) defect

N **E34.322** **Insulin-like growth factor-1 (IGF-1) resistance**
Including: Genetic syndrome with resistance to insulin-like growth factor-1, receptor (IGF-1R) defect, Post-insulin-like growth factor-1 receptor signaling defect

N **E34.328** **Other**
Including: Short stature due to: ACAN gene variant, aggrecan deficiency, NPR-2 gene variant

N **E34.329** **Unspecified**

N **E34.39** **Other**

 See Appendix A — Coding Reference Tables for lists of the ICD-10-CM Tabular indicators, HAC categories, and HCC codes.

Ch5
5. The Tabular List

OTHER NUTRITIONAL DEFICIENCIES (E5Ø-E64)

Excludes2:
nutritional anemias (D5Ø-D53)

E55- VITAMIN D DEFICIENCY
Excludes1:
adult osteomalacia (M83.-)
osteoporosis (M8Ø.-)
sequelae of rickets (E64.3)

E55.9 Unspecified
Including: Avitaminosis D

OVERWEIGHT, OBESITY AND OTHER HYPERALIMENTATION (E65-E68)

E66- OVERWEIGHT AND OBESITY
Code First:
obesity complicating pregnancy, childbirth and the puerperium, if applicable (O99.21-)
Use additional code to identify body mass index (BMI), if known (Z68.-)
Excludes1:
adiposogenital dystrophy (E23.6)
lipomatosis NOS (E88.2)
lipomatosis dolorosa [Dercum] (E88.2)
Prader-Willi syndrome (Q87.11)

E66.Ø- **Obesity due to excess calories**

E66.Ø1 Morbid (severe)
Excludes1:
morbid (severe) obesity with alveolar hypoventilation (E66.2)
Indicator(s): HAC: 11 | CMS22: 22 | CMS24: 22 | RxØ5: 43 | ESRD21: 22

E66.Ø9 Other
Indicator(s): QAdmit

E66.1 Drug-induced
Use additional code for adverse effect, if applicable, to identify drug (T36-T5Ø with fifth or sixth character 5)
Indicator(s): QAdmit

E66.2 Morbid (severe) obesity with alveolar hypoventilation
Including: Pickwickian syndrome
Indicator(s): CC | CMS22: 22 | CMS24: 22 | RxØ5: 43 | ESRD21: 22

E66.3 Overweight

E66.8 Other obesity
Indicator(s): QAdmit

E66.9 Obesity, unspecified
Including: Obesity NOS
Indicator(s): QAdmit | DSM-5

METABOLIC DISORDERS (E7Ø-E88)

Excludes1:
androgen insensitivity syndrome (E34.5-)
congenital adrenal hyperplasia (E25.Ø)
hemolytic anemias attributable to enzyme disorders (D55.-)
Marfan's syndrome (Q87.4)
5-alpha-reductase deficiency (E29.1)
Excludes2:
Ehlers-Danlos syndromes (Q79.6-)

E78- DISORDERS OF LIPOPROTEIN METABOLISM AND OTHER LIPIDEMIAS
Excludes1:
sphingolipidosis (E75.Ø-E75.3)

E78.Ø- **Pure hypercholesterolemia**
Including: Familial hypercholesterolemia; Fredrickson's hyperlipoproteinemia, type IIa; Hyperbetalipoproteinemia; Hyperlipidemia, Group A; Low-density-lipoprotein-type [LDL] hyperlipoproteinemia
Indicator(s): RxØ5: 45

E78.ØØ Unspecified
Including: Fredrickson's hyperlipoproteinemia, type IIa; Hyperbetalipoproteinemia; Low-density-lipoprotein-type [LDL] hyperlipoproteinemia; (Pure) hypercholesterolemia NOS

E78.Ø1 Familial

E78.1 Pure hyperglyceridemia
Including: Elevated fasting triglycerides, Endogenous, Fredrickson's hyperlipoproteinemia type IV, Hyperlipidemia group B, Hyperprebetalipoproteinemia, Very-low-density-lipoprotein-type [VLDL] hyperlipoproteinemia
Indicator(s): RxØ5: 45

E78.2 Mixed hyperlipidemia
Including: Broad- or floating-betalipoproteinemia, Combined hyperlipidemia NOS, Elevated cholesterol with elevated triglycerides NEC, Fredrickson's hyperlipoproteinemia type IIb or III, Hyperbetalipoproteinemia with prebetalipoproteinemia, Hypercholesteremia with endogenous hyperglyceridemia, Hyperlipidemia group C, Tubo-eruptive xanthoma, Xanthoma tuberosum
Excludes1:
cerebrotendinous cholesterosis [van Bogaert-Scherer-Epstein] (E75.5)
familial combined hyperlipidemia (E78.49)
Indicator(s): RxØ5: 45

E78.3 Hyperchylomicronemia
Including: Chylomicron retention disease, Fredrickson's hyperlipoproteinemia type I or V, Hyperlipidemia group D, Mixed hyperglyceridemia
Indicator(s): RxØ5: 45

E78.5 Hyperlipidemia, unspecified
Indicator(s): RxØ5: 45

E78.6 Lipoprotein deficiency
Including: Abetalipoproteinemia, Depressed HDL cholesterol, High-density lipoprotein deficiency, Hypoalphalipoproteinemia, Hypobetalipoproteinemia (familial), Lecithin cholesterol acyltransferase, Tangier disease
Indicator(s): RxØ5: 45

5. Mental, Behavioral and Neurodevelopmental disorders (FØ1-F99)

Includes:
disorders of psychological development
Excludes2:
symptoms, signs and abnormal clinical laboratory findings, not elsewhere classified (RØØ-R99)
See Guidelines: 1;C.2Ø.a.1

MENTAL DISORDERS DUE TO KNOWN PHYSIOLOGICAL CONDITIONS (FØ1-FØ9)

Notes:
This block comprises a range of mental disorders grouped together on the basis of their having in common a demonstrable etiology in cerebral disease, brain injury, or other insult leading to cerebral dysfunction. The dysfunction may be primary, as in diseases, injuries, and insults that affect the brain directly and selectively; or secondary, as in systemic diseases and disorders that attack the brain only as one of the multiple organs or systems of the body that are involved.

FØ7- PERSONALITY AND BEHAVIORAL DISORDERS DUE TO KNOWN PHYSIOLOGICAL CONDITION
Code First:
the underlying physiological condition

FØ7.8- **Other**

FØ7.81 Postconcussional syndrome
Including: Postcontusional syndrome (encephalopathy); Post-traumatic brain syndrome, nonpsychotic
Use additional code to identify associated post-traumatic headache, if applicable (G44.3-)
Excludes1:
current concussion (brain) (SØ6.Ø-)
postencephalitic syndrome (FØ7.89)

MENTAL AND BEHAVIORAL DISORDERS DUE TO PSYCHOACTIVE SUBSTANCE USE (F1Ø-F19)

See Guidelines: 1;C.5.b

F1Ø- ALCOHOL RELATED DISORDERS
Use additional code for blood alcohol level, if applicable (Y9Ø.-)
See Guidelines: 1;C.15.l.1

F1Ø.1- **Alcohol abuse**
Excludes1:
alcohol dependence (F1Ø.2-)
alcohol use, unspecified (F1Ø.9-)

F1Ø.1Ø Uncomplicated
Including: Alcohol use disorder, mild
Indicator(s): DSM-5

F1Ø.9- **Alcohol use, unspecified**
Excludes1:
alcohol abuse (F1Ø.1-)
alcohol dependence (F1Ø.2-)
See Guidelines: 1;C.5.b.3

N **F1Ø.9Ø Uncomplicated**

N **F1Ø.91 In remission**

F1Ø.99 With unspecified alcohol-induced disorder
Indicator(s): CC | DSM-5 | CMS22: 55 | CMS24: 55 | ESRD21: 55

F11- OPIOID RELATED DISORDERS
See Guidelines: 1;C.15.i.3

F11.1- **Opioid abuse**
Excludes1:
opioid dependence (F11.2-)
opioid use, unspecified (F11.9-)

F11.1Ø Uncomplicated
Including: Opioid use disorder, mild
Indicator(s): DSM-5 | CMS24: 56

F11.9- **Opioid use, unspecified**
Excludes1:
opioid abuse (F11.1-)
opioid dependence (F11.2-)
See Guidelines: 1;C.5.b.3

N **F11.91 In remission**

F11.99 With unspecified opioid-induced disorder
Indicator(s): DSM-5 | CMS22: 55 | CMS24: 55 | ESRD21: 55 | HHSØ7: 82

F12- CANNABIS RELATED DISORDERS
Includes:
marijuana
See Guidelines: 1;C.15.i.3

F12.1- **Cannabis abuse**
Excludes1:
cannabis dependence (F12.2-)
cannabis use, unspecified (F12.9-)

F12.1Ø Uncomplicated
Including: Cannabis use disorder (mild)
Indicator(s): DSM-5

F12.9- **Cannabis use, unspecified**
Excludes1:
cannabis abuse (F12.1-)
cannabis dependence (F12.2-)
See Guidelines: 1;C.5.b.3

N **F12.91 In remission**

F12.99 With unspecified cannabis-induced disorder
Indicator(s): DSM-5 | CMS22: 55 | CMS24: 55 | ESRD21: 55 | HHSØ7: 82

F13- SEDATIVE, HYPNOTIC, OR ANXIOLYTIC RELATED DISORDERS
See Guidelines: 1;C.15.i.3

F13.9- **Unspecified**
Excludes1:
sedative, hypnotic or anxiolytic-related abuse (F13.1-)
sedative, hypnotic or anxiolytic-related dependence (F13.2-)
See Guidelines: 1;C.5.b.3

N **F13.91 In remission**

F14- COCAINE RELATED DISORDERS
Excludes2:
other stimulant-related disorders (F15.-)
See Guidelines: 1;C.15.i.3

F14.9- **Cocaine use, unspecified**
Excludes1:
cocaine abuse (F14.1-)
cocaine dependence (F14.2-)
See Guidelines: 1;C.5.b.3

N **F14.91 In remission**

F15- OTHER STIMULANT RELATED DISORDERS

Includes:
amphetamine-related disorders
caffeine
Excludes2:
cocaine-related disorders (F14.-)
See Guidelines: 1;C.15.i.3

F15.9- **Other stimulant use, unspecified**
Excludes1:
other stimulant abuse (F15.1-)
other stimulant dependence (F15.2-)
See Guidelines: 1;C.5.b.3

N **F15.91** **In remission**

F16- HALLUCINOGEN RELATED DISORDERS

Includes:
ecstasy
PCP
phencyclidine
See Guidelines: 1;C.15.i.3

F16.9- **Hallucinogen use, unspecified**
Excludes1:
hallucinogen abuse (F16.1-)
hallucinogen dependence (F16.2-)
See Guidelines: 1;C.5.b.3

N **F16.91** **In remission**

F17- NICOTINE DEPENDENCE

Excludes1:
history of tobacco dependence (Z87.891)
tobacco use NOS (Z72.Ø)
Excludes2:
tobacco use (smoking) during pregnancy, childbirth and the puerperium (O99.33-)
toxic effect of nicotine (T65.2-)
See Guidelines: 1;C.15.I.2

F17.2- **Nicotine dependence**

F17.2Ø- **Unspecified**
Indicator(s): DSM-5

F17.2ØØ **Uncomplicated**
Including: Tobacco use disorder (mild, moderate, or severe)
Indicator(s): NoPDx/M

F18- INHALANT RELATED DISORDERS

Includes:
volatile solvents
See Guidelines: 1;C.15.i.3

F18.9- **Inhalant use, unspecified**
Excludes1:
inhalant abuse (F18.1-)
inhalant dependence (F18.2-)

N **F18.91** **In remission**

F19- OTHER PSYCHOACTIVE SUBSTANCE RELATED DISORDERS

Includes:
polysubstance drug use (indiscriminate drug use)
See Guidelines: 1;C.15.i.3

F19.9- **Other, unspecified**
Excludes1:
other psychoactive substance abuse (F19.1-)
other psychoactive substance dependence (F19.2-)

N **F19.91** **In remission**

ANXIETY, DISSOCIATIVE, STRESS-RELATED, SOMATOFORM AND OTHER NONPSYCHOTIC MENTAL DISORDERS (F4Ø-F48)

See Guidelines: 1;C.5.a

F45- SOMATOFORM DISORDERS

Excludes2:
dissociative and conversion disorders (F44.-)
factitious disorders (F68.1-, F68.A)
hair-plucking (F63.3)
lalling (F8Ø.Ø)
lisping (F8Ø.Ø)
malingering [conscious simulation] (Z76.5)
nail-biting (F98.8)
psychological or behavioral factors associated with disorders or diseases classified elsewhere (F54)
sexual dysfunction, not due to a substance or known physiological condition (F52.-)
thumb-sucking (F98.8)
tic disorders (in childhood and adolescence) (F95.-)
Tourette's syndrome (F95.2)
trichotillomania (F63.3)

F45.4- **Pain disorders related to psychological factors**
Excludes1:
pain NOS (R52)

F45.41 **Exclusively related to psychological factors**
Including: Somatoform pain disorder (persistent)

F45.42 **With related psychological factors**
Code Also
associated acute or chronic pain (G89.-)

F45.8 **Other**
Including: Psychogenic dysmenorrhea, Psychogenic dysphagia including 'globus hystericus', Psychogenic pruritus, Psychogenic torticollis, Somatoform autonomic dysfunction, Teeth grinding
Excludes1:
sleep related teeth grinding (G47.63)
Indicator(s): DSM-5 | RxØ5: 135

F45.9 **Unspecified**
Including: Psychosomatic disorder NOS
Indicator(s): DSM-5 | RxØ5: 135

BEHAVIORAL SYNDROMES ASSOCIATED WITH PHYSIOLOGICAL DISTURBANCES AND PHYSICAL FACTORS (F5Ø-F59)

F5Ø- EATING DISORDERS

Excludes1:
anorexia NOS (R63.Ø)
feeding problems of newborn (P92.-)
polyphagia (R63.2)
Excludes2:
feeding difficulties (R63.3)
feeding disorder in infancy or childhood (F98.2-)

F5Ø.Ø- **Anorexia nervosa**
Excludes1:
loss of appetite (R63.Ø)
psychogenic loss of appetite (F5Ø.89)
Indicator(s): CC | RxØ5: 133 | HHSØ5: 94 | HHSØ7: 94

F5Ø.ØØ **Unspecified**

F51- SLEEP DISORDERS NOT DUE TO A SUBSTANCE OR KNOWN PHYSIOLOGICAL CONDITION

Excludes2:
organic sleep disorders (G47.-)

F51.9 Unspecified
Including: Emotional sleep disorder NOS

F55- ABUSE OF NON-PSYCHOACTIVE SUBSTANCES

Excludes2:
abuse of psychoactive substances (F1Ø-F19)

F55.1 Herbal or folk remedies

INTELLECTUAL DISABILITIES (F7Ø-F79)

Code First:
any associated physical or developmental disorders
Excludes1:
borderline intellectual functioning, IQ above 7Ø to 84 (R41.83)

F7Ø Mild intellectual disabilities
Including: IQ level 5Ø-55 to approximately 7Ø, Mild mental subnormality
Indicator(s): DSM-5 | RxØ5: 148

F71 Moderate intellectual disabilities
Including: IQ level 35-4Ø to 5Ø-55, Moderate mental subnormality
Indicator(s): DSM-5 | RxØ5: 147

F72 Severe intellectual disabilities
Including: IQ 2Ø-25 to 35-4Ø, Severe mental subnormality
Indicator(s): CC | DSM-5 | RxØ5: 146

F73 Profound intellectual disabilities
Including: IQ level below 2Ø-25, Profound mental subnormality
Indicator(s): CC | DSM-5 | RxØ5: 146

F79 Unspecified intellectual disabilities
Including: Mental deficiency NOS, Mental subnormality NOS
Indicator(s): DSM-5 | RxØ5: 148

PERVASIVE AND SPECIFIC DEVELOPMENTAL DISORDERS (F8Ø-F89)

F84- PERVASIVE DEVELOPMENTAL DISORDERS

Code Also
any associated medical condition and intellectual disabilities
Indicator(s): CC | RxØ5: 145

F84.Ø Autistic disorder
Including: Autism spectrum disorder, Infantile autism, Infantile psychosis, Kanner's syndrome
Excludes1:
Asperger's syndrome (F84.5)
Indicator(s): DSM-5

F84.5 Asperger's syndrome
Including: Asperger's disorder, Autistic psychopathy, Schizoid disorder of childhood

F84.8 Other
Including: Overactive disorder associated with intellectual disabilities and stereotyped movements

F88 Other disorders of psychological development
Including: Developmental agnosia, Global developmental delay, Other specified neurodevelopmental disorder
Indicator(s): DSM-5

F89 Unspecified disorder of psychological development
Including: Developmental disorder NOS, Neurodevelopmental disorder NOS
Indicator(s): DSM-5

BEHAVIORAL AND EMOTIONAL DISORDERS WITH ONSET USUALLY OCCURRING IN CHILDHOOD AND ADOLESCENCE (F9Ø-F98)

Notes:
Codes within categories F9Ø-F98 may be used regardless of the age of a patient. These disorders generally have onset within the childhood or adolescent years, but may continue throughout life or not be diagnosed until adulthood

F9Ø- ATTENTION-DEFICIT HYPERACTIVITY DISORDERS

Includes:
attention deficit disorder with hyperactivity
attention deficit syndrome with hyperactivity
Excludes2:
anxiety disorders (F4Ø.-, F41.-)
mood [affective] disorders (F3Ø-F39)
pervasive developmental disorders (F84.-)
schizophrenia (F2Ø.-)
Indicator(s): DSM-5 | RxØ5: 133

F9Ø.9 Unspecified type
Including: disorder of childhood or adolescence NOS, disorder NOS

F91- CONDUCT DISORDERS

Excludes1:
antisocial behavior (Z72.81-)
antisocial personality disorder (F6Ø.2)
Excludes2:
conduct problems associated with attention-deficit hyperactivity disorder (F9Ø.-)
mood [affective] disorders (F3Ø-F39)
pervasive developmental disorders (F84.-)
schizophrenia (F2Ø.-)
Indicator(s): RxØ5: 133

F91.9 Unspecified
Including: Behavioral NOS, Conduct NOS, Disruptive behavior NOS
Indicator(s): DSM-5

F93- EMOTIONAL DISORDERS WITH ONSET SPECIFIC TO CHILDHOOD

F93.9 Unspecified

F94- DISORDERS OF SOCIAL FUNCTIONING WITH ONSET SPECIFIC TO CHILDHOOD AND ADOLESCENCE

F94.9 Unspecified

F98- OTHER BEHAVIORAL AND EMOTIONAL DISORDERS WITH ONSET USUALLY OCCURRING IN CHILDHOOD AND ADOLESCENCE

Excludes2:
breath-holding spells (RØ6.89)
gender identity disorder of childhood (F64.2)
Kleine-Levin syndrome (G47.13)
obsessive-compulsive disorder (F42.-)
sleep disorders not due to a substance or known physiological condition (F51.-)

F98.9 Unspecified

F99 UNSPECIFIED MENTAL DISORDER (F99) (F99-F99)

F99 Mental disorder, not otherwise specified
Including: Mental illness NOS
Excludes1:
unspecified mental disorder due to known physiological condition (FØ9)
Indicator(s): DSM-5

6. Diseases of the nervous system (GØØ-G99)

Excludes2:
certain conditions originating in the perinatal period (PØ4-P96)
certain infectious and parasitic diseases (AØØ-B99)
complications of pregnancy, childbirth and the puerperium (OØØ-O9A)
congenital malformations, deformations, and chromosomal abnormalities (QØØ-Q99)
endocrine, nutritional and metabolic diseases (EØØ-E88)
injury, poisoning and certain other consequences of external causes (SØØ-T88)
neoplasms (CØØ-D49)
symptoms, signs and abnormal clinical and laboratory findings, not elsewhere classified (RØØ-R94)
See Guidelines: 1;C.2Ø.a.1

SYSTEMIC ATROPHIES PRIMARILY AFFECTING THE CENTRAL NERVOUS SYSTEM (G1Ø-G14)

G1Ø Huntington's disease
Including: Huntington's chorea and dementia
Use additional code, if applicable, to identify:
dementia with anxiety (FØ2.84, FØ2.A4, FØ2.B4, FØ2.C4)
dementia with behavioral disturbance (FØ2.81-, FØ2.A1-, FØ2.B1-, FØ2.C1-)
dementia with mood disturbance (FØ2.83, FØ2.A3, FØ2.B3, FØ2.C3)
dementia with psychotic disturbance (FØ2.82, FØ2.A2, FØ2.B2, FØ2.C2)
dementia without behavioral disturbance (FØ2.8Ø, FØ2.AØ, FØ2.BØ, FØ2.CØ)
mild neurocognitive disorder due to known physiological condition (FØ6.7-)
Indicator(s): CC | DSM-5 | CMS22: 78 | CMS24: 78 | RxØ5: 161 | ESRD21: 78 | HHSØ5: 119

G12- SPINAL MUSCULAR ATROPHY AND RELATED SYNDROMES
Indicator(s): CC | HHSØ5: 111 | HHSØ7: 111

G12.Ø Infantile, type I [Werdnig-Hoffman]

G12.1 Other inherited
Including: Adult form; Childhood form, type II; Distal; Juvenile form, type III [Kugelberg-Welander]; Progressive bulbar palsy of childhood [Fazio-Londe]; Scapuloperoneal form

G12.2- **Motor neuron disease**

G12.2Ø Unspecified

G12.21 Amyotrophic lateral sclerosis
Indicator(s): Adult

G12.22 Progressive bulbar palsy

G12.23 Primary lateral sclerosis

G12.24 Familial

G12.25 Progressive spinal muscle atrophy

G12.29 Other

G12.8 Other

G12.9 Unspecified

G14 Postpolio syndrome
Includes:
postpolio myelitic syndrome
Excludes1:
sequelae of poliomyelitis (B91)

EXTRAPYRAMIDAL AND MOVEMENT DISORDERS (G2Ø-G26)

G2Ø Parkinson's disease
Including: Hemiparkinsonism, Idiopathic Parkinsonism, Paralysis agitans, Parkinsonism NOS, Primary Parkinsonism
Use additional code, if applicable, to identify:
dementia with anxiety (FØ2.84, FØ2.A4, FØ2.B4, FØ2.C4)
dementia with behavioral disturbance (FØ2.81-, FØ2.A1-, FØ2.B1-, FØ2.C1-)
dementia with mood disturbance (FØ2.83, FØ2.A3, FØ2.B3, FØ2.C3)
dementia with psychotic disturbance (FØ2.82, FØ2.A2, FØ2.B2, FØ2.C2)
dementia without behavioral disturbance (FØ2.8Ø, FØ2.AØ, FØ2.BØ, FØ2.CØ)
mild neurocognitive disorder due to known physiological condition (FØ6.7-)
Indicator(s): DSM-5 | CMS22: 78 | CMS24: 78 | RxØ5: 161 | ESRD21: 78 | HHSØ5: 119

G24- DYSTONIA
Includes:
dyskinesia
Excludes2:
athetoid cerebral palsy (G8Ø.3)

G24.Ø- **Drug induced dystonia**
Use additional code for adverse effect, if applicable, to identify drug (T36-T5Ø with fifth or sixth character 5)
Indicator(s): DSM-5

G24.Ø9 Other
Indicator(s): CC

G24.1 Genetic torsion
Including: Dystonia deformans progressiva, Dystonia musculorum deformans, Familial, Idiopathic familial, Idiopathic (torsion) dystonia NOS, (Schwalbe-) Ziehen-Oppenheim disease

G24.2 Idiopathic nonfamilial
Indicator(s): CC

G24.3 Spasmodic torticollis
Excludes1:
congenital torticollis (Q68.Ø)
hysterical torticollis (F44.4)
ocular torticollis (R29.891)
psychogenic torticollis (F45.8)
torticollis NOS (M43.6)
traumatic recurrent torticollis (S13.4)

G25- OTHER EXTRAPYRAMIDAL AND MOVEMENT DISORDERS
Excludes2:
sleep related movement disorders (G47.6-)

G25.Ø Essential tremor
Including: Familial tremor
Excludes1:
tremor NOS (R25.1)

G25.1 Drug-induced tremor
Use additional code for adverse effect, if applicable, to identify drug (T36-T5Ø with fifth or sixth character 5)
Indicator(s): DSM-5

G25.2 Other specified forms of tremor
Including: Intention tremor

G25.3 Myoclonus
Including: Drug-induced, Palatal myoclonus
Use additional code for adverse effect, if applicable, to identify drug (T36-T5Ø with fifth or sixth character 5)
Excludes1:
facial myokymia (G51.4)
myoclonic epilepsy (G4Ø.-)

G25.4 **Drug-induced chorea**
Use additional code for adverse effect, if applicable, to identify drug (T36-T5Ø with fifth or sixth character 5)

G25.5 **Other chorea**
Including: Chorea NOS
Excludes1:
chorea NOS with heart involvement (IØ2.Ø)
Huntington's chorea (G1Ø)
rheumatic chorea (IØ2.-)
Sydenham's chorea (IØ2.-)

G25.6- **Drug induced tics and other tics of organic origin**

G25.61 **Drug induced tics**
Use additional code for adverse effect, if applicable, to identify drug (T36-T5Ø with fifth or sixth character 5)

G25.69 **Other tics of organic origin**
Excludes1:
habit spasm (F95.9)
tic NOS (F95.9)
Tourette's syndrome (F95.2)

G25.7- **Other and unspecified drug induced movement disorders**
Use additional code for adverse effect, if applicable, to identify drug (T36-T5Ø with fifth or sixth character 5)

G25.7Ø **Unspecified**

G25.71 **Akathisia**
Including: Acathisia, Neuroleptic-induced acute akathisia, Tardive akathisia
Indicator(s): DSM-5

G25.79 **Other**
Indicator(s): DSM-5

G25.8- **Other specified extrapyramidal and movement disorders**

G25.81 **Restless legs syndrome**
Indicator(s): DSM-5

G25.82 **Stiff-man syndrome**
Indicator(s): CC

G25.83 **Benign shuddering attacks**

G25.89 **Other**

G25.9 **Unspecified**
Indicator(s): CC

OTHER DEGENERATIVE DISEASES OF THE NERVOUS SYSTEM (G3Ø-G32)

G3Ø- ALZHEIMER'S DISEASE

Includes:
Alzheimer's dementia senile and presenile forms
Use additional code, if applicable, to identify:
delirium, if applicable (FØ5)
dementia with anxiety (FØ2.84, FØ2.A4, FØ2.B4, FØ2.C4)
dementia with behavioral disturbance (FØ2.81-, FØ2.A1-, FØ2.B1-, FØ2.C1-)
dementia with mood disturbance (FØ2.83, FØ2.A3, FØ2.B3, FØ2.C3)
dementia with psychotic disturbance (FØ2.82, FØ2.A2, FØ2.B2, FØ2.C2)
dementia without behavioral disturbance (FØ2.8Ø, FØ2.AØ, FØ2.BØ, FØ2.CØ)
mild neurocognitive disorder due to known physiological condition (FØ6.7-)
Excludes1:
senile degeneration of brain NEC (G31.1)
senile dementia NOS (FØ3)
senility NOS (R41.81)
Indicator(s): CMS24: 52 | RxØ5: 111 | ESRD21: 52

G3Ø.9 **Unspecified**
Indicator(s): DSM-5

DEMYELINATING DISEASES OF THE CENTRAL NERVOUS SYSTEM (G35-G37)

G35 **Multiple sclerosis**
Including: Disseminated, Generalized, NOS, of brain stem, of cord
Indicator(s): CMS22: 77 | CMS24: 77 | RxØ5: 16Ø | ESRD21: 77 | HHSØ5: 118 | HHSØ7: 118

EPISODIC AND PAROXYSMAL DISORDERS (G4Ø-G47)

G4Ø- EPILEPSY AND RECURRENT SEIZURES

Notes:
the following terms are to be considered equivalent to intractable: pharmacoresistant (pharmacologically resistant), treatment resistant, refractory (medically) and poorly controlled
Excludes1:
conversion disorder with seizures (F44.5)
convulsions NOS (R56.9)
post traumatic seizures (R56.1)
seizure (convulsive) NOS (R56.9)
seizure of newborn (P9Ø)
Excludes2:
hippocampal sclerosis (G93.81)
mesial temporal sclerosis (G93.81)
temporal sclerosis (G93.81)
Todd's paralysis (G83.84)
Indicator(s): CMS22: 79 | ESRD21: 79 | HHSØ7: 12Ø

G4Ø.8- **Other epilepsy and recurrent seizures**
Including: Epilepsies and epileptic syndromes undetermined as to whether they are focal or generalized, Landau-Kleffner syndrome
Indicator(s): CC

G4Ø.89 **Other seizures**
Excludes1:
post traumatic seizures (R56.1)
recurrent seizures NOS (G4Ø.9Ø9)
seizure NOS (R56.9)

G4Ø.9- **Epilepsy, unspecified**

G4Ø.9Ø- **Not intractable**
Including: without intractability

G4Ø.9Ø1 **With status epilepticus**

G4Ø.9Ø9 **Without status epilepticus**
Including: Epilepsy NOS, Epileptic convulsions NOS, Epileptic fits NOS, Epileptic seizures NOS, Recurrent seizures NOS, Seizure disorder NOS

G4Ø.91- **Intractable**
Including: Intractable seizure disorder NOS
Indicator(s): CC

G4Ø.911 **With status epilepticus**

G4Ø.919 **Without status epilepticus**

G43- MIGRAINE

Notes:
the following terms are to be considered equivalent to intractable: pharmacoresistant (pharmacologically resistant), treatment resistant, refractory (medically) and poorly controlled
Use additional code for adverse effect, if applicable, to identify drug (T36-T5Ø with fifth or sixth character 5)
Excludes1:
headache NOS (R51.9)
lower half migraine (G44.ØØ)
Excludes2:
headache syndromes (G44.-)
Indicator(s): RxØ5: 166

G43.Ø- **Migraine without aura**
Including: Common migraine
Excludes1:
chronic migraine without aura (G43.7-)

G43.ØØ- **Not intractable**
Including: without mention of refractory migraine

G43.ØØ1 With status migrainosus

G43.ØØ9 Without status migrainosus
Including: without aura NOS

G43.Ø1- **Intractable**
Including: with refractory migraine

G43.Ø11 With status migrainosus

G43.Ø19 Without status migrainosus

G43.1- **Migraine with aura**
Including: Basilar migraine, Classical migraine, Migraine equivalents, Migraine preceded or accompanied by transient focal neurological phenomena, Migraine triggered seizures, Migraine with acute-onset aura, Migraine with aura without headache (migraine equivalents), Migraine with prolonged aura, Migraine with typical aura, Retinal migraine
Code Also
any associated seizure (G4Ø.-, R56.9)
Excludes1:
persistent migraine aura (G43.5-, G43.6-)

G43.1Ø- **Not intractable**
Including: without mention of refractory migraine

G43.1Ø1 With status migrainosus

G43.1Ø9 Without status migrainosus
Including: with aura NOS

G43.11- **Intractable**
Including: with refractory migraine

G43.111 With status migrainosus

G43.119 Without status migrainosus

G43.4- **Hemiplegic migraine**
Including: Familial, Sporadic

G43.4Ø- **Not intractable**
Including: without refractory migraine

G43.4Ø1 With status migrainosus

G43.4Ø9 Without status migrainosus
Including: Hemiplegic migraine NOS

G43.41- **Intractable**
Including: refractory migraine

G43.411 With status migrainosus

G43.419 Without status migrainosus

G43.5- **Persistent migraine aura without cerebral infarction**

G43.5Ø- **Not intractable**
Including: without refractory migraine

G43.5Ø1 With status migrainosus

G43.5Ø9 Without status migrainosus
Including: Persistent migraine aura NOS

G43.51- **Intractable**
Including: with refractory migraine

G43.511 With status migrainosus

G43.519 Without status migrainosus

G43.6- **Persistent migraine aura with cerebral infarction**
Code Also
the type of cerebral infarction (I63.-)
Indicator(s): *CC*

G43.6Ø- **Not intractable**
Including: without refractory migraine

G43.6Ø1 With status migrainosus

G43.6Ø9 Without status migrainosus

G43.61- **Intractable**
Including: with refractory migraine

G43.611 With status migrainosus

G43.619 Without status migrainosus

G43.7- **Chronic migraine without aura**
Including: Transformed migraine
Excludes1:
migraine without aura (G43.Ø-)

G43.7Ø- **Not intractable**
Including: without refractory migraine

G43.7Ø1 With status migrainosus

G43.7Ø9 Without status migrainosus
Including: Chronic migraine without aura NOS

G43.71- **Intractable**
Including: with refractory migraine

G43.711 With status migrainosus

G43.719 Witout status migrainosus

G43.8- **Other migraine**

G43.8Ø- **Other migraine, not intractable**
Including: without refractory migraine

G43.8Ø1 With status migrainosus

G43.8Ø9 Without status migrainosus

G43.81- **Other migraine, intractable**
Including: with refractory migraine

G43.811 With status migrainosus

G43.819 Without status migrainosus

G43.82- **Menstrual migraine, not intractable**
Including: Menstrual headache, without refractory migraine, Menstrually related migraine, Pre-menstrual headache, Pre-menstrual migraine, Pure menstrual migraine
Code Also
associated premenstrual tension syndrome (N94.3)

G43.821 With status migrainosus

G43.829 Without status migrainosus
Including: Menstrual migraine NOS

G43.83- **Menstrual migraine, intractable**
Including: Menstrual headache, with refractory migraine, Menstrually related migraine, Pre-menstrual headache, Pre-menstrual migraine, Pure menstrual migraine
Code Also
associated premenstrual tension syndrome (N94.3)

G43.831 With status migrainosus

G43.839 Without status migrainosus

G43.9- **Migraine, unspecified**

G43.9Ø- **Not intractable**
Including: without refractory migraine

G43.9Ø1 **With status migrainosus**
Including: Status migrainosus NOS

G43.9Ø9 **Without status migrainosus**
Including: Migraine NOS

G43.91- **Intractable**
Including: with refractory migraine

G43.911 **With status migrainosus**

G43.919 **Without status migrainosus**

G43.A- **Cyclical vomiting**
Excludes1:
cyclical vomiting syndrome unrelated to migraine (R11.15)

G43.AØ **In migraine, not intractable**
Including: without refractory migraine

G43.A1 **In migraine, intractable**
Including: with refractory migraine

G43.B- **Ophthalmoplegic migraine**

G43.BØ **Not intractable**
Including: without refractory migraine

G43.B1 **Intractable**
Including: with refractory migraine

G43.C- **Periodic headache syndromes in child or adult**

G43.CØ **Not intractable**
Including: without refractory migraine

G43.C1 **Intractable**
Including: with refractory migraine

G43.D- **Abdominal migraine**

G43.DØ **Not intractable**
Including: without refractory migraine

G43.D1 **Intractable**
Including: with refractory migraine

G44- OTHER HEADACHE SYNDROMES
Excludes1:
headache NOS (R51.9)
Excludes2:
atypical facial pain (G5Ø.1)
headache due to lumbar puncture (G97.1)
migraines (G43.-)
trigeminal neuralgia (G5Ø.Ø)

G44.Ø- **Cluster headaches and other trigeminal autonomic cephalgias (TAC)**

G44.ØØ- **Cluster headache syndrome, unspecified**
Including: Ciliary neuralgia, Cluster headache NOS, Histamine cephalgia, Lower half migraine, Migrainous neuralgia

G44.ØØ1 **Intractable**

G44.ØØ9 **Not intractable**
Including: Cluster headache syndrome NOS

G44.Ø1- **Episodic cluster headache**

G44.Ø11 **Intractable**

G44.Ø19 **Not intractable**
Including: Episodic cluster headache NOS

G44.Ø2- **Chronic cluster headache**

G44.Ø21 **Intractable**

G44.Ø29 **Not intractable**
Including: Chronic cluster headache NOS

G44.Ø3- **Episodic paroxysmal hemicrania**
Including: Paroxysmal hemicrania NOS

G44.Ø31 **Intractable**

G44.Ø39 **Not intractable**
Including: Episodic paroxysmal hemicrania NOS

G44.Ø4- **Chronic paroxysmal hemicrania**

G44.Ø41 **Intractable**

G44.Ø49 **Not intractable**
Including: Chronic paroxysmal hemicrania NOS

G44.Ø5- **Short lasting unilateral neuralgiform headache with conjunctival injection and tearing (SUNCT)**

G44.Ø51 **Intractable**

G44.Ø59 **Not intractable**
Including: NOS

G44.Ø9- **Other trigeminal autonomic cephalgias (TAC)**

G44.Ø91 **Intractable**

G44.Ø99 **Not intractable**

G44.1 **Vascular headache, NEC**
Excludes2:
cluster headache (G44.Ø)
complicated headache syndromes (G44.5-)
drug-induced headache (G44.4-)
migraine (G43.-)
other specified headache syndromes (G44.8-)
post-traumatic headache (G44.3-)
tension-type headache (G44.2-)

G44.2- **Tension-type headache**

G44.2Ø- **Tension-type headache, unspecified**

G44.2Ø1 **Intractable**

G44.2Ø9 **Not intractable**
Including: Tension headache NOS

G44.21- **Episodic tension-type headache**

G44.211 **Intractable**

G44.219 **Not intractable**
Including: Episodic tension-type headache NOS

G44.22- **Chronic tension-type headache**

G44.221 **Intractable**

G44.229 **Not intractable**
Including: Chronic tension-type headache NOS

G44.3- **Post-traumatic headache**

G44.3Ø- **Post-traumatic headache, unspecified**

G44.3Ø1 **Intractable**

G44.3Ø9 **Not intractable**
Including: Post-traumatic headache NOS

G44.31- **Acute post-traumatic headache**

G44.311 **Intractable**

G44.319 **Not intractable**
Including: Acute post-traumatic headache NOS

G44.32- **Chronic post-traumatic headache**

G44.321 **Intractable**

G44.329 **Not intractable**
Including: Chronic post-traumatic headache NOS

G44.4- **Drug-induced headache, not elsewhere classified**
Including: Medication overuse headache
Use additional code for adverse effect, if applicable, to identify drug (T36-T5Ø with fifth or sixth character 5)

G44.4Ø **Not intractable**

G44.41 **Intractable**

 See Appendix A — Coding Reference Tables for lists of the ICD-10-CM Tabular indicators, HAC categories, and HCC codes.

G44.5- **Complicated headache syndromes**

G44.51 **Hemicrania continua**

G44.52 **New daily persistent headache (NDPH)**

G44.53 **Primary thunderclap**

G44.59 **Other**

G44.8- **Other specified headache syndromes**

Excludes2:

headache with orthostatic or positional component, not elsewhere classified (R51.Ø)

G44.81 **Hypnic**

G44.82 **Associated with sexual activity**

Including: Orgasmic or Preorgasmic headache

G44.83 **Primary cough**

G44.84 **Primary exertional**

G44.85 **Primary stabbing**

G44.86 **Cervicogenic**

Code Also

associated cervical spinal condition, if known

G44.89 **Other**

G47- SLEEP DISORDERS

Excludes2:

nightmares (F51.5)

nonorganic sleep disorders (F51.-)

sleep terrors (F51.4)

sleepwalking (F51.3)

G47.Ø- **Insomnia**

Excludes2:

alcohol related insomnia (F1Ø.182, F1Ø.282, F1Ø.982)

drug-related insomnia (F11.182, F11.282, F11.982, F13.182, F13.282, F13.982, F14.182, F14.282, F14.982, F15.182, F15.282, F15.982, F19.182, F19.282, F19.982)

idiopathic insomnia (F51.Ø1)

insomnia due to a mental disorder (F51.Ø5)

insomnia not due to a substance or known physiological condition (F51.Ø-)

nonorganic insomnia (F51.Ø-)

primary insomnia (F51.Ø1)

sleep apnea (G47.3-)

G47.ØØ **Unspecified**

Including: Insomnia NOS

Indicator(s): *DSM-5*

G47.Ø1 **Due to medical condition**

Code Also

associated medical condition

G47.Ø9 **Other**

Indicator(s): *DSM-5*

G47.1- **Hypersomnia**

Excludes2:

alcohol-related hypersomnia (F1Ø.182, F1Ø.282, F1Ø.982)

drug-related hypersomnia (F11.182, F11.282, F11.982, F13.182, F13.282, F13.982, F14.182, F14.282, F14.982, F15.182, F15.282, F15.982, F19.182, F19.282, F19.982)

hypersomnia due to a mental disorder (F51.13)

hypersomnia not due to a substance or known physiological condition (F51.1-)

primary hypersomnia (F51.11)

sleep apnea (G47.3-)

G47.1Ø **Unspecified**

Including: Hypersomnia NOS

Indicator(s): *DSM-5*

G47.2- **Circadian rhythm sleep disorders**

Including: Disorders of the sleep wake schedule, Inversion of nyctohemeral rhythm, Inversion of sleep rhythm

G47.2Ø **Unspecified type**

Including: Sleep wake schedule disorder NOS

Indicator(s): *DSM-5*

G47.3- **Sleep apnea**

Code Also

any associated underlying condition

Excludes1:

apnea NOS (RØ6.81)

Cheyne-Stokes breathing (RØ6.3)

pickwickian syndrome (E66.2)

sleep apnea of newborn (P28.3-)

G47.3Ø **Unspecified**

Including: Sleep apnea NOS

G47.31 **Primary central**

Including: Idiopathic

Indicator(s): *DSM-5*

G47.32 **High altitude periodic breathing**

R **G47.33** **Obstructive (adult) (pediatric)**

Including: hypopnea

Excludes1:

obstructive sleep apnea of newborn (P28.3-)

Indicator(s): *DSM-5*

G47.34 **Idiopathic sleep related nonobstructive alveolar hypoventilation**

Including: Sleep related hypoxia

Indicator(s): *DSM-5*

G47.35 **Congenital central alveolar hypoventilation syndrome**

Indicator(s): *DSM-5*

G47.36 **Sleep related hypoventilation in conditions classified elsewhere**

Including: hypoxemia

Code First:

underlying condition

Indicator(s): *Manifestation | DSM-5*

G47.37 **Central, in conditions classified elsewhere**

Code First:

underlying condition

Indicator(s): *Manifestation | DSM-5*

G47.39 **Other**

G47.6- **Sleep related movement disorders**

Excludes2:

restless legs syndrome (G25.81)

G47.61 **Periodic limb movement**

G47.62 **Leg cramps**

G47.63 **Bruxism**

Excludes1:

psychogenic bruxism (F45.8)

G47.69 **Other**

G47.8 **Other**

Including: Other specified sleep-wake disorder

Indicator(s): *DSM-5*

G47.9 **Unspecified**

Including: Sleep disorder NOS, Unspecified sleep-wake disorder

Indicator(s): *DSM-5*

NERVE, NERVE ROOT AND PLEXUS DISORDERS (G5Ø-G59)

Excludes1:
current traumatic nerve, nerve root and plexus disorders - see Injury, nerve by body region
neuralgia NOS (M79.2)
neuritis NOS (M79.2)
peripheral neuritis in pregnancy (O26.82-)
radiculitis NOS (M54.1-)

G5Ø- DISORDERS OF TRIGEMINAL NERVE

Includes:
disorders of 5th cranial nerve
Indicator(s): RxØ5: 168

G5Ø.Ø Neuralgia
Including: Syndrome of paroxysmal facial pain, Tic douloureux

G5Ø.1 Atypical facial pain

G5Ø.8 Other

G5Ø.9 Unspecified

G51- FACIAL NERVE DISORDERS

Includes:
disorders of 7th cranial nerve

G51.Ø Bell's palsy
Including: Facial palsy

G51.1 Geniculate ganglionitis
Excludes1:
postherpetic geniculate ganglionitis (BØ2.21)

G51.2 Melkersson's syndrome
Including: Melkersson-Rosenthal

G51.3- **Clonic hemifacial spasm**

G51.31 Right

G51.32 Left

G51.33 Bilateral

G51.39 Unspecified

G51.4 Myokymia

G51.8 Other

G51.9 Unspecified

G52- DISORDERS OF OTHER CRANIAL NERVES

Excludes2:
disorders of acoustic [8th] nerve (H93.3)
disorders of optic [2nd] nerve (H46, H47.Ø)
paralytic strabismus due to nerve palsy (H49.Ø-H49.2)

G52.Ø Olfactory nerve
Including: 1st cranial nerve

G52.1 Glossopharyngeal nerve
Including: Disorder of 9th cranial nerve, Glossopharyngeal neuralgia

G52.2 Vagus nerve
Including: pneumogastric [1Øth] nerve

G52.3 Hypoglossal nerve
Including: 12th cranial nerve

G52.7 Multiple cranial nerves
Including: Polyneuritis cranialis

G52.8 Other specified

G52.9 Unspecified

G53 Cranial nerve disorders in diseases classified elsewhere
Code First:
underlying disease, such as:
neoplasm (CØØ-D49)
Excludes1:
multiple cranial nerve palsy in sarcoidosis (D86.82)
multiple cranial nerve palsy in syphilis (A52.15)
postherpetic geniculate ganglionitis (BØ2.21)
postherpetic trigeminal neuralgia (BØ2.22)
Indicator(s): Manifestation

G54- NERVE ROOT AND PLEXUS DISORDERS

Excludes1:
current traumatic nerve root and plexus disorders - see nerve injury by body region
intervertebral disc disorders (M5Ø-M51)
neuralgia or neuritis NOS (M79.2)
neuritis or radiculitis brachial NOS (M54.13)
neuritis or radiculitis lumbar NOS (M54.16)
neuritis or radiculitis lumbosacral NOS (M54.17)
neuritis or radiculitis thoracic NOS (M54.14)
radiculitis NOS (M54.1Ø)
radiculopathy NOS (M54.1Ø)
spondylosis (M47.-)

G54.Ø Brachial plexus
Including: Thoracic outlet syndrome

G54.1 Lumbosacral plexus

G54.2 Cervical root, NEC

G54.3 Thoracic root, NEC

G54.4 Lumbosacral root, NEC

G54.5 Neuralgic amyotrophy
Including: Parsonage-Aldren-Turner syndrome, Shoulder-girdle neuritis
Excludes1:
neuralgic amyotrophy in diabetes mellitus (EØ8-E13 with .44)

G54.6 Phantom limb syndrome with pain
Indicator(s): CMS22: 189 | CMS24: 189 | ESRD21: 189 | HHSØ5: 254 | HHSØ7: 254

G54.7 Phantom limb syndrome without pain
Including: Phantom limb syndrome NOS
Indicator(s): CMS22: 189 | CMS24: 189 | ESRD21: 189 | HHSØ5: 254 | HHSØ7: 254

G54.8 Other

G54.9 Unspecified

G55 Nerve root and plexus compressions in diseases classified elsewhere
Code First:
underlying disease, such as:
neoplasm (CØØ-D49)
Excludes1:
nerve root compression (due to) (in) ankylosing spondylitis (M45.-)
nerve root compression (due to) (in) dorsopathies (M53.-, M54.-)
nerve root compression (due to) (in) intervertebral disc disorders (M5Ø.1.-, M51.1.-)
nerve root compression (due to) (in) spondylopathies (M46.-, M48.-)
nerve root compression (due to) (in) spondylosis (M47.Ø-, M47.2.-)
Indicator(s): Manifestation

G56- MONONEUROPATHIES OF UPPER LIMB

Excludes1:

current traumatic nerve disorder - see nerve injury by body region

G56.Ø- **Carpal tunnel syndrome**

G56.ØØ Unspecified upper limb
G56.Ø1 Right upper limb
G56.Ø2 Left upper limb
G56.Ø3 Bilateral upper limbs

G56.1- **Other lesions of median nerve**

G56.1Ø Unspecified upper limb
G56.11 Right upper limb
G56.12 Left upper limb
G56.13 Bilateral upper limbs

G56.2- **Lesion of ulnar nerve**

Including: Tardy ulnar nerve palsy

G56.2Ø Unspecified upper limb
G56.21 Right upper limb
G56.22 Left upper limb
G56.23 Bilateral upper limbs

G56.3- **Lesion of radial nerve**

G56.3Ø Unspecified upper limb
G56.31 Right upper limb
G56.32 Left upper limb
G56.33 Bilateral upper limbs

G56.4- **Causalgia**

Including: Complex regional pain syndrome II

Excludes1:

complex regional pain syndrome I of lower limb (G9Ø.52-)
complex regional pain syndrome I of upper limb (G9Ø.51-)
complex regional pain syndrome II of lower limb (G57.7-)
reflex sympathetic dystrophy of lower limb (G9Ø.52-)
reflex sympathetic dystrophy of upper limb (G9Ø.51-)

G56.4Ø Unspecified upper limb
G56.41 Right upper limb
G56.42 Left upper limb
G56.43 Bilateral upper limb

G56.8- **Other specified mononeuropathies**

Including: Interdigital neuroma

G56.8Ø Unspecified upper limb
G56.81 Right upper limb
G56.82 Left upper limb
G56.83 Bilateral upper limb

G56.9- **Unspecified mononeuropathy**

G56.9Ø Unspecified upper limb
G56.91 Right upper limb
G56.92 Left upper limb
G56.93 Bilateral upper limb

G57- MONONEUROPATHIES OF LOWER LIMB

Excludes1:

current traumatic nerve disorder - see nerve injury by body region

G57.Ø- **Lesion of sciatic nerve**

Excludes1:

sciatica NOS (M54.3-)

Excludes2:

sciatica attributed to intervertebral disc disorder (M51.1.-)

G57.ØØ Unspecified lower limb
G57.Ø1 Right lower limb
G57.Ø2 Left lower limb
G57.Ø3 Bilateral lower limbs

G57.1- **Meralgia paresthetica**

Including: Lateral cutaneous nerve of thigh syndrome

G57.1Ø Unspecified lower limb
G57.11 Right lower limb
G57.12 Left lower limb
G57.13 Bilateral lower limbs

G57.2- **Lesion of femoral nerve**

G57.2Ø Unspecified lower limb
G57.21 Right lower limb
G57.22 Left lower limb
G57.23 Bilateral lower limbs

G57.3- **Lesion of lateral popliteal nerve**

Including: Peroneal nerve palsy

G57.3Ø Unspecified lower limb
G57.31 Right lower limb
G57.32 Left lower limb
G57.33 Bilateral lower limbs

G57.4- **Lesion of medial popliteal nerve**

G57.4Ø Unspecified lower limb
G57.41 Right lower limb
G57.42 Left lower limb
G57.43 Bilateral lower limbs

G57.5- **Tarsal tunnel syndrome**

G57.5Ø Unspecified lower limb
G57.51 Right lower limb
G57.52 Left lower limb
G57.53 Bilateral lower limbs

G57.6- **Lesion of plantar nerve**

Including: Morton's metatarsalgia

G57.6Ø Unspecified lower limb
G57.61 Right lower limb
G57.62 Left lower limb
G57.63 Bilateral lower limbs

G57.7- **Causalgia of lower limb**

Including: Complex regional pain syndrome II

Excludes1:

complex regional pain syndrome I of lower limb (G9Ø.52-)
complex regional pain syndrome I of upper limb (G9Ø.51-)
complex regional pain syndrome II of upper limb (G56.4-)
reflex sympathetic dystrophy of lower limb (G9Ø.52-)
reflex sympathetic dystrophy of upper limb (G9Ø.51-)

G57.7Ø Unspecified
G57.71 Right
G57.72 Left
G57.73 Bilateral

G57.8- **Other specified mononeuropathies**

Including: Interdigital neuroma

G57.8Ø Unspecified lower limb
G57.81 Right lower limb
G57.82 Left lower limb
G57.83 Bilateral lower limb

G57.9- **Unspecified mononeuropathy**

G57.9Ø Unspecified lower limb
G57.91 Right lower limb
G57.92 Left lower limb
G57.93 Bilateral lower limb

G58- OTHER MONONEUROPATHIES

G58.Ø **Intercostal neuropathy**

G58.7 **Mononeuritis multiplex**

G58.8 **Other specified**

G58.9 **Unspecified**

G59 **Mononeuropathy in diseases classified elsewhere**

Code First:
underlying disease
Excludes1:
diabetic mononeuropathy (EØ8-E13 with .41)
syphilitic nerve paralysis (A52.19)
syphilitic neuritis (A52.15)
tuberculous mononeuropathy (A17.83)
Indicator(s): Manifestation

POLYNEUROPATHIES AND OTHER DISORDERS OF THE PERIPHERAL NERVOUS SYSTEM (G6Ø-G65)

Excludes1:
neuralgia NOS (M79.2)
neuritis NOS (M79.2)
peripheral neuritis in pregnancy (O26.82-)
radiculitis NOS (M54.1Ø)

G6Ø- HEREDITARY AND IDIOPATHIC NEUROPATHY

Indicator(s): ESRD21: 75

G6Ø.Ø **Hereditary motor and sensory neuropathy**
Including: Charcôt-Marie-Tooth disease, Déjérine-Sottas disease, types I-IV, Hypertrophic neuropathy of infancy, Peroneal muscular atrophy (axonal type) (hypertrophic type), Roussy-Levy syndrome

G6Ø.1 **Refsum's disease**
Including: Infantile Refsum disease
Indicator(s): CC

G6Ø.2 **Neuropathy in association with hereditary ataxia**

G6Ø.3 **Idiopathic progressive neuropathy**

G6Ø.8 **Other**
Including: Dominantly inherited sensory neuropathy, Morvan's disease, Nelaton's syndrome, Recessively inherited sensory neuropathy

G6Ø.9 **Unspecified**

G61- INFLAMMATORY POLYNEUROPATHY

Indicator(s): CMS22: 75 | CMS24: 75 | RxØ5: 159 | HHSØ5: 115 | HHSØ7: 115

G61.Ø **Guillain-Barré syndrome**
Including: Acute (post-)infective polyneuritis, Miller Fisher
Indicator(s): CC

G62- OTHER AND UNSPECIFIED POLYNEUROPATHIES

Indicator(s): ESRD21: 75

G62.9 **Unspecified**
Including: Neuropathy NOS

G65- SEQUELAE OF INFLAMMATORY AND TOXIC POLYNEUROPATHIES

Code First:
condition resulting from (sequela) of inflammatory and toxic polyneuropathies
Indicator(s): CMS22: 75 | CMS24: 75 | RxØ5: 159 | ESRD21: 75 | HHSØ5: 115 | HHSØ7: 115

G65.Ø **Guillain-Barré syndrome**

G65.1 **Other inflammatory polyneuropathy**

G65.2 **Toxic polyneuropathy**

DISEASES OF MYONEURAL JUNCTION AND MUSCLE (G7Ø-G73)

G7Ø- MYASTHENIA GRAVIS AND OTHER MYONEURAL DISORDERS

Excludes1:
botulism (AØ5.1, A48.51-A48.52)
transient neonatal myasthenia gravis (P94.Ø)
Indicator(s): CMS22: 75 | CMS24: 75 | RxØ5: 156 | ESRD21: 75 | HHSØ5: 115 | HHSØ7: 115

G7Ø.Ø- **Myasthenia gravis**

G7Ø.ØØ **Without (acute) exacerbation**
Including: Myasthenia gravis NOS

G7Ø.Ø1 **With (acute) exacerbation**
Including: Myasthenia gravis in crisis
Indicator(s): MCC

G7Ø.1 **Toxic myoneural disorders**
Code First:
(T51-T65) to identify toxic agent

G7Ø.2 **Congenital and developmental myasthenia**

G7Ø.8- **Other specified myoneural disorders**

G7Ø.8Ø **Lambert-Eaton syndrome, unspecified**
Including: Lambert-Eaton syndrome NOS
Indicator(s): CC

G7Ø.81 **Lambert-Eaton syndrome in disease classified elsewhere**
Code First:
underlying disease
Excludes1:
Lambert-Eaton syndrome in neoplastic disease (G73.1)
Indicator(s): Manifestation | CC

G7Ø.89 **Other**

G7Ø.9 **Myoneural disorder, unspecified**

G71- PRIMARY DISORDERS OF MUSCLES

Excludes2:
arthrogryposis multiplex congenita (Q74.3)
metabolic disorders (E7Ø-E88)
myositis (M6Ø.-)

G71.Ø- **Muscular dystrophy**
Including: Autosomal recessive, childhood type, muscular dystrophy resembling Duchenne or Becker muscular dystrophy; Benign [Becker] muscular dystrophy; Benign scapuloperoneal muscular dystrophy with early contractures [Emery-Dreifuss]; Congenital muscular dystrophy NOS; Congenital muscular dystrophy with specific morphological abnormalities of the muscle fiber; Distal muscular dystrophy; Facioscapulohumeral muscular dystrophy; Limb-girdle muscular dystrophy; Ocular muscular dystrophy; Oculopharyngeal muscular dystrophy; Scapuloperoneal muscular dystrophy; Severe [Duchenne] muscular dystrophy

G71.ØØ **Unspecified**
Indicator(s): CMS22: 76 | CMS24: 76 | ESRD21: 76 | HHSØ5: 117 | HHSØ7: 117

G71.Ø1 **Duchenne or Becker**
Including: Autosomal recessive, childhood type, muscular dystrophy resembling Duchenne or Becker; Benign [Becker]; Severe [Duchenne]
Indicator(s): CMS22: 76 | CMS24: 76 | ESRD21: 76 | HHSØ5: 117 | HHSØ7: 117

G71.Ø2 **Facioscapulohumeral**
Including: Scapulohumeral
Indicator(s): CMS22: 76 | CMS24: 76 | ESRD21: 76 | HHSØ5: 117 | HHSØ7: 117

See Appendix A — Coding Reference Tables for lists of the ICD-10-CM Tabular indicators, HAC categories, and HCC codes.

G71.Ø3- **Limb girdle**

N **G71.Ø31 Autosomal dominant**

Including: LGMD D4 calpain-3-related, LGMD D5 collagen 6-related, Limb girdle muscular dystrophy type 1

N **G71.Ø32 Autosomal recessive due to calpain-3 dysfunction**

Including: Limb girdle muscular dystrophy type 2A, LGMD R1 calpain-3-related, Primary calpainopathy

N **G71.Ø33 Due to dysferlin dysfunction**

Including: Dysferlinopathy, LGMD R2 dysferlin-related, type 2B, Miyoshi Myopathy type 1

N **G71.Ø34Ø Unspecified**

Including: Sarcoglycanopathy, NOS

N **G71.Ø341 Alpha**

Including: Alpha sarcoglycanopathy, Limb-girdle muscular dystrophy due to alpha-sarcoglycan deficiency, type 2D

N **G71.Ø342 Beta**

Including: Beta sarcoglycanopathy, beta-sarcoglycan deficiency, type 2E

N **G71.Ø349 Other**

Including: Delta sarcoglycanopathy, Delta-sarcoglycan-related LGMD R6, Gamma sarcoglycanopathy, Gamma-sarcoglycan-related LGMD R5, type 2C, type 2F

N **G71.Ø35 Due to anoctamin-5 dysfunction**

Including: Anoctamin-5-related LGMD R12, Anoctaminopathy, Autosomal recessive limb girdle muscular dystrophy type 2L, Miyoshi myopathy type 3

N **G71.Ø38 Other**

Including: LGMD R9 FKRP-related, LGMD R22 collagen 6-related, due to fukutin related protein dysfunction, type 2I, autosomal recessive

N **G71.Ø39 Unspecified**

R **G71.Ø9 Other specified**

Including: Benign scapuloperoneal with early contractures [Emery-Dreifuss], Congenital NOS, Congenital with specific morphological abnormalities of the muscle fiber, Distal, Ocular, Oculopharyngeal, Scapuloperoneal

Indicator(s): CMS22: 76 | CMS24: 76 | ESRD21: 76 | HHSØ5: 117 | HHSØ7: 117

G71.9 Unspecified

Including: Hereditary myopathy NOS

Indicator(s): ESRD21: 75

G72- OTHER AND UNSPECIFIED MYOPATHIES

Excludes1:

arthrogryposis multiplex congenita (Q74.3)

dermatopolymyositis (M33.-)

ischemic infarction of muscle (M62.2-)

myositis (M6Ø.-)

polymyositis (M33.2.-)

Indicator(s): ESRD21: 75

G72.9 Unspecified

CEREBRAL PALSY AND OTHER PARALYTIC SYNDROMES (G8Ø-G83)

G8Ø- CEREBRAL PALSY

Excludes1:

hereditary spastic paraplegia (G11.4)

Indicator(s): CMS22: 74 | CMS24: 74 | ESRD21: 74

G8Ø.9 Unspecified

Including: Cerebral palsy NOS

G81- HEMIPLEGIA AND HEMIPARESIS

Notes:

This category is to be used only when hemiplegia (complete) (incomplete) is reported without further specification, or is stated to be old or longstanding but of unspecified cause. The category is also for use in multiple coding to identify these types of hemiplegia resulting from any cause.

Excludes1:

congenital cerebral palsy (G8Ø.-)

hemiplegia and hemiparesis due to sequela of cerebrovascular disease (I69.Ø5-, I69.15-, I69.25-, I69.35-, I69.85-, I69.95-)

See Guidelines: 1;C.6.a

Indicator(s): CC | CMS22: 1Ø3 | CMS24: 1Ø3 | ESRD21: 1Ø3 | HHSØ5: 15Ø | HHSØ7: 15Ø

G81.Ø- **Flaccid hemiplegia**

G81.ØØ Affecting unspecified side

G81.Ø1 Affecting right dominant side

G81.Ø2 Affecting left dominant side

G81.Ø3 Affecting right nondominant side

G81.Ø4 Affecting left nondominant side

G81.1- **Spastic hemiplegia**

G81.1Ø Affecting unspecified side

G81.11 Affecting right dominant side

G81.12 Affecting left dominant side

G81.13 Affecting right nondominant side

G81.14 Affecting left nondominant side

G81.9- **Hemiplegia, unspecified**

G81.9Ø Affecting unspecified side

G81.91 Affecting right dominant side

G81.92 Affecting left dominant side

G81.93 Affecting right nondominant side

G81.94 Affecting left nondominant side

G82- PARAPLEGIA (PARAPARESIS) AND QUADRIPLEGIA (QUADRIPARESIS)

Notes:

This category is to be used only when the listed conditions are reported without further specification, or are stated to be old or longstanding but of unspecified cause. The category is also for use in multiple coding to identify these conditions resulting from any cause

Excludes1:

congenital cerebral palsy (G8Ø.-)

functional quadriplegia (R53.2)

hysterical paralysis (F44.4)

See Guidelines: 1;C.6.a

G82.2- **Paraplegia**

Including: Paralysis of both lower limbs NOS, Paraparesis (lower) NOS, Paraplegia (lower) NOS

Indicator(s): CC | CMS22: 71 | CMS24: 71 | ESRD21: 71 | HHSØ5: 1Ø9 | HHSØ7: 1Ø9

G82.2Ø Unspecified

G82.21 Complete

G82.22 Incomplete

G82.5- **Quadriplegia**
See Guidelines: 1;C.18.f
Indicator(s): MCC | CMS22: 70 | CMS24: 70 | ESRD21: 70 | HHS05: 107 | HHS07: 107

G82.50 Unspecified

G82.51 C1-C4 complete

G82.52 C1-C4 incomplete

G82.53 C5-C7 complete

G82.54 C5-C7 incomplete

G83- OTHER PARALYTIC SYNDROMES

Notes:
This category is to be used only when the listed conditions are reported without further specification, or are stated to be old or longstanding but of unspecified cause. The category is also for use in multiple coding to identify these conditions resulting from any cause.
Includes:
paralysis (complete) (incomplete), except as in G80-G82
See Guidelines: 1;C.6.a

G83.0 Diplegia of upper limbs
Including: Diplegia (upper), Paralysis of both upper limbs
Indicator(s): CC | CMS22: 104 | CMS24: 104 | ESRD21: 104 | HHS05: 151 | HHS07: 151

G83.1- **Monoplegia of lower limb**
Including: Paralysis of lower limb
Excludes1:
monoplegia of lower limbs due to sequela of cerebrovascular disease (I69.04-, I69.14-, I69.24-, I69.34-, I69.84-, I69.94-)
Indicator(s): CMS22: 104 | CMS24: 104 | ESRD21: 104 | HHS05: 151 | HHS07: 151

G83.10 Affecting unspecified side

G83.11 Affecting right dominant side

G83.12 Affecting left dominant side

G83.13 Affecting right nondominant side

G83.14 Affecting left nondominant side

G83.2- **Monoplegia of upper limb**
Including: Paralysis of upper limb
Excludes1:
monoplegia of upper limbs due to sequela of cerebrovascular disease (I69.03-, I69.13-, I69.23-, I69.33-, I69.83-, I69.93-)
Indicator(s): CMS22: 104 | CMS24: 104 | ESRD21: 104 | HHS05: 151 | HHS07: 151

G83.20 Affecting unspecified side

G83.21 Affecting right dominant side

G83.22 Affecting left dominant side

G83.23 Affecting right nondominant side

G83.24 Affecting left nondominant side

G83.3- **Monoplegia, unspecified**
Indicator(s): CMS22: 104 | CMS24: 104 | ESRD21: 104 | HHS05: 151 | HHS07: 151

G83.30 Affecting unspecified side

G83.31 Affecting right dominant side

G83.32 Affecting left dominant side

G83.33 Affecting right nondominant side

G83.34 Affecting left nondominant side

G83.4 Cauda equina syndrome
Including: Neurogenic bladder due to cauda equina syndrome
Excludes1:
cord bladder NOS (G95.89)
neurogenic bladder NOS (N31.9)
Indicator(s): CC | CMS22: 72 | CMS24: 72 | Rx05: 157 | ESRD21: 72 | HHS05: 110 | HHS07: 110

G83.5 Locked-in state
Indicator(s): MCC | CMS22: 104 | CMS24: 104 | ESRD21: 104 | HHS05: 122 | HHS07: 122

G83.8- **Other specified paralytic syndromes**
Excludes1:
paralytic syndromes due to current spinal cord injury-code to spinal cord injury (S14, S24, S34)
Indicator(s): CMS22: 104 | CMS24: 104 | ESRD21: 104 | HHS05: 151 | HHS07: 151

G83.81 Brown-Séquard

G83.82 Anterior cord

G83.83 Posterior cord

G83.84 Todd's paralysis (postepileptic)

G83.89 Other

G83.9 Unspecified
Indicator(s): CMS22: 104 | CMS24: 104 | ESRD21: 104 | HHS05: 151 | HHS07: 151

OTHER DISORDERS OF THE NERVOUS SYSTEM (G89-G99)

G89- PAIN, NOT ELSEWHERE CLASSIFIED

Code Also
related psychological factors associated with pain (F45.42)
Excludes1:
generalized pain NOS (R52)
pain disorders exclusively related to psychological factors (F45.41)
pain NOS (R52)
Excludes2:
atypical face pain (G50.1)
headache syndromes (G44.-)
localized pain, unspecified type - code to pain by site, such as:
abdomen pain (R10.-)
back pain (M54.9)
breast pain (N64.4)
chest pain (R07.1-R07.9)
ear pain (H92.0-)
eye pain (H57.1)
headache (R51.9)
joint pain (M25.5-)
limb pain (M79.6-)
lumbar region pain (M54.5-)
painful urination (R30.9)
pelvic and perineal pain (R10.2)
shoulder pain (M25.51-)
spine pain (M54.-)
throat pain (R07.0)
tongue pain (K14.6)
tooth pain (K08.8)
renal colic (N23)
migraines (G43.-)
myalgia (M79.1-)
pain from prosthetic devices, implants, and grafts (T82.84, T83.84, T84.84, T85.84-)
phantom limb syndrome with pain (G54.6)
vulvar vestibulitis (N94.810)
vulvodynia (N94.81-)
See Guidelines: 1;C.5.a | 1;C.6.b | 1;C.6.b.1 | 1;C.6.b.1.b | 1;C.6.b.3.a | 1;C.19.g.2

G89.0 Central pain syndrome
Including: Déjérine-Roussy syndrome, Myelopathic pain syndrome, Thalamic pain syndrome (hyperesthetic)
See Guidelines: 1;C.6.b.6

G89.1- **Acute pain, not elsewhere classified**

G89.11 **Due to trauma**
See Guidelines: 1;C.6.b.1.b

G89.12 **Post-thoracotomy**
Including: Post-thoracotomy pain NOS

G89.18 **Other postprocedural**
Including: Postoperative pain NOS, Postprocedural pain NOS

G89.2- **Chronic pain, not elsewhere classified**
Excludes1:
causalgia, lower limb (G57.7-)
causalgia, upper limb (G56.4-)
central pain syndrome (G89.Ø)
chronic pain syndrome (G89.4)
complex regional pain syndrome II, lower limb (G57.7-)
complex regional pain syndrome II, upper limb (G56.4-)
neoplasm related chronic pain (G89.3)
reflex sympathetic dystrophy (G9Ø.5-)
See Guidelines: 1;C.6.b.4

G89.21 **Due to trauma**

G89.22 **Post-thoracotomy**

G89.28 **Other postprocedural**
Including: postoperative

G89.29 **Other**

G89.3 **Neoplasm related pain (acute) (chronic)**
Including: Cancer associated pain, Pain due to malignancy (primary) (secondary), Tumor associated pain
See Guidelines: 1;C.6.b.5

G89.4 **Chronic pain syndrome**
Including: Chronic pain associated with significant psychosocial dysfunction
See Guidelines: 1;C.6.b.6

G9Ø- DISORDERS OF AUTONOMIC NERVOUS SYSTEM
Excludes1:
dysfunction of the autonomic nervous system due to alcohol (G31.2)

G9Ø.Ø- **Idiopathic peripheral autonomic neuropathy**
Indicator(s): ESRD21: 75

G9Ø.Ø1 **Carotid sinus syncope**
Including: Carotid sinus syndrome

G9Ø.Ø9 **Other**
Including: Idiopathic peripheral autonomic neuropathy NOS

G9Ø.1 **Familial dysautonomia [Riley-Day]**
Indicator(s): CMS22: 72 | CMS24: 72 | RxØ5: 157 | ESRD21: 72 | HHSØ5: 114 | HHSØ7: 114

G9Ø.2 **Horner's syndrome**
Including: Bernard(-Horner) syndrome, Cervical sympathetic dystrophy or paralysis
Indicator(s): ESRD21: 75

G9Ø.3 **Multi-system degeneration of the autonomic nervous system**
Including: Neurogenic orthostatic hypotension [Shy-Drager]
Excludes1:
orthostatic hypotension NOS (I95.1)
Indicator(s): CC | CMS22: 78 | CMS24: 78 | ESRD21: 78 | HHSØ5: 119

G9Ø.4 **Autonomic dysreflexia**
Use additional code to identify the cause, such as:
fecal impaction (K56.41)
pressure ulcer (pressure area) (L89.-)
urinary tract infection (N39.Ø)
Indicator(s): ESRD21: 75

G9Ø.5- **Complex regional pain syndrome I (CRPS I)**
Including: Reflex sympathetic dystrophy
Excludes1:
causalgia of lower limb (G57.7-)
causalgia of upper limb (G56.4-)
complex regional pain syndrome II of lower limb (G57.7-)
complex regional pain syndrome II of upper limb (G56.4-)
Indicator(s): CC | ESRD21: 75

G9Ø.5Ø **Unspecified**

G9Ø.51- **Upper limb**

G9Ø.511 **Right**

G9Ø.512 **Left**

G9Ø.513 **Bilateral**

G9Ø.519 **Unspecified**

G9Ø.52- **Lower limb**

G9Ø.521 **Right**

G9Ø.522 **Left**

G9Ø.523 **Bilateral**

G9Ø.529 **Unspecified**

G9Ø.59 **Other specified site**

G9Ø.8 **Other**
Indicator(s): ESRD21: 75

G9Ø.9 **Unspecified**
Indicator(s): ESRD21: 75

N **G9Ø.A** **Postural orthostatic tachycardia syndrome [POTS]**
Including: Chronic orthostatic intolerance, tachycardia syndrome

G93- OTHER DISORDERS OF BRAIN

G93.2 **Benign intracranial hypertension**
Including: Pseudotumor
Excludes1:
hypertensive encephalopathy (I67.4)
obstructive hydrocephalus (G91.1)

G93.3- **Postviral and related fatigue syndromes**
Including: Benign myalgic encephalomyelitis
Excludes1:
chronic fatigue syndrome NOS (R53.82)

N **G93.31** **Postviral fatigue syndrome**

N **G93.32** **Myalgic encephalomyelitis/chronic fatigue syndrome**
Including: Chronic fatigue syndrome, ME/CFS, Myalgic encephalomyelitis

N **G93.39** **Other post infection**

G93.5 **Compression**
Including: Arnold-Chiari type 1; brain (stem); Herniation of brain (stem)
Excludes1:
traumatic compression of brain (SØ6.A-)
Indicator(s): MCC | CMS22: 8Ø | CMS24: 8Ø | ESRD21: 8Ø | HHSØ5: 122 | HHSØ7: 122

G93.6 Cerebral edema

Excludes1:

cerebral edema due to birth injury (P11.Ø)

traumatic cerebral edema (SØ6.1-)

Indicator(s): *MCC | CMS22: 8Ø | CMS24: 8Ø | ESRD21: 8Ø | HHSØ5: 122 | HHSØ7: 122*

G93.7 Reye's syndrome

Code First:

poisoning due to salicylates, if applicable (T39.Ø-, with sixth character 1-4)

Use additional *code for adverse effect due to salicylates, if applicable (T39.Ø-, with sixth character 5)*

Indicator(s): *Pediatric | MCC | CMS24: 52 | RxØ5: 112 | ESRD21: 52 | HHSØ5: 119*

G95- OTHER AND UNSPECIFIED DISEASES OF SPINAL CORD

Excludes2:

myelitis (GØ4.-)

Indicator(s): *CMS22: 72 | CMS24: 72 | RxØ5: 157 | ESRD21: 72 | HHSØ5: 11Ø | HHSØ7: 11Ø*

G95.2- **Other and unspecified cord compression**

Indicator(s): *CC*

G95.2Ø Unspecified

G95.29 Other

G95.8- **Other specified diseases of spinal cord**

Excludes1:

neurogenic bladder NOS (N31.9)

neurogenic bladder due to cauda equina syndrome (G83.4)

neuromuscular dysfunction of bladder without spinal cord lesion (N31.-)

Indicator(s): *CC*

G95.81 Conus medullaris syndrome

G95.89 Other

Including: Cord bladder NOS, Drug-induced myelopathy, Radiation-induced myelopathy

Excludes1:

myelopathy NOS (G95.9)

G95.9 Unspecified

Including: Myelopathy NOS

Indicator(s): *CC*

Ch5

5. The Tabular List

7. Diseases of the eye and adnexa (HØØ-H59)

This Chapter was not included in this common codes list. For a complete listing of ICD-10-CM codes see FindACode.com

8. Diseases of the ear and mastoid process (H6Ø-H95)

Notes:
Use an external cause code following the code for the ear condition, if applicable, to identify the cause of the ear condition

Excludes2:
certain conditions originating in the perinatal period (PØ4-P96)
certain infectious and parasitic diseases (AØØ-B99)
complications of pregnancy, childbirth and the puerperium (OØØ-O9A)
congenital malformations, deformations and chromosomal abnormalities (QØØ-Q99)
endocrine, nutritional and metabolic diseases (EØØ-E88)
injury, poisoning and certain other consequences of external causes (SØØ-T88)
neoplasms (CØØ-D49)
symptoms, signs and abnormal clinical and laboratory findings, not elsewhere classified (RØØ-R94)

See Guidelines: *1;C.2Ø.a.1*

DISEASES OF EXTERNAL EAR (H6Ø-H62)

H6Ø- OTITIS EXTERNA

H6Ø.Ø- **Abscess of external ear**
Including: Boil, Carbuncle of auricle or external auditory canal, Furuncle

H6Ø.ØØ Unspecified ear
H6Ø.Ø1 Right ear
H6Ø.Ø2 Left ear
H6Ø.Ø3 Bilateral

H6Ø.1- **Cellulitis of external ear**
Including: auricle, external auditory canal

H6Ø.1Ø Unspecified ear
H6Ø.11 Right ear
H6Ø.12 Left ear
H6Ø.13 Bilateral

H6Ø.2- **Malignant otitis externa**
Indicator(s): *CC*

H6Ø.2Ø Unspecified ear
H6Ø.21 Right ear
H6Ø.22 Left ear
H6Ø.23 Bilateral

H6Ø.3- **Other infective otitis externa**

H6Ø.31- **Diffuse otitis externa**

H6Ø.311 Right ear
H6Ø.312 Left ear
H6Ø.313 Bilateral
H6Ø.319 Unspecified ear

H6Ø.32- **Hemorrhagic otitis externa**

H6Ø.321 Right ear
H6Ø.322 Left ear
H6Ø.323 Bilateral
H6Ø.329 Unspecified ear

H6Ø.33- **Swimmer's ear**

H6Ø.331 Right ear
H6Ø.332 Left ear
H6Ø.333 Bilateral
H6Ø.339 Unspecified ear

H6Ø.39- **Other infective otitis externa**

H6Ø.391 Right ear
H6Ø.392 Left ear
H6Ø.393 Bilateral
H6Ø.399 Unspecified ear

H6Ø.4- **Cholesteatoma of external ear**
Including: Keratosis obturans of external ear (canal)
Excludes2:
cholesteatoma of middle ear (H71.-)
recurrent cholesteatoma of postmastoidectomy cavity (H95.Ø-)

H6Ø.4Ø Unspecified ear
H6Ø.41 Right ear
H6Ø.42 Left ear
H6Ø.43 Bilateral

H6Ø.5- **Acute noninfective otitis externa**

H6Ø.5Ø- **Unspecified acute noninfective otitis externa**
Including: Acute otitis externa NOS

H6Ø.5Ø1 Right ear
H6Ø.5Ø2 Left ear
H6Ø.5Ø3 Bilateral
H6Ø.5Ø9 Unspecified ear

H6Ø.51- **Acute actinic otitis externa**

H6Ø.511 Right ear
H6Ø.512 Left ear
H6Ø.513 Bilateral
H6Ø.519 Unspecified ear

H6Ø.52- **Acute chemical otitis externa**

H6Ø.521 Right ear
H6Ø.522 Left ear
H6Ø.523 Bilateral
H6Ø.529 Unspecified ear

H6Ø.53- **Acute contact otitis externa**

H6Ø.531 Right ear
H6Ø.532 Left ear
H6Ø.533 Bilateral
H6Ø.539 Unspecified ear

H6Ø.54- **Acute eczematoid otitis externa**

H6Ø.541 Right ear
H6Ø.542 Left ear
H6Ø.543 Bilateral
H6Ø.549 Unspecified ear

H6Ø.55- **Acute reactive otitis externa**

H6Ø.551 Right ear
H6Ø.552 Left ear
H6Ø.553 Bilateral
H6Ø.559 Unspecified ear

H6Ø.59- **Other noninfective acute otitis externa**

H6Ø.591 Right ear
H6Ø.592 Left ear
H6Ø.593 Bilateral
H6Ø.599 Unspecified ear

H6Ø.6- **Unspecified chronic otitis externa**
- **H6Ø.6Ø** **Unspecified ear**
- **H6Ø.61** **Right ear**
- **H6Ø.62** **Left ear**
- **H6Ø.63** **Bilateral**

H6Ø.8- **Other otitis externa**
- **H6Ø.8x1** **Right ear**
- **H6Ø.8x2** **Left ear**
- **H6Ø.8x3** **Bilateral**
- **H6Ø.8x9** **Unspecified ear**

H6Ø.9- **Unspecified otitis externa**
- **H6Ø.9Ø** **Unspecified ear**
- **H6Ø.91** **Right ear**
- **H6Ø.92** **Left ear**
- **H6Ø.93** **Bilateral**

H61- OTHER DISORDERS OF EXTERNAL EAR

H61.Ø- **Chondritis and perichondritis of external ear**
Including: Chondrodermatitis nodularis chronica helicis, Perichondritis of auricle, Perichondritis of pinna

H61.ØØ- **Unspecified perichondritis of external ear**
- **H61.ØØ1** **Right ear**
- **H61.ØØ2** **Left ear**
- **H61.ØØ3** **Bilateral**
- **H61.ØØ9** **Unspecified ear**

H61.Ø1- **Acute perichondritis of external ear**
- **H61.Ø11** **Right ear**
- **H61.Ø12** **Left ear**
- **H61.Ø13** **Bilateral**
- **H61.Ø19** **Unspecified ear**

H61.Ø2- **Chronic perichondritis of external ear**
- **H61.Ø21** **Right ear**
- **H61.Ø22** **Left ear**
- **H61.Ø23** **Bilateral**
- **H61.Ø29** **Unspecified ear**

H61.Ø3- **Chondritis of external ear**
Including: auricle, pinna
- **H61.Ø31** **Right ear**
- **H61.Ø32** **Left ear**
- **H61.Ø33** **Bilateral**
- **H61.Ø39** **Unspecified ear**

H61.1- **Noninfective disorders of pinna**
Excludes2:
cauliflower ear (M95.1-)
gouty tophi of ear (M1A.-)

H61.1Ø- **Unspecified noninfective disorders of pinna**
Including: Disorder of pinna NOS
- **H61.1Ø1** **Right ear**
- **H61.1Ø2** **Left ear**
- **H61.1Ø3** **Bilateral**
- **H61.1Ø9** **Unspecified ear**

H61.11- **Acquired deformity of pinna**
Including: Acquired deformity of auricle
Excludes2:
cauliflower ear (M95.1-)
- **H61.111** **Right ear**
- **H61.112** **Left ear**
- **H61.113** **Bilateral**
- **H61.119** **Unspecified ear**

H61.12- **Hematoma of pinna**
Including: Hematoma of auricle
- **H61.121** **Right ear**
- **H61.122** **Left ear**
- **H61.123** **Bilateral**
- **H61.129** **Unspecified ear**

H61.19- **Other noninfective disorders of pinna**
- **H61.191** **Right ear**
- **H61.192** **Left ear**
- **H61.193** **Bilateral**
- **H61.199** **Unspecified ear**

H61.2- **Impacted cerumen**
Including: Wax in ear
Indicator(s): *QAdmit*
- **H61.2Ø** **Unspecified ear**
- **H61.21** **Right ear**
- **H61.22** **Left ear**
- **H61.23** **Bilateral**

H61.3- **Acquired stenosis of external ear canal**
Including: Collapse of external ear canal
Excludes1:
postprocedural stenosis of external ear canal (H95.81-)

H61.3Ø- **Unspecified**
- **H61.3Ø1** **Right ear**
- **H61.3Ø2** **Left ear**
- **H61.3Ø3** **Bilateral**
- **H61.3Ø9** **Unspecified ear**

H61.31- **Secondary to trauma**
- **H61.311** **Right ear**
- **H61.312** **Left ear**
- **H61.313** **Bilateral**
- **H61.319** **Unspecified ear**

H61.32- **Secondary to inflammation and infection**
- **H61.321** **Right ear**
- **H61.322** **Left ear**
- **H61.323** **Bilateral**
- **H61.329** **Unspecified ear**

H61.39- **Other**
- **H61.391** **Right ear**
- **H61.392** **Left ear**
- **H61.393** **Bilateral ear**
- **H61.399** **Unspecified**

H61.8- **Other specified disorders of external ear**

H61.81- **Exostosis of external canal**

H61.811 **Right ear**

H61.812 **Left ear**

H61.813 **Bilateral**

H61.819 **Unspecified ear**

H61.89- **Other specified disorders of external ear**

H61.891 **Right ear**

H61.892 **Left ear**

H61.893 **Bilateral**

H61.899 **Unspecified ear**

H61.9- **Disorder of external ear, unspecified**

H61.90 **Unspecified ear**

H61.91 **Right ear**

H61.92 **Left ear**

H61.93 **Bilateral**

DISEASES OF MIDDLE EAR AND MASTOID (H65-H75)

H65- NONSUPPURATIVE OTITIS MEDIA

Includes:

nonsuppurative otitis media with myringitis

Use additional code for any associated perforated tympanic membrane (H72.-)

Use additional code, if applicable, to identify:

exposure to environmental tobacco smoke (Z77.22)

exposure to tobacco smoke in the perinatal period (P96.81)

history of tobacco dependence (Z87.891)

infectious agent (B95-B97)

occupational exposure to environmental tobacco smoke (Z57.31)

tobacco dependence (F17.-)

tobacco use (Z72.0)

H65.0- **Acute serous otitis media**

Including: Acute and subacute secretory otitis

H65.00 **Unspecified ear**

H65.01 **Right ear**

H65.02 **Left ear**

H65.03 **Bilateral**

H65.04 **Recurrent, right ear**

H65.05 **Recurrent, left ear**

H65.06 **Recurrent, bilateral**

H65.07 **Recurrent, unspecified ear**

H65.1- **Other acute nonsuppurative otitis media**

Excludes1:

otitic barotrauma (T70.0)

otitis media (acute) NOS (H66.9)

H65.11- **Acute and subacute allergic otitis media (mucoid) (sanguinous) (serous)**

H65.111 **Right ear**

H65.112 **Left ear**

H65.113 **Bilateral**

H65.114 **Recurrent, right ear**

H65.115 **Recurrent, left ear**

H65.116 **Recurrent, bilateral**

H65.117 **Recurrent, unspecified ear**

H65.119 **Unspecified ear**

H65.19- **Other acute nonsuppurative otitis media**

Including: Acute and subacute mucoid, Acute and subacute nonsuppurative otitis media NOS, Acute and subacute sanguinous, Acute and subacute seromucinous

H65.191 **Right ear**

H65.192 **Left ear**

H65.193 **Bilateral**

H65.194 **Recurrent, right ear**

H65.195 **Recurrent, left ear**

H65.196 **Recurrent, bilateral**

H65.197 **Recurrent, unspecified ear**

H65.199 **Unspecified ear**

H65.2- **Chronic serous otitis media**

Including: Chronic tubotympanal catarrh

H65.20 **Unspecified ear**

H65.21 **Right ear**

H65.22 **Left ear**

H65.23 **Bilateral**

H65.3- **Chronic mucoid otitis media**

Including: Chronic mucinous, Chronic secretory, Chronic transudative, Glue ear

Excludes1:

adhesive middle ear disease (H74.1)

H65.30 **Unspecified ear**

H65.31 **Right ear**

H65.32 **Left ear**

H65.33 **Bilateral**

H65.4- **Other chronic nonsuppurative otitis media**

H65.41- **Chronic allergic otitis media**

H65.411 **Right ear**

H65.412 **Left ear**

H65.413 **Bilateral**

H65.419 **Unspecified ear**

H65.49- **Other chronic nonsuppurative otitis media**

Including: Chronic exudative, Chronic nonsuppurative otitis media NOS, Chronic otitis media with effusion (nonpurulent), Chronic seromucinous

H65.491 **Right ear**

H65.492 **Left ear**

H65.493 **Bilateral**

H65.499 **Unspecified ear**

H65.9- **Unspecified nonsuppurative otitis media**

Including: Allergic otitis media NOS, Catarrhal otitis media NOS, Exudative otitis media NOS, Mucoid otitis media NOS, Otitis media with effusion (nonpurulent) NOS, Secretory otitis media NOS, Seromucinous otitis media NOS, Serous otitis media NOS, Transudative otitis media NOS

H65.90 **Unspecified ear**

H65.91 **Right ear**

H65.92 **Left ear**

H65.93 **Bilateral**

See Appendix A — Coding Reference Tables for lists of the ICD-10-CM Tabular indicators, HAC categories, and HCC codes.

H66- SUPPURATIVE AND UNSPECIFIED OTITIS MEDIA

Includes:
suppurative and unspecified otitis media with myringitis
Use additional code to identify:
exposure to environmental tobacco smoke (Z77.22)
exposure to tobacco smoke in the perinatal period (P96.81)
history of tobacco dependence (Z87.891)
occupational exposure to environmental tobacco smoke (Z57.31)
tobacco dependence (F17.-)
tobacco use (Z72.Ø)

H66.Ø- **Acute suppurative otitis media**

H66.ØØ- **Acute suppurative otitis media without spontaneous rupture of ear drum**

H66.ØØ1 Right ear
H66.ØØ2 Left ear
H66.ØØ3 Bilateral
H66.ØØ4 Recurrent, right ear
H66.ØØ5 Recurrent, left ear
H66.ØØ6 Recurrent, bilateral
H66.ØØ7 Recurrent, unspecified ear
H66.ØØ9 Unspecified ear

H66.Ø1- **Acute suppurative otitis media with spontaneous rupture of ear drum**

H66.Ø11 Right ear
H66.Ø12 Left ear
H66.Ø13 Bilateral
H66.Ø14 Recurrent, right ear
H66.Ø15 Recurrent, left ear
H66.Ø16 Recurrent, bilateral
H66.Ø17 Recurrent, unspecified ear
H66.Ø19 Unspecified ear

H66.1- **Chronic tubotympanic suppurative otitis media**

Including: Benign chronic, Chronic tubotympanic disease
Use additional code for any associated perforated tympanic membrane (H72.-)

H66.1Ø Unspecified
H66.11 Right ear
H66.12 Left ear
H66.13 Bilateral

H66.2- **Chronic atticoantral suppurative otitis media**

Including: Chronic atticoantral disease
Use additional code for any associated perforated tympanic membrane (H72.-)

H66.2Ø Unspecified ear
H66.21 Right ear
H66.22 Left ear
H66.23 Bilateral

H66.3- **Other chronic suppurative otitis media**

Including: Chronic suppurative otitis media NOS
Use additional code for any associated perforated tympanic membrane (H72.-)
Excludes1:
tuberculous otitis media (A18.6)

H66.3x1 Right ear
H66.3x2 Left ear
H66.3x3 Bilateral
H66.3x9 Unspecified ear

H66.4- **Suppurative otitis media, unspecified**

Including: Purulent otitis media NOS
Use additional code for any associated perforated tympanic membrane (H72.-)

H66.4Ø Unspecified ear
H66.41 Right ear
H66.42 Left ear
H66.43 Bilateral

H66.9- **Otitis media, unspecified**

Including: Otitis media NOS, Acute NOS, Chronic NOS
Use additional code for any associated perforated tympanic membrane (H72.-)

H66.9Ø Unspecified ear
H66.91 Right ear
H66.92 Left ear
H66.93 Bilateral

DISEASES OF INNER EAR (H8Ø-H83)

H81- DISORDERS OF VESTIBULAR FUNCTION

Excludes1:
epidemic vertigo (A88.1)
vertigo NOS (R42)

H81.Ø- **Ménière's disease**

Including: Labyrinthine hydrops, Ménière's syndrome or vertigo

H81.Ø1 Right ear
H81.Ø2 Left ear
H81.Ø3 Bilateral
H81.Ø9 Unspecified ear

H81.1- **Benign paroxysmal vertigo**

H81.1Ø Unspecified ear
H81.11 Right ear
H81.12 Left ear
H81.13 Bilateral

H81.2- **Vestibular neuronitis**

H81.2Ø Unspecified ear
H81.21 Right ear
H81.22 Left ear
H81.23 Bilateral

H81.3- **Other peripheral vertigo**

H81.31- **Aural vertigo**

H81.311 Right ear
H81.312 Left ear
H81.313 Bilateral
H81.319 Unspecified ear

H81.39- **Other peripheral vertigo**

Including: Lermoyez' syndrome, Otogenic vertigo, Peripheral vertigo NOS

H81.391 Right ear
H81.392 Left ear
H81.393 Bilateral
H81.399 Unspecified ear

H81.4 Vertigo of central origin

Including: Central positional nystagmus

H81.8- **Other disorders of vestibular function**

- **H81.8x1** **Right ear**
- **H81.8x2** **Left ear**
- **H81.8x3** **Bilateral**
- **H81.8x9** **Unspecified ear**

H81.9- **Unspecified disorder of vestibular function**

Including: Vertiginous syndrome NOS

- **H81.9Ø** **Unspecified ear**
- **H81.91** **Right ear**
- **H81.92** **Left ear**
- **H81.93** **Bilateral**

H83- OTHER DISEASES OF INNER EAR

H83.Ø- **Labyrinthitis**

- **H83.Ø1** **Right ear**
- **H83.Ø2** **Left ear**
- **H83.Ø3** **Bilateral**
- **H83.Ø9** **Unspecified ear**

H83.1- **Labyrinthine fistula**

- **H83.11** **Right ear**
- **H83.12** **Left ear**
- **H83.13** **Bilateral**
- **H83.19** **Unspecified ear**

H83.2- **Labyrinthine dysfunction**

Including: hypersensitivity, hypofunction, loss of function

- **H83.2x1** **Right ear**
- **H83.2x2** **Left ear**
- **H83.2x3** **Bilateral**
- **H83.2x9** **Unspecified ear**

H83.3- **Noise effects on inner ear**

Including: Acoustic trauma, Noise-induced hearing loss

- **H83.3x1** **Right ear**
- **H83.3x2** **Left ear**
- **H83.3x3** **Bilateral**
- **H83.3x9** **Unspecified ear**

H83.8- **Other specified diseases of inner ear**

- **H83.8x1** **Right ear**
- **H83.8x2** **Left ear**
- **H83.8x3** **Bilateral**
- **H83.8x9** **Unspecified ear**

H83.9- **Unspecified disease of inner ear**

- **H83.9Ø** **Unspecified ear**
- **H83.91** **Right ear**
- **H83.92** **Left ear**
- **H83.93** **Bilateral**

OTHER DISORDERS OF EAR (H9Ø-H94)

H93- OTHER DISORDERS OF EAR, NOT ELSEWHERE CLASSIFIED

H93.1- **Tinnitus**

- **H93.11** **Right ear**
- **H93.12** **Left ear**
- **H93.13** **Bilateral**
- **H93.19** **Unspecified ear**

See Appendix A — Coding Reference Tables for lists of the ICD-10-CM Tabular indicators, HAC categories, and HCC codes.

9. Diseases of the circulatory system (I00-I99)

Excludes2:
certain conditions originating in the perinatal period (P04-P96)
certain infectious and parasitic diseases (A00-B99)
complications of pregnancy, childbirth and the puerperium (O00-O9A)
congenital malformations, deformations, and chromosomal abnormalities (Q00-Q99)
endocrine, nutritional and metabolic diseases (E00-E88)
injury, poisoning and certain other consequences of external causes (S00-T88)
neoplasms (C00-D49)
symptoms, signs and abnormal clinical and laboratory findings, not elsewhere classified (R00-R94)
systemic connective tissue disorders (M30-M36)
transient cerebral ischemic attacks and related syndromes (G45.-)
See Guidelines: 1;C.20.a.1

HYPERTENSIVE DISEASES (I10-I16)

Use additional code to identify:
exposure to environmental tobacco smoke (Z77.22)
history of tobacco dependence (Z87.891)
occupational exposure to environmental tobacco smoke (Z57.31)
tobacco dependence (F17.-)
tobacco use (Z72.0)
Excludes1:
neonatal hypertension (P29.2)
primary pulmonary hypertension (I27.0)
Excludes2:
hypertensive disease complicating pregnancy, childbirth and the puerperium (O10-O11, O13-O16)
See Guidelines: 1;C.9.a | 1;C.15.d

I10 Essential (primary) hypertension
Includes:
high blood pressure
hypertension (arterial) (benign) (essential) (malignant) (primary) (systemic)
Excludes1:
hypertensive disease complicating pregnancy, childbirth and the puerperium (O10-O11, O13-O16)
Excludes2:
essential (primary) hypertension involving vessels of brain (I60-I69)
essential (primary) hypertension involving vessels of eye (H35.0-)
See Guidelines: 1;C.9.a.8 | 1;C.9.a.9
Indicator(s): QAdmit | Rx05: 187

I15- SECONDARY HYPERTENSION
Code Also
underlying condition
Excludes1:
postprocedural hypertension (I97.3)
Excludes2:
secondary hypertension involving vessels of brain (I60-I69)
secondary hypertension involving vessels of eye (H35.0-)
See Guidelines: 1;C.9.a.8 | 1;C.9.a.9
Indicator(s): Rx05: 187

I15.0 Renovascular
I15.1 Secondary to other renal disorders
I15.2 Secondary to endocrine disorders
I15.8 Other
I15.9 Unspecified

CEREBROVASCULAR DISEASES (I60-I69)

Use additional code to identify presence of:
alcohol abuse and dependence (F10.-)
exposure to environmental tobacco smoke (Z77.22)
history of tobacco dependence (Z87.891)
hypertension (I10-I16)
occupational exposure to environmental tobacco smoke (Z57.31)
tobacco dependence (F17.-)
tobacco use (Z72.0)
Excludes1:
traumatic intracranial hemorrhage (S06.-)
See Guidelines: 1;C.9.a.4 | 1;C.9.c | 1;C.9.d | 1;C.18.e

I69- SEQUELAE OF CEREBROVASCULAR DISEASE
Notes:
Category I69 is to be used to indicate conditions in I60-I67 as the cause of sequelae. The 'sequelae' include conditions specified as such or as residuals which may occur at any time after the onset of the causal condition
Excludes1:
personal history of cerebral infarction without residual deficit (Z86.73)
personal history of prolonged reversible ischemic neurologic deficit (PRIND) (Z86.73)
personal history of reversible ischemic neurologcial deficit (RIND) (Z86.73)
sequelae of traumatic intracranial injury (S06.-)
See Guidelines: 1;C.9.d.1-3

I69.3- **Cerebral infarction**
Including: Sequelae of stroke NOS
Indicator(s): POAEx

I69.30 Unspecified
I69.31- **Cognitive deficits following**
I69.310 Attention and concentration deficit
I69.311 Memory deficit
I69.312 Visuospatial deficit and spatial neglect
I69.313 Psychomotor deficit
I69.314 Frontal lobe and executive function deficit
I69.315 Social or emotional deficit
I69.318 Other symptoms and signs involving cognitive functions
I69.319 Unspecified symptoms and signs involving cognitive functions
I69.32- **Apeech and language deficits following**
I69.320 Aphasia
I69.321 Dysphasia
I69.322 Dysarthria
Excludes2:
transient ischemic attack (TIA) (G45.9)
I69.323 Fluency disorder
Including: Stuttering
I69.328 Other
I69.33- **Monoplegia of upper limb following**
Indicator(s): CMS22: 104 | CMS24: 104 | ESRD21: 104 | HHS05: 151 | HHS07: 151
I69.331 Affecting right dominant side
I69.332 Affecting left dominant side
I69.333 Affecting right non-dominant side
I69.334 Affecting left non-dominant side
I69.339 Affecting unspecified side

I69.34- **Monoplegia of lower limb following**
Indicator(s): CMS22: 1Ø4 | CMS24: 1Ø4 | ESRD21: 1Ø4 | HHSØ5: 151 | HHSØ7: 151

- **I69.341 Affecting right dominant side**
- **I69.342 Affecting left dominant side**
- **I69.343 Affecting right non-dominant side**
- **I69.344 Affecting left non-dominant side**
- **I69.349 Affecting unspecified side**

I69.35- **Hemiplegia and hemiparesis following**
Indicator(s): CC | CMS22: 1Ø3 | CMS24: 1Ø3 | ESRD21: 1Ø3 | HHSØ5: 15Ø | HHSØ7: 15Ø

- **I69.351 Affecting right dominant side**
  Excludes2:
  transient ischemic attack (TIA) (G45.9)
- **I69.352 Affecting left dominant side**
- **I69.353 Affecting right non-dominant side**
- **I69.354 Affecting left non-dominant side**
- **I69.359 Affecting unspecified side**

I69.36- **Other paralytic syndrome following**
Use additional code to identify type of paralytic syndrome, such as:
locked-in state (G83.5)
quadriplegia (G82.5-)
Excludes1:
hemiplegia/hemiparesis following cerebral infarction (I69.35-)
monoplegia of lower limb following cerebral infarction (I69.34-)
monoplegia of upper limb following cerebral infarction (I69.33-)
Indicator(s): CMS22: 1Ø4 | CMS24: 1Ø4 | ESRD21: 1Ø4 | HHSØ5: 151 | HHSØ7: 151

- **I69.361 Affecting right dominant side**
- **I69.362 Affecting left dominant side**
- **I69.363 Affecting right non-dominant side**
- **I69.364 Affecting left non-dominant side**
- **I69.365 Bilateral**
- **I69.369 Affecting unspecified side**

I69.39- **Other sequelae**

- **I69.39Ø Apraxia**
- R **I69.391 Dysphagia**
  Use additional code to identify the type of dysphagia, if known (R13.11-R13.19)
- **I69.392 Facial weakness**
  Including: Facial droop
- **I69.393 Ataxia**
- **I69.398 Other**
  Including: Alteration of sensation; Disturbance of vision
  Use additional code to identify the sequelae

DISEASES OF VEINS, LYMPHATIC VESSELS AND LYMPH NODES, NOT ELSEWHERE CLASSIFIED (I8Ø-I89)

I83- VARICOSE VEINS OF LOWER EXTREMITIES

Excludes2:
varicose veins complicating pregnancy (O22.Ø-)
varicose veins complicating the puerperium (O87.4)

I83.Ø- **Varicose veins of lower extremities with ulcer**
Use additional code to identify severity of ulcer (L97.-)
Indicator(s): CMS22: 1Ø7 | CMS24: 1Ø7 | ESRD21: 1Ø7 | HHSØ5: 217 | HHSØ7: 217

I83.ØØ- **Unspecified lower extremity**

- **I83.ØØ1 Thigh**
- **I83.ØØ2 Calf**
- **I83.ØØ3 Ankle**
- **I83.ØØ4 Heel and midfoot**
  Including: Plantar surface of midfoot
- **I83.ØØ5 Other part of foot**
  Including: Toe
- **I83.ØØ8 Other part lower leg**
- **I83.ØØ9 Unspecified site**

I83.Ø1- **Right lower extremity**

- **I83.Ø11 Thigh**
- **I83.Ø12 Calf**
- **I83.Ø13 Ankle**
- **I83.Ø14 Heel and midfoot**
  Including: Plantar surface of midfoot
- **I83.Ø15 Other part of foot**
  Including: Toe
- **I83.Ø18 Other part of lower leg**
- **I83.Ø19 Unspecified site**

I83.Ø2- **Left lower extremity**

- **I83.Ø21 Thigh**
- **I83.Ø22 Calf**
- **I83.Ø23 Ankle**
- **I83.Ø24 Heel and midfoot**
  Including: Plantar surface of midfoot
- **I83.Ø25 Other part of foot**
  Including: Toe
- **I83.Ø28 Other part of lower leg**
- **I83.Ø29 Unspecified site**

I83.1- **Varicose veins of lower extremities with inflammation**

- **I83.1Ø Unspecified**
- **I83.11 Right**
- **I83.12 Left**

I83.2- **Varicose veins of lower extremities with both ulcer and inflammation**
Use additional code to identify severity of ulcer (L97.-)
Indicator(s): CC | CMS22: 1Ø7 | CMS24: 1Ø7 | ESRD21: 1Ø7 | HHSØ5: 217 | HHSØ7: 217

I83.2Ø- **Unspecified lower extremity**

- **I83.2Ø1 Thigh**
- **I83.2Ø2 Calf**
- **I83.2Ø3 Ankle**
- **I83.2Ø4 Heel and midfoot**
  Including: Plantar surface of midfoot
- **I83.2Ø5 Other part of foot**
  Including: Toe
- **I83.2Ø8 Other part of lower extremity**
- **I83.2Ø9 Unspecified site**

I83.21- **Right lower extremity**

I83.211 Thigh

I83.212 Calf

I83.213 Ankle

I83.214 Heel and midfoot
Including: Plantar surface of midfoot

I83.215 Other part of foot
Including: Toe

I83.218 Other part of lower extremity

I83.219 Unspecified site

I83.22- **Left lower extremity**

I83.221 Thigh

I83.222 Calf

I83.223 Ankle

I83.224 Heel and midfoot
Including: Plantar surface of midfoot

I83.225 Other part of foot
Including: Toe

I83.228 Other part of lower extremity

I83.229 Unspecified site

I83.8- **Varicose veins of lower extremities with other complications**

I83.81- **With pain**

I83.811 Right extremity

I83.812 Left extremity

I83.813 Bilateral extremities

I83.819 Unspecified extremity

I83.89- **With other complications**
Including: With edema; With swelling

I83.891 Right extremity

I83.892 Left extremity

I83.893 Bilateral extremities

I83.899 Unspecified extremity

I83.9- **Asymptomatic varicose veins of lower extremities**
Including: Phlebectasia of lower extremities; Varicose veins or Varix of lower extremities

I83.9Ø Unspecified extremity
Including: Varicose veins NOS

I83.91 Right extremity

I83.92 Left extremity

I83.93 Bilateral extremities

OTHER AND UNSPECIFIED DISORDERS OF THE CIRCULATORY SYSTEM (I95-I99)

I95- HYPOTENSION

Excludes1:
cardiovascular collapse (R57.9)
maternal hypotension syndrome (O26.5-)
nonspecific low blood pressure reading NOS (RØ3.1)

I95.Ø Idiopathic

I95.1 Orthostatic
Including: Hypotension, postural
Excludes1:
neurogenic orthostatic hypotension [Shy-Drager] (G9Ø.3)
orthostatic hypotension due to drugs (I95.2)

I95.9 Unspecified

Ch5

5. The Tabular List

1Ø. Diseases of the respiratory system (JØØ-J99)

Notes:
When a respiratory condition is described as occurring in more than one site and is not specifically indexed, it should be classified to the lower anatomic site (e.g. tracheobronchitis to bronchitis in J4Ø).
Use additional code, where applicable, to identify:
exposure to environmental tobacco smoke (Z77.22)
exposure to tobacco smoke in the perinatal period (P96.81)
history of tobacco dependence (Z87.891)
occupational exposure to environmental tobacco smoke (Z57.31)
tobacco dependence (F17.-)
tobacco use (Z72.Ø)
Excludes2:
certain conditions originating in the perinatal period (PØ4-P96)
certain infectious and parasitic diseases (AØØ-B99)
complications of pregnancy, childbirth and the puerperium (OØØ-O9A)
congenital malformations, deformations and chromosomal abnormalities (QØØ-Q99)
endocrine, nutritional and metabolic diseases (EØØ-E88)
injury, poisoning and certain other consequences of external causes (SØØ-T88)
neoplasms (CØØ-D49)
smoke inhalation (T59.81-)
symptoms, signs and abnormal clinical and laboratory findings, not elsewhere classified (RØØ-R94)
See Guidelines: 1;C.2Ø.a.1

ACUTE UPPER RESPIRATORY INFECTIONS (JØØ-JØ6)

Excludes1:
chronic obstructive pulmonary disease with acute lower respiratory infection (J44.Ø)

JØØ Acute nasopharyngitis [common cold]
Including: Acute rhinitis; Coryza (acute); Infective nasopharyngitis NOS; Infective rhinitis; Nasal catarrh, acute; Nasopharyngitis NOS
Excludes1:
acute pharyngitis (JØ2.-)
acute sore throat NOS (JØ2.9)
influenza virus with other respiratory manifestations (JØ9.X2, J1Ø.1, J11.1)
pharyngitis NOS (JØ2.9)
rhinitis NOS (J31.Ø)
sore throat NOS (JØ2.9)
Excludes2:
allergic rhinitis (J3Ø.1-J3Ø.9)
chronic pharyngitis (J31.2)
chronic rhinitis (J31.Ø)
chronic sore throat (J31.2)
nasopharyngitis, chronic (J31.1)
vasomotor rhinitis (J3Ø.Ø)

JØ1- ACUTE SINUSITIS
Includes:
acute abscess of sinus
acute empyema of sinus
acute infection of sinus
acute inflammation of sinus
acute suppuration of sinus
Use additional code (B95-B97) to identify infectious agent.
Excludes1:
sinusitis NOS (J32.9)
Excludes2:
chronic sinusitis (J32.Ø-J32.8)

JØ1.Ø- **Acute maxillary sinusitis**
Including: Acute antritis
JØ1.ØØ Unspecified
JØ1.Ø1 Recurrent

JØ1.1- **Acute frontal sinusitis**
JØ1.1Ø Unspecified
JØ1.11 Recurrent

JØ1.2- **Acute ethmoidal sinusitis**
JØ1.2Ø Unspecified
JØ1.21 Recurrent

JØ1.3- **Acute sphenoidal sinusitis**
JØ1.3Ø Unspecified
JØ1.31 Recurrent

JØ1.4- **Acute pansinusitis**
JØ1.4Ø Unspecified
JØ1.41 Recurrent

JØ1.8- **Other acute sinusitis**
JØ1.8Ø Other
Including: Acute sinusitis involving more than one sinus but not pansinusitis
JØ1.81 Recurrent
Including: Acute recurrent sinusitis involving more than one sinus but not pansinusitis

JØ1.9- **Acute sinusitis, unspecified**
JØ1.9Ø Unspecified
JØ1.91 Recurrent

JØ2- ACUTE PHARYNGITIS
Includes:
acute sore throat
Excludes1:
acute laryngopharyngitis (JØ6.Ø)
peritonsillar abscess (J36)
pharyngeal abscess (J39.1)
retropharyngeal abscess (J39.Ø)
Excludes2:
chronic pharyngitis (J31.2)

JØ2.Ø Streptococcal
Including: Septic pharyngitis; Streptococcal sore throat
Excludes2:
scarlet fever (A38.-)

JØ2.8 Due to other specified organisms
Use additional code (B95-B97) to identify infectious agent
Excludes1:
acute pharyngitis due to coxsackie virus (BØ8.5)
acute pharyngitis due to gonococcus (A54.5)
acute pharyngitis due to herpes [simplex] virus (BØØ.2)
acute pharyngitis due to infectious mononucleosis (B27.-)
enteroviral vesicular pharyngitis (BØ8.5)

JØ2.9 Unspecified
Including: Gangrenous pharyngitis (acute); Infective pharyngitis (acute) NOS; Pharyngitis (acute) NOS; Sore throat (acute) NOS; Suppurative pharyngitis (acute); Ulcerative pharyngitis (acute)
Excludes1:
influenza virus with other respiratory manifestations (JØ9.X2, J1Ø.1, J11.1)

J06- ACUTE UPPER RESPIRATORY INFECTIONS OF MULTIPLE AND UNSPECIFIED SITES

Excludes1:
acute respiratory infection NOS (J22)
influenza virus with other respiratory manifestations (J09.X2, J10.1, J11.1)
streptococcal pharyngitis (J02.0)

J06.0 **Acute laryngopharyngitis**

J06.9 **Unspecified**
Including: Upper respiratory disease, acute; Upper respiratory infection NOS
Use additional code (B95-B97) to identify infectious agent, if known, such as:
respiratory syncytial virus (RSV) (B97.4)

OTHER ACUTE LOWER RESPIRATORY INFECTIONS (J20-J22)

Excludes2:
chronic obstructive pulmonary disease with acute lower respiratory infection (J44.0)

J20- ACUTE BRONCHITIS

Includes:
acute and subacute bronchitis (with) bronchospasm
acute and subacute bronchitis (with) tracheitis
acute and subacute bronchitis (with) tracheobronchitis, acute
acute and subacute fibrinous bronchitis
acute and subacute membranous bronchitis
acute and subacute purulent bronchitis
acute and subacute septic bronchitis

Excludes1:
bronchitis NOS (J40)
tracheobronchitis NOS (J40)

Excludes2:
acute bronchitis with bronchiectasis (J47.0)
acute bronchitis with chronic obstructive asthma (J44.0)
acute bronchitis with chronic obstructive pulmonary disease (J44.0)
allergic bronchitis NOS (J45.909-)
bronchitis due to chemicals, fumes and vapors (J68.0)
chronic bronchitis NOS (J42)
chronic mucopurulent bronchitis (J41.1)
chronic obstructive bronchitis (J44.-)
chronic obstructive tracheobronchitis (J44.-)
chronic simple bronchitis (J41.0)
chronic tracheobronchitis (J42)

J20.0 **Due to Mycoplasma pneumoniae**

J20.1 **Due to Hemophilus influenzae**

J20.2 **Due to streptococcus**

J20.3 **Due to coxsackievirus**

J20.4 **Due to parainfluenza virus**

J20.5 **Due to respiratory syncytial virus**
Including: Acute bronchitis due to RSV

J20.6 **Due to rhinovirus**

J20.7 **Due to echovirus**

J20.8 **Due to other specified organisms**

J20.9 **Unspecified**

J21- ACUTE BRONCHIOLITIS

Includes:
acute bronchiolitis with bronchospasm

Excludes2:
respiratory bronchiolitis interstitial lung disease (J84.115)

Indicator(s): CC

J21.9 **Unspecified**
Including: Bronchiolitis (acute)
Excludes1:
chronic bronchiolitis (J44.-)

J22 **Unspecified acute lower respiratory infection**
Including: Acute (lower) respiratory (tract) infection NOS
Excludes1:
upper respiratory infection (acute) (J06.9)

OTHER DISEASES OF UPPER RESPIRATORY TRACT (J30-J39)

J30- VASOMOTOR AND ALLERGIC RHINITIS

Includes:
spasmodic rhinorrhea

Excludes1:
allergic rhinitis with asthma (bronchial) (J45.909)
rhinitis NOS (J31.0)

J30.0 **Vasomotor rhinitis**

J30.1 **Allergic rhinitis due to pollen**
Including: Allergy NOS due to pollen, Hay fever, Pollinosis

J30.2 **Other seasonal allergic rhinitis**

J30.5 **Allergic rhinitis due to food**

J30.8- **Other allergic rhinitis**

J30.81 **Due to animal (cat) (dog) hair and dander**

J30.89 **Other**
Including: Perennial allergic rhinitis

J30.9 **Allergic rhinitis, unspecified**

J31- CHRONIC RHINITIS, NASOPHARYNGITIS AND PHARYNGITIS

Use additional code to identify:
exposure to environmental tobacco smoke (Z77.22)
exposure to tobacco smoke in the perinatal period (P96.81)
history of tobacco dependence (Z87.891)
occupational exposure to environmental tobacco smoke (Z57.31)
tobacco dependence (F17.-)
tobacco use (Z72.0)

J31.0 **Rhinitis**
Including: Atrophic, Granulomatous, Hypertrophic, Obstructive, Purulent, NOS, Ulcerative rhinitis (chronic); Ozena
Excludes1:
allergic rhinitis (J30.1-J30.9)
vasomotor rhinitis (J30.0)

J31.1 **Nasopharyngitis**
Excludes2:
acute nasopharyngitis (J00)

J31.2 **Pharyngitis**
Including: Chronic sore throat; Atrophic, Granular, Hypertrophic pharyngitis (chronic)
Excludes2:
acute pharyngitis (J02.9)

J32- CHRONIC SINUSITIS

Includes:
sinus abscess
sinus empyema
sinus infection
sinus suppuration
Use additional code to identify:
exposure to environmental tobacco smoke (Z77.22)
exposure to tobacco smoke in the perinatal period (P96.81)
history of tobacco dependence (Z87.891)
infectious agent (B95-B97)
occupational exposure to environmental tobacco smoke (Z57.31)
tobacco dependence (F17.-)
tobacco use (Z72.Ø)
Excludes2:
acute sinusitis (JØ1.-)

J32.Ø Maxillary
Including: Antritis (chronic), Maxillary sinusitis NOS

J32.1 Frontal
Including: Frontal sinusitis NOS

J32.2 Ethmoidal
Including: Ethmoidal sinusitis NOS
Excludes1:
Woakes' ethmoiditis (J33.1)

J32.3 Sphenoidal
Including: Sphenoidal sinusitis NOS

J32.4 Pansinusitis
Including: Pansinusitis NOS

J32.8 Other
Including: Sinusitis (chronic) involving more than one sinus but not pansinusitis

J32.9 Unspecified
Including: Sinusitis (chronic) NOS

CHRONIC LOWER RESPIRATORY DISEASES (J4Ø-J47)

Excludes1:
bronchitis due to chemicals, gases, fumes and vapors (J68.Ø)
Excludes2:
cystic fibrosis (E84.-)

J4Ø Bronchitis, not specified as acute or chronic
Including: Bronchitis NOS, with tracheitis NOS, Catarrhal bronchitis, Tracheobronchitis NOS
Use additional code to identify:
exposure to environmental tobacco smoke (Z77.22)
exposure to tobacco smoke in the perinatal period (P96.81)
history of tobacco dependence (Z87.891)
occupational exposure to environmental tobacco smoke (Z57.31)
tobacco dependence (F17.-)
tobacco use (Z72.Ø)
Excludes1:
acute bronchitis (J2Ø.-)
allergic bronchitis NOS (J45.9Ø9-)
asthmatic bronchitis NOS (J45.9-)
bronchitis due to chemicals, gases, fumes and vapors (J68.Ø)

J43- EMPHYSEMA

Use additional code to identify:
exposure to environmental tobacco smoke (Z77.22)
history of tobacco dependence (Z87.891)
occupational exposure to environmental tobacco smoke (Z57.31)
tobacco dependence (F17.-)
tobacco use (Z72.Ø)
Excludes1:
compensatory emphysema (J98.3)
emphysema due to inhalation of chemicals, gases, fumes or vapors (J68.4)
emphysema with chronic (obstructive) bronchitis (J44.-)
emphysematous (obstructive) bronchitis (J44.-)
interstitial emphysema (J98.2)
mediastinal emphysema (J98.2)
neonatal interstitial emphysema (P25.Ø)
surgical (subcutaneous) emphysema (T81.82)
Excludes2:
traumatic subcutaneous emphysema (T79.7)
Indicator(s): CMS22: 111 | CMS24: 111 | RxØ5: 226 | ESRD21: 111 | HHSØ5: 16Ø | HHSØ7: 16Ø

J43.9 Unspecified
Including: Bullous, Vesicular, NOS emphysema (lung) (pulmonary); Emphysematous bleb

J44- OTHER CHRONIC OBSTRUCTIVE PULMONARY DISEASE

Includes:
asthma with chronic obstructive pulmonary disease
chronic asthmatic (obstructive) bronchitis
chronic bronchitis with airway obstruction
chronic bronchitis with emphysema
chronic emphysematous bronchitis
chronic obstructive asthma
chronic obstructive bronchitis
chronic obstructive tracheobronchitis
Code Also
type of asthma, if applicable (J45.-)
Use additional code to identify:
exposure to environmental tobacco smoke (Z77.22)
history of tobacco dependence (Z87.891)
occupational exposure to environmental tobacco smoke (Z57.31)
tobacco dependence (F17.-)
tobacco use (Z72.Ø)
Excludes1:
bronchiectasis (J47.-)
chronic bronchitis NOS (J42)
chronic simple and mucopurulent bronchitis (J41.-)
chronic tracheitis (J42)
chronic tracheobronchitis (J42)
emphysema without chronic bronchitis (J43.-)
See Guidelines: 1;C.1Ø.a | 1;C.1Ø.a.1
Indicator(s): CMS22: 111 | CMS24: 111 | RxØ5: 226 | ESRD21: 111 | HHSØ5: 16Ø | HHSØ7: 16Ø

J44.9 Unspecified
Including: Chronic obstructive airway disease NOS; Chronic obstructive lung disease NOS
Excludes2:
lung diseases due to external agents (J6Ø-J7Ø)

J45- ASTHMA

Includes:
allergic (predominantly) asthma
allergic bronchitis NOS
allergic rhinitis with asthma
atopic asthma
extrinsic allergic asthma
hay fever with asthma
idiosyncratic asthma
intrinsic nonallergic asthma
nonallergic asthma
Use additional code to identify:
eosinophilic asthma (J82.83)
exposure to environmental tobacco smoke (Z77.22)
exposure to tobacco smoke in the perinatal period (P96.81)
history of tobacco dependence (Z87.891)
occupational exposure to environmental tobacco smoke (Z57.31)
tobacco dependence (F17.-)
tobacco use (Z72.Ø)
Excludes1:
detergent asthma (J69.8)
miner's asthma (J6Ø)
wheezing NOS (RØ6.2)
wood asthma (J67.8)
Excludes2:
asthma with chronic obstructive pulmonary disease (J44.9)
chronic asthmatic (obstructive) bronchitis (J44.9)
chronic obstructive asthma (J44.9)
See Guidelines: 1;C.1Ø.a | 1;C.1Ø.a.1
Indicator(s): RxØ5: 226 | HHSØ5: 161

J45.9- **Other and unspecified asthma**

J45.9Ø- **Unspecified asthma**
Including: Asthmatic bronchitis NOS; Childhood asthma NOS; Late onset asthma

J45.9Ø9 **Uncomplicated**
Including: Asthma NOS
Excludes2:
lung diseases due to external agents (J6Ø-J7Ø)

OTHER DISEASES OF THE RESPIRATORY SYSTEM (J96-J99)

J98- OTHER RESPIRATORY DISORDERS

Use additional code to identify:
exposure to environmental tobacco smoke (Z77.22)
exposure to tobacco smoke in the perinatal period (P96.81)
history of tobacco dependence (Z87.891)
occupational exposure to environmental tobacco smoke (Z57.31)
tobacco dependence (F17.-)
tobacco use (Z72.Ø)
Excludes1:
newborn apnea (P28.4-)
newborn sleep apnea (P28.3-)
Excludes2:
apnea NOS (RØ6.81)
sleep apnea (G47.3-)

J98.9 **Unspecified**
Including: Respiratory disease (chronic) NOS

11. Diseases of the digestive system (KØØ-K95)

Excludes2:
certain conditions originating in the perinatal period (PØ4-P96)
certain infectious and parasitic diseases (AØØ-B99)
complications of pregnancy, childbirth and the puerperium (OØØ-O9A)
congenital malformations, deformations and chromosomal abnormalities (QØØ-Q99)
endocrine, nutritional and metabolic diseases (EØØ-E88)
injury, poisoning and certain other consequences of external causes (SØØ-T88)
neoplasms (CØØ-D49)
symptoms, signs and abnormal clinical and laboratory findings, not elsewhere classified (RØØ-R94)
See Guidelines: 1;C.2Ø.a.1

DISEASES OF ESOPHAGUS, STOMACH AND DUODENUM (K2Ø-K31)

Excludes2:
hiatus hernia (K44.-)

K31- OTHER DISEASES OF STOMACH AND DUODENUM
Includes:
functional disorders of stomach
Excludes2:
diabetic gastroparesis (EØ8.43, EØ9.43, E1Ø.43, E11.43, E13.43)
diverticulum of duodenum (K57.ØØ-K57.13)

K31.9 Unspecified

NONINFECTIVE ENTERITIS AND COLITIS (K5Ø-K52)

Includes:
noninfective inflammatory bowel disease
Excludes1:
irritable bowel syndrome (K58.-)
megacolon (K59.3-)

K5Ø- CROHN'S DISEASE [REGIONAL ENTERITIS]
Includes:
granulomatous enteritis
Use additional code to identify manifestations, such as:
pyoderma gangrenosum (L88)
Excludes1:
ulcerative colitis (K51.-)
Indicator(s): CMS22: 35 | CMS24: 35 | RxØ5: 67 | ESRD21: 35 | HHSØ5: 48

K5Ø.9- **Crohn's disease, unspecified**
Indicator(s): CC

K5Ø.9Ø Without complications
Including: Crohn's NOS, Regional enteritis NOS

K51- ULCERATIVE COLITIS
Use additional code to identify manifestations, such as:
pyoderma gangrenosum (L88)
Excludes1:
Crohn's disease [regional enteritis] (K5Ø.-)
Indicator(s): CMS22: 35 | CMS24: 35 | RxØ5: 67 | ESRD21: 35 | HHSØ5: 48

K51.9- **Ulcerative colitis, unspecified**
Indicator(s): CC

K51.9Ø Without complications

K52- OTHER AND UNSPECIFIED NONINFECTIVE GASTROENTERITIS AND COLITIS

K52.9 Unspecified
Including: Colitis NOS, Enteritis NOS, Gastroenteritis NOS, Ileitis NOS, Jejunitis NOS, Sigmoiditis NOS
Excludes1:
diarrhea NOS (R19.7)
functional diarrhea (K59.1)
infectious gastroenteritis and colitis NOS (AØ9)
neonatal diarrhea (noninfective) (P78.3)
psychogenic diarrhea (F45.8)

OTHER DISEASES OF INTESTINES (K55-K64)

K58- IRRITABLE BOWEL SYNDROME
Includes:
irritable colon
spastic colon

K58.Ø With diarrhea

K58.1 With constipation

K58.9 Without diarrhea
Including: Irritable bowel syndrome NOS

K59- OTHER FUNCTIONAL INTESTINAL DISORDERS
Excludes1:
change in bowel habit NOS (R19.4)
intestinal malabsorption (K9Ø.-)
psychogenic intestinal disorders (F45.8)
Excludes2:
functional disorders of stomach (K31.-)

K59.Ø- **Constipation**
Excludes1:
fecal impaction (K56.41)
incomplete defecation (R15.Ø)

K59.ØØ Unspecified

K59.Ø9 Other
Including: Chronic constipation

K59.1 Functional diarrhea
Excludes1:
diarrhea NOS (R19.7)
irritable bowel syndrome with diarrhea (K58.Ø)

K64- HEMORRHOIDS AND PERIANAL VENOUS THROMBOSIS
Includes:
piles
Excludes1:
hemorrhoids complicating childbirth and the puerperium (O87.2)
hemorrhoids complicating pregnancy (O22.4)

K64.9 Unspecified
Including: Hemorrhoids (bleeding) NOS, Hemorrhoids (bleeding) without mention of degree

DISEASES OF LIVER (K7Ø-K77)

Excludes1:
jaundice NOS (R17)
Excludes2:
hemochromatosis (E83.11-)
Reye's syndrome (G93.7)
viral hepatitis (B15-B19)
Wilson's disease (E83.Ø)

See Appendix A — Coding Reference Tables for lists of the ICD-10-CM Tabular indicators, HAC categories, and HCC codes.

K7Ø- ALCOHOLIC LIVER DISEASE

Use additional code to identify:
alcohol abuse and dependence (F1Ø.-)

K7Ø.9 Unspecified

Indicator(s): CMS22: 28 | CMS24: 28 | ESRD21: 28 | HHSØ5: 36

K76- OTHER DISEASES OF LIVER

Excludes2:
alcoholic liver disease (K7Ø.-)
amyloid degeneration of liver (E85.-)
cystic disease of liver (congenital) (Q44.6)
hepatic vein thrombosis (I82.Ø)
hepatomegaly NOS (R16.Ø)
pigmentary cirrhosis (of liver) (E83.11Ø)
portal vein thrombosis (I81)
toxic liver disease (K71.-)

K76.9 Unspecified

12. Diseases of the skin and subcutaneous tissue (LØØ-L99)

Excludes2:
certain conditions originating in the perinatal period (PØ4-P96)
certain infectious and parasitic diseases (AØØ-B99)
complications of pregnancy, childbirth and the puerperium (OØØ-O9A)
congenital malformations, deformations, and chromosomal abnormalities (QØØ-Q99)
endocrine, nutritional and metabolic diseases (EØØ-E88)
lipomelanotic reticulosis (I89.8)
neoplasms (CØØ-D49)
symptoms, signs and abnormal clinical and laboratory findings, not elsewhere classified (RØØ-R94)
systemic connective tissue disorders (M3Ø-M36)
viral warts (BØ7.-)
See Guidelines: 1;C.2Ø.a.1

DERMATITIS AND ECZEMA (L2Ø-L3Ø)

Notes:
In this block the terms dermatitis and eczema are used synonymously and interchangeably.
Excludes2:
chronic (childhood) granulomatous disease (D71)
dermatitis gangrenosa (LØ8.Ø)
dermatitis herpetiformis (L13.Ø)
dry skin dermatitis (L85.3)
factitial dermatitis (L98.1)
perioral dermatitis (L71.Ø)
radiation-related disorders of the skin and subcutaneous tissue (L55-L59)
stasis dermatitis (I87.2)

L2Ø- ATOPIC DERMATITIS

L2Ø.9 Unspecified

L22 Diaper dermatitis
Including: Diaper erythema, rash; Psoriasiform diaper rash

L23- ALLERGIC CONTACT DERMATITIS

Excludes1:
allergy NOS (T78.4Ø)
contact dermatitis NOS (L25.9)
dermatitis NOS (L3Ø.9)
Excludes2:
dermatitis due to substances taken internally (L27.-)
dermatitis of eyelid (HØ1.1-)
diaper dermatitis (L22)
eczema of external ear (H6Ø.5-)
irritant contact dermatitis (L24.-)
perioral dermatitis (L71.Ø)
radiation-related disorders of the skin and subcutaneous tissue (L55-L59)

L23.Ø Due to metals
Including: chromium, nickel

L23.1 Due to adhesives

L23.2 Due to cosmetics

L23.3 Due to drugs in contact with skin
Use additional code for adverse effect, if applicable, to identify drug (T36-T5Ø with fifth or sixth character 5)
Excludes2:
dermatitis due to ingested drugs and medicaments (L27.Ø-L27.1)

L23.4 Due to dyes

L23.5 Due to other chemical products
Including: cement, insecticide, plastic, rubber

L23.6 Due to food in contact with the skin
Excludes2:
dermatitis due to ingested food (L27.2)

L23.7 Due to plants, except food
Excludes2:
allergy NOS due to pollen (J3Ø.1)

L23.8- **Due to other agents**

L23.81 Animal (cat) (dog) dander
Including: due to animal (cat) (dog) hair

L23.89 Other

L23.9 Unspecified cause
Including: Allergic contact eczema NOS

L24- IRRITANT CONTACT DERMATITIS

Excludes1:
allergy NOS (T78.4Ø)
contact dermatitis NOS (L25.9)
dermatitis NOS (L3Ø.9)
Excludes2:
allergic contact dermatitis (L23.-)
dermatitis due to substances taken internally (L27.-)
dermatitis of eyelid (HØ1.1-)
diaper dermatitis (L22)
eczema of external ear (H6Ø.5-)
perioral dermatitis (L71.Ø)
radiation-related disorders of the skin and subcutaneous tissue (L55-L59)

L24.Ø Due to detergents

L24.1 Due to oils and greases

L24.2 Due to solvents
Including: chlorocompound, cyclohexane, ester, glycol, hydrocarbon, ketone

L24.3 Due to cosmetics

L24.4 Due to drugs in contact with skin
Use additional code for adverse effect, if applicable, to identify drug (T36-T5Ø with fifth or sixth character 5)

L24.5 Due to other chemical products
Including: cement, insecticide, plastic, rubber

L24.6 Due to food in contact with skin
Excludes2:
dermatitis due to ingested food (L27.2)

L24.7 Due to plants, except food
Excludes2:
allergy NOS to pollen (J3Ø.1)

L24.8- **Due to other agents**

L24.81 Metals
Including: chromium, nickel

L24.89 Other
Including: dyes

L24.9 Unspecified cause
Including: Irritant contact eczema NOS

L25- UNSPECIFIED CONTACT DERMATITIS

Excludes1:
allergic contact dermatitis (L23.-)
allergy NOS (T78.4Ø)
dermatitis NOS (L3Ø.9)
irritant contact dermatitis (L24.-)
Excludes2:
dermatitis due to ingested substances (L27.-)
dermatitis of eyelid (HØ1.1-)
eczema of external ear (H6Ø.5-)
perioral dermatitis (L71.Ø)
radiation-related disorders of the skin and subcutaneous tissue (L55-L59)

L25.Ø Due to cosmetics

L25.1 Due to drugs in contact with skin
Use additional code for adverse effect, if applicable, to identify drug (T36-T5Ø with fifth or sixth character 5)
Excludes2:
dermatitis due to ingested drugs and medicaments (L27.Ø-L27.1)

L25.2 Due to dyes

L25.3 Due to other chemical products
Including: cement, insecticide

L25.4 Due to food in contact with skin
Excludes2:
dermatitis due to ingested food (L27.2)

L25.5 Due to plants, except food
Excludes1:
nettle rash (L5Ø.9)
Excludes2:
allergy NOS due to pollen (J3Ø.1)

L25.8 Due to other agents

L25.9 Unspecified cause
Including: Contact dermatitis (occupational) NOS, Contact eczema (occupational) NOS

L26 Exfoliative dermatitis
Including: Hebra's pityriasis
Excludes1:
Ritter's disease (LØØ)

L27- DERMATITIS DUE TO SUBSTANCES TAKEN INTERNALLY

Excludes1:
allergy NOS (T78.4Ø)
Excludes2:
adverse food reaction, except dermatitis (T78.Ø-T78.1)
contact dermatitis (L23-L25)
drug photoallergic response (L56.1)
drug phototoxic response (L56.Ø)
urticaria (L5Ø.-)

L27.Ø Generalized skin eruption due to drugs and medicaments
Use additional code for adverse effect, if applicable, to identify drug (T36-T5Ø with fifth or sixth character 5)

L27.1 Localized skin eruption due to drugs and medicaments
Use additional code for adverse effect, if applicable, to identify drug (T36-T5Ø with fifth or sixth character 5)

L27.2 Ingested food
Excludes2:
dermatitis due to food in contact with skin (L23.6, L24.6, L25.4)

L27.8 Other substances

L27.9 Unspecified substance

L29- PRURITUS

Excludes1:
neurotic excoriation (L98.1)
psychogenic pruritus (F45.8)

L29.9 Unspecified
Including: Itch NOS

L3Ø- OTHER AND UNSPECIFIED DERMATITIS

Excludes2:
contact dermatitis (L23-L25)
dry skin dermatitis (L85.3)
small plaque parapsoriasis (L41.3)
stasis dermatitis (I87.2)

L3Ø.9 Unspecified
Including: Eczema NOS

PAPULOSQUAMOUS DISORDERS (L4Ø-L45)

L4Ø- PSORIASIS

L4Ø.9 Unspecified
Indicator(s): RxØ5: 316

URTICARIA AND ERYTHEMA (L49-L54)

Excludes1:
Lyme disease (A69.2-)
rosacea (L71.-)

L5Ø- URTICARIA

Excludes1:
allergic contact dermatitis (L23.-)
angioneurotic edema (T78.3)
giant urticaria (T78.3)
hereditary angio-edema (D84.1)
Quincke's edema (T78.3)
serum urticaria (T8Ø.6-)
solar urticaria (L56.3)
urticaria neonatorum (P83.8)
urticaria papulosa (L28.2)
urticaria pigmentosa (D47.Ø1)

L5Ø.9 Unspecified

L51- ERYTHEMA MULTIFORME

Use additional code for adverse effect, if applicable, to identify drug (T36-T5Ø with fifth or sixth character 5)
Use additional code to identify associated manifestations, such as:
arthropathy associated with dermatological disorders (M14.8-)
conjunctival edema (H11.42)
conjunctivitis (H1Ø.22-)
corneal scars and opacities (H17.-)
corneal ulcer (H16.Ø-)
edema of eyelid (HØ2.84-)
inflammation of eyelid (HØ1.8)
keratoconjunctivitis sicca (H16.22-)
mechanical lagophthalmos (HØ2.22-)
stomatitis (K12.-)
symblepharon (H11.23-)
Use additional code to identify percentage of skin exfoliation (L49.-)
Excludes1:
staphylococcal scalded skin syndrome (LØØ)
Ritter's disease (LØØ)

L51.9 Unspecified
Including: Erythema iris, multiforme major NOS, multiforme minor NOS; Herpes iris

L52 Erythema nodosum
Excludes1:
tuberculous erythema nodosum (A18.4)

Ch5

5. The Tabular List

L53- OTHER ERYTHEMATOUS CONDITIONS

Excludes1:
erythema ab igne (L59.Ø)
erythema due to external agents in contact with skin (L23-L25)
erythema intertrigo (L3Ø.4)

L53.9 **Unspecified**
Including: Erythema NOS, Erythroderma NOS

RADIATION-RELATED DISORDERS OF THE SKIN AND SUBCUTANEOUS TISSUE (L55-L59)

L55- SUNBURN

L55.Ø **First degree**

L55.1 **Second degree**

L55.2 **Third degree**
Indicator(s): HHSØ7: 219

L55.9 **Unspecified**

DISORDERS OF SKIN APPENDAGES (L6Ø-L75)

Excludes1:
congenital malformations of integument (Q84.-)

L6Ø- NAIL DISORDERS

Excludes2:
clubbing of nails (R68.3)
onychia and paronychia (LØ3.Ø-)

L6Ø.9 **Unspecified**

L7Ø- ACNE

Excludes2:
acne keloid (L73.Ø)

L7Ø.Ø **Vulgaris**

L7Ø.9 **Unspecified**

L71- ROSACEA

Use additional code for adverse effect, if applicable, to identify drug (T36-T5Ø with fifth or sixth character 5)

L71.9 **Unspecified**

OTHER DISORDERS OF THE SKIN AND SUBCUTANEOUS TISSUE (L8Ø-L99)

L84 **Corns and callosities**
Including: Callus, Clavus

L98- OTHER DISORDERS OF SKIN AND SUBCUTANEOUS TISSUE, NOT ELSEWHERE CLASSIFIED

L98.9 **Unspecified**

13. Diseases of the musculoskeletal system and connective tissue (MØØ-M99)

Notes:

Use an external cause code following the code for the musculoskeletal condition, if applicable, to identify the cause of the musculoskeletal condition

Excludes2:

arthropathic psoriasis (L4Ø.5-)
certain conditions originating in the perinatal period (PØ4-P96)
certain infectious and parasitic diseases (AØØ-B99)
compartment syndrome (traumatic) (T79.A-)
complications of pregnancy, childbirth and the puerperium (OØØ-O9A)
congenital malformations, deformations, and chromosomal abnormalities (QØØ-Q99)
endocrine, nutritional and metabolic diseases (EØØ-E88)
injury, poisoning and certain other consequences of external causes (SØØ-T88)
neoplasms (CØØ-D49)
symptoms, signs and abnormal clinical and laboratory findings, not elsewhere classified (RØØ-R94)

See Guidelines: 1;C.13.a-b | 1;C.2Ø.a.1

ARTHROPATHIES (MØØ-M25)

Includes:

Disorders affecting predominantly peripheral (limb) joints

INFECTIOUS ARTHROPATHIES (MØØ-MØ2)

Notes:

This block comprises arthropathies due to microbiological agents. Distinction is made between the following types of etiological relationship:
a) direct infection of joint, where organisms invade synovial tissue and microbial antigen is present in the joint;
b) indirect infection, which may be of two types: a reactive arthropathy, where microbial infection of the body is established but neither organisms nor antigens can be identified in the joint, and a postinfective arthropathy, where microbial antigen is present but recovery of an organism is inconstant and evidence of local multiplication is lacking.

MØ2- POSTINFECTIVE AND REACTIVE ARTHROPATHIES

Code First:

underlying disease, such as:
congenital syphilis [Clutton's joints] (A5Ø.5)
enteritis due to Yersinia enterocolitica (AØ4.6)
infective endocarditis (I33.Ø)
viral hepatitis (B15-B19)

Excludes1:

Behçet's disease (M35.2)
direct infections of joint in infectious and parasitic diseases classified elsewhere (MØ1.-)
postmeningococcal arthritis (A39.84)
mumps arthritis (B26.85)
rubella arthritis (BØ6.82)
syphilis arthritis (late) (A52.77)
rheumatic fever (IØØ)
tabetic arthropathy [Charcôt's] (A52.16)

MØ2.3- **Reiter's disease**
Including: Reactive arthritis
Indicator(s): CC | CMS22: 4Ø | CMS24: 4Ø | RxØ5: 83 | ESRD21: 4Ø | HHSØ5: 57 | HHSØ7: 57

MØ2.3Ø Unspecified site
MØ2.31- **Shoulder**
MØ2.311 Right
MØ2.312 Left
MØ2.319 Unspecified
MØ2.32- **Elbow**
MØ2.321 Right
MØ2.322 Left
MØ2.329 Unspecified
MØ2.33- **Wrist**
Including: Carpal bones
MØ2.331 Right
MØ2.332 Left
MØ2.339 Unspecified
MØ2.34- **Hand**
Including: Metacarpus and phalanges
MØ2.341 Right
MØ2.342 Left
MØ2.349 Unspecified
MØ2.35- **Hip**
MØ2.351 Right
MØ2.352 Left
MØ2.359 Unspecified
MØ2.36- **Knee**
MØ2.361 Right
MØ2.362 Left
MØ2.369 Unspecified
MØ2.37- **Ankle and foot**
Including: Tarsus, metatarsus and phalanges
MØ2.371 Right
MØ2.372 Left
MØ2.379 Unspecified
MØ2.38 Vertebrae
MØ2.39 Multiple sites

INFLAMMATORY POLYARTHROPATHIES (MØ5-M14)

MØ5- RHEUMATOID ARTHRITIS WITH RHEUMATOID FACTOR

Excludes1:

rheumatic fever (IØØ)
juvenile rheumatoid arthritis (MØ8.-)
rheumatoid arthritis of spine (M45.-)

Indicator(s): CMS22: 4Ø | HHSØ7: 56

MØ5.Ø- **Felty's syndrome**
Including: Rheumatoid arthritis with splenoadenomegaly and leukopenia

MØ5.ØØ Unspecified site
MØ5.Ø1- **Shoulder**
MØ5.Ø11 Right
MØ5.Ø12 Left
MØ5.Ø19 Unspecified

MØ5.Ø2- **Elbow**
- **MØ5.Ø21** **Right**
- **MØ5.Ø22** **Left**
- **MØ5.Ø29** **Unspecified**

MØ5.Ø3- **Wrist**
Including: Carpal bones
- **MØ5.Ø31** **Right**
- **MØ5.Ø32** **Left**
- **MØ5.Ø39** **Unspecified**

MØ5.Ø4- **Hand**
Including: Metacarpus and phalanges
- **MØ5.Ø41** **Right**
- **MØ5.Ø42** **Left**
- **MØ5.Ø49** **Unspecified**

MØ5.Ø5- **Hip**
- **MØ5.Ø51** **Right**
- **MØ5.Ø52** **Left**
- **MØ5.Ø59** **Unspecified**

MØ5.Ø6- **Knee**
- **MØ5.Ø61** **Right**
- **MØ5.Ø62** **Left**
- **MØ5.Ø69** **Unspecified**

MØ5.Ø7- **Ankle and foot**
Including: Tarsus, metatarsus and phalanges
- **MØ5.Ø71** **Right**
- **MØ5.Ø72** **Left**
- **MØ5.Ø79** **Unspecified**

MØ5.Ø9 **Multiple sites**

MØ5.1- **Rheumatoid lung disease with rheumatoid arthritis**

MØ5.1Ø **Unspecified site**

MØ5.11- **Shoulder**
- **MØ5.111** **Right**
- **MØ5.112** **Left**
- **MØ5.119** **Unspecified**

MØ5.12- **Elbow**
- **MØ5.121** **Right**
- **MØ5.122** **Left**
- **MØ5.129** **Unspecified**

MØ5.13- **Wrist**
Including: Carpal bones
- **MØ5.131** **Right**
- **MØ5.132** **Left**
- **MØ5.139** **Unspecified**

MØ5.14- **Hand**
Including: Metacarpus and phalanges
- **MØ5.141** **Right**
- **MØ5.142** **Left**
- **MØ5.149** **Unspecified**

MØ5.15- **Hip**
- **MØ5.151** **Right**
- **MØ5.152** **Left**
- **MØ5.159** **Unspecified**

MØ5.16- **Knee**
- **MØ5.161** **Right**
- **MØ5.162** **Left**
- **MØ5.169** **Unspecified**

MØ5.17- **Ankle and foot**
Including: Tarsus, metatarsus and phalanges
- **MØ5.171** **Right**
- **MØ5.172** **Left**
- **MØ5.179** **Unspecified**

MØ5.19 **Multiple sites**

MØ5.2- **Rheumatoid vasculitis with rheumatoid arthritis**

MØ5.2Ø **Unspecified site**

MØ5.21- **Shoulder**
- **MØ5.211** **Right**
- **MØ5.212** **Left**
- **MØ5.219** **Unspecified**

MØ5.22- **Elbow**
- **MØ5.221** **Right**
- **MØ5.222** **Left**
- **MØ5.229** **Unspecified**

MØ5.23- **Wrist**
Including: Carpal bones
- **MØ5.231** **Right**
- **MØ5.232** **Left**
- **MØ5.239** **Unspecified**

MØ5.24- **Hand**
Including: Metacarpus and phalanges
- **MØ5.241** **Right**
- **MØ5.242** **Left**
- **MØ5.249** **Unspecified**

MØ5.25- **Hip**
- **MØ5.251** **Right**
- **MØ5.252** **Left**
- **MØ5.259** **Unspecified**

MØ5.26- **Knee**
- **MØ5.261** **Right**
- **MØ5.262** **Left**
- **MØ5.269** **Unspecified**

MØ5.27- **Ankle and foot**
Including: Tarsus, metatarsus and phalanges
- **MØ5.271** **Right**
- **MØ5.272** **Left**
- **MØ5.279** **Unspecified**

MØ5.29 **Multiple sites**

MØ5.3- **Rheumatoid heart disease with rheumatoid arthritis**
Including: Carditis, endocarditis, myocarditis, pericarditis

MØ5.3Ø **Unspecified site**

MØ5.31- **Shoulder**
- **MØ5.311** **Right**
- **MØ5.312** **Left**
- **MØ5.319** **Unspecified**

MØ5.32- **Elbow**
- **MØ5.321** **Right**
- **MØ5.322** **Left**
- **MØ5.329** **Unspecified**

MØ5.33- **Wrist**
Including: Carpal bones
MØ5.331 Right
MØ5.332 Left
MØ5.339 Unspecified
MØ5.34- **Hand**
Including: Metacarpus and phalanges
MØ5.341 Right
MØ5.342 Left
MØ5.349 Unspecified
MØ5.35- **Hip**
MØ5.351 Right
MØ5.352 Left
MØ5.359 Unspecified
MØ5.36- **Knee**
MØ5.361 Right
MØ5.362 Left
MØ5.369 Unspecified
MØ5.37- **Ankle and foot**
Including: Tarsus, metatarsus and phalanges
MØ5.371 Right
MØ5.372 Left
MØ5.379 Unspecified
MØ5.39 Multiple sites

MØ5.4- **Rheumatoid myopathy with rheumatoid arthritis**
Indicator(s): CC
MØ5.4Ø Unspecified site
MØ5.41- **Shoulder**
MØ5.411 Right
MØ5.412 Left
MØ5.419 Unspecified
MØ5.42- **Elbow**
MØ5.421 Right
MØ5.422 Left
MØ5.429 Unspecified
MØ5.43- **Wrist**
Including: Carpal bones
MØ5.431 Right
MØ5.432 Left
MØ5.439 Unspecified
MØ5.44- **Hand**
Including: Metacarpus and phalanges
MØ5.441 Right
MØ5.442 Left
MØ5.449 Unspecified
MØ5.45- **Hip**
MØ5.451 Right
MØ5.452 Left
MØ5.459 Unspecified
MØ5.46- **Knee**
MØ5.461 Right
MØ5.462 Left
MØ5.469 Unspecified
MØ5.47- **Ankle and foot**
Including: Tarsus, metatarsus and phalanges
MØ5.471 Right
MØ5.472 Left
MØ5.479 Unspecified
MØ5.49 Multiple sites

MØ5.5- **Rheumatoid polyneuropathy with rheumatoid arthritis**
MØ5.5Ø Unspecified site
MØ5.51- **Shoulder**
MØ5.511 Right
MØ5.512 Left
MØ5.519 Unspecified
MØ5.52- **Elbow**
MØ5.521 Right
MØ5.522 Left
MØ5.529 Unspecified
MØ5.53- **Wrist**
Including: Carpal bones
MØ5.531 Right
MØ5.532 Left
MØ5.539 Unspecified
MØ5.54- **Hand**
Including: Metacarpus and phalanges
MØ5.541 Right
MØ5.542 Left
MØ5.549 Unspecified
MØ5.55- **Hip**
MØ5.551 Right
MØ5.552 Left
MØ5.559 Unspecified
MØ5.56- **Knee**
MØ5.561 Right
MØ5.562 Left
MØ5.569 Unspecified
MØ5.57- **Ankle and foot**
Including: Tarsus, metatarsus and phalanges
MØ5.571 Right
MØ5.572 Left
MØ5.579 Unspecified
MØ5.59 Multiple sites

MØ5.6- **Rheumatoid arthritis with involvement of other organs and systems**
MØ5.6Ø Unspecified site
MØ5.61- **Shoulder**
MØ5.611 Right
MØ5.612 Left
MØ5.619 Unspecified
MØ5.62- **Elbow**
MØ5.621 Right
MØ5.622 Left
MØ5.629 Unspecified
MØ5.63- **Wrist**
Including: Carpal bones
MØ5.631 Right
MØ5.632 Left
MØ5.639 Unspecified

M05.64- **Hand**
Including: Metacarpus and phalanges
M05.641 Right
M05.642 Left
M05.649 Unspecified
M05.65- **Hip**
M05.651 Right
M05.652 Left
M05.659 Unspecified
M05.66- **Knee**
M05.661 Right
M05.662 Left
M05.669 Unspecified
M05.67- **Ankle and foot**
Including: Metatarsus and phalanges
M05.671 Right
M05.672 Left
M05.679 Unspecified
M05.69 Multiple sites

M05.7- **Rheumatoid arthritis with rheumatoid factor without organ or systems involvement**
M05.70 Unspecified site
M05.71- **Shoulder**
M05.711 Right
M05.712 Left
M05.719 Unspecified
M05.72- **Elbow**
M05.721 Right
M05.722 Left
M05.729 Unspecified
M05.73- **Wrist**
M05.731 Right
M05.732 Left
M05.739 Unspecified
M05.74- **Hand**
M05.741 Right
M05.742 Left
M05.749 Unspecified
M05.75- **Hip**
M05.751 Right
M05.752 Left
M05.759 Unspecified
M05.76- **Knee**
M05.761 Right
M05.762 Left
M05.769 Unspecified
M05.77- **Ankle and foot**
M05.771 Right
M05.772 Left
M05.779 Unspecified
M05.79 Multiple sites
M05.7A Other specified site

M05.8- **Other rheumatoid arthritis with rheumatoid factor**
M05.80 Unspecified site
M05.81- **Shoulder**
M05.811 Right
M05.812 Left
M05.819 Unspecified
M05.82- **Elbow**
M05.821 Right
M05.822 Left
M05.829 Unspecified
M05.83- **Wrist**
M05.831 Right
M05.832 Left
M05.839 Unspecified
M05.84- **Hand**
M05.841 Right
M05.842 Left
M05.849 Unspecified
M05.85- **Hip**
M05.851 Right
M05.852 Left
M05.859 Unspecified
M05.86- **Knee**
M05.861 Right
M05.862 Left
M05.869 Unspecified
M05.87- **Ankle and foot**
M05.871 Right
M05.872 Left
M05.879 Unspecified
M05.89 Multiple sites
M05.8A Other specified site

M05.9 Unspecified

M14- ARTHROPATHIES IN OTHER DISEASES CLASSIFIED ELSEWHERE

Excludes1:
arthropathy in:
diabetes mellitus (E08-E13 with .61-)
hematological disorders (M36.2-M36.3)
hypersensitivity reactions (M36.4)
neoplastic disease (M36.1)
neurosyphillis (A52.16)
sarcoidosis (D86.86)
enteropathic arthropathies (M07.-)
juvenile psoriatic arthropathy (L40.54)
lipoid dermatoarthritis (E78.81)

M14.8- **Arthropathies in other specified diseases classified elsewhere**
Code First:
underlying disease, such as:
amyloidosis (E85.-)
erythema multiforme (L51.-)
erythema nodosum (L52)
hemochromatosis (E83.11-)
hyperparathyroidism (E21.-)
hypothyroidism (E00-E03)
sickle-cell disorders (D57.-)
thyrotoxicosis [hyperthyroidism] (E05.-)
Whipple's disease (K90.81)
M14.80 Unspecified site
M14.88 Vertebrae
M14.89 Multiple sites

See Appendix A — Coding Reference Tables for lists of the ICD-10-CM Tabular indicators, HAC categories, and HCC codes.

MØ6- OTHER RHEUMATOID ARTHRITIS

Indicator(s): CMS22: 4Ø | ESRD21: 4Ø

MØ6.Ø- **Rheumatoid arthritis without rheumatoid factor**

MØ6.ØØ Unspecified site

MØ6.Ø1- **Shoulder**

MØ6.Ø11 Right

MØ6.Ø12 Left

MØ6.Ø19 Unspecified

MØ6.Ø2- **Elbow**

MØ6.Ø21 Right

MØ6.Ø22 Left

MØ6.Ø29 Unspecified

MØ6.Ø3- **Wrist**

MØ6.Ø31 Right

MØ6.Ø32 Left

MØ6.Ø39 Unspecified

MØ6.Ø4- **Hand**

MØ6.Ø41 Right

MØ6.Ø42 Left

MØ6.Ø49 Unspecified

MØ6.Ø5- **Hip**

MØ6.Ø51 Right

MØ6.Ø52 Left

MØ6.Ø59 Unspecified

MØ6.Ø6- **Knee**

MØ6.Ø61 Right

MØ6.Ø62 Left

MØ6.Ø69 Unspecified

MØ6.Ø7- **Ankle and foot**

MØ6.Ø71 Right

MØ6.Ø72 Left

MØ6.Ø79 Unspecified

MØ6.Ø8 Vertebrae

MØ6.Ø9 Multiple sites

MØ6.ØA Other specified site

MØ6.1 Adult-onset Still's disease

Excludes1:

Still's disease NOS (MØ8.2-)

Indicator(s): Adult

MØ6.2- **Rheumatoid bursitis**

MØ6.2Ø Unspecified site

MØ6.21- **Shoulder**

MØ6.211 Right

MØ6.212 Left

MØ6.219 Unspecified

MØ6.22- **Elbow**

MØ6.221 Right

MØ6.222 Left

MØ6.229 Unspecified

MØ6.23- **Wrist**

MØ6.231 Right

MØ6.232 Left

MØ6.239 Unspecified

MØ6.24- **Hand**

MØ6.241 Right

MØ6.242 Left

MØ6.249 Unspecified

MØ6.25- **Hip**

MØ6.251 Right

MØ6.252 Left

MØ6.259 Unspecified

MØ6.26- **Knee**

MØ6.261 Right

MØ6.262 Left

MØ6.269 Unspecified

MØ6.27- **Ankle and foot**

MØ6.271 Right

MØ6.272 Left

MØ6.279 Unspecified

MØ6.28 Vertebrae

MØ6.29 Multiple sites

MØ6.3- **Rheumatoid nodule**

MØ6.3Ø Unspecified site

MØ6.31- **Shoulder**

MØ6.311 Right

MØ6.312 Left

MØ6.319 Unspecified

MØ6.32- **Elbow**

MØ6.321 Right

MØ6.322 Left

MØ6.329 Unspecified

MØ6.33- **Wrist**

MØ6.331 Right

MØ6.332 Left

MØ6.339 Unspecified

MØ6.34- **Hand**

MØ6.341 Right

MØ6.342 Left

MØ6.349 Unspecified

MØ6.35- **Hip**

MØ6.351 Right

MØ6.352 Left

MØ6.359 Unspecified

MØ6.36- **Knee**

MØ6.361 Right

MØ6.362 Left

MØ6.369 Unspecified

MØ6.37- **Ankle and foot**

MØ6.371 Right

MØ6.372 Left

MØ6.379 Unspecified

MØ6.38 Vertebrae

MØ6.39 Multiple sites

MØ6.8- **Other specified rheumatoid arthritis**

MØ6.88 Vertebrae

MØ6.89 Multiple sites

MØ6.8A Other specified site

MØ6.9 Unspecified

MØ8- JUVENILE ARTHRITIS

<u>*Code Also*</u>

any associated underlying condition, such as:

regional enteritis [Crohn's disease] (K5Ø.-)

ulcerative colitis (K51.-)

<u>*Excludes1:*</u>

arthropathy in Whipple's disease (M14.8)

Felty's syndrome (MØ5.Ø)

juvenile dermatomyositis (M33.Ø-)

psoriatic juvenile arthropathy (L4Ø.54)

<u>*Indicator(s):*</u> *CMS22: 4Ø | ESRD21: 4Ø | HHSØ7: 56*

MØ8.Ø- **Unspecified juvenile rheumatoid arthritis**

Including: Juvenile rheumatoid arthritis with or without rheumatoid factor

MØ8.ØØ Unspecified site

MØ8.Ø1- **Shoulder**

MØ8.Ø11 Right

MØ8.Ø12 Left

MØ8.Ø19 Unspecified

MØ8.Ø2- **Elbow**

MØ8.Ø21 Right

MØ8.Ø22 Left

MØ8.Ø29 Unspecified

MØ8.Ø3- **Wrist**

MØ8.Ø31 Right

MØ8.Ø32 Left

MØ8.Ø39 Unspecified

MØ8.Ø4- **Hand**

MØ8.Ø41 Right

MØ8.Ø42 Left

MØ8.Ø49 Unspecified

MØ8.Ø5- **Hip**

MØ8.Ø51 Right

MØ8.Ø52 Left

MØ8.Ø59 Unspecified

MØ8.Ø6- **Knee**

MØ8.Ø61 Right

MØ8.Ø62 Left

MØ8.Ø69 Unspecified

MØ8.Ø7- **Ankle and foot**

MØ8.Ø71 Right

MØ8.Ø72 Left

MØ8.Ø79 Unspecified

MØ8.Ø8 Vertebrae

MØ8.Ø9 Multiple sites

MØ8.ØA Other specified site

MØ8.1 Ankylosing spondylitis

<u>*Excludes1:*</u>

ankylosing spondylitis in adults (M45.Ø-)

MØ8.2- **Juvenile rheumatoid arthritis with systemic onset**

Including: Still's disease NOS

<u>*Excludes1:*</u>

adult-onset Still's disease (MØ6.1-)

MØ8.2Ø Unspecified site

MØ8.21- **Shoulder**

MØ8.211 Right

MØ8.212 Left

MØ8.219 Unspecified

MØ8.22- **Elbow**

MØ8.221 Right

MØ8.222 Left

MØ8.229 Unspecified

MØ8.23- **Wrist**

MØ8.231 Right

MØ8.232 Left

MØ8.239 Unspecified

MØ8.24- **Hand**

MØ8.241 Right

MØ8.242 Left

MØ8.249 Unspecified

MØ8.25- **Hip**

MØ8.251 Right

MØ8.252 Left

MØ8.259 Unspecified

MØ8.26- **Knee**

MØ8.261 Right

MØ8.262 Left

MØ8.269 Unspecified

MØ8.27- **Ankle and foot**

MØ8.271 Right

MØ8.272 Left

MØ8.279 Unspecified

MØ8.28 Vertebrae

MØ8.29 Multiple sites

MØ8.2A Other specified site

MØ8.3 Rheumatoid polyarthritis (seronegative)

MØ8.4- **Pauciarticular juvenile rheumatoid arthritis**

MØ8.4Ø Unspecified site

MØ8.41- **Shoulder**

MØ8.411 Right

MØ8.412 Left

MØ8.419 Unspecified

MØ8.42- **Elbow**

MØ8.421 Right

MØ8.422 Left

MØ8.429 Unspecified

MØ8.43- **Wrist**

MØ8.431 Right

MØ8.432 Left

MØ8.439 Unspecified

MØ8.44- **Hand**

MØ8.441 Right

MØ8.442 Left

MØ8.449 Unspecified

MØ8.45- **Hip**

MØ8.451 Right

MØ8.452 Left

MØ8.459 Unspecified

M08.46- **Knee**
- **M08.461** **Right**
- **M08.462** **Left**
- **M08.469** **Unspecified**

M08.47- **Ankle and foot**
- **M08.471** **Right**
- **M08.472** **Left**
- **M08.479** **Unspecified**

M08.48 **Vertebrae**

M08.4A **Other specified site**

M08.8- **Other juvenile arthritis**

M08.80 **Unspecified site**

M08.81- **Shoulder**
- **M08.811** **Right**
- **M08.812** **Left**
- **M08.819** **Unspecified**

M08.82- **Elbow**
- **M08.821** **Right**
- **M08.822** **Left**
- **M08.829** **Unspecified**

M08.83- **Wrist**
- **M08.831** **Right**
- **M08.832** **Left**
- **M08.839** **Unspecified**

M08.84- **Hand**
- **M08.841** **Right**
- **M08.842** **Left**
- **M08.849** **Unspecified**

M08.85- **Hip**
- **M08.851** **Right**
- **M08.852** **Left**
- **M08.859** **Unspecified**

M08.86- **Knee**
- **M08.861** **Right**
- **M08.862** **Left**
- **M08.869** **Unspecified**

M08.87- **Ankle and foot**
- **M08.871** **Right**
- **M08.872** **Left**
- **M08.879** **Unspecified**

M08.88 **Other specified site**
Including: Vertebrae

M08.89 **Multiple sites**

M08.9- **Juvenile arthritis, unspecified**
Excludes1:
juvenile rheumatoid arthritis, unspecified (M08.0-)

M08.90 **Unspecified site**

M08.91- **Shoulder**
- **M08.911** **Right**
- **M08.912** **Left**
- **M08.919** **Unspecified**

M08.92- **Elbow**
- **M08.921** **Right**
- **M08.922** **Left**
- **M08.929** **Unspecified**

M08.93- **Wrist**
- **M08.931** **Right**
- **M08.932** **Left**
- **M08.939** **Unspecified**

M08.94- **Hand**
- **M08.941** **Right**
- **M08.942** **Left**
- **M08.949** **Unspecified**

M08.95- **Hip**
- **M08.951** **Right**
- **M08.952** **Left**
- **M08.959** **Unspecified**

M08.96- **Knee**
- **M08.961** **Right**
- **M08.962** **Left**
- **M08.969** **Unspecified**

M08.97- **Ankle and foot**
- **M08.971** **Right**
- **M08.972** **Left**
- **M08.979** **Unspecified**

M08.98 **Vertebrae**

M08.99 **Multiple sites**

M08.9A **Other specified site**

M1A- CHRONIC GOUT

Use additional code to identify:
Autonomic neuropathy in diseases classified elsewhere (G99.0)
Calculus of urinary tract in diseases classified elsewhere (N22)
Cardiomyopathy in diseases classified elsewhere (I43)
Disorders of external ear in diseases classified elsewhere (H61.1-, H62.8-)
Disorders of iris and ciliary body in diseases classified elsewhere (H22)
Glomerular disorders in diseases classified elsewhere (N08)
Excludes1:
gout NOS (M10.-)
Excludes2:
acute gout (M10.-)

The appropriate 7th character is to be added to each code from category M1A
0 - without tophus (tophi)
1 - with tophus (tophi)

M1A.0- **Idiopathic chronic gout**
Including: Chronic gouty bursitis, Primary chronic gout

M1A.00x_ **Unspecified site**

M1A.01- **Shoulder**
- **M1A.011_** **Right**
- **M1A.012_** **Left**
- **M1A.019_** **Unspecified**

M1A.02- **Elbow**
- **M1A.021_** **Right**
- **M1A.022_** **Left**
- **M1A.029_** **Unspecified**

M1A.03- **Wrist**
- **M1A.031_** **Right**
- **M1A.032_** **Left**
- **M1A.039_** **Unspecified**

Ch5

5. The Tabular List

M1A.Ø4- **Hand**
M1A.Ø41_ Right
M1A.Ø42_ Left
M1A.Ø49_ Unspecified
M1A.Ø5- **Hip**
M1A.Ø51_ Right
M1A.Ø52_ Left
M1A.Ø59_ Unspecified
M1A.Ø6- **Knee**
M1A.Ø61_ Right
M1A.Ø62_ Left
M1A.Ø69_ Unspecified
M1A.Ø7- **Ankle and foot**
M1A.Ø71_ Right
M1A.Ø72_ Left
M1A.Ø79_ Unspecified
M1A.Ø8x_ Vertebrae
M1A.Ø9x_ Multiple sites

M1A.1- **Lead-induced chronic gout**
Code First:
toxic effects of lead and its compounds (T56.Ø-)
M1A.1Øx_ Unspecified site
M1A.11- **Shoulder**
M1A.111_ Right
M1A.112_ Left
M1A.119_ Unspecified
M1A.12- **Elbow**
M1A.121_ Right
M1A.122_ Left
M1A.129_ Unspecified
M1A.13- **Wrist**
M1A.131_ Right
M1A.132_ Left
M1A.139_ Unspecified
M1A.14- **Hand**
M1A.141_ Right
M1A.142_ Left
M1A.149_ Unspecified
M1A.15- **Hip**
M1A.151_ Right
M1A.152_ Left
M1A.159_ Unspecified
M1A.16- **Knee**
M1A.161_ Right
M1A.162_ Left
M1A.169_ Unspecified
M1A.17- **Ankle and foot**
M1A.171_ Right
M1A.172_ Left
M1A.179_ Unspecified
M1A.18x_ Vertebrae
M1A.19x_ Multiple sites

M1A.2- **Drug-induced chronic gout**
Use additional code for adverse effect, if applicable, to identify drug (T36-T5Ø with fifth or sixth character 5)
M1A.2Øx_ Unspecified site
M1A.21- **Shoulder**
M1A.211_ Right
M1A.212_ Left
M1A.219_ Unspecified
M1A.22- **Elbow**
M1A.221_ Right
M1A.222_ Left
M1A.229_ Unspecified
M1A.23- **Wrist**
M1A.231_ Right
M1A.232_ Left
M1A.239_ Unspecified
M1A.24- **Hand**
M1A.241_ Right
M1A.242_ Left
M1A.249_ Unspecified
M1A.25- **Hip**
M1A.251_ Right
M1A.252_ Left
M1A.259_ Unspecified
M1A.26- **Knee**
M1A.261_ Right
M1A.262_ Left
M1A.269_ Unspecified
M1A.27- **Ankle and foot**
M1A.271_ Right
M1A.272_ Left
M1A.279_ Unspecified
M1A.28x_ Vertebrae
M1A.29x_ Multiple sites

M1A.3- **Chronic gout due to renal impairment**
Code First:
associated renal disease
M1A.3Øx_ Unspecified site
M1A.31- **Shoulder**
M1A.311_ Right
M1A.312_ Left
M1A.319_ Unspecified
M1A.32- **Elbow**
M1A.321_ Right
M1A.322_ Left
M1A.329_ Unspecified
M1A.33- **Wrist**
M1A.331_ Right
M1A.332_ Left
M1A.339_ Unspecified
M1A.34- **Hand**
M1A.341_ Right
M1A.342_ Left
M1A.349_ Unspecified

M1A.35- **Hip**
- **M1A.351_ Right**
- **M1A.352_ Left**
- **M1A.359_ Unspecified**

M1A.36- **Knee**
- **M1A.361_ Right**
- **M1A.362_ Left**
- **M1A.369_ Unspecified**

M1A.37- **Ankle and foot**
- **M1A.371_ Right**
- **M1A.372_ Left**
- **M1A.379_ Unspecified**

M1A.38x_ Vertebrae

M1A.39x_ Multiple sites

M1A.4- **Other secondary chronic gout**

Code First:
associated condition

M1A.40x_ Unspecified site

M1A.41- **Shoulder**
- **M1A.411_ Right**
- **M1A.412_ Left**
- **M1A.419_ Unspecified**

M1A.42- **Elbow**
- **M1A.421_ Right**
- **M1A.422_ Left**
- **M1A.429_ Unspecified**

M1A.43- **Wrist**
- **M1A.431_ Right**
- **M1A.432_ Left**
- **M1A.439_ Unspecified**

M1A.44- **Hand**
- **M1A.441_ Right**
- **M1A.442_ Left**
- **M1A.449_ Unspecified**

M1A.45- **Hip**
- **M1A.451_ Right**
- **M1A.452_ Left**
- **M1A.459_ Unspecified**

M1A.46- **Knee**
- **M1A.461_ Right**
- **M1A.462_ Left**
- **M1A.469_ Unspecified**

M1A.47- **Ankle and foot**
- **M1A.471_ Right**
- **M1A.472_ Left**
- **M1A.479_ Unspecified**

M1A.48x_ Vertebrae

M1A.49x_ Multiple sites

M1A.9xx_ Chronic gout, unspecified

M1Ø- GOUT

Including: Acute, Gout attack, Gout flare, Podagra

Use additional code to identify:
Autonomic neuropathy in diseases classified elsewhere (G99.Ø)
Calculus of urinary tract in diseases classified elsewhere (N22)
Cardiomyopathy in diseases classified elsewhere (I43)
Disorders of external ear in diseases classified elsewhere (H61.1-, H62.8-)
Disorders of iris and ciliary body in diseases classified elsewhere (H22)
Glomerular disorders in diseases classified elsewhere (NØ8)

Excludes2:
chronic gout (M1A.-)

M1Ø.Ø- **Idiopathic gout**

Including: Gouty bursitis, Primary gout

M1Ø.ØØ Unspecified site

M1Ø.Ø1- **Idiopathic gout, shoulder**
- **M1Ø.Ø11 Right**
- **M1Ø.Ø12 Left**
- **M1Ø.Ø19 Unspecified**

M1Ø.Ø2- **Idiopathic gout, elbow**
- **M1Ø.Ø21 Right**
- **M1Ø.Ø22 Left**
- **M1Ø.Ø29 Unspecified**

M1Ø.Ø3- **Idiopathic gout, wrist**
- **M1Ø.Ø31 Right**
- **M1Ø.Ø32 Left**
- **M1Ø.Ø39 Unspecified**

M1Ø.Ø4- **Idiopathic gout, hand**
- **M1Ø.Ø41 Right**
- **M1Ø.Ø42 Left**
- **M1Ø.Ø49 Unspecified**

M1Ø.Ø5- **Idiopathic gout, hip**
- **M1Ø.Ø51 Right**
- **M1Ø.Ø52 Left**
- **M1Ø.Ø59 Unspecified**

M1Ø.Ø6- **Idiopathic gout, knee**
- **M1Ø.Ø61 Right**
- **M1Ø.Ø62 Left**
- **M1Ø.Ø69 Unspecified**

M1Ø.Ø7- **Idiopathic gout, ankle and foot**
- **M1Ø.Ø71 Right**
- **M1Ø.Ø72 Left**
- **M1Ø.Ø79 Unspecified**

M1Ø.Ø8 Vertebrae

M1Ø.Ø9 Multiple sites

M1Ø.1- **Lead-induced gout**

Code First:
toxic effects of lead and its compounds (T56.Ø-)

M1Ø.1Ø Unspecified site

M1Ø.11- **Shoulder**
- **M1Ø.111 Right**
- **M1Ø.112 Left**
- **M1Ø.119 Unspecified**

M1Ø.12- **Elbow**
- **M1Ø.121 Right**
- **M1Ø.122 Left**
- **M1Ø.129 Unspecified**

M1Ø.13- **Wrist**
- **M1Ø.131** **Right**
- **M1Ø.132** **Left**
- **M1Ø.139** **Unspecified**

M1Ø.14- **Hand**
- **M1Ø.141** **Right**
- **M1Ø.142** **Left**
- **M1Ø.149** **Unspecified**

M1Ø.15- **Hip**
- **M1Ø.151** **Right**
- **M1Ø.152** **Left**
- **M1Ø.159** **Unspecified**

M1Ø.16- **Knee**
- **M1Ø.161** **Right**
- **M1Ø.162** **Left**
- **M1Ø.169** **Unspecified**

M1Ø.17- **Lead-induced gout, ankle and foot**
- **M1Ø.171** **Right**
- **M1Ø.172** **Left**
- **M1Ø.179** **Unspecified**

M1Ø.18 **Vertebrae**

M1Ø.19 **Multiple sites**

Ch5

M1Ø.2- **Drug-induced gout**

Use additional code for adverse effect, if applicable, to identify drug (T36-T5Ø with fifth or sixth character 5)

M1Ø.2Ø **Unspecified site**

M1Ø.21- **Shoulder**
- **M1Ø.211** **Right**
- **M1Ø.212** **Left**
- **M1Ø.219** **Unspecified**

M1Ø.22- **Elbow**
- **M1Ø.221** **Right**
- **M1Ø.222** **Left**
- **M1Ø.229** **Unspecified**

M1Ø.23- **Wrist**
- **M1Ø.231** **Right**
- **M1Ø.232** **Left**
- **M1Ø.239** **Unspecified**

M1Ø.24- **Hand**
- **M1Ø.241** **Right**
- **M1Ø.242** **Left**
- **M1Ø.249** **Unspecified**

M1Ø.25- **Hip**
- **M1Ø.251** **Right**
- **M1Ø.252** **Left**
- **M1Ø.259** **Unspecified**

M1Ø.26- **Knee**
- **M1Ø.261** **Right**
- **M1Ø.262** **Left**
- **M1Ø.269** **Unspecified**

M1Ø.27- **Ankle and foot**
- **M1Ø.271** **Right**
- **M1Ø.272** **Left**
- **M1Ø.279** **Unspecified**

M1Ø.28 **Vertebrae**

M1Ø.29 **Multiple sites**

M1Ø.3- **Gout due to renal impairment**

Code First:
associated renal disease

M1Ø.3Ø **Unspecified site**

M1Ø.31- **Shoulder**
- **M1Ø.311** **Right**
- **M1Ø.312** **Left**
- **M1Ø.319** **Unspecified**

M1Ø.32- **Elbow**
- **M1Ø.321** **Right**
- **M1Ø.322** **Left**
- **M1Ø.329** **Unspecified**

M1Ø.33- **Wrist**
- **M1Ø.331** **Right**
- **M1Ø.332** **Left**
- **M1Ø.339** **Unspecified**

M1Ø.34- **Hand**
- **M1Ø.341** **Right**
- **M1Ø.342** **Left**
- **M1Ø.349** **Unspecified**

M1Ø.35- **Hip**
- **M1Ø.351** **Right**
- **M1Ø.352** **Left**
- **M1Ø.359** **Unspecified**

M1Ø.36- **Knee**
- **M1Ø.361** **Right**
- **M1Ø.362** **Left**
- **M1Ø.369** **Unspecified**

M1Ø.37- **Ankle and foot**
- **M1Ø.371** **Right**
- **M1Ø.372** **Left**
- **M1Ø.379** **Unspecified**

M1Ø.38 **Vertebrae**

M1Ø.39 **Multiple sites**

M1Ø.4- **Other secondary gout**

Code First:
associated condition

M1Ø.4Ø **Unspecified site**

M1Ø.41- **Shoulder**
- **M1Ø.411** **Right**
- **M1Ø.412** **Left**
- **M1Ø.419** **Unspecified**

M1Ø.42- **Elbow**
- **M1Ø.421** **Right**
- **M1Ø.422** **Left**
- **M1Ø.429** **Unspecified**

M1Ø.43- **Wrist**
- **M1Ø.431** **Right**
- **M1Ø.432** **Left**
- **M1Ø.439** **Unspecified**

M1Ø.44- **Hand**
- **M1Ø.441** **Right**
- **M1Ø.442** **Left**
- **M1Ø.449** **Unspecified**

See Appendix A — Coding Reference Tables for lists of the ICD-10-CM Tabular indicators, HAC categories, and HCC codes.

M1Ø.45- **Hip**
- **M1Ø.451** **Right**
- **M1Ø.452** **Left**
- **M1Ø.459** **Unspecified**

M1Ø.46- **Knee**
- **M1Ø.461** **Right**
- **M1Ø.462** **Left**
- **M1Ø.469** **Unspecified**

M1Ø.47- **Ankle and foot**
- **M1Ø.471** **Right**
- **M1Ø.472** **Left**
- **M1Ø.479** **Unspecified**

M1Ø.48 **Vertebrae**

M1Ø.49 **Multiple sites**

M1Ø.9 **Unspecified**
Including: Gout NOS

M11- OTHER CRYSTAL ARTHROPATHIES

M11.Ø- **Hydroxyapatite deposition disease**
- **M11.ØØ** **Unspecified site**
- **M11.Ø8** **Vertebrae**
- **M11.Ø9** **Multiple sites**

M11.1- **Familial chondrocalcinosis**
- **M11.1Ø** **Unspecified site**
- **M11.18** **Vertebrae**
- **M11.19** **Multiple sites**

M11.2- **Other chondrocalcinosis**
Including: Chondrocalcinosis NOS
- **M11.2Ø** **Unspecified site**
- **M11.28** **Vertebrae**
- **M11.29** **Multiple sites**

M11.8- **Other specified crystal arthropathies**
- **M11.8Ø** **Unspecified site**
- **M11.88** **Vertebrae**
- **M11.89** **Multiple sites**

M11.9 **Unspecified**

M12- OTHER AND UNSPECIFIED ARTHROPATHY

Excludes1:
arthrosis (M15-M19)
cricoarytenoid arthropathy (J38.7)

M12.Ø- **Chronic postrheumatic arthropathy [Jaccoud]**
Indicator(s): CMS22: 4Ø | CMS24: 4Ø | RxØ5: 83 | ESRD21: 4Ø | HHSØ5: 57 | HHSØ7: 57
- **M12.ØØ** **Unspecified site**
- **M12.Ø8** **Other specified site**
  Including: Vertebrae
- **M12.Ø9** **Multiple sites**

M12.5- **Traumatic arthropathy**
Excludes1:
current injury-see Alphabetic Index
post-traumatic osteoarthritis of first carpometacarpal joint (M18.2-M18.3)
post-traumatic osteoarthritis of hip (M16.4-M16.5)
post-traumatic osteoarthritis of knee (M17.2-M17.3)
post-traumatic osteoarthritis NOS (M19.1-)
post-traumatic osteoarthritis of other single joints (M19.1-)
- **M12.5Ø** **Unspecified site**

M12.51- **Shoulder**
- **M12.511** **Right**
- **M12.512** **Left**
- **M12.519** **Unspecified**

M12.52- **Elbow**
- **M12.521** **Right**
- **M12.522** **Left**
- **M12.529** **Unspecified**

M12.53- **Wrist**
- **M12.531** **Right**
- **M12.532** **Left**
- **M12.539** **Unspecified**

M12.54- **Hand**
- **M12.541** **Right**
- **M12.542** **Left**
- **M12.549** **Unspecified**

M12.55- **Hip**
- **M12.551** **Right**
- **M12.552** **Left**
- **M12.559** **Unspecified**

M12.56- **Knee**
- **M12.561** **Right**
- **M12.562** **Left**
- **M12.569** **Unspecified**

M12.57- **Ankle and foot**
- **M12.571** **Right**
- **M12.572** **Left**
- **M12.579** **Unspecified**

M12.58 **Other specified site**
Including: Vertebrae

M12.59 **Multiple sites**

M12.8- **Other specific arthropathies, not elsewhere classified**
Including: Transient arthropathy
- **M12.8Ø** **Unspecified site**

M12.81- **Shoulder**
- **M12.811** **Right**
- **M12.812** **Left**
- **M12.819** **Unspecified**

M12.82- **Elbow**
- **M12.821** **Right**
- **M12.822** **Left**
- **M12.829** **Unspecified**

M12.83- **Wrist**
- **M12.831** **Right**
- **M12.832** **Left**
- **M12.839** **Unspecified**

M12.84- **Hand**
- **M12.841** **Right**
- **M12.842** **Left**
- **M12.849** **Unspecified**

M12.85- **Hip**
- **M12.851** **Right**
- **M12.852** **Left**
- **M12.859** **Unspecified**

M12.86- **Knee**
- **M12.861** **Right**
- **M12.862** **Left**
- **M12.869** **Unspecified**

M12.87- **Ankle and foot**
- **M12.871** **Right**
- **M12.872** **Left**
- **M12.879** **Unspecified**

M12.88 **Other specified site**
Including: Vertebrae

M12.89 **Multiple sites**

M12.9 **Unspecified**

M13- OTHER ARTHRITIS

Excludes1:
arthrosis (M15-M19)
osteoarthritis (M15-M19)

M13.Ø **Polyarthritis, unspecified**

M13.1- **Monoarthritis, not elsewhere classified**

M13.1Ø **Unspecified site**

M13.11- **Shoulder**
- **M13.111** **Right**
- **M13.112** **Left**
- **M13.119** **Unspecified**

M13.12- **Elbow**
- **M13.121** **Right**
- **M13.122** **Left**
- **M13.129** **Unspecified**

M13.13- **Wrist**
- **M13.131** **Right**
- **M13.132** **Left**
- **M13.139** **Unspecified**

M13.14- **Hand**
- **M13.141** **Right**
- **M13.142** **Left**
- **M13.149** **Unspecified**

M13.15- **Hip**
- **M13.151** **Right**
- **M13.152** **Left**
- **M13.159** **Unspecified**

M13.16- **Knee**
- **M13.161** **Right**
- **M13.162** **Left**
- **M13.169** **Unspecified**

M13.17- **Ankle and foot**
- **M13.171** **Right**
- **M13.172** **Left**
- **M13.179** **Unspecified**

M13.8- **Other specified arthritis**
Including: Allergic arthritis
Excludes1:
osteoarthritis (M15-M19)

- **M13.8Ø** **Unspecified site**
- **M13.88** **Other site**
- **M13.89** **Multiple sites**

OSTEOARTHRITIS (M15-M19)

Excludes2:
osteoarthritis of spine (M47.-)

M15- POLYOSTEOARTHRITIS

Includes:
arthritis of multiple sites
Excludes1:
bilateral involvement of single joint (M16-M19)

M15.Ø **Primary generalized (osteo)arthritis**

M15.1 **Heberden's nodes (with arthropathy)**
Including: Interphalangeal distal osteoarthritis

M15.2 **Bouchard's nodes (with arthropathy)**
Including: Juxtaphalangeal distal osteoarthritis

M15.3 **Secondary multiple arthritis**
Including: Post-traumatic polyosteoarthritis

M15.4 **Erosive (osteo)arthritis**

M15.8 **Other**

M15.9 **Unspecified**
Including: Generalized osteoarthritis NOS

M16- OSTEOARTHRITIS OF HIP

M16.Ø **Bilateral primary**

M16.1- **Unilateral primary**
Including: Primary osteoarthritis of hip NOS
- **M16.1Ø** **Unspecified hip**
- **M16.11** **Right**
- **M16.12** **Left**

M16.2 **Bilateral, resulting from hip dysplasia**

M16.3- **Unilateral, resulting from hip dysplasia**
Including: Dysplastic osteoarthritis of hip NOS
- **M16.3Ø** **Unspecified hip**
- **M16.31** **Right**
- **M16.32** **Left**

M16.4 **Bilateral post-traumatic**

M16.5- **Unilateral post-traumatic**
Including: Post-traumatic osteoarthritis of hip NOS
- **M16.5Ø** **Unspecified hip**
- **M16.51** **Right**
- **M16.52** **Left**

M16.6 **Other bilateral secondary**

M16.7 **Other unilateral secondary**
Including: Secondary osteoarthritis of hip NOS

M16.9 **Unspecified**

M17- OSTEOARTHRITIS OF KNEE

M17.Ø **Bilateral primary**

M17.1- **Unilateral primary**
Including: Primary osteoarthritis of knee NOS
- **M17.1Ø** **Unspecified**
- **M17.11** **Right**
- **M17.12** **Left**

M17.2 **Bilateral post-traumatic**

M17.3- **Unilateral post-traumatic**
Including: Post-traumatic osteoarthritis of knee NOS
- **M17.3Ø** **Unspecified**
- **M17.31** **Right**
- **M17.32** **Left**

M17.4 **Other bilateral secondary**

M17.5 **Other unilateral secondary**
Including: Secondary osteoarthritis of knee NOS

M17.9 **Unspecified**

M18- OSTEOARTHRITIS OF FIRST CARPOMETACARPAL JOINT

M18.Ø **Bilateral primary**

M18.1- **Unilateral primary**
Including: Primary osteoarthritis of first carpometacarpal joint NOS

M18.1Ø **Unspecified hand**
M18.11 **Right hand**
M18.12 **Left hand**

M18.2 **Bilateral post-traumatic**

M18.3- **Unilateral post-traumatic**
Including: Post-traumatic osteoarthritis of first carpometacarpal joint NOS

M18.3Ø **Unspecified hand**
M18.31 **Right hand**
M18.32 **Left hand**

M18.4 **Other bilateral secondary**

M18.5- **Other unilateral secondary**
Including: Secondary osteoarthritis of first carpometacarpal joint NOS

M18.5Ø **Unspecified hand**
M18.51 **Right hand**
M18.52 **Left hand**

M18.9 **Unspecified**

M19- OTHER AND UNSPECIFIED OSTEOARTHRITIS

Excludes1:
polyarthritis (M15.-)
Excludes2:
arthrosis of spine (M47.-)
hallux rigidus (M2Ø.2)
osteoarthritis of spine (M47.-)

M19.Ø- **Primary osteoarthritis of other joints**

M19.Ø1- **Shoulder**
M19.Ø11 **Right**
M19.Ø12 **Left**
M19.Ø19 **Unspecified**

M19.Ø2- **Elbow**
M19.Ø21 **Right**
M19.Ø22 **Left**
M19.Ø29 **Unspecified**

M19.Ø3- **Wrist**
M19.Ø31 **Right**
M19.Ø32 **Left**
M19.Ø39 **Unspecified**

M19.Ø4- **Hand**
Excludes2:
primary osteoarthritis of first carpometacarpal joint (M18.Ø-, M18.1-)
M19.Ø41 **Right**
M19.Ø42 **Left**
M19.Ø49 **Unspecified**

M19.Ø7- **Ankle and foot**
M19.Ø71 **Right**
M19.Ø72 **Left**
M19.Ø79 **Unspecified**

M19.Ø9 **Other specified site**

M19.1- **Post-traumatic osteoarthritis of other joints**

M19.11- **Shoulder**
M19.111 **Right**
M19.112 **Left**
M19.119 **Unspecified**

M19.12- **Elbow**
M19.121 **Right**
M19.122 **Left**
M19.129 **Unspecified**

M19.13- **Wrist**
M19.131 **Right**
M19.132 **Left**
M19.139 **Unspecified**

M19.14- **Hand**
Excludes2:
post-traumatic osteoarthritis of first carpometacarpal joint (M18.2-, M18.3-)
M19.141 **Right**
M19.142 **Left**
M19.149 **Unspecified**

M19.17- **Ankle and foot**
M19.171 **Right**
M19.172 **Left**
M19.179 **Unspecified**

M19.19 **Other specified site**

M19.2- **Secondary osteoarthritis of other joints**

M19.21- **Shoulder**
M19.211 **Right**
M19.212 **Left**
M19.219 **Unspecified**

M19.22- **Elbow**
M19.221 **Right**
M19.222 **Left**
M19.229 **Unspecified**

M19.23- **Wrist**
M19.231 **Right**
M19.232 **Left**
M19.239 **Unspecified**

M19.24- **Hand**
M19.241 **Right**
M19.242 **Left**
M19.249 **Unspecified**

M19.27- **Ankle and foot**
M19.271 **Right**
M19.272 **Left**
M19.279 **Unspecified**

M19.29 **Other specified site**

M19.9- **Osteoarthritis, unspecified site**

M19.9Ø **Unspecified**
Including: Arthrosis NOS, Arthritis NOS, Osteoarthritis NOS

M19.91 **Primary**
Including: Primary osteoarthritis NOS

M19.92 **Post-traumatic**
Including: Post-traumatic osteoarthritis NOS

M19.93 **Secondary**
Including: Secondary osteoarthritis NOS

OTHER JOINT DISORDERS (M2Ø-M25)

Excludes2:
joints of the spine (M4Ø-M54)

M2Ø- ACQUIRED DEFORMITIES OF FINGERS AND TOES

Excludes1:
acquired absence of fingers and toes (Z89.-)
congenital absence of fingers and toes (Q71.3-, Q72.3-)
congenital deformities and malformations of fingers and toes (Q66.-, Q68-Q7Ø, Q74.-)

M2Ø.Ø- **Deformity of finger(s)**
Excludes1:
clubbing of fingers (R68.3)
palmar fascial fibromatosis [Dupuytren] (M72.Ø)
trigger finger (M65.3)

M2Ø.ØØ- **Unspecified deformity of finger(s)**
M2Ø.ØØ1 Right
M2Ø.ØØ2 Left
M2Ø.ØØ9 Unspecified

M2Ø.Ø1- **Mallet finger**
M2Ø.Ø11 Right finger(s)
M2Ø.Ø12 Left finger(s)
M2Ø.Ø19 Unspecified finger(s)

M2Ø.Ø2- **Boutonnière deformity**
M2Ø.Ø21 Right finger(s)
M2Ø.Ø22 Left finger(s)
M2Ø.Ø29 Unspecified finger(s)

M2Ø.Ø3- **Swan-neck deformity**
M2Ø.Ø31 Right finger(s)
M2Ø.Ø32 Left finger(s)
M2Ø.Ø39 Unspecified finger(s)

M2Ø.Ø9- **Other deformity of finger(s)**
M2Ø.Ø91 Right
M2Ø.Ø92 Left
M2Ø.Ø99 Unspecified

M2Ø.1- **Hallux valgus (acquired)**
M2Ø.1Ø Unspecified foot
M2Ø.11 Right foot
M2Ø.12 Left foot

M2Ø.2- **Hallux rigidus**
M2Ø.2Ø Unspecified foot
M2Ø.21 Right foot
M2Ø.22 Left foot

M2Ø.3- **Hallux varus (acquired)**
M2Ø.3Ø Unspecified foot
M2Ø.31 Right foot
M2Ø.32 Left foot

M2Ø.4- **Other hammer toe(s) (acquired)**
M2Ø.4Ø Unspecified foot
M2Ø.41 Right foot
M2Ø.42 Left foot

M2Ø.5- **Other deformities of toe(s) (acquired)**
M2Ø.5x1 Right foot
M2Ø.5x2 Left foot
M2Ø.5x9 Unspecified foot

M2Ø.6- **Acquired deformities of toe(s), unspecified**
M2Ø.6Ø Unspecified foot
M2Ø.61 Right foot
M2Ø.62 Left foot

M21- OTHER ACQUIRED DEFORMITIES OF LIMBS

Excludes1:
acquired absence of limb (Z89.-)
congenital absence of limbs (Q71-Q73)
congenital deformities and malformations of limbs (Q65-Q66, Q68-Q74)
Excludes2:
acquired deformities of fingers or toes (M2Ø.-)
coxa plana (M91.2)

M21.Ø- **Valgus deformity, not elsewhere classified**
Excludes1:
metatarsus valgus (Q66.6)
talipes calcaneovalgus (Q66.4-)

M21.ØØ Unspecified site

M21.Ø2- **Elbow**
Including: Cubitus valgus
M21.Ø21 Right
M21.Ø22 Left
M21.Ø29 Unspecified

M21.Ø5- **Hip**
M21.Ø51 Right
M21.Ø52 Left
M21.Ø59 Unspecified

M21.Ø6- **Knee**
Including: Genu valgum, Knock knee
M21.Ø61 Right
M21.Ø62 Left
M21.Ø69 Unspecified

M21.Ø7- **Ankle**
M21.Ø71 Right
M21.Ø72 Left
M21.Ø79 Unspecified

M21.1- **Varus deformity, not elsewhere classified**
Excludes1:
metatarsus varus (Q66.22-)
tibia vara (M92.51-)

M21.1Ø Unspecified site

M21.12- **Elbow**
Including: Cubitus varus, elbow
M21.121 Right
M21.122 Left
M21.129 Unspecified

M21.15- **Hip**
M21.151 Right
M21.152 Left
M21.159 Unspecified

M21.16- **Knee**
Including: Bow leg, Genu varum
M21.161 Right
M21.162 Left
M21.169 Unspecified

M21.17- **Ankle**
M21.171 Right
M21.172 Left
M21.179 Unspecified

M21.2- **Flexion deformity**
- **M21.2Ø** **Unspecified site**
- M21.21- **Shoulder**
  - **M21.211** **Right**
  - **M21.212** **Left**
  - **M21.219** **Unspecified**
- M21.22- **Elbow**
  - **M21.221** **Right**
  - **M21.222** **Left**
  - **M21.229** **Unspecified**
- M21.23- **Wrist**
  - **M21.231** **Right**
  - **M21.232** **Left**
  - **M21.239** **Unspecified**
- M21.24- **Finger joints**
  - **M21.241** **Right**
  - **M21.242** **Left**
  - **M21.249** **Unspecified**
- M21.25- **Hip**
  - **M21.251** **Right**
  - **M21.252** **Left**
  - **M21.259** **Unspecified**
- M21.26- **Knee**
  - **M21.261** **Right**
  - **M21.262** **Left**
  - **M21.269** **Unspecified**
- M21.27- **Ankle and toes**
  - **M21.271** **Right**
  - **M21.272** **Left**
  - **M21.279** **Unspecified**

M21.3- **Wrist or foot drop (acquired)**
- M21.33- **Wrist drop (acquired)**
  - **M21.331** **Right**
  - **M21.332** **Left**
  - **M21.339** **Unspecified**
- M21.37- **Foot drop (acquired)**
  - **M21.371** **Right**
  - **M21.372** **Left**
  - **M21.379** **Unspecified**

M21.4- **Flat foot [pes planus] (acquired)**

Excludes1:
congenital pes planus (Q66.5-)

- **M21.4Ø** **Unspecified foot**
- **M21.41** **Right**
- **M21.42** **Left**

M21.5- **Acquired clawhand, clubhand, clawfoot and clubfoot**

Excludes1:
clubfoot, not specified as acquired (Q66.89)

- M21.51- **Acquired clawhand**
  - **M21.511** **Right hand**
  - **M21.512** **Left hand**
  - **M21.519** **Unspecified hand**
- M21.52- **Acquired clubhand**
  - **M21.521** **Right hand**
  - **M21.522** **Left hand**
  - **M21.529** **Unspecified hand**
- M21.53- **Acquired clawfoot**
  - **M21.531** **Right foot**
  - **M21.532** **Left foot**
  - **M21.539** **Unspecified foot**
- M21.54- **Acquired clubfoot**
  - **M21.541** **Right foot**
  - **M21.542** **Left foot**
  - **M21.549** **Unspecified foot**

M21.6- **Other acquired deformities of foot**

Excludes2:
deformities of toe (acquired) (M2Ø.1-M2Ø.6-)

- M21.61- **Bunion**
  - **M21.611** **Right foot**
  - **M21.612** **Left foot**
  - **M21.619** **Unspecified foot**
- M21.62- **Bunionette**
  - **M21.621** **Right foot**
  - **M21.622** **Left foot**
  - **M21.629** **Unspecified foot**
- M21.6X- **Other acquired deformities of foot**
  - **M21.6x1** **Right**
  - **M21.6x2** **Left**
  - **M21.6x9** **Unspecified**

M21.7- **Unequal limb length (acquired)**

Notes:
The site used should correspond to the shorter limb

- **M21.7Ø** **Unspecified site**
- M21.72- **Humerus**
  - **M21.721** **Right**
  - **M21.722** **Left**
  - **M21.729** **Unspecified**
- M21.73- **Ulna and radius**
  - **M21.731** **Right ulna**
  - **M21.732** **Left ulna**
  - **M21.733** **Right radius**
  - **M21.734** **Left radius**
  - **M21.739** **Unspecified ulna and radius**
- M21.75- **Femur**
  - **M21.751** **Right**
  - **M21.752** **Left**
  - **M21.759** **Unspecified**
- M21.76- **Tibia and fibula**
  - **M21.761** **Right tibia**
  - **M21.762** **Left tibia**
  - **M21.763** **Right fibula**
  - **M21.764** **Left fibula**
  - **M21.769** **Unspecified tibia and fibula**

M21.8- **Other specified acquired deformities of limbs**

Excludes2:
coxa plana (M91.2)

- **M21.8Ø** **Unspecified limb**
- M21.82- **Upper arm**
  - **M21.821** **Right**
  - **M21.822** **Left**
  - **M21.829** **Unspecified**

M21.83- **Forearm**
- **M21.831 Right**
- **M21.832 Left**
- **M21.839 Unspecified**

M21.85- **Thigh**
- **M21.851 Right**
- **M21.852 Left**
- **M21.859 Unspecified**

M21.86- **Lower leg**
- **M21.861 Right**
- **M21.862 Left**
- **M21.869 Unspecified**

M21.9- **Unspecified acquired deformity of limb and hand**
- **M21.9Ø Unspecified limb**

M21.92- **Upper arm**
- **M21.921 Right**
- **M21.922 Left**
- **M21.929 Unspecified**

M21.93- **Forearm**
- **M21.931 Right**
- **M21.932 Left**
- **M21.939 Unspecified**

M21.94- **Hand**
- **M21.941 Right**
- **M21.942 Left**
- **M21.949 Unspecified**

M21.95- **Thigh**
- **M21.951 Right**
- **M21.952 Left**
- **M21.959 Unspecified**

M21.96- **Lower leg**
- **M21.961 Right**
- **M21.962 Left**
- **M21.969 Unspecified**

M22- DISORDER OF PATELLA

Excludes2:
traumatic dislocation of patella (S83.Ø-)

M22.Ø- **Recurrent dislocation of patella**
- **M22.ØØ Unspecified knee**
- **M22.Ø1 Right knee**
- **M22.Ø2 Left knee**

M22.1- **Recurrent subluxation of patella**
Including: Incomplete dislocation
- **M22.1Ø Unspecified knee**
- **M22.11 Right knee**
- **M22.12 Left knee**

M22.2- **Patellofemoral disorders**
- **M22.2x1 Right knee**
- **M22.2x2 Left knee**
- **M22.2x9 Unspecified knee**

M22.3- **Other derangements of patella**
- **M22.3x1 Right knee**
- **M22.3x2 Left knee**
- **M22.3x9 Unspecified knee**

M22.4- **Chondromalacia patellae**
- **M22.4Ø Unspecified knee**
- **M22.41 Right knee**
- **M22.42 Left knee**

M22.8- **Other disorders of patella**
- **M22.8x1 Right knee**
- **M22.8x2 Left knee**
- **M22.8x9 Unspecified knee**

M22.9- **Unspecified disorder of patella**
- **M22.9Ø Unspecified knee**
- **M22.91 Right knee**
- **M22.92 Left knee**

M23- INTERNAL DERANGEMENT OF KNEE

Excludes1:
ankylosis (M24.66)
deformity of knee (M21.-)
osteochondritis dissecans (M93.2)
Excludes2:
current injury - see injury of knee and lower leg (S8Ø-S89)
recurrent dislocation or subluxation of joints (M24.4)
recurrent dislocation or subluxation of patella (M22.Ø-M22.1)

M23.Ø- **Cystic meniscus**

M23.ØØ- **Unspecified meniscus**
Including: Unspecified lateral meniscus, medial meniscus
- **M23.ØØØ Lateral meniscus, right knee**
- **M23.ØØ1 Lateral meniscus, left knee**
- **M23.ØØ2 Lateral meniscus, unspecified knee**
- **M23.ØØ3 Medial meniscus, right knee**
- **M23.ØØ4 Medial meniscus, left knee**
- **M23.ØØ5 Medial meniscus, unspecified knee**
- **M23.ØØ6 Unspecified meniscus, right knee**
- **M23.ØØ7 Unspecified meniscus, left knee**
- **M23.ØØ9 Unspecified meniscus, unspecified knee**

M23.Ø1- **Anterior horn of medial meniscus**
- **M23.Ø11 Right knee**
- **M23.Ø12 Left knee**
- **M23.Ø19 Unspecified knee**

M23.Ø2- **Posterior horn of medial meniscus**
- **M23.Ø21 Right knee**
- **M23.Ø22 Left knee**
- **M23.Ø29 Unspecified knee**

M23.Ø3- **Other medial meniscus**
- **M23.Ø31 Right knee**
- **M23.Ø32 Left knee**
- **M23.Ø39 Unspecified knee**

M23.Ø4- **Anterior horn of lateral meniscus**
- **M23.Ø41 Right knee**
- **M23.Ø42 Left knee**
- **M23.Ø49 Unspecified knee**

M23.Ø5- **Posterior horn of lateral meniscus**
- **M23.Ø51 Right knee**
- **M23.Ø52 Left knee**
- **M23.Ø59 Unspecified knee**

M23.Ø6- **Other lateral meniscus**
- **M23.Ø61 Right knee**
- **M23.Ø62 Left knee**
- **M23.Ø69 Unspecified knee**

M23.2- **Derangement of meniscus due to old tear or injury**
Including: Old bucket-handle tear

M23.2Ø- **Unspecified meniscus**
Including: Unspecified lateral, medial meniscus

M23.2ØØ **Lateral meniscus, right knee**
M23.2Ø1 **Lateral meniscus, left knee**
M23.2Ø2 **Lateral meniscus, unspecified knee**
M23.2Ø3 **Medial meniscus, right knee**
M23.2Ø4 **Medial meniscus, left knee**
M23.2Ø5 **Medial meniscus, unspecified knee**
M23.2Ø6 **Unspecified meniscus, right knee**
M23.2Ø7 **Unspecified meniscus, left knee**
M23.2Ø9 **Unspecified meniscus, unspecified knee**

M23.21- **Anterior horn of medial meniscus**

M23.211 **Right knee**
M23.212 **Left knee**
M23.219 **Unspecified knee**

M23.22- **Posterior horn of medial meniscus**

M23.221 **Right knee**
M23.222 **Left knee**
M23.229 **Unspecified knee**

M23.23- **Other medial meniscus**

M23.231 **Right knee**
M23.232 **Left knee**
M23.239 **Unspecified knee**

M23.24- **Anterior horn of lateral meniscus**

M23.241 **Right knee**
M23.242 **Left knee**
M23.249 **Unspecified knee**

M23.25- **Posterior horn of lateral meniscus**

M23.251 **Right knee**
M23.252 **Left knee**
M23.259 **Unspecified knee**

M23.26- **Other lateral meniscus**

M23.261 **Right knee**
M23.262 **Left knee**
M23.269 **Unspecified knee**

M23.3- **Other meniscus derangements**
Including: Degenerate, Detached, Retained meniscus

M23.3Ø- **Unspecified meniscus**
Including: Unspecified lateral, medial meniscus

M23.3ØØ **Lateral meniscus, right knee**
M23.3Ø1 **Lateral meniscus, left knee**
M23.3Ø2 **Lateral meniscus, unspecified knee**
M23.3Ø3 **Medial meniscus, right knee**
M23.3Ø4 **Medial meniscus, left knee**
M23.3Ø5 **Medial meniscus, unspecified kne**
M23.3Ø6 **Unspecified meniscus, right knee**
M23.3Ø7 **Unspecified meniscus, left knee**
M23.3Ø9 **Unspecified meniscus, unspecified knee**

M23.31- **Anterior horn of medial meniscus**

M23.311 **Right knee**
M23.312 **Left knee**
M23.319 **Unspecified knee**

M23.32- **Posterior horn of medial meniscus**

M23.321 **Right knee**
M23.322 **Left knee**
M23.329 **Unspecified knee**

M23.33- **Other medial meniscus**

M23.331 **Right knee**
M23.332 **Left knee**
M23.339 **Unspecified knee**

M23.34- **Anterior horn of lateral meniscus**

M23.341 **Right knee**
M23.342 **Left knee**
M23.349 **Unspecified knee**

M23.35- **Posterior horn of lateral meniscus**

M23.351 **Right knee**
M23.352 **Left knee**
M23.359 **Unspecified knee**

M23.36- **Other lateral meniscus**

M23.361 **Right knee**
M23.362 **Left knee**
M23.369 **Unspecified knee**

M23.4- **Loose body in knee**

M23.4Ø **Unspecified knee**
M23.41 **Right knee**
M23.42 **Left knee**

M23.5- **Chronic instability of knee**

M23.5Ø **Unspecified knee**
M23.51 **Right knee**
M23.52 **Left knee**

M23.6- **Other spontaneous disruption of ligament(s) of knee**

M23.6Ø- **Unspecified ligament**

M23.6Ø1 **Right knee**
M23.6Ø2 **Left knee**
M23.6Ø9 **Unspecified knee**

M23.61- **Anterior cruciate ligament**

M23.611 **Right knee**
M23.612 **Left knee**
M23.619 **Unspecified knee**

M23.62- **Posterior cruciate ligament**

M23.621 **Right knee**
M23.622 **Left knee**
M23.629 **Unspecified knee**

M23.63- **Medial collateral ligament**

M23.631 **Right knee**
M23.632 **Left knee**
M23.639 **Unspecified knee**

M23.64- **Lateral collateral ligament**

M23.641 **Right knee**
M23.642 **Left knee**
M23.649 **Unspecified knee**

M23.67- **Capsular ligament**
- **M23.671** **Right knee**
- **M23.672** **Left knee**
- **M23.679** **Unspecified knee**

M23.8- **Other internal derangements of knee**
Including: Laxity of ligament, Snapping knee
- **M23.8x1** **Right knee**
- **M23.8x2** **Left knee**
- **M23.8x9** **Unspecified knee**

M23.9- **Unspecified internal derangement of knee**
- **M23.90** **Unspecified knee**
- **M23.91** **Right knee**
- **M23.92** **Left knee**

M24- OTHER SPECIFIC JOINT DERANGEMENTS
Excludes1:
current injury - see injury of joint by body region
Excludes2:
ganglion (M67.4)
snapping knee (M23.8-)
temporomandibular joint disorders (M26.6-)

M24.0- **Loose body in joint**
Excludes2:
loose body in knee (M23.4)
- **M24.00** **Unspecified joint**

M24.01- **Loose body in shoulder**
- **M24.011** **Right**
- **M24.012** **Left**
- **M24.019** **Unspecified**

M24.02- **Loose body in elbow**
- **M24.021** **Right**
- **M24.022** **Left**
- **M24.029** **Unspecified**

M24.03- **Loose body in wrist**
- **M24.031** **Right**
- **M24.032** **Left**
- **M24.039** **Unspecified**

M24.04- **Loose body in finger joints**
- **M24.041** **Right joint(s)**
- **M24.042** **Left joint(s)**
- **M24.049** **Unspecified joint(s)**

M24.05- **Loose body in hip**
- **M24.051** **Right**
- **M24.052** **Left**
- **M24.059** **Unspecified**

M24.07- **Loose body in ankle and toe joints**
- **M24.071** **Right ankle**
- **M24.072** **Left ankle**
- **M24.073** **Unspecified ankle**
- **M24.074** **Right toe joint(s)**
- **M24.075** **Left toe joint(s)**
- **M24.076** **Unspecified toe joints**

M24.08 **Other site**

M24.1- **Other articular cartilage disorders**
Excludes2:
chondrocalcinosis (M11.1, M11.2-)
internal derangement of knee (M23.-)
metastatic calcification (E83.5)
ochronosis (E70.2)
- **M24.10** **Unspecified site**

M24.11- **Shoulder**
- **M24.111** **Right**
- **M24.112** **Left**
- **M24.119** **Unspecified**

M24.12- **Elbow**
- **M24.121** **Right**
- **M24.122** **Left**
- **M24.129** **Unspecified**

M24.13- **Wrist**
- **M24.131** **Right**
- **M24.132** **Left**
- **M24.139** **Unspecified**

M24.14- **Hand**
- **M24.141** **Right**
- **M24.142** **Left**
- **M24.149** **Unspecified**

M24.15- **Hip**
- **M24.151** **Right**
- **M24.152** **Left**
- **M24.159** **Unspecified**

M24.17- **Ankle and foot**
- **M24.171** **Right ankle**
- **M24.172** **Left ankle**
- **M24.173** **Unspecified ankle**
- **M24.174** **Right foot**
- **M24.175** **Left foot**
- **M24.176** **Unspecified foot**

M24.2- **Disorder of ligament**
Including: Instability secondary to old ligament injury, Ligamentous laxity NOS
Excludes1:
familial ligamentous laxity (M35.7)
Excludes2:
internal derangement of knee (M23.5-M23.8X9)
- **M24.20** **Unspecified site**

M24.21- **Shoulder**
- **M24.211** **Right**
- **M24.212** **Left**
- **M24.219** **Unspecified**

M24.22- **Elbow**
- **M24.221** **Right**
- **M24.222** **Left**
- **M24.229** **Unspecified**

M24.23- **Wrist**
- **M24.231** **Right**
- **M24.232** **Left**
- **M24.239** **Unspecified**

M24.24- **Hand**
- **M24.241 Right**
- **M24.242 Left**
- **M24.249 Unspecified**

M24.25- **Hip**
- **M24.251 Right**
- **M24.252 Left**
- **M24.259 Unspecified**

M24.27- **Ankle and foot**
- **M24.271 Right ankle**
- **M24.272 Left ankle**
- **M24.273 Unspecified ankle**
- **M24.274 Right foot**
- **M24.275 Left foot**
- **M24.276 Unspecified foot**

M24.28 Vertebrae

M24.29 Other specified site

M24.3- **Pathological dislocation of joint, not elsewhere classified**

Excludes1:
congenital dislocation or displacement of joint- see congenital malformations and deformations of the musculoskeletal system (Q65-Q79)
current injury - see injury of joints and ligaments by body region
recurrent dislocation of joint (M24.4-)

M24.3Ø Unspecified joint

M24.31- **Shoulder**
- **M24.311 Right**
- **M24.312 Left**
- **M24.319 Unspecified**

M24.32- **Elbow**
- **M24.321 Right**
- **M24.322 Left**
- **M24.329 Unspecified**

M24.33- **Wrist**
- **M24.331 Right**
- **M24.332 Left**
- **M24.339 Unspecified**

M24.34- **Hand**
- **M24.341 Right**
- **M24.342 Left**
- **M24.349 Unspecified**

M24.35- **Hip**
- **M24.351 Right**
- **M24.352 Left**
- **M24.359 Unspecified**

M24.36- **Knee**
- **M24.361 Right**
- **M24.362 Left**
- **M24.369 Unspecified**

M24.37- **Ankle and foot**
- **M24.371 Right ankle**
- **M24.372 Left ankle**
- **M24.373 Unspecified ankle**
- **M24.374 Right foot**
- **M24.375 Left foot**
- **M24.376 Unspecified foot**

M24.39 Other specified

M24.4- **Recurrent dislocation of joint**

Including: Recurrent subluxation

Excludes2:
recurrent dislocation of patella (M22.Ø-M22.1)
recurrent vertebral dislocation (M43.3-, M43.4, M43.5-)

M24.4Ø Unspecified joint

M24.41- **Shoulder**
- **M24.411 Right**
- **M24.412 Left**
- **M24.419 Unspecified**

M24.42- **Elbow**
- **M24.421 Right**
- **M24.422 Left**
- **M24.429 Unspecified**

M24.43- **Wrist**
- **M24.431 Right**
- **M24.432 Left**
- **M24.439 Unspecified**

M24.44- **Hand and finger(s)**
- **M24.441 Right hand**
- **M24.442 Left hand**
- **M24.443 Unspecified hand**
- **M24.444 Right finger**
- **M24.445 Left finger**
- **M24.446 Unspecified finger**

M24.45- **Hip**
- **M24.451 Right**
- **M24.452 Left**
- **M24.459 Unspecified**

M24.46- **Knee**
- **M24.461 Right**
- **M24.462 Left**
- **M24.469 Unspecified**

M24.47- **Ankle, foot and toes**
- **M24.471 Right ankle**
- **M24.472 Left ankle**
- **M24.473 Unspecified ankle**
- **M24.474 Right foot**
- **M24.475 Left foot**
- **M24.476 Unspecified foot**
- **M24.477 Right toe(s)**
- **M24.478 Left toe(s)**
- **M24.479 Unspecified toe(s)**

M24.49 Other specified

M24.5- **Contracture of joint**

Excludes1:
contracture of muscle without contracture of joint (M62.4-)
contracture of tendon (sheath) without contracture of joint (M62.4-)
Dupuytren's contracture (M72.Ø)

Excludes2:
acquired deformities of limbs (M2Ø-M21)

M24.5Ø Unspecified joint

M24.51- **Shoulder**
- **M24.511 Right**
- **M24.512 Left**
- **M24.519 Unspecified**

M24.52- **Elbow**
- **M24.521 Right**
- **M24.522 Left**
- **M24.529 Unspecified**

M24.53- **Wrist**
- **M24.531 Right**
- **M24.532 Left**
- **M24.539 Unspecified**

M24.54- **Hand**
- **M24.541 Right**
- **M24.542 Left**
- **M24.549 Unspecified**

M24.55- **Hip**
- **M24.551 Right**
- **M24.552 Left**
- **M24.559 Unspecified**

M24.56- **Knee**
- **M24.561 Right**
- **M24.562 Left**
- **M24.569 Unspecified**

M24.57- **Ankle and foot**
- **M24.571 Right ankle**
- **M24.572 Left ankle**
- **M24.573 Unspecified ankle**
- **M24.574 Right foot**
- **M24.575 Left foot**
- **M24.576 Unspecified foot**

M24.59 Other specified

M24.6- **Ankylosis of joint**

Excludes1:
stiffness of joint without ankylosis (M25.6-)
Excludes2:
spine (M43.2-)

M24.6Ø Unspecified joint

M24.61- **Shoulder**
- **M24.611 Right**
- **M24.612 Left**
- **M24.619 Unspecified**

M24.62- **Elbow**
- **M24.621 Right**
- **M24.622 Left**
- **M24.629 Unspecified**

M24.63- **Wrist**
- **M24.631 Right**
- **M24.632 Left**
- **M24.639 Unspecified**

M24.64- **Hand**
- **M24.641 Right**
- **M24.642 Left**
- **M24.649 Unspecified**

M24.65- **Hip**
- **M24.651 Right**
- **M24.652 Left**
- **M24.659 Unspecified**

M24.66- **Knee**
- **M24.661 Right**
- **M24.662 Left**
- **M24.669 Unspecified**

M24.67- **Ankle and foot**
- **M24.671 Right ankle**
- **M24.672 Left ankle**
- **M24.673 Unspecified ankle**
- **M24.674 Right foot**
- **M24.675 Left foot**
- **M24.676 Unspecified foot**

M24.69 Other specified

M24.7 Protrusio acetabuli

M24.8- **Other specific joint derangements, not elsewhere classified**

Excludes2:
iliotibial band syndrome (M76.3)

M24.8Ø Unspecified joint

M24.81- **Shoulder**
- **M24.811 Right**
- **M24.812 Left**
- **M24.819 Unspecified**

M24.82- **Elbow**
- **M24.821 Right**
- **M24.822 Left**
- **M24.829 Unspecified**

M24.83- **Wrist**
- **M24.831 Right**
- **M24.832 Left**
- **M24.839 Unspecified**

M24.84- **Hand**
- **M24.841 Right**
- **M24.842 Left**
- **M24.849 Unspecified**

M24.85- **Hip**

Including: Irritable hip
- **M24.851 Right**
- **M24.852 Left**
- **M24.859 Unspecified**

M24.87- **Ankle and foot**
- **M24.871 Right ankle**
- **M24.872 Left ankle**
- **M24.873 Unspecified ankle**
- **M24.874 Right foot**
- **M24.875 Left foot**
- **M24.876 Unspecified foot**

M24.89 Other specified joint

M24.9 Joint derangement, unspecified

M25- OTHER JOINT DISORDER, NOT ELSEWHERE CLASSIFIED

Excludes2:
abnormality of gait and mobility (R26.-)
acquired deformities of limb (M2Ø-M21)
calcification of bursa (M71.4-)
calcification of shoulder (joint) (M75.3)
calcification of tendon (M65.2-)
difficulty in walking (R26.2)
temporomandibular joint disorder (M26.6-)

M25.Ø- **Hemarthrosis**

Excludes1:
current injury - see injury of joint by body region
hemophilic arthropathy (M36.2)
Indicator(s): CC

M25.ØØ Unspecified joint
M25.Ø1- **Shoulder**
M25.Ø11 Right
M25.Ø12 Left
M25.Ø19 Unspecified
M25.Ø2- **Elbow**
M25.Ø21 Right
M25.Ø22 Left
M25.Ø29 Unspecified
M25.Ø3- **Wrist**
M25.Ø31 Right
M25.Ø32 Left
M25.Ø39 Unspecified
M25.Ø4- **Hand**
M25.Ø41 Right
M25.Ø42 Left
M25.Ø49 Unspecified
M25.Ø5- **Hip**
M25.Ø51 Right
M25.Ø52 Left
M25.Ø59 Unspecified
M25.Ø6- **Knee**
M25.Ø61 Right
M25.Ø62 Left
M25.Ø69 Unspecified
M25.Ø7- **Ankle and foot**
M25.Ø71 Right ankle
M25.Ø72 Left ankle
M25.Ø73 Unspecified ankle
M25.Ø74 Right foot
M25.Ø75 Left foot
M25.Ø76 Unspecified foot
M25.Ø8 Other specified site
Including: Vertebrae

M25.1- **Fistula of joint**

M25.1Ø Unspecified joint
M25.11- **Shoulder**
M25.111 Right
M25.112 Left
M25.119 Unspecified
M25.12- **Elbow**
M25.121 Right
M25.122 Left
M25.129 Unspecified
M25.13- **Wrist**
M25.131 Right
M25.132 Left
M25.139 Unspecified
M25.14- **Hand**
M25.141 Right
M25.142 Left
M25.149 Unspecified
M25.15- **Hip**
M25.151 Right
M25.152 Left
M25.159 Unspecified
M25.16- **Knee**
M25.161 Right
M25.162 Left
M25.169 Unspecified
M25.17- **Ankle and foot**
M25.171 Right ankle
M25.172 Left ankle
M25.173 Unspecified ankle
M25.174 Right foot
M25.175 Left foot
M25.176 Unspecified foot
M25.18 Other specified site
Including: Vertebrae

M25.2- **Flail joint**

M25.2Ø Unspecified joint
M25.21- **Shoulder**
M25.211 Right
M25.212 Left
M25.219 Unspecified
M25.22- **Elbow**
M25.221 Right
M25.222 Left
M25.229 Unspecified
M25.23- **Wrist**
M25.231 Right
M25.232 Left
M25.239 Unspecified
M25.24- **Hand**
M25.241 Right
M25.242 Left
M25.249 Unspecified
M25.25- **Hip**
M25.251 Right
M25.252 Left
M25.259 Unspecified
M25.26- **Knee**
M25.261 Right
M25.262 Left
M25.269 Unspecified
M25.27- **Ankle and foot**
M25.271 Right
M25.272 Left
M25.279 Unspecified
M25.28 Other site

M25.3- **Other instability of joint**
<u>*Excludes1:*</u>
instability of joint secondary to old ligament injury (M24.2-)
instability of joint secondary to removal of joint prosthesis (M96.8-)
<u>*Excludes2:*</u>
spinal instabilities (M53.2-)

M25.3Ø Unspecified joint
M25.31- **Shoulder**
M25.311 Right
M25.312 Left
M25.319 Unspecified
M25.32- **Elbow**
M25.321 Right
M25.322 Left
M25.329 Unspecified
M25.33- **Wrist**
M25.331 Right
M25.332 Left
M25.339 Unspecified
M25.34- **Hand**
M25.341 Right
M25.342 Left
M25.349 Unspecified
M25.35- **Hip**
M25.351 Right
M25.352 Left
M25.359 Unspecified
M25.36- **Knee**
M25.361 Right
M25.362 Left
M25.369 Unspecified
M25.37- **Ankle and foot**
M25.371 Right ankle
M25.372 Left ankle
M25.373 Unspecified ankle
M25.374 Right foot
M25.375 Left foot
M25.376 Unspecified foot
M25.39 Other specified joint

M25.4- **Effusion of joint**
<u>*Excludes1:*</u>
hydrarthrosis in yaws (A66.6)
intermittent hydrarthrosis (M12.4-)
other infective (teno)synovitis (M65.1-)

M25.4Ø Unspecified joint
M25.41- **Shoulder**
M25.411 Right
M25.412 Left
M25.419 Unspecified
M25.42- **Elbow**
M25.421 Right
M25.422 Left
M25.429 Unspecified
M25.43- **Wrist**
M25.431 Right
M25.432 Left
M25.439 Unspecified
M25.44- **Hand**
M25.441 Right
M25.442 Left
M25.449 Unspecified
M25.45- **Hip**
M25.451 Right
M25.452 Left
M25.459 Unspecified
M25.46- **Knee**
M25.461 Right
M25.462 Left
M25.469 Unspecified
M25.47- **Ankle and foot**
M25.471 Right ankle
M25.472 Left ankle
M25.473 Unspecified ankle
M25.474 Right foot
M25.475 Left foot
M25.476 Unspecified foot
M25.48 Other site

M25.5- **Pain in joint**
<u>*Excludes2:*</u>
pain in hand (M79.64-)
pain in fingers (M79.64-)
pain in foot (M79.67-)
pain in limb (M79.6-)
pain in toes (M79.67-)

M25.5Ø Unspecified joint
M25.51- **Shoulder**
M25.511 Right
M25.512 Left
M25.519 Unspecified
M25.52- **Elbow**
M25.521 Right
M25.522 Left
M25.529 Unspecified
M25.53- **Wrist**
M25.531 Right
M25.532 Left
M25.539 Unspecified
M25.54- **Joints of hand**
M25.541 Right
M25.542 Left
M25.549 Unspecified
Including: Pain in joints of hand NOS
M25.55- **Hip**
M25.551 Right
M25.552 Left
M25.559 Unspecified
M25.56- **Knee**
M25.561 Right
M25.562 Left
M25.569 Unspecified

See Appendix A — Coding Reference Tables for lists of the ICD-10-CM Tabular indicators, HAC categories, and HCC codes.

M25.57- **Ankle and joints of foot**
- **M25.571 Right**
- **M25.572 Left**
- **M25.579 Unspecified**

M25.59 Other specified joint

M25.6- **Stiffness of joint, not elsewhere classified**

Excludes1:
ankylosis of joint (M24.6-)
contracture of joint (M24.5-)

M25.60 Unspecified joint

M25.61- **Shoulder**
- **M25.611 Right**
- **M25.612 Left**
- **M25.619 Unspecified**

M25.62- **Elbow**
- **M25.621 Right**
- **M25.622 Left**
- **M25.629 Unspecified**

M25.63- **Wrist**
- **M25.631 Right**
- **M25.632 Left**
- **M25.639 Unspecified**

M25.64- **Hand**
- **M25.641 Right**
- **M25.642 Left**
- **M25.649 Unspecified**

M25.65- **Hip**
- **M25.651 Right**
- **M25.652 Left**
- **M25.659 Unspecified**

M25.66- **Knee**
- **M25.661 Right**
- **M25.662 Left**
- **M25.669 Unspecified**

M25.67- **Ankle and foot**
- **M25.671 Right ankle**
- **M25.672 Left ankle**
- **M25.673 Unspecified ankle**
- **M25.674 Right foot**
- **M25.675 Left foot**
- **M25.676 Unspecified foot**

M25.69 Other specified joint

M25.7- **Osteophyte**

M25.70 Unspecified joint

M25.71- **Shoulder**
- **M25.711 Right**
- **M25.712 Left**
- **M25.719 Unspecified**

M25.72- **Elbow**
- **M25.721 Right**
- **M25.722 Left**
- **M25.729 Unspecified**

M25.73- **Wrist**
- **M25.731 Right**
- **M25.732 Left**
- **M25.739 Unspecified**

M25.74- **Hand**
- **M25.741 Right**
- **M25.742 Left**
- **M25.749 Unspecified**

M25.75- **Hip**
- **M25.751 Right**
- **M25.752 Left**
- **M25.759 Unspecified**

M25.76- **Knee**
- **M25.761 Right**
- **M25.762 Left**
- **M25.769 Unspecified**

M25.77- **Ankle and foot**
- **M25.771 Right ankle**
- **M25.772 Left ankle**
- **M25.773 Unspecified ankle**
- **M25.774 Right foot**
- **M25.775 Left foot**
- **M25.776 Unspecified foot**

M25.78 Vertebrae

M25.8- **Other specified joint disorders**

M25.80 Unspecified joint

M25.81- **Shoulder**
- **M25.811 Right**
- **M25.812 Left**
- **M25.819 Unspecified**

M25.82- **Elbow**
- **M25.821 Right**
- **M25.822 Left**
- **M25.829 Unspecified**

M25.83- **Wrist**
- **M25.831 Right**
- **M25.832 Left**
- **M25.839 Unspecified**

M25.84- **Hand**
- **M25.841 Right**
- **M25.842 Left**
- **M25.849 Unspecified**

M25.85- **Hip**
- **M25.851 Right**
- **M25.852 Left**
- **M25.859 Unspecified**

M25.86- **Knee**
- **M25.861 Right**
- **M25.862 Left**
- **M25.869 Unspecified**

M25.87- **Ankle and foot**
- **M25.871 Right**
- **M25.872 Left**
- **M25.879 Unspecified**

M25.9 Joint disorder, unspecified

DENTOFACIAL ANOMALIES [INCLUDING MALOCCLUSION] AND OTHER DISORDERS OF JAW (M26-M27)

Excludes1:
hemifacial atrophy or hypertrophy (Q67.4)
unilateral condylar hyperplasia or hypoplasia (M27.8)

M26- DENTOFACIAL ANOMALIES [INCLUDING MALOCCLUSION]

M26.6- **Temporomandibular joint disorders**
Excludes2:
current temporomandibular joint dislocation (SØ3.Ø)
current temporomandibular joint sprain (SØ3.4)

M26.6Ø- **Temporomandibular joint disorder, unspecified**
M26.6Ø1 Right
M26.6Ø2 Left
M26.6Ø3 Bilateral
M26.6Ø9 Unspecified side
Including: Temporomandibular joint disorder NOS

M26.61- **Adhesions and ankylosis of temporomandibular joint**
M26.611 Right
M26.612 Left
M26.613 Bilateral
M26.619 Unspecified side

M26.62- **Arthralgia of temporomandibular joint**
M26.621 Right
M26.622 Left
M26.623 Bilateral
M26.629 Unspecified side

M26.63- **Articular disc disorder of temporomandibular joint**
M26.631 Right
M26.632 Left
M26.633 Bilateral
M26.639 Unspecified side

M26.64- **Arthritis of temporomandibular joint**
M26.641 Right
M26.642 Left
M26.643 Bilateral
M26.649 Unspecified

M26.65- **Arthropathy of temporomandibular joint**
M26.651 Right
M26.652 Left
M26.653 Bilateral
M26.659 Unspecified

M26.69 Other specified

M27- OTHER DISEASES OF JAWS

M27.Ø Developmental disorders
Including: Latent bone cyst of jaw, Stafne's cyst, Torus mandibularis, Torus palatinus

M27.9 Unspecified

SYSTEMIC CONNECTIVE TISSUE DISORDERS (M3Ø-M36)

Includes:
autoimmune disease NOS
collagen (vascular) disease NOS
systemic autoimmune disease
systemic collagen (vascular) disease
Excludes1:
autoimmune disease, single organ or single cell-type -code to relevant condition category

M32- SYSTEMIC LUPUS ERYTHEMATOSUS (SLE)

Excludes1:
lupus erythematosus (discoid) (NOS) (L93.Ø)
Indicator(s): CMS22: 4Ø | CMS24: 4Ø | RxØ5: 84 | ESRD21: 4Ø | HHSØ5: 57 | HHSØ7: 57

M32.9 Unspecified
Including: SLE NOS; Systemic lupus erythematosus NOS, without organ involvement

M33- DERMATOPOLYMYOSITIS

Indicator(s): CC | CMS24: 4Ø | RxØ5: 84 | HHSØ5: 56 | HHSØ7: 56

M33.Ø- **Juvenile dermatomyositis**
M33.ØØ Organ involvement unspecified
M33.Ø1 With respiratory involvement
M33.Ø2 With myopathy
M33.Ø9 With other organ involvement

M33.1- **Other dermatomyositis**
Including: Adult dermatomyositis
M33.1Ø Organ involvement unspecified
M33.11 With respiratory involvement
M33.12 With myopathy
M33.19 With other organ involvement

M33.2- **Polymyositis**
M33.2Ø Organ involvement unspecified
M33.21 With respiratory involvement
M33.22 With myopathy
M33.29 With other organ involvement

M33.9- **Dermatopolymyositis, unspecified**
M33.9Ø Organ involvement unspecified
M33.91 With respiratory involvement
M33.92 With myopathy
M33.99 With other organ involvement

M34- SYSTEMIC SCLEROSIS [SCLERODERMA]

Excludes1:
circumscribed scleroderma (L94.Ø)
neonatal scleroderma (P83.88)
Indicator(s): CMS22: 4Ø | CMS24: 4Ø | RxØ5: 82 | HHSØ5: 56 | HHSØ7: 56

M34.Ø Progressive

M34.1 CR(E)ST syndrome
Including: Combination of calcinosis, Raynaud's phenomenon, esophageal dysfunction, sclerodactyly, telangiectasia

M34.2 Induced by drug and chemical
Code First:
poisoning due to drug or toxin, if applicable (T36-T65 with fifth or sixth character 1-4 or 6)
Use additional code for adverse effect, if applicable, to identify drug (T36-T5Ø with fifth or sixth character 5)

See Appendix A — Coding Reference Tables for lists of the ICD-10-CM Tabular indicators, HAC categories, and HCC codes.

M34.8- **Other forms of systemic sclerosis**

M34.81 **With lung involvement**
Code Also
if applicable:
other interstitial pulmonary diseases (J84.89)
secondary pulmonary arterial hypertension (I27.21)
Indicator(s): CC

M34.82 **With myopathy**
Indicator(s): CC

M34.83 **With polyneuropathy**

M34.89 **Other**

M34.9 **Unspecified**

M35- OTHER SYSTEMIC INVOLVEMENT OF CONNECTIVE TISSUE
Excludes1:
reactive perforating collagenosis (L87.1)

M35.Ø- **Sjögren syndrome**
Including: Sicca
Use additional *code to identify associated manifestations*
Excludes1:
dry mouth, unspecified (R68.2)
Indicator(s): CMS24: 4Ø

M35.ØØ **Unspecified**

M35.Ø1 **With keratoconjunctivitis**

M35.Ø2 **With lung involvement**

M35.Ø3 **With myopathy**
Indicator(s): CC

M35.Ø4 **With tubulo-interstitial nephropathy**
Including: Renal tubular acidosis in sicca syndrome

M35.Ø9 **With other organ involvement**

M35.1 **Other overlap syndromes**
Including: Mixed connective tissue disease
Excludes1:
polyangiitis overlap syndrome (M3Ø.8)
Indicator(s): CC | CMS22: 4Ø | CMS24: 4Ø | RxØ5: 84 | ESRD21: 4Ø | HHSØ5: 57 | HHSØ7: 57

M35.2 **Behçet's disease**
Indicator(s): CC | CMS22: 4Ø | CMS24: 4Ø | RxØ5: 83 | ESRD21: 4Ø | HHSØ5: 56 | HHSØ7: 56

M35.3 **Polymyalgia rheumatica**
Excludes1:
polymyalgia rheumatica with giant cell arteritis (M31.5)
Indicator(s): CMS22: 4Ø | CMS24: 4Ø | ESRD21: 4Ø | HHSØ5: 57 | HHSØ7: 57

M35.4 **Diffuse (eosinophilic) fasciitis**

M35.5 **Multifocal fibrosclerosis**
Indicator(s): CC | CMS22: 4Ø | CMS24: 4Ø | RxØ5: 84 | ESRD21: 4Ø | HHSØ5: 57 | HHSØ7: 57

M35.6 **Relapsing panniculitis [Weber-Christian]**
Excludes1:
lupus panniculitis (L93.2)
panniculitis NOS (M79.3-)

M35.7 **Hypermobility syndrome**
Including: Familial ligamentous laxity
Excludes1:
ligamentous laxity, NOS (M24.2-)
Excludes2:
Ehlers-Danlos syndromes (Q79.6-)

M35.9 **Unspecified**
Including: Autoimmune disease (systemic) NOS, Collagen (vascular) disease NOS
Indicator(s): CMS22: 4Ø | CMS24: 4Ø | RxØ5: 84 | ESRD21: 4Ø | HHSØ5: 57 | HHSØ7: 57

M36- SYSTEMIC DISORDERS OF CONNECTIVE TISSUE IN DISEASES CLASSIFIED ELSEWHERE
Excludes2:
arthropathies in diseases classified elsewhere (M14.-)

M36.Ø **Dermato(poly)myositis in neoplastic disease**
Code First:
underlying neoplasm (CØØ-D49)
Indicator(s): CC | CMS22: 4Ø | CMS24: 4Ø | RxØ5: 84 | ESRD21: 4Ø | HHSØ5: 56 | HHSØ7: 56

M36.1 **Arthropathy in neoplastic disease**
Code First:
underlying neoplasm, such as:
leukemia (C91-C95)
malignant histiocytosis (C96.A)
multiple myeloma (C9Ø.Ø)

R **M36.2** **Hemophilic arthropathy**
Including: Hemarthrosis in hemophilic arthropathy
Code First:
underlying disease, such as:
factor VIII deficiency (D66)
with vascular defect (D68.Ø-)
factor IX deficiency (D67)
hemophilia (classical) (D66)
hemophilia B (D67)
hemophilia C (D68.1)

M36.3 **Arthropathy in other blood disorders**

M36.4 **Arthropathy in hypersensitivity reactions classified elsewhere**
Code First:
underlying disease, such as:
Henoch (-Schönlein) purpura (D69.Ø)
serum sickness (T8Ø.6-)

M36.8 **Other**
Code First:
underlying disease, such as:
alkaptonuria (E7Ø.2)
hypogammaglobulinemia (D8Ø.-)
ochronosis (E7Ø.2)
Indicator(s): CMS22: 4Ø | CMS24: 4Ø | RxØ5: 84 | ESRD21: 4Ø | HHSØ5: 57 | HHSØ7: 57

DORSOPATHIES (M4Ø-M54)

DEFORMING DORSOPATHIES (M4Ø-M43)

M4Ø- KYPHOSIS AND LORDOSIS
Code First:
underlying disease
Excludes1:
congenital kyphosis and lordosis (Q76.4)
kyphoscoliosis (M41.-)
postprocedural kyphosis and lordosis (M96.-)

M4Ø.Ø- **Postural kyphosis**
Excludes1:
osteochondrosis of spine (M42.-)

M4Ø.ØØ **Site unspecified**

M4Ø.Ø3 **Cervicothoracic region**

M4Ø.Ø4 **Thoracic region**

M4Ø.Ø5 **Thoracolumbar region**

M4Ø.1- **Other secondary kyphosis**
Indicator(s): NoPDx/M
- **M4Ø.1Ø** Site unspecified
- **M4Ø.12** Cervical region
- **M4Ø.13** Cervicothoracic region
- **M4Ø.14** Thoracic region
- **M4Ø.15** Thoracolumbar region

M4Ø.2- **Other and unspecified kyphosis**

M4Ø.2Ø- **Unspecified kyphosis**
- **M4Ø.2Ø2** Cervical region
- **M4Ø.2Ø3** Cervicothoracic region
- **M4Ø.2Ø4** Thoracic region
- **M4Ø.2Ø5** Thoracolumbar region
- **M4Ø.2Ø9** Site unspecified

M4Ø.29- **Other kyphosis**
- **M4Ø.292** Cervical region
- **M4Ø.293** Cervicothoracic region
- **M4Ø.294** Thoracic region
- **M4Ø.295** Thoracolumbar region
- **M4Ø.299** Site unspecified

M4Ø.3- **Flatback syndrome**
- **M4Ø.3Ø** Site unspecified
- **M4Ø.35** Thoracolumbar region
- **M4Ø.36** Lumbar region
- **M4Ø.37** Lumbosacral region

M4Ø.4- **Postural lordosis**
Including: Acquired lordosis
- **M4Ø.4Ø** Site unspecified
- **M4Ø.45** Thoracolumbar region
- **M4Ø.46** Lumbar region
- **M4Ø.47** Lumbosacral region

M4Ø.5- **Lordosis, unspecified**
- **M4Ø.5Ø** Site unspecified
- **M4Ø.55** Thoracolumbar region
- **M4Ø.56** Lumbar region
- **M4Ø.57** Lumbosacral region

M41- SCOLIOSIS

Includes:
kyphoscoliosis
Excludes1:
congenital scoliosis NOS (Q67.5)
congenital scoliosis due to bony malformation (Q76.3)
postural congenital scoliosis (Q67.5)
kyphoscoliotic heart disease (I27.1)
Excludes2:
postprocedural scoliosis (M96.-)

M41.Ø- **Infantile idiopathic scoliosis**
- **M41.ØØ** Site unspecified
- **M41.Ø2** Cervical region
- **M41.Ø3** Cervicothoracic region
- **M41.Ø4** Thoracic region
- **M41.Ø5** Thoracolumbar region
- **M41.Ø6** Lumbar region
- **M41.Ø7** Lumbosacral region
- **M41.Ø8** Sacral and sacrococcygeal region

M41.1- **Juvenile and adolescent idiopathic scoliosis**

M41.11- **Juvenile idiopathic scoliosis**
- **M41.112** Cervical region
- **M41.113** Cervicothoracic region
- **M41.114** Thoracic region
- **M41.115** Thoracolumbar region
- **M41.116** Lumbar region
- **M41.117** Lumbosacral region
- **M41.119** Site unspecified

M41.12- **Adolescent scoliosis**
- **M41.122** Idiopathic, cervical region
- **M41.123** Idiopathic, cervicothoracic region
- **M41.124** Idiopathic, thoracic region
- **M41.125** Idiopathic, thoracolumbar region
- **M41.126** Idiopathic, lumbar region
- **M41.127** Idiopathic, lumbosacral region
- **M41.129** Idiopathic, site unspecified

M41.2- **Other idiopathic scoliosis**
- **M41.2Ø** Site unspecified
- **M41.22** Cervical region
- **M41.23** Cervicothoracic region
- **M41.24** Thoracic region
- **M41.25** Thoracolumbar region
- **M41.26** Lumbar region
- **M41.27** Lumbosacral region

M41.3- **Thoracogenic scoliosis**
- **M41.3Ø** Site unspecified
- **M41.34** Thoracic region
- **M41.35** Thoracolumbar region

M41.4- **Neuromuscular scoliosis**
Including: Scoliosis secondary to cerebral palsy, Friedreich's ataxia, poliomyelitis and other neuromuscular disorders
Code Also
underlying condition
- **M41.4Ø** Site unspecified
- **M41.41** Occipito-atlanto-axial region
- **M41.42** Cervical region
- **M41.43** Cervicothoracic region
- **M41.44** Thoracic region
- **M41.45** Thoracolumbar region
- **M41.46** Lumbar region
- **M41.47** Lumbosacral region

M41.5- **Other secondary scoliosis**
Code First:
underlying disease
Indicator(s): NoPDx/M
- **M41.5Ø** Site unspecified
- **M41.52** Cervical region
- **M41.53** Cervicothoracic region
- **M41.54** Thoracic region
- **M41.55** Thoracolumbar region
- **M41.56** Lumbar region
- **M41.57** Lumbosacral region

M41.8- **Other forms of scoliosis**

M41.8Ø **Site unspecified**

M41.82 **Cervical region**

M41.83 **Cervicothoracic region**

M41.84 **Thoracic region**

M41.85 **Thoracolumbar region**

M41.86 **Lumbar region**

M41.87 **Lumbosacral**

M41.9 **Scoliosis, unspecified**

M42- SPINAL OSTEOCHONDROSIS

M42.Ø- **Juvenile osteochondrosis of spine**

Including: Calvé's disease, Scheuermann's disease

Excludes1:

postural kyphosis (M4Ø.Ø)

Indicator(s): *HHSØ5: 62 | HHSØ7: 62*

M42.ØØ **Site unspecified**

M42.Ø1 **Occipito-atlanto-axial region**

M42.Ø2 **Cervical region**

M42.Ø3 **Cervicothoracic region**

M42.Ø4 **Thoracic region**

M42.Ø5 **Thoracolumbar region**

M42.Ø6 **Lumbar region**

M42.Ø7 **Lumbosacral region**

M42.Ø8 **Sacral and sacrococcygeal region**

M42.Ø9 **Multiple sites in spine**

M42.1- **Adult osteochondrosis of spine**

M42.1Ø **Site unspecified**

M42.11 **Occipito-atlanto-axial region**

M42.12 **Cervical region**

M42.13 **Cervicothoracic region**

M42.14 **Thoracic region**

M42.15 **Thoracolumbar region**

M42.16 **Lumbar region**

M42.17 **Lumbosacral region**

M42.18 **Sacral and sacrococcygeal region**

M42.19 **Multiple sites in spine**

M42.9 **Unspecified**

M43- OTHER DEFORMING DORSOPATHIES

Excludes1:

congenital spondylolysis and spondylolisthesis (Q76.2)
hemivertebra (Q76.3-Q76.4)
Klippel-Feil syndrome (Q76.1)
lumbarization and sacralization (Q76.4)
platyspondylisis (Q76.4)
spina bifida occulta (Q76.Ø)
spinal curvature in osteoporosis (M8Ø.-)
spinal curvature in Paget's disease of bone [osteitis deformans] (M88.-)

M43.Ø- **Spondylolysis**

Excludes1:

congenital spondylolysis (Q76.2)
spondylolisthesis (M43.1)

M43.ØØ **Site unspecified**

M43.Ø1 **Occipito-atlanto-axial region**

M43.Ø2 **Cervical region**

M43.Ø3 **Cervicothoracic region**

M43.Ø4 **Thoracic region**

M43.Ø5 **Thoracolumbar region**

M43.Ø6 **Lumbar region**

M43.Ø7 **Lumbosacral region**

M43.Ø8 **Sacral and sacrococcygeal region**

M43.Ø9 **Multiple sites in spine region**

M43.1- **Spondylolisthesis**

Excludes1:

acute traumatic of lumbosacral region (S33.1)
acute traumatic of sites other than lumbosacral- code to Fracture, vertebra, by region
congenital spondylolisthesis (Q76.2)

M43.1Ø **Site unspecified**

M43.11 **Occipito-atlanto-axial region**

M43.12 **Cervical region**

M43.13 **Cervicothoracic region**

M43.14 **Thoracic region**

M43.15 **Thoracolumbar region**

M43.16 **Lumbar region**

M43.17 **Lumbosacral region**

M43.18 **Sacral and sacrococcygeal region**

M43.19 **Multiple sites in spine**

M43.2- **Fusion of spine**

Including: Ankylosis of spinal joint

Excludes1:

ankylosing spondylitis (M45.Ø-)
congenital fusion of spine (Q76.4)

Excludes2:

arthrodesis status (Z98.1)
pseudoarthrosis after fusion or arthrodesis (M96.Ø)

M43.2Ø **Site unspecified**

M43.21 **Occipito-atlanto-axial region**

M43.22 **Cervical region**

M43.23 **Cervicothoracic region**

M43.24 **Thoracic region**

M43.25 **Thoracolumbar region**

M43.26 **Lumbar region**

M43.27 **Lumbosacral region**

M43.28 **Sacral and sacrococcygeal region**

M43.3 **Recurrent atlantoaxial dislocation with myelopathy**

M43.4 **Other recurrent atlantoaxial dislocation**

M43.5- **Other recurrent vertebral dislocation**

Excludes1:

biomechanical lesions NEC (M99.-)

M43.5x2 **Cervical region**

M43.5x3 **Cervicothoracic region**

M43.5x4 **Thoracic region**

M43.5x5 **Thoracolumbar region**

M43.5x6 **Lumbar region**

M43.5x7 **Lumbosacral region**

M43.5x8 **Sacral and sacrococcygeal region**

M43.5x9 **Site unspecified**

M43.6 **Torticollis**

Excludes1:

congenital (sternomastoid) torticollis (Q68.Ø)
current injury - see Injury, of spine, by body region
ocular torticollis (R29.891)
psychogenic torticollis (F45.8)
spasmodic torticollis (G24.3)
torticollis due to birth injury (P15.2)

M43.8- **Other specified deforming dorsopathies**
Excludes2:
kyphosis and lordosis (M4Ø.-)
scoliosis (M41.-)
M43.8x1 Occipito-atlanto-axial region
M43.8x2 Cervical region
M43.8x3 Cervicothoracic region
M43.8x4 Thoracic region
M43.8x5 Thoracolumbar region
M43.8x6 Lumbar region
M43.8x7 Lumbosacral region
M43.8x8 Sacral and sacrococcygeal region
M43.8x9 Site unspecified
M43.9 Deforming dorsopathy, unspecified
Including: Curvature of spine NOS

SPONDYLOPATHIES (M45-M49)

M45- ANKYLOSING SPONDYLITIS

Including: Rheumatoid arthritis of spine
Excludes1:
arthropathy in Reiter's disease (MØ2.3-)
juvenile (ankylosing) spondylitis (MØ8.1)
Excludes2:
Behçet's disease (M35.2)
Indicator(s): CMS24: 4Ø
M45.Ø Multiple sites in spine
M45.1 Occipito-atlanto-axial region
M45.2 Cervical region
M45.3 Cervicothoracic region
M45.4 Thoracic region
M45.5 Thoracolumbar region
M45.6 Lumbar region
M45.7 Lumbosacral region
M45.8 Sacral and sacrococcygeal region
M45.9 Unspecified sites in spine
M45.A- **Non-radiographic axial spondyloarthritis**
M45.AØ Unspecified sites in spine
M45.A1 Occipito-atlanto-axial region
M45.A2 Cervical region
M45.A3 Cervicothoracic region
M45.A4 Thoracic region
M45.A5 Thoracolumbar region
M45.A6 Lumbar region
M45.A7 Lumbosacral region
M45.A8 Sacral and sacrococcygeal region
M45.AB Multiple sites in spine

M46- OTHER INFLAMMATORY SPONDYLOPATHIES

M46.Ø- **Spinal enthesopathy**
Including: Disorder of ligamentous or muscular attachments of spine
Indicator(s): CMS22: 4Ø | CMS24: 4Ø | RxØ5: 84 | ESRD21: 4Ø
M46.ØØ Site unspecified
M46.Ø1 Occipito-atlanto-axial region
M46.Ø2 Cervical region
M46.Ø3 Cervicothoracic region
M46.Ø4 Thoracic region
M46.Ø5 Thoracolumbar region
M46.Ø6 Lumbar region
M46.Ø7 Lumbosacral region
M46.Ø8 Sacral and sacrococcygeal region
M46.Ø9 Multiple sites in spine
M46.1 Sacroiliitis, NEC
Indicator(s): CMS22: 4Ø | CMS24: 4Ø | RxØ5: 84 | ESRD21: 4Ø
M46.2- **Osteomyelitis of vertebra**
Indicator(s): CC | CMS22: 39 | CMS24: 39 | ESRD21: 39 | HHSØ5: 55 | HHSØ7: 55
M46.2Ø Site unspecified
M46.21 Occipito-atlanto-axial region
M46.22 Cervical region
M46.23 Cervicothoracic region
M46.24 Thoracic region
M46.25 Thoracolumbar region
M46.26 Lumbar region
M46.27 Lumbosacral region
M46.28 Sacral and sacrococcygeal region
M46.3- **Infection of intervertebral disc (pyogenic)**
Use additional code (B95-B97) to identify infectious agent.
Indicator(s): CC | CMS22: 39 | CMS24: 39 | ESRD21: 39 | HHSØ5: 55 | HHSØ7: 55
M46.3Ø Site unspecified
M46.31 Occipito-atlanto-axial region
M46.32 Cervical region
M46.33 Cervicothoracic region
M46.34 Thoracic region
M46.35 Thoracolumbar region
M46.36 Lumbar region
M46.37 Lumbosacral region
M46.38 Sacral and sacrococcygeal region
M46.39 Multiple sites in spine
M46.4- **Discitis, unspecified**
M46.4Ø Site unspecified
M46.41 Occipito-atlanto-axial region
M46.42 Cervical region
M46.43 Cervicothoracic region
M46.44 Thoracic region
M46.45 Thoracolumbar region
M46.46 Lumbar region
M46.47 Lumbosacral region
M46.48 Sacral and sacrococcygeal region
M46.49 Multiple sites in spine
M46.5- **Other infective spondylopathies**
Indicator(s): CMS22: 4Ø | CMS24: 4Ø | RxØ5: 84 | ESRD21: 4Ø
M46.5Ø Site unspecified
M46.51 Occipito-atlanto-axial region
M46.52 Cervical region
M46.53 Cervicothoracic region
M46.54 Thoracic region
M46.55 Thoracolumbar region
M46.56 Lumbar region
M46.57 Lumbosacral region
M46.58 Sacral and sacrococcygeal region
M46.59 Multiple sites in spine

M46.8- **Other specified inflammatory spondylopathies**
<u>Indicator(s):</u> *CMS22: 4Ø | CMS24: 4Ø | RxØ5: 84 | ESRD21: 4Ø*

M46.8Ø **Site unspecified**
M46.81 **Occipito-atlanto-axial region**
M46.82 **Cervical region**
M46.83 **Cervicothoracic region**
M46.84 **Thoracic region**
M46.85 **Thoracolumbar region**
M46.86 **Lumbar region**
M46.87 **Lumbosacral region**
M46.88 **Sacral and sacrococcygeal region**
M46.89 **Multiple sites in spine**

M46.9- **Unspecified inflammatory spondylopathy**
<u>Indicator(s):</u> *CMS22: 4Ø | CMS24: 4Ø | RxØ5: 84 | ESRD21: 4Ø*

M46.9Ø **Site unspecified**
M46.91 **Occipito-atlanto-axial region**
M46.92 **Cervical region**
M46.93 **Cervicothoracic region**
M46.94 **Thoracic region**
M46.95 **Thoracolumbar region**
M46.96 **Lumbar region**
M46.97 **Lumbosacral region**
M46.98 **Sacral and sacrococcygeal region**
M46.99 **Multiple sites in spine**

M47- SPONDYLOSIS

<u>Includes:</u>
arthrosis or osteoarthritis of spine
degeneration of facet joints

M47.Ø- **Anterior spinal and vertebral artery compression syndromes**
<u>Indicator(s):</u> *CC*

M47.Ø1- **Anterior spinal artery compression syndromes**

M47.Ø11 **Occipito-atlanto-axial region**
M47.Ø12 **Cervical region**
M47.Ø13 **Cervicothoracic region**
M47.Ø14 **Thoracic region**
M47.Ø15 **Thoracolumbar region**
M47.Ø16 **Lumbar region**
M47.Ø19 **Site unspecified**

M47.Ø2- **Vertebral artery compression syndromes**

M47.Ø21 **Occipito-atlanto-axial region**
M47.Ø22 **Cervical region**
M47.Ø29 **Site unspecified**

M47.1- **Other spondylosis with myelopathy**
Including: Spondylogenic compression of spinal cord
<u>Excludes1:</u>
vertebral subluxation (M43.3-M43.5X9)
<u>Indicator(s):</u> *CC*

M47.1Ø **Site unspecified**
M47.11 **Occipito-atlanto-axial region**
M47.12 **Cervical region**
M47.13 **Cervicothoracic region**
M47.14 **Thoracic region**
M47.15 **Thoracolumbar region**
M47.16 **Lumbar region**

M47.2- **Other spondylosis with radiculopathy**

M47.2Ø **Site unspecified**
M47.21 **Occipito-atlanto-axial region**
M47.22 **Cervical region**
M47.23 **Cervicothoracic region**
M47.24 **Thoracic region**
M47.25 **Thoracolumbar region**
M47.26 **Lumbar region**
M47.27 **Lumbosacral region**
M47.28 **Sacral and sacrococcygeal region**

M47.8- **Other spondylosis**

M47.81- **Spondylosis without myelopathy or radiculopathy**

M47.811 **Occipito-atlanto-axial region**
M47.812 **Cervical region**
M47.813 **Cervicothoracic region**
M47.814 **Thoracic region**
M47.815 **Thoracolumbar region**
M47.816 **Lumbar region**
M47.817 **Lumbosacral region**
M47.818 **Sacral and sacrococcygeal region**
M47.819 **Site unspecified**

M47.89- **Other spondylosis**

M47.891 **Occipito-atlanto-axial region**
M47.892 **Cervical region**
M47.893 **Cervicothoracic region**
M47.894 **Thoracic region**
M47.895 **Thoracolumbar region**
M47.896 **Lumbar region**
M47.897 **Lumbosacral region**
M47.898 **Sacral and sacrococcygeal region**
M47.899 **Site unspecified**

M47.9 **Spondylosis, unspecified**

M48- OTHER SPONDYLOPATHIES

M48.Ø- **Spinal stenosis**
Including: Caudal stenosis

M48.ØØ **Site unspecified**
M48.Ø1 **Occipito-atlanto-axial region**
M48.Ø2 **Cervical region**
M48.Ø3 **Cervicothoracic region**
M48.Ø4 **Thoracic region**
M48.Ø5 **Thoracolumbar region**

M48.Ø6- **Lumbar region**

M48.Ø61 **Without neurogenic claudication**
Including: Spinal stenosis, lumbar region NOS
M48.Ø62 **With neurogenic claudication**

M48.Ø7 **Lumbosacral region**
M48.Ø8 **Sacral and sacrococcygeal region**

M48.1- **Ankylosing hyperostosis [Forestier]**
Including: Diffuse idiopathic skeletal hyperostosis [DISH]

M48.1Ø **Site unspecified**
M48.11 **Occipito-atlanto-axial region**
M48.12 **Cervical region**
M48.13 **Cervicothoracic region**
M48.14 **Thoracic region**
M48.15 **Thoracolumbar region**
M48.16 **Lumbar region**
M48.17 **Lumbosacral region**
M48.18 **Sacral and sacrococcygeal region**
M48.19 **Multiple sites in spine**

M48.2- **Kissing spine**

M48.2Ø **Site unspecified**
M48.21 **Occipito-atlanto-axial region**
M48.22 **Cervical region**
M48.23 **Cervicothoracic region**
M48.24 **Thoracic region**
M48.25 **Thoracolumbar region**
M48.26 **Lumbar region**
M48.27 **Lumbosacral region**

Ch5

M48.3- **Traumatic spondylopathy**
Indicator(s): CC

M48.3Ø **Site unspecified**
M48.31 **Occipito-atlanto-axial region**
M48.32 **Cervical region**
M48.33 **Cervicothoracic region**
M48.34 **Thoracic region**
M48.35 **Thoracolumbar region**
M48.36 **Lumbar region**
M48.37 **Lumbosacral region**
M48.38 **Sacral and sacrococcygeal region**

M48.4- **Fatigue fracture of vertebra**
Including: Stress fracture of vertebra
Excludes1:
pathological fracture NOS (M84.4-)
pathological fracture of vertebra due to neoplasm (M84.58)
pathological fracture of vertebra due to other diagnosis (M84.68)
pathological fracture of vertebra due to osteoporosis (M8Ø.-)
traumatic fracture of vertebrae (S12.Ø-S12.3-, S22.Ø-, S32.Ø-)

The appropriate 7th character is to be added to each code from subcategory M48.4:
A - initial encounter for fracture
D - subsequent encounter for fracture with routine healing
G - subsequent encounter for fracture with delayed healing
S - sequela of fracture

M48.4Øx_ **Site unspecified**
M48.41x_ **Occipito-atlanto-axial region**
M48.42x_ **Cervical region**
M48.43x_ **Cervicothoracic region**
M48.44x_ **Thoracic region**
M48.45x_ **Thoracolumbar region**
M48.46x_ **Lumbar region**
M48.47x_ **Lumbosacral region**
M48.48x_ **Sacral and sacrococcygeal region**

M48.5- **Collapsed vertebra, not elsewhere classified**
Including: Collapsed vertebra NOS, Compression fracture of vertebra NOS, Wedging of vertebra NOS
Excludes1:
current injury - see Injury of spine, by body region
fatigue fracture of vertebra (M48.4)
pathological fracture of vertebra due to neoplasm (M84.58)
pathological fracture of vertebra due to other diagnosis (M84.68)
pathological fracture of vertebra due to osteoporosis (M8Ø.-)
pathological fracture NOS (M84.4-)
stress fracture of vertebra (M48.4-)
traumatic fracture of vertebra (S12.-, S22.-, S32.-)

The appropriate 7th character is to be added to each code from subcategory M48.5:
A - initial encounter for fracture
D - subsequent encounter for fracture with routine healing
G - subsequent encounter for fracture with delayed healing
S - sequela of fracture

Indicator(s): CC (7th A) | CMS22: 169 (7th A) | CMS24: 169 (7th A) | RxØ5: 87 (7th A) | ESRD21: 169 (7th A) | HHSØ5: 226 (7th A) | HHSØ7: 228 (7th A)

M48.5Øx_ **Site unspecified**
M48.51x_ **Occipito-atlanto-axial region**
M48.52x_ **Cervical region**
M48.53x_ **Cervicothoracic region**
M48.54x_ **Thoracic region**
M48.55x_ **Thoracolumbar region**
M48.56x_ **Lumbar region**
M48.57x_ **Lumbosacral region**
M48.58x_ **Sacral and sacrococcygeal region**

M48.8- **Other specified spondylopathies**
Including: Ossification of posterior longitudinal ligament
Indicator(s): CMS22: 4Ø | CMS24: 4Ø | RxØ5: 84 | ESRD21: 4Ø | HHSØ5: 56 | HHSØ7: 56

M48.8X- **Other specified**

M48.8x1 **Occipito-atlanto-axial region**
M48.8x2 **Cervical region**
M48.8x3 **Cervicothoracic region**
M48.8x4 **Thoracic region**
M48.8x5 **Thoracolumbar region**
M48.8x6 **Lumbar region**
M48.8x7 **Lumbosacral region**
M48.8x8 **Sacral and sacrococcygeal region**
M48.8x9 **Site unspecified**

M48.9 **Spondylopathy, unspecified**

M49- SPONDYLOPATHIES IN DISEASES CLASSIFIED ELSEWHERE

Includes:
curvature of spine in diseases classified elsewhere
deformity of spine in diseases classified elsewhere
kyphosis in diseases classified elsewhere
scoliosis in diseases classified elsewhere
spondylopathy in diseases classified elsewhere
Code First:
underlying disease, such as:
brucellosis (A23.-)
Charcot-Marie-Tooth disease (G6Ø.Ø)
enterobacterial infections (AØ1-AØ4)
osteitis fibrosa cystica (E21.Ø)

5. The Tabular List

Excludes1:
curvature of spine in tuberculosis [Pott's] (A18.Ø1)
enteropathic arthropathies (MØ7.-)
gonococcal spondylitis (A54.41)
neuropathic [tabes dorsalis] spondylitis (A52.11)
neuropathic spondylopathy in syringomyelia (G95.Ø)
neuropathic spondylopathy in tabes dorsalis (A52.11)
nonsyphilitic neuropathic spondylopathy NEC (G98.Ø)
spondylitis in syphilis (acquired) (A52.77)
tuberculous spondylitis (A18.Ø1)
typhoid fever spondylitis (AØ1.Ø5)
Indicator(s): CMS22: 4Ø | CMS24: 4Ø | RxØ5: 84 | ESRD21: 4Ø

M49.8- **Spondylopathy in diseases classified elsewhere**
M49.8Ø Site unspecified
M49.81 Occipito-atlanto-axial region
M49.82 Cervical region
M49.83 Cervicothoracic region
M49.84 Thoracic region
M49.85 Thoracolumbar region
M49.86 Lumbar region
M49.87 Lumbosacral region
M49.88 Sacral and sacrococcygeal region
M49.89 Multiple sites in spine

OTHER DORSOPATHIES (M5Ø-M54)

Excludes1:
current injury - see injury of spine by body region
discitis NOS (M46.4-)

M5Ø- CERVICAL DISC DISORDERS

Includes:
cervicothoracic disc disorders with cervicalgia
cervicothoracic disc disorders

M5Ø.Ø- **Cervical disc disorder with myelopathy**
Indicator(s): CC
M5Ø.ØØ Unspecified cervical region
M5Ø.Ø1 High cervical region
Including: C2-C3, C3-C4
M5Ø.Ø2- **Mid-cervical region**
M5Ø.Ø2Ø Unspecified level
M5Ø.Ø21 At C4-C5 level
Including: C4-C5 disc disorder
M5Ø.Ø22 At C5-C6 level
Including: C5-C6 disc disorder
M5Ø.Ø23 At C6-C7 level
Including: C6-C7 disc disorder
M5Ø.Ø3 Cervicothoracic region
Including: C7-T1 disc disorder with myelopathy

M5Ø.1- **Cervical disc disorder with radiculopathy**
Excludes2:
brachial radiculitis NOS (M54.13)
M5Ø.1Ø Unspecified cervical region
M5Ø.11 High cervical region
Including: C2-C3, C3-C4 disc disorder with radiculopathy; C3, C4 radiculopathy due to disc disorder
M5Ø.12- **Mid-cervical region**
M5Ø.12Ø Unspecified level
M5Ø.121 C4-C5 level
Including: C4-C5 disc disorder, C5 radiculopathy due to disc disorder
M5Ø.122 C5-C6 level
Including: C5-C6 disc disorder, C6 radiculopathy due to disc disorder
M5Ø.123 C6-C7 level
Including: C6-C7 disc disorder, C7 radiculopathy due to disc disorder
M5Ø.13 Cervicothoracic region
Including: C7-T1, C8 radiculopathy due to disc disorder

M5Ø.2- **Other cervical disc displacement**
M5Ø.2Ø Unspecified cervical region
M5Ø.21 High cervical region
Including: C2-C3, C3-C4
M5Ø.22- **Mid-cervical region**
M5Ø.22Ø Unspecified level
M5Ø.221 C4-C5 level
Including: C4-C5 cervical disc displacement
M5Ø.222 C5-C6 level
Including: C5-C6 cervical disc displacement
M5Ø.223 C6-C7 level
Including: C6-C7 cervical disc displacement
M5Ø.23 Cervicothoracic region
Including: C7-T1 cervical disc displacement

M5Ø.3- **Other cervical disc degeneration**
M5Ø.3Ø Unspecified cervical region
M5Ø.31 High cervical region
Including: C2-C3, C3-C4
M5Ø.32- **Mid-cervical region**
M5Ø.32Ø Unspecified level
M5Ø.321 C4-C5 level
Including: C4-C5 cervical disc degeneration
M5Ø.322 C5-C6 level
Including: C5-C6 cervical disc degeneration
M5Ø.323 C6-C7 level
Including: C6-C7 cervical disc degeneration
M5Ø.33 Cervicothoracic region
Including: C7-T1 cervical disc degeneration

M5Ø.8- **Other cervical disc disorders**
M5Ø.8Ø Unspecified cervical region
M5Ø.81 High cervical region
Including: C2-C3, C3-C4
M5Ø.82- **Mid-cervical region**
M5Ø.82Ø Unspecified level
M5Ø.821 C4-C5 level
Including: C4-C5 cervical disc disorders
M5Ø.822 C5-C6 level
Including: C5-C6 cervical disc disorders
M5Ø.823 C6-C7 level
Including: C6-C7 cervical disc disorders
M5Ø.83 Cervicothoracic region
Including: C7-T1 cervical disc disorders

M5Ø.9- **Cervical disc disorder, unspecified**

- **M5Ø.9Ø** **Unspecified cervical region**
- **M5Ø.91** **High cervical region**
  Including: C2-C3, C3-C4
- M5Ø.92- **Mid-cervical region**
  - **M5Ø.92Ø** **Unspecified level**
  - **M5Ø.921** **C4-C5 level**
    Including: C4-C5 cervical disc disorder
  - **M5Ø.922** **C5-C6 level**
    Including: C5-C6 cervical disc disorder
  - **M5Ø.923** **C6-C7 level**
    Including: C6-C7 cervical disc disorder
- **M5Ø.93** **Cervicothoracic region**
  Including: C7-T1 cervical disc disorder, unspecified

M51- THORACIC, THORACOLUMBAR, AND LUMBOSACRAL INTERVERTEBRAL DISC DISORDERS

Excludes2:
cervical and cervicothoracic disc disorders (M5Ø.-)
sacral and sacrococcygeal disorders (M53.3)

M51.Ø- **With myelopathy**
Indicator(s): *CC*

- **M51.Ø4** **Thoracic region**
- **M51.Ø5** **Thoracolumbar region**
- **M51.Ø6** **Lumbar region**

M51.1- **With radiculopathy**
Including: Sciatica due to intervertebral disc disorder
Excludes1:
lumbar radiculitis NOS (M54.16)
sciatica NOS (M54.3)

- **M51.14** **Thoracic region**
- **M51.15** **Thoracolumbar region**
- **M51.16** **Lumbar region**
- **M51.17** **Lumbosacral region**

M51.2- **Other, disc displacement**
Including: Lumbago due to displacement of intervertebral disc

- **M51.24** **Thoracic region**
- **M51.25** **Thoracolumbar region**
- **M51.26** **Lumbar region**
- **M51.27** **Lumbosacral region**

M51.3- **Other, disc degeneration**

- **M51.34** **Thoracic region**
- **M51.35** **Thoracolumbar region**
- **M51.36** **Lumbar region**
- **M51.37** **Lumbosacral region**

M51.4- **Schmorl's nodes**

- **M51.44** **Thoracic region**
- **M51.45** **Thoracolumbar region**
- **M51.46** **Lumbar region**
- **M51.47** **Lumbosacral region**

M51.8- **Other**

- **M51.84** **Thoracic region**
- **M51.85** **Thoracolumbar region**
- **M51.86** **Lumbar region**
- **M51.87** **Lumbosacral region**

M51.9 **Unspecified**

M51.A- **Other lumbar and lumbosacral annulus fibrosus disc defects**

- N **M51.AØ** **Lumbar region, unspecified size**
  Code First:
  if applicable, lumbar disc herniation (M51.Ø6, M51.16, M51.26)
- N **M51.A1** **Small, lumbar region**
  Code First:
  if applicable, lumbar disc herniation (M51.Ø6, M51.16, M51.26)
- N **M51.A2** **Large, lumbar region**
  Code First:
  if applicable, lumbar disc herniation (M51.Ø6, M51.16, M51.26)
- N **M51.A3** **Lumbosacral region, unspecified size**
  Code First:
  if applicable, lumbosacral disc herniation (M51.17, M51.27)
- N **M51.A4** **Small, lumbosacral region**
  Code First:
  if applicable, lumbosacral disc herniation (M51.17, M51.27)
- N **M51.A5** **Large, lumbosacral region**
  Code First:
  if applicable, lumbosacral disc herniation (M51.17, M51.27)

M53- OTHER AND UNSPECIFIED DORSOPATHIES, NOT ELSEWHERE CLASSIFIED

M53.Ø **Cervicocranial syndrome**
Including: Posterior cervical sympathetic syndrome

M53.1 **Cervicobrachial syndrome**
Excludes2:
cervical disc disorder (M5Ø.-)
thoracic outlet syndrome (G54.Ø)

M53.2- **Spinal instabilities**

- **M53.2x1** **Occipito-atlanto-axial region**
- **M53.2x2** **Cervical region**
- **M53.2x3** **Cervicothoracic region**
- **M53.2x4** **Thoracic region**
- **M53.2x5** **Thoracolumbar region**
- **M53.2x6** **Lumbar region**
- **M53.2x7** **Lumbosacral region**
- **M53.2x8** **Sacral and sacrococcygeal region**
- **M53.2x9** **Site unspecified**

M53.3 **Sacrococcygeal disorders**
Including: Coccygodynia

M53.8- **Other specified dorsopathies**

- **M53.8Ø** **Site unspecified**
- **M53.81** **Occipito-atlanto-axial region**
- **M53.82** **Cervical region**
- **M53.83** **Cervicothoracic region**
- **M53.84** **Thoracic region**
- **M53.85** **Thoracolumbar region**
- **M53.86** **Lumbar region**
- **M53.87** **Lumbosacral region**
- **M53.88** **Sacral and sacrococcygeal region**

M53.9 **Dorsopathy, unspecified**

M54- DORSALGIA

Excludes1:
psychogenic dorsalgia (F45.41)

M54.Ø- **Panniculitis affecting regions of neck and back**
Excludes1:
lupus panniculitis (L93.2)
panniculitis NOS (M79.3)
relapsing [Weber-Christian] panniculitis (M35.6)

M54.ØØ Site unspecified
M54.Ø1 Occipito-atlanto-axial region
M54.Ø2 Cervical region
M54.Ø3 Cervicothoracic region
M54.Ø4 Thoracic region
M54.Ø5 Thoracolumbar region
M54.Ø6 Lumbar region
M54.Ø7 Lumbosacral region
M54.Ø8 Sacral and sacrococcygeal region
M54.Ø9 Multiple sites in spine

M54.1- **Radiculopathy**
Including: Brachial, Lumbar, Lumbosacral, Thoracic neuritis or radiculitis NOS; Radiculitis NOS
Excludes1:
neuralgia and neuritis NOS (M79.2)
radiculopathy with cervical disc disorder (M5Ø.1)
radiculopathy with lumbar and other intervertebral disc disorder (M51.1-)
radiculopathy with spondylosis (M47.2-)

M54.1Ø Site unspecified
M54.11 Occipito-atlanto-axial region
M54.12 Cervical region
M54.13 Cervicothoracic region
M54.14 Thoracic region
M54.15 Thoracolumbar region
M54.16 Lumbar region
M54.17 Lumbosacral region
M54.18 Sacral and sacrococcygeal region

M54.2 Cervicalgia
Excludes1:
cervicalgia due to intervertebral cervical disc disorder (M5Ø.-)
See Guidelines: 1;C.6.b.1.b

M54.3- **Sciatica**
Excludes1:
lesion of sciatic nerve (G57.Ø)
sciatica due to intervertebral disc disorder (M51.1-)
sciatica with lumbago (M54.4-)

M54.3Ø Unspecified side
M54.31 Right side
M54.32 Left side

M54.4- **Lumbago with sciatica**
Excludes1:
lumbago with sciatica due to intervertebral disc disorder (M51.1-)

M54.4Ø Unspecified side
M54.41 Right side
M54.42 Left side

M54.5- **Low back pain**

M54.5Ø Unspecified
Including: Loin pain, Lumbago NOS
M54.51 Vertebrogenic
Including: Low back vertebral endplate
M54.59 Other

M54.6 Pain in thoracic spine
Excludes1:
pain in thoracic spine due to intervertebral disc disorder (M51.-)

M54.8- **Other dorsalgia**
Excludes1:
dorsalgia in thoracic region (M54.6)
low back pain (M54.5-)

M54.81 Occipital neuralgia
M54.89 Other

M54.9 Dorsalgia, unspecified
Including: Backache NOS, Back pain NOS

SOFT TISSUE DISORDERS (M6Ø-M79)

DISORDERS OF MUSCLES (M6Ø-M63)

Excludes1:
dermatopolymyositis (M33.-)
myopathy in amyloidosis (E85.-)
myopathy in polyarteritis nodosa (M3Ø.Ø)
myopathy in rheumatoid arthritis (MØ5.32)
myopathy in scleroderma (M34.-)
myopathy in Sjögren's syndrome (M35.Ø3)
myopathy in systemic lupus erythematosus (M32.-)
Excludes2:
muscular dystrophies and myopathies (G71-G72)

M6Ø- MYOSITIS

Excludes2:
inclusion body myositis [IBM] (G72.41)

M6Ø.Ø- **Infective myositis**
Including: Tropical pyomyositis
Use additional code (B95-B97) to identify infectious agent
Indicator(s): CC

M6Ø.ØØ- **Unspecified site**
M6Ø.ØØ9 Unspecified site

M6Ø.1- **Interstitial myositis**
M6Ø.1Ø Unspecified site

M6Ø.2- **Foreign body granuloma of soft tissue, not elsewhere classified**
Use additional code to identify the type of retained foreign body (Z18.-)
Excludes1:
foreign body granuloma of skin and subcutaneous tissue (L92.3)

M6Ø.2Ø Unspecified site

M6Ø.21- **Shoulder**
M6Ø.211 Right
M6Ø.212 Left
M6Ø.219 Unspecified

M6Ø.22- **Upper arm**
M6Ø.221 Right
M6Ø.222 Left
M6Ø.229 Unspecified

M6Ø.23- **Forearm**
- **M6Ø.231** **Right**
- **M6Ø.232** **Left**
- **M6Ø.239** **Unspecified**

M6Ø.24- **Hand**
- **M6Ø.241** **Right**
- **M6Ø.242** **Left**
- **M6Ø.249** **Unspecified**

M6Ø.25- **Thigh**
- **M6Ø.251** **Right**
- **M6Ø.252** **Left**
- **M6Ø.259** **Unspecified**

M6Ø.26- **Lower leg**
- **M6Ø.261** **Right**
- **M6Ø.262** **Left**
- **M6Ø.269** **Unspecified**

M6Ø.27- **Ankle and foot**
- **M6Ø.271** **Right**
- **M6Ø.272** **Left**
- **M6Ø.279** **Unspecified**

M6Ø.28 **Other site**

M6Ø.8- **Other myositis**

M6Ø.8Ø **Unspecified site**

M6Ø.81- **Shoulder**
- **M6Ø.811** **Right**
- **M6Ø.812** **Left**
- **M6Ø.819** **Unspecified**

M6Ø.82- **Upper arm**
- **M6Ø.821** **Right**
- **M6Ø.822** **Left**
- **M6Ø.829** **Unspecified**

M6Ø.83- **Forearm**
- **M6Ø.831** **Right**
- **M6Ø.832** **Left**
- **M6Ø.839** **Unspecified**

M6Ø.84- **Hand**
- **M6Ø.841** **Right**
- **M6Ø.842** **Left**
- **M6Ø.849** **Unspecified**

M6Ø.85- **Thigh**
- **M6Ø.851** **Right**
- **M6Ø.852** **Left**
- **M6Ø.859** **Unspecified**

M6Ø.86- **Lower leg**
- **M6Ø.861** **Right**
- **M6Ø.862** **Left**
- **M6Ø.869** **Unspecified**

M6Ø.87- **Ankle and foot**
- **M6Ø.871** **Right**
- **M6Ø.872** **Left**
- **M6Ø.879** **Unspecified**

M6Ø.88 **Other site**

M6Ø.89 **Multiple sites**

M6Ø.9 **Myositis, unspecified**

M61- CALCIFICATION AND OSSIFICATION OF MUSCLE

M61.Ø- **Myositis ossificans traumatica**

M61.ØØ **Unspecified site**

M61.Ø1- **Shoulder**
- **M61.Ø11** **Right**
- **M61.Ø12** **Left**
- **M61.Ø19** **Unspecified**

M61.Ø2- **Upper arm**
- **M61.Ø21** **Right**
- **M61.Ø22** **Left**
- **M61.Ø29** **Unspecified**

M61.Ø3- **Forearm**
- **M61.Ø31** **Right**
- **M61.Ø32** **Left**
- **M61.Ø39** **Unspecified**

M61.Ø4- **Hand**
- **M61.Ø41** **Right**
- **M61.Ø42** **Left**
- **M61.Ø49** **Unspecified**

M61.Ø5- **Thigh**
- **M61.Ø51** **Right**
- **M61.Ø52** **Left**
- **M61.Ø59** **Unspecified**

M61.Ø6- **Lower leg**
- **M61.Ø61** **Right**
- **M61.Ø62** **Left**
- **M61.Ø69** **Unspecified**

M61.Ø7- **Ankle and foot**
- **M61.Ø71** **Right**
- **M61.Ø72** **Left**
- **M61.Ø79** **Unspecified**

M61.Ø8 **Other site**

M61.Ø9 **Multiple sites**

M61.1- **Myositis ossificans progressiva**

Including: Fibrodysplasia ossificans progressiva

M61.1Ø **Unspecified site**

M61.11- **Shoulder**
- **M61.111** **Right**
- **M61.112** **Left**
- **M61.119** **Unspecified**

M61.12- **Upper arm**
- **M61.121** **Right**
- **M61.122** **Left**
- **M61.129** **Unspecified**

M61.13- **Forearm**
- **M61.131** **Right**
- **M61.132** **Left**
- **M61.139** **Unspecified**

M61.14- **Hand and finger(s)**
- **M61.141** **Right hand**
- **M61.142** **Left hand**
- **M61.143** **Unspecified hand**
- **M61.144** **Right finger(s)**
- **M61.145** **Left finger(s)**
- **M61.146** **Unspecified finger(s)**

See Appendix A — Coding Reference Tables for lists of the ICD-10-CM Tabular indicators, HAC categories, and HCC codes.

M61.15- **Thigh**
- **M61.151 Right**
- **M61.152 Left**
- **M61.159 Unspecified**

M61.16- **Lower leg**
- **M61.161 Right**
- **M61.162 Left**
- **M61.169 Unspecified**

M61.17- **Ankle, foot and toe(s)**
- **M61.171 Right ankle**
- **M61.172 Left ankle**
- **M61.173 Unspecified ankle**
- **M61.174 Right foot**
- **M61.175 Left foot**
- **M61.176 Unspecified foot**
- **M61.177 Right toe(s)**
- **M61.178 Left toe(s)**
- **M61.179 Unspecified toe(s)**

M61.18 Other site

M61.19 Multiple sites

M61.2- **Paralytic calcification and ossification of muscle**
Including: Myositis ossificans associated with quadriplegia or paraplegia

M61.2Ø Unspecified site

M61.21- **Shoulder**
- **M61.211 Right**
- **M61.212 Left**
- **M61.219 Unspecified**

M61.22- **Upper arm**
- **M61.221 Right**
- **M61.222 Left**
- **M61.229 Unspecified**

M61.23- **Forearm**
- **M61.231 Right**
- **M61.232 Left**
- **M61.239 Unspecified**

M61.24- **Hand**
- **M61.241 Right**
- **M61.242 Left**
- **M61.249 Unspecified**

M61.25- **Thigh**
- **M61.251 Right**
- **M61.252 Left**
- **M61.259 Unspecified**

M61.26- **Lower leg**
- **M61.261 Right**
- **M61.262 Left**
- **M61.269 Unspecified**

M61.27- **Ankle and foot**
- **M61.271 Right**
- **M61.272 Left**
- **M61.279 Unspecified**

M61.28 Other site

M61.29 Multiple sites

M61.3- **Calcification and ossification of muscles associated with burns**
Including: Myositis ossificans

M61.3Ø Unspecified site

M61.31- **Shoulder**
- **M61.311 Right**
- **M61.312 Left**
- **M61.319 Unspecified**

M61.32- **Upper arm**
- **M61.321 Right**
- **M61.322 Left**
- **M61.329 Unspecified**

M61.33- **Forearm**
- **M61.331 Right**
- **M61.332 Left**
- **M61.339 Unspecified**

M61.34- **Hand**
- **M61.341 Right**
- **M61.342 Left**
- **M61.349 Unspecified**

M61.35- **Thigh**
- **M61.351 Right**
- **M61.352 Left**
- **M61.359 Unspecified**

M61.36- **Lower leg**
- **M61.361 Right**
- **M61.362 Left**
- **M61.369 Unspecified**

M61.37- **Ankle and foot**
- **M61.371 Right**
- **M61.372 Left**
- **M61.379 Unspecified**

M61.38 Other site

M61.39 Multiple sites

M61.4- **Other calcification of muscle**
Excludes1:
calcific tendinitis NOS (M65.2-)
calcific tendinitis of shoulder (M75.3)

M61.4Ø Unspecified site

M61.41- **Shoulder**
- **M61.411 Right**
- **M61.412 Left**
- **M61.419 Unspecified**

M61.42- **Upper arm**
- **M61.421 Right**
- **M61.422 Left**
- **M61.429 Unspecified**

M61.43- **Forearm**
- **M61.431 Right**
- **M61.432 Left**
- **M61.439 Unspecified**

M61.44- **Hand**
- **M61.441 Right**
- **M61.442 Left**
- **M61.449 Unspecified**

M61.45- **Thigh**
M61.451 **Right**
M61.452 **Left**
M61.459 **Unspecified**
M61.46- **Lower leg**
M61.461 **Right**
M61.462 **Left**
M61.469 **Unspecified**
M61.47- **Ankle and foot**
M61.471 **Right**
M61.472 **Left**
M61.479 **Unspecified**
M61.48 **Other site**
M61.49 **Multiple sites**

M61.5- **Other ossification of muscle**
M61.5Ø **Unspecified site**
M61.51- **Shoulder**
M61.511 **Right**
M61.512 **Left**
M61.519 **Unspecified**
M61.52- **Upper arm**
M61.521 **Right**
M61.522 **Left**
M61.529 **Unspecified**
M61.53- **Forearm**
M61.531 **Right**
M61.532 **Left**
M61.539 **Unspecified**
M61.54- **Hand**
M61.541 **Right**
M61.542 **Left**
M61.549 **Unspecified**
M61.55- **Thigh**
M61.551 **Right**
M61.552 **Left**
M61.559 **Unspecified**
M61.56- **Lower leg**
M61.561 **Right**
M61.562 **Left**
M61.569 **Unspecified**
M61.57- **Ankle and foot**
M61.571 **Right**
M61.572 **Left**
M61.579 **Unspecified**
M61.58 **Other site**
M61.59 **Multiple sites**

M61.9 **Calcification and ossification of muscle, unspecified**

M62- OTHER DISORDERS OF MUSCLE

Excludes1:
alcoholic myopathy (G72.1)
cramp and spasm (R25.2)
drug-induced myopathy (G72.Ø)
myalgia (M79.1-)
stiff-man syndrome (G25.82)
Excludes2:
nontraumatic hematoma of muscle (M79.81)

M62.Ø- **Separation of muscle (nontraumatic)**
Including: Diastasis of muscle
Excludes1:
diastasis recti complicating pregnancy, labor and delivery (O71.8)
traumatic separation of muscle- see strain of muscle by body region
M62.ØØ **Unspecified site**
M62.Ø1- **Shoulder**
M62.Ø11 **Right**
M62.Ø12 **Left**
M62.Ø19 **Unspecified**
M62.Ø2- **Upper arm**
M62.Ø21 **Right**
M62.Ø22 **Left**
M62.Ø29 **Unspecified**
M62.Ø3- **Forearm**
M62.Ø31 **Right**
M62.Ø32 **Left**
M62.Ø39 **Unspecified**
M62.Ø4- **Hand**
M62.Ø41 **Right**
M62.Ø42 **Left**
M62.Ø49 **Unspecified**
M62.Ø5- **Thigh**
M62.Ø51 **Right**
M62.Ø52 **Left**
M62.Ø59 **Unspecified**
M62.Ø6- **Lower leg**
M62.Ø61 **Right**
M62.Ø62 **Left**
M62.Ø69 **Unspecified**
M62.Ø7- **Ankle and foot**
M62.Ø71 **Right**
M62.Ø72 **Left**
M62.Ø79 **Unspecified**
M62.Ø8 **Other site**

M62.1- **Other rupture of muscle (nontraumatic)**
Excludes1:
traumatic rupture of muscle - see strain of muscle by body region
Excludes2:
rupture of tendon (M66.-)
M62.1Ø **Unspecified site**
M62.11- **Shoulder**
M62.111 **Right**
M62.112 **Left**
M62.119 **Unspecified**
M62.12- **Upper arm**
M62.121 **Right**
M62.122 **Left**
M62.129 **Unspecified**
M62.13- **Forearm**
M62.131 **Right**
M62.132 **Left**
M62.139 **Unspecified**

M62.14- **Hand**
- **M62.141** **Right**
- **M62.142** **Left**
- **M62.149** **Unspecified**

M62.15- **Thigh**
- **M62.151** **Right**
- **M62.152** **Left**
- **M62.159** **Unspecified**

M62.16- **Lower leg**
- **M62.161** **Right**
- **M62.162** **Left**
- **M62.169** **Unspecified**

M62.17- **Ankle and foot**
- **M62.171** **Right**
- **M62.172** **Left**
- **M62.179** **Unspecified**

M62.18 **Other site**

M62.2- **Nontraumatic ischemic infarction of muscle**

Excludes1:
compartment syndrome (traumatic) (T79.A-)
nontraumatic compartment syndrome (M79.A-)
traumatic ischemia of muscle (T79.6)
rhabdomyolysis (M62.82)
Volkmann's ischemic contracture (T79.6)

M62.2Ø **Unspecified site**

M62.21- **Shoulder**
- **M62.211** **Right**
- **M62.212** **Left**
- **M62.219** **Unspecified**

M62.22- **Upper arm**
- **M62.221** **Right**
- **M62.222** **Left**
- **M62.229** **Unspecified**

M62.23- **Forearm**
- **M62.231** **Right**
- **M62.232** **Left**
- **M62.239** **Unspecified**

M62.24- **Hand**
- **M62.241** **Right**
- **M62.242** **Left**
- **M62.249** **Unspecified**

M62.25- **Thigh**
- **M62.251** **Right**
- **M62.252** **Left**
- **M62.259** **Unspecified**

M62.26- **Lower leg**
- **M62.261** **Right**
- **M62.262** **Left**
- **M62.269** **Unspecified**

M62.27- **Ankle and foot**
- **M62.271** **Right**
- **M62.272** **Left**
- **M62.279** **Unspecified**

M62.28 **Other site**

M62.3 **Immobility syndrome (paraplegic)**

M62.4- **Contracture of muscle**

Including: Tendon (sheath)

Excludes1:
contracture of joint (M24.5-)

M62.4Ø **Unspecified site**

M62.41- **Shoulder**
- **M62.411** **Right**
- **M62.412** **Left**
- **M62.419** **Unspecified**

M62.42- **Upper arm**
- **M62.421** **Right**
- **M62.422** **Left**
- **M62.429** **Unspecified**

M62.43- **Forearm**
- **M62.431** **Right**
- **M62.432** **Left**
- **M62.439** **Unspecified**

M62.44- **Hand**
- **M62.441** **Right**
- **M62.442** **Left**
- **M62.449** **Unspecified**

M62.45- **Thigh**
- **M62.451** **Right**
- **M62.452** **Left**
- **M62.459** **Unspecified**

M62.46- **Lower leg**
- **M62.461** **Right**
- **M62.462** **Left**
- **M62.469** **Unspecified**

M62.47- **Ankle and foot**
- **M62.471** **Right**
- **M62.472** **Left**
- **M62.479** **Unspecified**

M62.48 **Other site**

M62.49 **Multiple sites**

M62.5- **Muscle wasting and atrophy, NEC**

Including: Disuse atrophy NEC

Excludes1:
neuralgic amyotrophy (G54.5)
progressive muscular atrophy (G12.29)
sarcopenia (M62.84)

Excludes2:
pelvic muscle wasting (N81.84)

M62.5Ø **Unspecified site**

M62.51- **Shoulder**
- **M62.511** **Right**
- **M62.512** **Left**
- **M62.519** **Unspecified**

M62.52- **Upper arm**
- **M62.521** **Right**
- **M62.522** **Left**
- **M62.529** **Unspecified**

M62.53- **Forearm**
- **M62.531** **Right**
- **M62.532** **Left**
- **M62.539** **Unspecified**

Ch5

5. The Tabular List

M62.54- **Hand**
M62.541 **Right**
M62.542 **Left**
M62.549 **Unspecified**
M62.55- **Thigh**
M62.551 **Right**
M62.552 **Left**
M62.559 **Unspecified**
M62.56- **Lower leg**
M62.561 **Right**
M62.562 **Left**
M62.569 **Unspecified**
M62.57- **Ankle and foot**
M62.571 **Right**
M62.572 **Left**
M62.579 **Unspecified**
M62.58 **Other site**
M62.59 **Multiple sites**
M62.5A- **Back**
N **M62.5A0** **Cervical**
N **M62.5A1** **Thoracic**
N **M62.5A2** **Lumbosacral**
N **M62.5A9** **Unspecified level**

M62.8- **Other specified disorders of muscle**
Excludes2:
nontraumatic hematoma of muscle (M79.81)
M62.81 **Muscle weakness (generalized)**
Excludes1:
muscle weakness in sarcopenia (M62.84)
M62.82 **Rhabdomyolysis**
Excludes1:
traumatic rhabdomyolysis (T79.6)
Indicator(s): CC
M62.83- **Muscle spasm**
M62.830 **Back**
M62.831 **Calf**
Including: Charley-horse
M62.838 **Other**
M62.84 **Sarcopenia**
Including: Age-related sarcopenia
Code First:
underlying disease, if applicable, such as:
disorders of myoneural junction and muscle disease in diseases classified elsewhere (G73.-)
other and unspecified myopathies (G72.-)
primary disorders of muscles (G71.-)
M62.89 **Other**
Including: Muscle (sheath) hernia

M62.9 **Disorder of muscle, unspecified**

M63- DISORDERS OF MUSCLE IN DISEASES CLASSIFIED ELSEWHERE
Code First:
underlying disease, such as:
leprosy (A30.-)
neoplasm (C49.-, C79.89, D21.-, D48.1)
schistosomiasis (B65.-)
trichinellosis (B75)
Excludes1:
myopathy in cysticercosis (B69.81)
myopathy in endocrine diseases (G73.7)
myopathy in metabolic diseases (G73.7)
myopathy in sarcoidosis (D86.87)
myopathy in secondary syphilis (A51.49)
myopathy in syphilis (late) (A52.78)
myopathy in toxoplasmosis (B58.82)
myopathy in tuberculosis (A18.09)
M63.80 **Unspecified site**
M63.81- **Shoulder**
M63.811 **Right**
M63.812 **Left**
M63.819 **Unspecified**
M63.82- **Upper arm**
M63.821 **Right**
M63.822 **Left**
M63.829 **Unspecified**
M63.83- **Forearm**
M63.831 **Right**
M63.832 **Left**
M63.839 **Unspecified**
M63.84- **Hand**
M63.841 **Right**
M63.842 **Left**
M63.849 **Unspecified**
M63.85- **Thigh**
M63.851 **Right**
M63.852 **Left**
M63.859 **Unspecified**
M63.86- **Lower leg**
M63.861 **Right**
M63.862 **Left**
M63.869 **Unspecified**
M63.87- **Ankle and foot**
M63.871 **Right**
M63.872 **Left**
M63.879 **Unspecified**
M63.88 **Other site**
M63.89 **Multiple sites**

DISORDERS OF SYNOVIUM AND TENDON (M65-M67)

M65- SYNOVITIS AND TENOSYNOVITIS
Excludes1:
chronic crepitant synovitis of hand and wrist (M70.0-)
current injury - see injury of ligament or tendon by body region
soft tissue disorders related to use, overuse and pressure (M70.-)

M65.0- **Abscess of tendon sheath**
Use additional code (B95-B96) to identify bacterial agent.
M65.00 **Unspecified site**
M65.01- **Shoulder**
M65.011 **Right**
M65.012 **Left**
M65.019 **Unspecified**

M65.Ø2- **Upper arm**
M65.Ø21 Right
M65.Ø22 Left
M65.Ø29 Unspecified
M65.Ø3- **Forearm**
M65.Ø31 Right
M65.Ø32 Left
M65.Ø39 Unspecified
M65.Ø4- **Hand**
M65.Ø41 Right
M65.Ø42 Left
M65.Ø49 Unspecified
M65.Ø5- **Thigh**
M65.Ø51 Right
M65.Ø52 Left
M65.Ø59 Unspecified
M65.Ø6- **Lower leg**
M65.Ø61 Right
M65.Ø62 Left
M65.Ø69 Unspecified
M65.Ø7- **Ankle and foot**
M65.Ø71 Right
M65.Ø72 Left
M65.Ø79 Unspecified
M65.Ø8 Other site

M65.1- **Other infective (teno)synovitis**
M65.1Ø Unspecified site
M65.11- **Shoulder**
M65.111 Right
M65.112 Left
M65.119 Unspecified
M65.12- **Elbow**
M65.121 Right
M65.122 Left
M65.129 Unspecified
M65.13- **Wrist**
M65.131 Right
M65.132 Left
M65.139 Unspecified
M65.14- **Hand**
M65.141 Right
M65.142 Left
M65.149 Unspecified
M65.15- **Hip**
M65.151 Right
M65.152 Left
M65.159 Unspecified
M65.16- **Knee**
M65.161 Right
M65.162 Left
M65.169 Unspecified
M65.17- **Ankle and foot**
M65.171 Right
M65.172 Left
M65.179 Unspecified
M65.18 Other site
M65.19 Multiple sites

M65.2- **Calcific tendinitis**
Excludes1:
tendinitis as classified in M75-M77
calcified tendinitis of shoulder (M75.3)
M65.2Ø Unspecified site
M65.22- **Upper arm**
M65.221 Right
M65.222 Left
M65.229 Unspecified
M65.23- **Forearm**
M65.231 Right
M65.232 Left
M65.239 Unspecified
M65.24- **Hand**
M65.241 Right
M65.242 Left
M65.249 Unspecified
M65.25- **Thigh**
M65.251 Right
M65.252 Left
M65.259 Unspecified
M65.26- **Lower leg**
M65.261 Right
M65.262 Left
M65.269 Unspecified
M65.27- **Ankle and foot**
M65.271 Right
M65.272 Left
M65.279 Unspecified
M65.28 Other site
M65.29 Multiple sites

M65.3- **Trigger finger**
Including: Nodular tendinous disease
M65.3Ø Unspecified finger
M65.31- **Trigger thumb**
M65.311 Right
M65.312 Left
M65.319 Unspecified
M65.32- **Trigger finger, index finger**
M65.321 Right
M65.322 Left
M65.329 Unspecified
M65.33- **Trigger finger, middle finger**
M65.331 Right
M65.332 Left
M65.339 Unspecified
M65.34- **Trigger finger, ring finger**
M65.341 Right
M65.342 Left
M65.349 Unspecified
M65.35- **Trigger finger, little finger**
M65.351 Right
M65.352 Left
M65.359 Unspecified

M65.4 **Radial styloid tenosynovitis [de Quervain]**
M65.8- **Other synovitis and tenosynovitis**
M65.8Ø **Unspecified site**
M65.81- **Shoulder**
M65.811 **Right**
M65.812 **Left**
M65.819 **Unspecified**
M65.82- **Upper arm**
M65.821 **Right**
M65.822 **Left**
M65.829 **Unspecified**
M65.83- **Forearm**
M65.831 **Right**
M65.832 **Left**
M65.839 **Unspecified**
M65.84- **Hand**
M65.841 **Right**
M65.842 **Left**
M65.849 **Unspecified**
M65.85- **Thigh**
M65.851 **Right**
M65.852 **Left**
M65.859 **Unspecified**
M65.86- **Lower leg**
M65.861 **Right**
M65.862 **Left**
M65.869 **Unspecified**
M65.87- **Ankle and foot**
M65.871 **Right**
M65.872 **Left**
M65.879 **Unspecified**
M65.88 **Other site**
M65.89 **Multiple sites**
M65.9 **Synovitis and tenosynovitis, unspecified**

M66- SPONTANEOUS RUPTURE OF SYNOVIUM AND TENDON

Includes:
rupture that occurs when a normal force is applied to tissues that are inferred to have less than normal strength
Excludes2:
rotator cuff syndrome (M75.1-)
rupture where an abnormal force is applied to normal tissue - see injury of tendon by body region

M66.Ø **Popliteal cyst**
M66.1- **Rupture of synovium**
Including: Rupture of synovial cyst
Excludes2:
rupture of popliteal cyst (M66.Ø)
M66.1Ø **Unspecified joint**
M66.11- **Shoulder**
M66.111 **Right**
M66.112 **Left**
M66.119 **Unspecified**
M66.12- **Elbow**
M66.121 **Right**
M66.122 **Left**
M66.129 **Unspecified**
M66.13- **Wrist**
M66.131 **Right**
M66.132 **Left**
M66.139 **Unspecified**
M66.14- **Hand and fingers**
M66.141 **Right hand**
M66.142 **Left hand**
M66.143 **Unspecified hand**
M66.144 **Right finger(s)**
M66.145 **Left finger(s)**
M66.146 **Unspecified finger(s)**
M66.15- **Hip**
M66.151 **Right**
M66.152 **Left**
M66.159 **Unspecified**
M66.17- **Ankle, foot and toes**
M66.171 **Right ankle**
M66.172 **Left ankle**
M66.173 **Unspecified ankle**
M66.174 **Right foot**
M66.175 **Left foot**
M66.176 **Unspecified foot**
M66.177 **Right toe(s)**
M66.178 **Left toe(s)**
M66.179 **Unspecified toe(s)**
M66.18 **Other site**
M66.2- **Spontaneous rupture of extensor tendons**
M66.2Ø **Unspecified site**
M66.21- **Shoulder**
M66.211 **Right**
M66.212 **Left**
M66.219 **Unspecified**
M66.22- **Upper arm**
M66.221 **Right**
M66.222 **Left**
M66.229 **Unspecified**
M66.23- **Forearm**
M66.231 **Right**
M66.232 **Left**
M66.239 **Unspecified**
M66.24- **Hand**
M66.241 **Right**
M66.242 **Left**
M66.249 **Unspecified**
M66.25- **Thigh**
M66.251 **Right**
M66.252 **Left**
M66.259 **Unspecified**
M66.26- **Lower leg**
M66.261 **Right**
M66.262 **Left**
M66.269 **Unspecified**

M66.27- **Ankle and foot**
- **M66.271 Right**
- **M66.272 Left**
- **M66.279 Unspecified**

M66.28 Other site

M66.29 Multiple sites

M66.3- **Spontaneous rupture of flexor tendons**

M66.3Ø Unspecified site

M66.31- **Shoulder**
- **M66.311 Right**
- **M66.312 Left**
- **M66.319 Unspecified**

M66.32- **Upper arm**
- **M66.321 Right**
- **M66.322 Left**
- **M66.329 Unspecified**

M66.33- **Forearm**
- **M66.331 Right**
- **M66.332 Left**
- **M66.339 Unspecified**

M66.34- **Hand**
- **M66.341 Right**
- **M66.342 Left**
- **M66.349 Unspecified**

M66.35- **Thigh**
- **M66.351 Right**
- **M66.352 Left**
- **M66.359 Unspecified**

M66.36- **Lower leg**
- **M66.361 Right**
- **M66.362 Left**
- **M66.369 Unspecified**

M66.37- **Ankle and foot**
- **M66.371 Right**
- **M66.372 Left**
- **M66.379 Unspecified**

M66.38 Other site

M66.39 Multiple sites

M66.8- **Spontaneous rupture of other tendons**

M66.8Ø Unspecified site

M66.81- **Shoulder**
- **M66.811 Right**
- **M66.812 Left**
- **M66.819 Unspecified**

M66.82- **Upper arm**
- **M66.821 Right**
- **M66.822 Left**
- **M66.829 Unspecified**

M66.83- **Forearm**
- **M66.831 Right**
- **M66.832 Left**
- **M66.839 Unspecified**

M66.84- **Hand**
- **M66.841 Right**
- **M66.842 Left**
- **M66.849 Unspecified**

M66.85- **Thigh**
- **M66.851 Right**
- **M66.852 Left**
- **M66.859 Unspecified**

M66.86- **Lower leg**
- **M66.861 Right**
- **M66.862 Left**
- **M66.869 Unspecified**

M66.87- **Ankle and foot**
- **M66.871 Right**
- **M66.872 Left**
- **M66.879 Unspecified**

M66.88 Other sites

M66.89 Multiple sites

M66.9 Spontaneous rupture of unspecified tendon

Including: Rupture at musculotendinous junction, nontraumatic

M67- OTHER DISORDERS OF SYNOVIUM AND TENDON

<u>*Excludes1:*</u>

palmar fascial fibromatosis [Dupuytren] (M72.Ø)

tendinitis NOS (M77.9-)

xanthomatosis localized to tendons (E78.2)

M67.Ø- **Short Achilles tendon (acquired)**
- **M67.ØØ Unspecified ankle**
- **M67.Ø1 Right ankle**
- **M67.Ø2 Left ankle**

M67.2- **Synovial hypertrophy, not elsewhere classified**

<u>*Excludes1:*</u>

villonodular synovitis (pigmented) (M12.2-)

M67.2Ø Unspecified site

M67.21- **Shoulder**
- **M67.211 Right**
- **M67.212 Left**
- **M67.219 Unspecified**

M67.22- **Upper arm**
- **M67.221 Right**
- **M67.222 Left**
- **M67.229 Unspecified**

M67.23- **Forearm**
- **M67.231 Right**
- **M67.232 Left**
- **M67.239 Unspecified**

M67.24- **Hand**
- **M67.241 Right**
- **M67.242 Left**
- **M67.249 Unspecified**

M67.25- **Thigh**
- **M67.251 Right**
- **M67.252 Left**
- **M67.259 Unspecified**

M67.26- **Lower leg**
- **M67.261 Right**
- **M67.262 Left**
- **M67.269 Unspecified**

M67.27- **Ankle and foot**
- **M67.271 Right**
- **M67.272 Left**
- **M67.279 Unspecified**

M67.28 Other site

M67.29 Multiple sites

M67.3- **Transient synovitis**

Including: Toxic synovitis

Excludes1:

palindromic rheumatism (M12.3-)

M67.3Ø Unspecified site

M67.31- **Shoulder**
- **M67.311 Right**
- **M67.312 Left**
- **M67.319 Unspecified**

M67.32- **Elbow**
- **M67.321 Right**
- **M67.322 Left**
- **M67.329 Unspecified**

M67.33- **Wrist**
- **M67.331 Right**
- **M67.332 Left**
- **M67.339 Unspecified**

M67.34- **Hand**
- **M67.341 Right**
- **M67.342 Left**
- **M67.349 Unspecified**

M67.35- **Hip**
- **M67.351 Right**
- **M67.352 Left**
- **M67.359 Unspecified**

M67.36- **Knee**
- **M67.361 Right**
- **M67.362 Left**
- **M67.369 Unspecified**

M67.37- **Ankle and foot**
- **M67.371 Right**
- **M67.372 Left**
- **M67.379 Unspecified**

M67.38 Other site

M67.39 Multiple sites

M67.4- **Ganglion**

Including: Ganglion of joint or tendon (sheath)

Excludes1:

ganglion in yaws (A66.6)

Excludes2:

cyst of bursa (M71.2-M71.3)

cyst of synovium (M71.2-M71.3)

M67.4Ø Unspecified site

M67.41- **Shoulder**
- **M67.411 Right**
- **M67.412 Left**
- **M67.419 Unspecified**

M67.42- **Elbow**
- **M67.421 Right**
- **M67.422 Left**
- **M67.429 Unspecified**

M67.43- **Wrist**
- **M67.431 Right**
- **M67.432 Left**
- **M67.439 Unspecified**

M67.44- **Hand**
- **M67.441 Right**
- **M67.442 Left**
- **M67.449 Unspecified**

M67.45- **Hip**
- **M67.451 Right**
- **M67.452 Left**
- **M67.459 Unspecified**

M67.46- **Knee**
- **M67.461 Right**
- **M67.462 Left**
- **M67.469 Unspecified**

M67.47- **Ankle and foot**
- **M67.471 Right**
- **M67.472 Left**
- **M67.479 Unspecified**

M67.48 Other site

M67.49 Multiple sites

M67.5- **Plica syndrome**

Including: Plica knee

M67.5Ø Unspecified knee

M67.51 Right knee

M67.52 Left knee

M67.8- **Other specified disorders of synovium and tendon**

M67.8Ø Unspecified site

M67.81- **Shoulder**
- **M67.811 Synovium, right**
- **M67.812 Synovium, left**
- **M67.813 Tendon, right**
- **M67.814 Tendon, left**
- **M67.819 Synovium and tendon, unspecified**

M67.82- **Elbow**
- **M67.821 Synovium, right**
- **M67.822 Synovium, left**
- **M67.823 Tendon, right**
- **M67.824 Tendon, left**
- **M67.829 Synovium and tendon, unspecified**

M67.83- **Wrist**
- **M67.831 Synovium, right**
- **M67.832 Synovium, left**
- **M67.833 Tendon, right**
- **M67.834 Tendon, left**
- **M67.839 Unspecified wrist**

M67.84- **Hand**
- **M67.841** **Synovium, right**
- **M67.842** **Synovium, left**
- **M67.843** **Tendon, right**
- **M67.844** **Tendon, left**
- **M67.849** **Synovium and tendon, unspecified**

M67.85- **Hip**
- **M67.851** **Synovium, right**
- **M67.852** **Synovium, left**
- **M67.853** **Tendon, right**
- **M67.854** **Tendon, left**
- **M67.859** **Synovium and tendon, unspecified**

M67.86- **Knee**
- **M67.861** **Synovium, right**
- **M67.862** **Synovium, left**
- **M67.863** **Tendon, right**
- **M67.864** **Tendon, left**
- **M67.869** **Synovium and tendon, unspecified**

M67.87- **Ankle and foot**
- **M67.871** **Synovium, right**
- **M67.872** **Synovium, left**
- **M67.873** **Tendon, right**
- **M67.874** **Tendon, left**
- **M67.879** **Synovium and tendon, unspecified**

M67.88 **Other site**

M67.89 **Multiple sites**

M67.9- **Unspecified disorder of synovium and tendon**

M67.9Ø **Unspecified site**

M67.91- **Shoulder**
- **M67.911** **Right**
- **M67.912** **Left**
- **M67.919** **Unspecified**

M67.92- **Upper arm**
- **M67.921** **Right**
- **M67.922** **Left**
- **M67.929** **Unspecified**

M67.93- **Forearm**
- **M67.931** **Right**
- **M67.932** **Left**
- **M67.939** **Unspecified**

M67.94- **Hand**
- **M67.941** **Right**
- **M67.942** **Left**
- **M67.949** **Unspecified**

M67.95- **Thigh**
- **M67.951** **Right**
- **M67.952** **Left**
- **M67.959** **Unspecified**

M67.96- **Lower leg**
- **M67.961** **Right**
- **M67.962** **Left**
- **M67.969** **Unspecified**

M67.97- **Ankle and foot**
- **M67.971** **Right**
- **M67.972** **Left**
- **M67.979** **Unspecified**

M67.98 **Other site**

M67.99 **Multiple sites**

OTHER SOFT TISSUE DISORDERS (M7Ø-M79)

M7Ø- SOFT TISSUE DISORDERS RELATED TO USE, OVERUSE AND PRESSURE

Includes:
soft tissue disorders of occupational origin
Use additional external cause code to identify activity causing disorder (Y93.-)
Excludes1:
bursitis NOS (M71.9-)
Excludes2:
bursitis of shoulder (M75.5)
enthesopathies (M76-M77)
pressure ulcer (pressure area) (L89.-)

M7Ø.Ø- **Crepitant synovitis (acute) (chronic) of hand and wrist**

M7Ø.Ø3- **Wrist**
- **M7Ø.Ø31** **Right**
- **M7Ø.Ø32** **Left**
- **M7Ø.Ø39** **Unspecified**

M7Ø.Ø4- **Hand**
- **M7Ø.Ø41** **Right**
- **M7Ø.Ø42** **Left**
- **M7Ø.Ø49** **Unspecified**

M7Ø.1- **Bursitis of hand**
- **M7Ø.1Ø** **Unspecified**
- **M7Ø.11** **Right**
- **M7Ø.12** **Left**

M7Ø.2- **Olecranon bursitis**
- **M7Ø.2Ø** **Unspecified**
- **M7Ø.21** **Right elbow**
- **M7Ø.22** **Left elbow**

M7Ø.3- **Other bursitis of elbow**
- **M7Ø.3Ø** **Unspecified**
- **M7Ø.31** **Right**
- **M7Ø.32** **Left**

M7Ø.4- **Prepatellar bursitis**
- **M7Ø.4Ø** **Unspecified**
- **M7Ø.41** **Right**
- **M7Ø.42** **Left**

M7Ø.5- **Other bursitis of knee**
- **M7Ø.5Ø** **Unspecified**
- **M7Ø.51** **Right**
- **M7Ø.52** **Left**

M7Ø.6- **Trochanteric bursitis**

Including: Trochanteric tendinitis
- **M7Ø.6Ø** **Unspecified**
- **M7Ø.61** **Right**
- **M7Ø.62** **Left**

M7Ø.7- **Other bursitis of hip**
Including: Ischial bursitis
M7Ø.7Ø Unspecified
M7Ø.71 Right
M7Ø.72 Left

M7Ø.8- **Other soft tissue disorders related to use, overuse and pressure**
M7Ø.8Ø Unspecified site
M7Ø.81- **Shoulder**
M7Ø.811 Right
M7Ø.812 Left
M7Ø.819 Unspecified
M7Ø.82- **Upper arm**
M7Ø.821 Right
M7Ø.822 Left
M7Ø.829 Unspecified
M7Ø.83- **Forearm**
M7Ø.831 Right
M7Ø.832 Left
M7Ø.839 Unspecified
M7Ø.84- **Hand**
M7Ø.841 Right
M7Ø.842 Left
M7Ø.849 Unspecified
M7Ø.85- **Thigh**
M7Ø.851 Right
M7Ø.852 Left
M7Ø.859 Unspecified
M7Ø.86- **Lower leg**
M7Ø.861 Right
M7Ø.862 Left
M7Ø.869 Unspecified
M7Ø.87- **Ankle and foot**
M7Ø.871 Right
M7Ø.872 Left
M7Ø.879 Unspecified
M7Ø.88 Other site
M7Ø.89 Multiple sites

M7Ø.9- **Unspecified soft tissue disorder related to use, overuse and pressure**
M7Ø.9Ø Unspecified site
M7Ø.91- **Shoulder**
M7Ø.911 Right
M7Ø.912 Left
M7Ø.919 Unspecified
M7Ø.92- **Upper arm**
M7Ø.921 Right
M7Ø.922 Left
M7Ø.929 Unspecified
M7Ø.93- **Forearm**
M7Ø.931 Right
M7Ø.932 Left
M7Ø.939 Unspecified
M7Ø.94- **Hand**
M7Ø.941 Right
M7Ø.942 Left
M7Ø.949 Unspecified
M7Ø.95- **Thigh**
M7Ø.951 Right
M7Ø.952 Left
M7Ø.959 Unspecified
M7Ø.96- **Lower leg**
M7Ø.961 Right
M7Ø.962 Left
M7Ø.969 Unspecified
M7Ø.97- **Ankle and foot**
M7Ø.971 Right
M7Ø.972 Left
M7Ø.979 Unspecified
M7Ø.98 Other
M7Ø.99 Multiple sites

M71- OTHER BURSOPATHIES

Excludes1:
bunion (M2Ø.1)
bursitis related to use, overuse or pressure (M7Ø.-)
enthesopathies (M76-M77)

M71.Ø- **Abscess of bursa**
Use additional code (B95.-, B96.-) to identify causative organism
M71.ØØ Unspecified site
M71.Ø1- **Shoulder**
M71.Ø11 Right
M71.Ø12 Left
M71.Ø19 Unspecified
M71.Ø2- **Elbow**
M71.Ø21 Right
M71.Ø22 Left
M71.Ø29 Unspecified
M71.Ø3- **Wrist**
M71.Ø31 Right
M71.Ø32 Left
M71.Ø39 Unspecified
M71.Ø4- **Hand**
M71.Ø41 Right
M71.Ø42 Left
M71.Ø49 Unspecified
M71.Ø5- **Hip**
M71.Ø51 Right
M71.Ø52 Left
M71.Ø59 Unspecified
M71.Ø6- **Knee**
M71.Ø61 Right
M71.Ø62 Left
M71.Ø69 Unspecified
M71.Ø7- **Ankle and foot**
M71.Ø71 Right
M71.Ø72 Left
M71.Ø79 Unspecified
M71.Ø8 Other site
M71.Ø9 Multiple sites

Ch5

5. The Tabular List

M71.1- **Other infective bursitis**
Use additional code (B95.-, B96.-) to identify causative organism
M71.1Ø Unspecified site
M71.11- **Shoulder**
M71.111 Right
M71.112 Left
M71.119 Unspecified
M71.12- **Elbow**
M71.121 Right
M71.122 Left
M71.129 Unspecified
M71.13- **Wrist**
M71.131 Right
M71.132 Left
M71.139 Unspecified
M71.14- **Hand**
M71.141 Right
M71.142 Left
M71.149 Unspecified
M71.15- **Hip**
M71.151 Right
M71.152 Left
M71.159 Unspecified
M71.16- **Knee**
M71.161 Right
M71.162 Left
M71.169 Unspecified
M71.17- **Ankle and foot**
M71.171 Right
M71.172 Left
M71.179 Unspecified
M71.18 Other site
M71.19 Multiple sites
M71.2- **Synovial cyst of popliteal space [Baker]**
Excludes1:
synovial cyst of popliteal space with rupture (M66.Ø)
M71.2Ø Unspecified
M71.21 Right
M71.22 Left
M71.3- **Other bursal cyst**
Including: Synovial cyst NOS
Excludes1:
synovial cyst with rupture (M66.1-)
M71.3Ø Unspecified site
M71.31- **Shoulder**
M71.311 Right
M71.312 Left
M71.319 Unspecified
M71.32- **Elbow**
M71.321 Right
M71.322 Left
M71.329 Unspecified
M71.33- **Wrist**
M71.331 Right
M71.332 Left
M71.339 Unspecified
M71.34- **Hand**
M71.341 Right
M71.342 Left
M71.349 Unspecified
M71.35- **Hip**
M71.351 Right
M71.352 Left
M71.359 Unspecified
M71.37- **Ankle and foot**
M71.371 Right
M71.372 Left
M71.379 Unspecified
M71.38 Other site
M71.39 Multiple sites
M71.4- **Calcium deposit in bursa**
Excludes2:
calcium deposit in bursa of shoulder (M75.3)
M71.4Ø Unspecified site
M71.42- **Elbow**
M71.421 Right
M71.422 Left
M71.429 Unspecified
M71.43- **Wrist**
M71.431 Right
M71.432 Left
M71.439 Unspecified
M71.44- **Hand**
M71.441 Right
M71.442 Left
M71.449 Unspecified
M71.45- **Hip**
M71.451 Right
M71.452 Left
M71.459 Unspecified
M71.46- **Knee**
M71.461 Right
M71.462 Left
M71.469 Unspecified
M71.47- **Ankle and foot**
M71.471 Right
M71.472 Left
M71.479 Unspecified
M71.48 Other site
M71.49 Multiple sites
M71.5- **Other bursitis, not elsewhere classified**
Excludes1:
bursitis NOS (M71.9-)
Excludes2:
bursitis of shoulder (M75.5)
bursitis of tibial collateral [Pellegrini-Stieda] (M76.4-)
M71.5Ø Unspecified site
M71.52- **Elbow**
M71.521 Right
M71.522 Left
M71.529 Unspecified

M71.53- **Wrist**
M71.531 Right
M71.532 Left
M71.539 Unspecified
M71.54- **Hand**
M71.541 Right
M71.542 Left
M71.549 Unspecified
M71.55- **Hip**
M71.551 Right
M71.552 Left
M71.559 Unspecified
M71.56- **Knee**
M71.561 Right
M71.562 Left
M71.569 Unspecified
M71.57- **Ankle and foot**
M71.571 Right
M71.572 Left
M71.579 Unspecified
M71.58 Other site

M71.8- **Other specified bursopathies**
M71.8Ø Unspecified site
M71.81- **Shoulder**
M71.811 Right
M71.812 Left
M71.819 Unspecified
M71.82- **Elbow**
M71.821 Right
M71.822 Left
M71.829 Unspecified
M71.83- **Wrist**
M71.831 Right
M71.832 Left
M71.839 Unspecified
M71.84- **Hand**
M71.841 Right
M71.842 Left
M71.849 Unspecified
M71.85- **Hip**
M71.851 Right
M71.852 Left
M71.859 Unspecified
M71.86- **Knee**
M71.861 Right
M71.862 Left
M71.869 Unspecified
M71.87- **Ankle and foot**
M71.871 Right
M71.872 Left
M71.879 Unspecified
M71.88 Other site
M71.89 Multiple sites

M71.9 Bursopathy, unspecified
Including: Bursitis NOS

M72- FIBROBLASTIC DISORDERS
Excludes2:
retroperitoneal fibromatosis (D48.3)

M72.Ø Palmar fascial fibromatosis [Dupuytren]
Indicator(s): Adult

M72.1 Knuckle pads

M72.2 Plantar fascial fibromatosis
Including: Plantar fasciitis

M72.4 Pseudosarcomatous fibromatosis
Including: Nodular fasciitis

M72.6 Necrotizing fasciitis
Use additional code (B95.-, B96.-) to identify causative organism
Indicator(s): MCC | CMS22: 39 | CMS24: 39 | ESRD21: 39 | HHSØ5: 54 | HHSØ7: 54

M72.8 Other
Including: Abscess of fascia, Fasciitis NEC, Other infective fasciitis
Use additional code to (B95.-, B96.-) identify causative organism
Excludes1:
diffuse (eosinophilic) fasciitis (M35.4)
necrotizing fasciitis (M72.6)
nodular fasciitis (M72.4)
perirenal fasciitis NOS (N13.5)
perirenal fasciitis with infection (N13.6)
plantar fasciitis (M72.2)

M72.9 Unspecified
Including: Fasciitis NOS, Fibromatosis NOS

M75- SHOULDER LESIONS
Excludes2:
shoulder-hand syndrome (M89.Ø-)

M75.Ø- **Adhesive capsulitis of shoulder**
Including: Frozen shoulder, Periarthritis of shoulder
M75.ØØ Unspecified
M75.Ø1 Right
M75.Ø2 Left

M75.1- **Rotator cuff tear or rupture, not specified as traumatic**
Including: Rotator cuff syndrome, Supraspinatus tear or rupture not specified as traumatic, Supraspinatus syndrome
Excludes1:
tear of rotator cuff, traumatic (S46.Ø1-)
M75.1Ø- **Unspecified tear or rupture**
M75.1ØØ Unspecified shoulder
M75.1Ø1 Right shoulder
M75.1Ø2 Left shoulder
M75.11- **Incomplete tear or rupture**
M75.11Ø Unspecified shoulder
M75.111 Right shoulder
M75.112 Left shoulder
M75.12- **Complete tear or rupture**
M75.12Ø Unspecified shoulder
M75.121 Right shoulder
M75.122 Left shoulder

M75.2- **Bicipital tendinitis**
M75.2Ø Unspecified shoulder
M75.21 Right shoulder
M75.22 Left shoulder

M75.3- **Calcific tendinitis of shoulder**
Including: Calcified bursa
- **M75.30** **Unspecified**
- **M75.31** **Right**
- **M75.32** **Left**

M75.4- **Impingement syndrome of shoulder**
- **M75.40** **Unspecified**
- **M75.41** **Right**
- **M75.42** **Left**

M75.5- **Bursitis of shoulder**
- **M75.50** **Unspecified**
- **M75.51** **Right**
- **M75.52** **Left**

M75.8- **Other shoulder lesions**
- **M75.80** **Unspecified**
- **M75.81** **Right**
- **M75.82** **Left**

M75.9- **Shoulder lesion, unspecified**
- **M75.90** **Unspecified**
- **M75.91** **Right**
- **M75.92** **Left**

M76- ENTHESOPATHIES, LOWER LIMB, EXCLUDING FOOT

Excludes2:
bursitis due to use, overuse and pressure (M70.-)
enthesopathies of ankle and foot (M77.5-)

M76.0- **Gluteal tendinitis**
- **M76.00** **Unspecified hip**
- **M76.01** **Right hip**
- **M76.02** **Left hip**

M76.1- **Psoas tendinitis**
- **M76.10** **Unspecified hip**
- **M76.11** **Right hip**
- **M76.12** **Left hip**

M76.2- **Iliac crest spur**
- **M76.20** **Unspecified hip**
- **M76.21** **Right hip**
- **M76.22** **Left hip**

M76.3- **Iliotibial band syndrome**
- **M76.30** **Unspecified leg**
- **M76.31** **Right leg**
- **M76.32** **Left leg**

M76.4- **Tibial collateral bursitis [Pellegrini-Stieda]**
- **M76.40** **Unspecified leg**
- **M76.41** **Right leg**
- **M76.42** **Left leg**

M76.5- **Patellar tendinitis**
- **M76.50** **Unspecified knee**
- **M76.51** **Right knee**
- **M76.52** **Left knee**

M76.6- **Achilles tendinitis**
Including: Achilles bursitis
- **M76.60** **Unspecified leg**
- **M76.61** **Right leg**
- **M76.62** **Left leg**

M76.7- **Peroneal tendinitis**
- **M76.70** **Unspecified leg**
- **M76.71** **Right leg**
- **M76.72** **Left leg**

M76.8- **Other specified enthesopathies of lower limb, excluding foot**

M76.81- **Anterior tibial syndrome**
- **M76.811** **Right leg**
- **M76.812** **Left leg**
- **M76.819** **Unspecified leg**

M76.82- **Posterior tibial tendinitis**
- **M76.821** **Right leg**
- **M76.822** **Left leg**
- **M76.829** **Unspecified leg**

M76.89- **Other specified enthesopathies of lower limb, excluding foot**
- **M76.891** **Right leg**
- **M76.892** **Left leg**
- **M76.899** **Unspecified leg**

M76.9 **Unspecified**

M77- OTHER ENTHESOPATHIES

Excludes1:
bursitis NOS (M71.9-)
Excludes2:
bursitis due to use, overuse and pressure (M70.-)
osteophyte (M25.7)
spinal enthesopathy (M46.0-)

M77.0- **Medial epicondylitis**
- **M77.00** **Unspecified elbow**
- **M77.01** **Right elbow**
- **M77.02** **Left elbow**

M77.1- **Lateral epicondylitis**
Including: Tennis elbow
- **M77.10** **Unspecified elbow**
- **M77.11** **Right elbow**
- **M77.12** **Left elbow**

M77.2- **Periarthritis of wrist**
- **M77.20** **Unspecified wrist**
- **M77.21** **Right wrist**
- **M77.22** **Left wrist**

M77.3- **Calcaneal spur**
- **M77.30** **Unspecified foot**
- **M77.31** **Right foot**
- **M77.32** **Left foot**

M77.4- **Metatarsalgia**
Excludes1:
Morton's metatarsalgia (G57.6)
- **M77.40** **Unspecified foot**
- **M77.41** **Right foot**
- **M77.42** **Left foot**

M77.5- **Other enthesopathy of foot and ankle**
- **M77.50** **Unspecified foot and ankle**
- **M77.51** **Right foot and ankle**
- **M77.52** **Left foot and ankle**

M77.8 **NEC**

M77.9 **Unspecified**
Including: Bone spur NOS, Capsulitis NOS, Periarthritis NOS, Tendinitis NOS

Ch5

5. The Tabular List

M79- OTHER AND UNSPECIFIED SOFT TISSUE DISORDERS, NOT ELSEWHERE CLASSIFIED

Excludes1:
psychogenic rheumatism (F45.8)
soft tissue pain, psychogenic (F45.41)

M79.Ø **Rheumatism, unspecified**
Excludes1:
fibromyalgia (M79.7)
palindromic rheumatism (M12.3-)

M79.1- **Myalgia**
Including: Myofascial pain syndrome
Excludes1:
fibromyalgia (M79.7)
myositis (M6Ø.-)

M79.1Ø **Unspecified site**
M79.11 **Mastication muscle**
M79.12 **Auxiliary muscles, head and neck**
M79.18 **Other site**

M79.2 **Neuralgia and neuritis, unspecified**
Excludes1:
brachial radiculitis NOS (M54.1)
lumbosacral radiculitis NOS (M54.1)
mononeuropathies (G56-G58)
radiculitis NOS (M54.1)
sciatica (M54.3-M54.4)

M79.3 **Panniculitis, unspecified**
Excludes1:
lupus panniculitis (L93.2)
neck and back panniculitis (M54.Ø-)
relapsing [Weber-Christian] panniculitis (M35.6)

M79.4 **Hypertrophy of (infrapatellar) fat pad**

M79.5 **Residual foreign body in soft tissue**
Excludes1:
foreign body granuloma of skin and subcutaneous tissue (L92.3)
foreign body granuloma of soft tissue (M6Ø.2-)

M79.6- **Pain in limb, hand, foot, fingers and toes**
Excludes2:
pain in joint (M25.5-)

M79.6Ø- **Pain in limb, unspecified**
M79.6Ø1 **Right arm**
Including: Pain in right upper limb NOS
M79.6Ø2 **Left arm**
Including: Pain in left upper limb NOS
M79.6Ø3 **Unspecified arm**
Including: Pain in upper limb NOS
M79.6Ø4 **Right leg**
Including: Pain in right lower limb NOS
M79.6Ø5 **Left leg**
Including: Pain in left lower limb NOS
M79.6Ø6 **Unspecified leg**
Including: Pain in lower limb NOS
M79.6Ø9 **Unspecified limb**
Including: Pain in limb NOS

M79.62- **Pain in upper arm**
Including: Pain in axillary region
M79.621 **Right**
M79.622 **Left**
M79.629 **Unspecified**

M79.63- **Pain in forearm**
M79.631 **Right**
M79.632 **Left**
M79.639 **Unspecified**

M79.64- **Pain in hand and fingers**
M79.641 **Right hand**
M79.642 **Left hand**
M79.643 **Unspecified hand**
M79.644 **Right finger(s)**
M79.645 **Left finger(s)**
M79.646 **Unspecified finger(s)**

M79.65- **Pain in thigh**
M79.651 **Right**
M79.652 **Left**
M79.659 **Unspecified**

M79.66- **Pain in lower leg**
M79.661 **Right**
M79.662 **Left**
M79.669 **Unspecified**

M79.67- **Pain in foot and toes**
M79.671 **Right foot**
M79.672 **Left foot**
M79.673 **Unspecified foot**
M79.674 **Right toe(s)**
M79.675 **Left toe(s)**
M79.676 **Unspecified toe(s)**

M79.7 **Fibromyalgia**
Including: Fibromyositis, Fibrositis, Myofibrositis

M79.8- **Other specified soft tissue disorders**
M79.81 **Nontraumatic hematoma**
Including: Nontraumatic hematoma of muscle, Nontraumatic seroma of muscle and soft tissue
M79.89 **Other**
Including: Polyalgia

M79.9 **Soft tissue disorder, unspecified**

M79.A- **Nontraumatic compartment syndrome**
Code First:
if applicable, associated postprocedural complication
Excludes1:
compartment syndrome NOS (T79.A-)
fibromyalgia (M79.7)
nontraumatic ischemic infarction of muscle (M62.2-)
traumatic compartment syndrome (T79.A-)
Indicator(s): CC

M79.A1- **Nontraumatic compartment syndrome of upper extremity**
Including: Shoulder, arm, forearm, wrist, hand, and fingers
M79.A11 **Right**
M79.A12 **Left**
M79.A19 **Unspecified**

M79.A2- **Nontraumatic compartment syndrome of lower extremity**
Including: Hip, buttock, thigh, leg, foot, and toes
M79.A21 **Right**
M79.A22 **Left**
M79.A29 **Unspecified**

M79.A3 **Abdomen**
M79.A9 **Other sites**

OSTEOPATHIES AND CHONDROPATHIES (M8Ø-M94)

DISORDERS OF BONE DENSITY AND STRUCTURE (M8Ø-M85)

M81- OSTEOPOROSIS WITHOUT CURRENT PATHOLOGICAL FRACTURE

Use additional code to identify:
major osseous defect, if applicable (M89.7-)
personal history of (healed) osteoporosis fracture, if applicable (Z87.31Ø)
Excludes1:
osteoporosis with current pathological fracture (M8Ø.-)
Sudeck's atrophy (M89.Ø)
See Guidelines: 1;C.13.a.1 | 1;C.13.d
Indicator(s): RxØ5: 87

M81.Ø **Age-related**
Including: Involutional, Postmenopausal, Senile osteoporosis; Osteoporosis NOS
Indicator(s): Adult

M81.6 **Localized [Lequesne]**
Excludes1:
Sudeck's atrophy (M89.Ø)

M81.8 **Other**
Including: Drug-induced, Idiopathic, Osteoporosis of disuse, Postoophorectomy, Postsurgical malabsorption, Post-traumatic osteoporosis
Use additional code for adverse effect, if applicable, to identify drug (T36-T5Ø with fifth or sixth character 5)

M83- ADULT OSTEOMALACIA

Excludes1:
infantile and juvenile osteomalacia (E55.Ø)
renal osteodystrophy (N25.Ø)
rickets (active) (E55.Ø)
rickets (active) sequelae (E64.3)
vitamin D-resistant osteomalacia (E83.3)
vitamin D-resistant rickets (active) (E83.3)
Indicator(s): RxØ5: 87

M83.Ø **Puerperal**
Indicator(s): Female

M83.1 **Senile**
Indicator(s): Adult

M83.2 **Due to malabsorption**
Including: Postsurgical malabsorption osteomalacia in adults
Indicator(s): Adult

M83.3 **Due to malnutrition**
Indicator(s): Adult

M83.4 **Aluminum bone disease**

M83.5 **Other drug-induced**
Use additional code for adverse effect, if applicable, to identify drug (T36-T5Ø with fifth or sixth character 5)
Indicator(s): Adult

M83.8 **Other**
Indicator(s): Adult

M83.9 **Unspecified**
Indicator(s): Adult

M84- DISORDER OF CONTINUITY OF BONE

Excludes2:
traumatic fracture of bone-see fracture, by site

M84.3- **Stress fracture**
Including: Fatigue, March, Stress fracture NOS, Stress reaction
Use additional external cause code(s) to identify the cause of the stress fracture
Excludes1:
pathological fracture NOS (M84.4.-)
pathological fracture due to osteoporosis (M8Ø.-)
traumatic fracture (S12.-, S22.-, S32.-, S42.-, S52.-, S62.-, S72.-, S82.-, S92.-)
Excludes2:
personal history of (healed) stress (fatigue) fracture (Z87.312)
stress fracture of vertebra (M48.4-)

The appropriate 7th character is to be added to each code from subcategory M84.3:
A - initial encounter for fracture
D - subsequent encounter for fracture with routine healing
G - subsequent encounter for fracture with delayed healing
K - subsequent encounter for fracture with nonunion
P - subsequent encounter for fracture with malunion
S - sequela

Indicator(s): CC (7th K/P)

M84.3Øx_ **Unspecified site**

M84.31- **Shoulder**
M84.311_ **Right**
M84.312_ **Left**
M84.319_ **Unspecified**

M84.32- **Humerus**
M84.321_ **Right**
M84.322_ **Left**
M84.329_ **Unspecified**

M84.33- **Ulna and radius**
M84.331_ **Right**
M84.332_ **Left**
M84.333_ **Right**
M84.334_ **Left**
M84.339_ **Unspecified**

M84.34- **Hand and fingers**
M84.341_ **Right**
M84.342_ **Left**
M84.343_ **Unspecified**
M84.344_ **Right finger(s)**
M84.345_ **Left finger(s)**
M84.346_ **Unspecified finger(s)**

M84.35- **Pelvis and femur**
Including: Stress fracture, hip
M84.35Ø_ **Pelvis**
M84.351_ **Right**
M84.352_ **Left**
M84.353_ **Unspecified**
M84.359_ **Hip, unspecified**

M84.36- **Tibia and fibula**
M84.361_ **Right**
M84.362_ **Left**
M84.363_ **Right**
M84.364_ **Left**
M84.369_ **Unspecified**

M84.37- **Ankle, foot and toes**
M84.371_ Right
M84.372_ Left
M84.373_ Unspecified
M84.374_ Right
M84.375_ Left
M84.376_ Unspecified
M84.377_ Right toe(s)
M84.378_ Left toe(s)
M84.379_ Unspecified toe(s)
M84.38x_ Other site
Excludes2:
stress fracture of vertebra (M48.4-)

M84.4- **Pathological fracture, not elsewhere classified**
Including: Chronic fracture, Pathological fracture NOS
Excludes1:
collapsed vertebra NEC (M48.5)
pathological fracture in neoplastic disease (M84.5-)
pathological fracture in osteoporosis (M8Ø.-)
pathological fracture in other disease (M84.6-)
stress fracture (M84.3-)
traumatic fracture (S12.-, S22.-, S32.-, S42.-, S52.-, S62.-, S72.-, S82.-, S92.-)
Excludes2:
personal history of (healed) pathological fracture (Z87.311)

The appropriate 7th character is to be added to each code from subcategory M84.4:
A - initial encounter for fracture
D - subsequent encounter for fracture with routine healing
G - subsequent encounter for fracture with delayed healing
K - subsequent encounter for fracture with nonunion
P - subsequent encounter for fracture with malunion
S - sequela

See Guidelines: *1;C.13.c*
Indicator(s): *CC (7th A/K/P) | RxØ5: 87 (7th A)*
M84.4Øx_ Unspecified site
M84.9 Disorder of continuity of bone, unspecified

M85- OTHER DISORDERS OF BONE DENSITY AND STRUCTURE
Excludes1:
osteogenesis imperfecta (Q78.Ø)
osteopetrosis (Q78.2)
osteopoikilosis (Q78.8)
polyostotic fibrous dysplasia (Q78.1)

M85.Ø- **Fibrous dysplasia (monostotic)**
Excludes2:
fibrous dysplasia of jaw (M27.8)
M85.ØØ Unspecified site

M85.1- **Skeletal fluorosis**
M85.1Ø Unspecified site

M85.3- **Osteitis condensans**
M85.3Ø Unspecified site

M85.4- **Solitary bone cyst**
Excludes2:
solitary cyst of jaw (M27.4)
M85.4Ø Unspecified site
M85.41- **Shoulder**
M85.411 Right
M85.412 Left
M85.419 Unspecified
M85.42- **Humerus**
M85.421 Right
M85.422 Left
M85.429 Unspecified
M85.43- **Ulna and radius**
M85.431 Right
M85.432 Left
M85.439 Unspecified
M85.44- **Hand**
M85.441 Right
M85.442 Left
M85.449 Unspecified
M85.45- **Pelvis**
M85.451 Right
M85.452 Left
M85.459 Unspecified
M85.46- **Tibia and fibula**
M85.461 Right
M85.462 Left
M85.469 Unspecified
M85.47- **Ankle and foot**
M85.471 Right
M85.472 Left
M85.479 Unspecified
M85.48 Other site

M85.5- **Aneurysmal bone cyst**
Excludes2:
aneurysmal cyst of jaw (M27.4)
M85.5Ø Unspecified site
M85.51- **Shoulder**
M85.511 Right
M85.512 Left
M85.519 Unspecified
M85.52- **Upper arm**
M85.521 Right
M85.522 Left
M85.529 Unspecified
M85.53- **Forearm**
M85.531 Right
M85.532 Left
M85.539 Unspecified
M85.54- **Hand**
M85.541 Right
M85.542 Left
M85.549 Unspecified
M85.55- **Thigh**
M85.551 Right
M85.552 Left
M85.559 Unspecified
M85.56- **Lower leg**
M85.561 Right
M85.562 Left
M85.569 Unspecified

M85.57- **Ankle and foot**
M85.571 Right
M85.572 Left
M85.579 Unspecified
M85.58 Other site
M85.59 Multiple sites

M85.6- **Other cyst of bone**
Excludes1:
cyst of jaw NEC (M27.4)
osteitis fibrosa cystica generalisata [von Recklinghausen's disease of bone] (E21.Ø)
M85.6Ø Unspecified site
M85.61- **Shoulder**
M85.611 Right
M85.612 Left
M85.619 Unspecified
M85.62- **Upper arm**
M85.621 Right
M85.622 Left
M85.629 Unspecified
M85.63- **Forearm**
M85.631 Right
M85.632 Left
M85.639 Unspecified
M85.64- **Hand**
M85.641 Right
M85.642 Left
M85.649 Unspecified
M85.65- **Thigh**
M85.651 Right
M85.652 Left
M85.659 Unspecified
M85.66- **Lower leg**
M85.661 Right
M85.662 Left
M85.669 Unspecified
M85.67- **Ankle and foot**
M85.671 Right
M85.672 Left
M85.679 Unspecified
M85.68 Other site
M85.69 Multiple sites

M85.8- **Other specified disorders of bone density and structure**
Including: Hyperostosis of bones except skull; Osteosclerosis acquired
Excludes1:
diffuse idiopathic skeletal hyperostosis [DISH] (M48.1)
osteosclerosis congenita (Q77.4)
osteosclerosis fragilitas (generalista) (Q78.2)
osteosclerosis myelofibrosis (D75.81)
M85.8Ø Unspecified site
M85.81- **Shoulder**
M85.811 Right
M85.812 Left
M85.819 Unspecified
M85.82- **Upper arm**
M85.821 Right
M85.822 Left
M85.829 Unspecified
M85.83- **Forearm**
M85.831 Right
M85.832 Left
M85.839 Unspecified
M85.84- **Hand**
M85.841 Right
M85.842 Left
M85.849 Unspecified
M85.85- **Thigh**
M85.851 Right
M85.852 Left
M85.859 Unspecified
M85.86- **Lower leg**
M85.861 Right
M85.862 Left
M85.869 Unspecified
M85.87- **Ankle and foot**
M85.871 Right
M85.872 Left
M85.879 Unspecified
M85.88 Other site
M85.89 Multiple sites

M85.9 Disorder of bone density and structure, unspecified

OTHER OSTEOPATHIES (M86-M9Ø)

Excludes1:
postprocedural osteopathies (M96.-)

M86- OSTEOMYELITIS

Use additional code (B95-B97) to identify infectious agent
Use additional code to identify major osseous defect, if applicable (M89.7-)
Excludes1:
osteomyelitis due to:
echinococcus (B67.2)
gonococcus (A54.43)
salmonella (AØ2.24)
Excludes2:
ostemyelitis of:
orbit (HØ5.Ø-)
petrous bone (H7Ø.2-)
vertebra (M46.2-)
Indicator(s): CC | CMS22: 39 | CMS24: 39 | ESRD21: 39 | HHSØ5: 55 | HHSØ7: 55

M86.9 Osteomyelitis, unspecified
Including: Infection of bone NOS, Periostitis without osteomyelitis

M87- OSTEONECROSIS

Includes:
avascular necrosis of bone
Use additional code to identify major osseous defect, if applicable (M89.7-)
Excludes1:
juvenile osteonecrosis (M91-M92)
osteochondropathies (M9Ø-M93)
See Guidelines: 1;C.13.a.1
Indicator(s): CC | CMS22: 39 | CMS24: 39 | RxØ5: 8Ø | ESRD21: 39 | HHSØ5: 55 | HHSØ7: 55

M87.2- **Osteonecrosis due to previous trauma**
Indicator(s): CC

M87.2Ø Unspecified bone

M87.21- **Shoulder**
M87.211 Right
M87.212 Left
M87.219 Unspecified

M87.22- **Humerus**
M87.221 Right
M87.222 Left
M87.229 Unspecified

M87.23- **Radius, ulna and carpus**
M87.231 Right radius
M87.232 Left radius
M87.233 Unspecified radius
M87.234 Right ulna
M87.235 Left ulna
M87.236 Unspecified ulna
M87.237 Right carpus
M87.238 Left carpus
M87.239 Unspecified carpus

M87.24- **Hand and fingers**
M87.241 Right hand
M87.242 Left hand
M87.243 Unspecified hand
M87.244 Right finger(s)
M87.245 Left finger(s)
M87.246 Unspecified finger(s)

M87.25- **Pelvis and femur**
M87.25Ø Pelvis
M87.251 Right femur
M87.252 Left femur
M87.256 Unspecified femur

M87.26- **Tibia and fibula**
M87.261 Right tibia
M87.262 Left tibia
M87.263 Unspecified tibia
M87.264 Right fibula
M87.265 Left fibula
M87.266 Unspecified fibula

M87.27- **Ankle, foot and toes**
M87.271 Right ankle
M87.272 Left ankle
M87.273 Unspecified ankle
M87.274 Right foot
M87.275 Left foot
M87.276 Unspecified foot
M87.277 Right toe(s)
M87.278 Left toe(s)
M87.279 Unspecified toe(s)

M87.28 Other site
M87.29 Multiple sites

M88- OSTEITIS DEFORMANS [PAGET'S DISEASE OF BONE]

Excludes1:
osteitis deformans in neoplastic disease (M9Ø.6)

M88.Ø Skull
M88.1 Vertebrae
M88.8- **Osteitis deformans of other bones**
M88.89 Multiple sites
M88.9 Unspecified bone

M89- OTHER DISORDERS OF BONE

M89.3- **Hypertrophy of bone**
M89.3Ø Unspecified site

M89.31- **Shoulder**
M89.311 Right
M89.312 Left
M89.319 Unspecified

M89.32- **Humerus**
M89.321 Right
M89.322 Left
M89.329 Unspecified

M89.33- **Ulna and radius**
M89.331 Right ulna
M89.332 Left ulna
M89.333 Right radius
M89.334 Left radius
M89.339 Unspecified ulna and radius

M89.34- **Hand**
M89.341 Right
M89.342 Left
M89.349 Unspecified

M89.35- **Femur**
M89.351 Right
M89.352 Left
M89.359 Unspecified

M89.36- **Tibia and fibula**
M89.361 Right tibia
M89.362 Left tibia
M89.363 Right fibula
M89.364 Left fibula
M89.369 Unspecified tibia and fibula

M89.37- **Ankle and foot**
M89.371 **Right**
M89.372 **Left**
M89.379 **Unspecified**
M89.38 **Other site**
M89.39 **Multiple sites**

M89.5- **Osteolysis**
Use additional code to identify major osseous defect, if applicable (M89.7-)
Excludes2:
periprosthetic osteolysis of internal prosthetic joint (T84.Ø5-)
M89.5Ø **Unspecified site**
M89.51- **Shoulder**
M89.511 **Right**
M89.512 **Left**
M89.519 **Unspecified**
M89.52- **Upper arm**
M89.521 **Right**
M89.522 **Left**
M89.529 **Unspecified**
M89.53- **Forearm**
M89.531 **Right**
M89.532 **Left**
M89.539 **Unspecified**
M89.54- **Hand**
M89.541 **Right**
M89.542 **Left**
M89.549 **Unspecified**
M89.55- **Thigh**
M89.551 **Right**
M89.552 **Left**
M89.559 **Unspecified**
M89.56- **Lower leg**
M89.561 **Right**
M89.562 **Left**
M89.569 **Unspecified**
M89.57- **Ankle and foot**
M89.571 **Right**
M89.572 **Left**
M89.579 **Unspecified**
M89.58 **Other site**
M89.59 **Multiple sites**

M89.7- **Major osseous defect**
Code First:
underlying disease, if known, such as:
aseptic necrosis of bone (M87.-)
malignant neoplasm of bone (C4Ø.-)
osteolysis (M89.5)
osteomyelitis (M86.-)
osteonecrosis (M87.-)
osteoporosis (M8Ø.-, M81.-)
periprosthetic osteolysis (T84.Ø5-)
M89.7Ø **Unspecified site**
M89.71- **Shoulder region**
Including: Clavicle or scapula
M89.711 **Right**
M89.712 **Left**
M89.719 **Unspecified**
M89.72- **Humerus**
M89.721 **Right**
M89.722 **Left**
M89.729 **Unspecified**
M89.73- **Forearm**
Including: Radius and ulna
M89.731 **Right**
M89.732 **Left**
M89.739 **Unspecified**
M89.74- **Hand**
Including: Carpus, fingers, metacarpus
M89.741 **Right**
M89.742 **Left**
M89.749 **Unspecified**
M89.75- **Pelvic region and thigh**
Including: Femur and pelvis
M89.751 **Right**
M89.752 **Left**
M89.759 **Unspecified**
M89.76- **Lower leg**
Including: Fibula and tibia
M89.761 **Right**
M89.762 **Left**
M89.769 **Unspecified**
M89.77- **Ankle and foot**
Including: Metatarsus, tarsus, toes
M89.771 **Right**
M89.772 **Left**
M89.779 **Unspecified**
M89.78 **Other site**
M89.79 **Multiple sites**

M89.9 **Disorder of bone, unspecified**

CHONDROPATHIES (M91-M94)

Excludes1:
postprocedural chondropathies (M96.-)

M91- JUVENILE OSTEOCHONDROSIS OF HIP AND PELVIS

Excludes1:
slipped upper femoral epiphysis (nontraumatic) (M93.Ø-)
Indicator(s): HHSØ5: 62 | HHSØ7: 62

M91.Ø **Pelvis**
Including: Acetabulum, iliac crest [Buchanan], ischiopubic synchondrosis [van Neck], symphysis pubis [Pierson]

M91.1- **Juvenile osteochondrosis of head of femur [Legg-Calvé-Perthes]**
M91.1Ø **Unspecified leg**
M91.11 **Right leg**
M91.12 **Left leg**

M91.2- **Coxa plana**
Including: Hip deformity due to previous juvenile osteochondrosis
M91.2Ø **Unspecified hip**
M91.21 **Right hip**
M91.22 **Left hip**

M91.3- **Pseudocoxalgia**
- **M91.3Ø** **Unspecified hip**
- **M91.31** **Right hip**
- **M91.32** **Left hip**

M91.4- **Coxa magna**
- **M91.4Ø** **Unspecified hip**
- **M91.41** **Right hip**
- **M91.42** **Left hip**

M91.8- **Other juvenile osteochondrosis of hip and pelvis**
Including: after reduction of congenital dislocation of hip
- **M91.8Ø** **Unspecified leg**
- **M91.81** **Right leg**
- **M91.82** **Left leg**

M91.9- **Juvenile osteochondrosis of hip and pelvis, unspecified**
- **M91.9Ø** **Unspecified leg**
- **M91.91** **Right leg**
- **M91.92** **Left leg**

M92- OTHER JUVENILE OSTEOCHONDROSIS

M92.Ø- **Juvenile osteochondrosis of humerus**
Including: Capitulum of humerus [Panner], head of humerus [Haas]
- **M92.ØØ** **Unspecified arm**
- **M92.Ø1** **Right arm**
- **M92.Ø2** **Left arm**

M92.1- **Juvenile osteochondrosis of radius and ulna**
Including: Lower ulna [Burns], radial head [Brailsford]
- **M92.1Ø** **Unspecified arm**
- **M92.11** **Right arm**
- **M92.12** **Left arm**

M92.2- **Juvenile osteochondrosis, hand**
- M92.2Ø- **Unspecified juvenile osteochondrosis, hand**
  - **M92.2Ø1** **Right hand**
  - **M92.2Ø2** **Left hand**
  - **M92.2Ø9** **Unspecified hand**
- M92.21- **Osteochondrosis (juvenile) of carpal lunate [Kienböck]**
  - **M92.211** **Right hand**
  - **M92.212** **Left hand**
  - **M92.219** **Unspecified hand**
- M92.22- **Osteochondrosis (juvenile) of metacarpal heads [Mauclaire]**
  - **M92.221** **Right hand**
  - **M92.222** **Left hand**
  - **M92.229** **Unspecified hand**
- M92.29- **Other juvenile osteochondrosis, hand**
  - **M92.291** **Right hand**
  - **M92.292** **Left hand**
  - **M92.299** **Unspecified hand**

M92.3- **Other juvenile osteochondrosis, upper limb**
- **M92.3Ø** **Unspecified**
- **M92.31** **Right**
- **M92.32** **Left**

M92.4- **Juvenile osteochondrosis of patella**
Including: Primary patellar center [Köhler], Secondary patellar centre [Sinding Larsen]
- **M92.4Ø** **Unspecified knee**
- **M92.41** **Right knee**
- **M92.42** **Left knee**

M92.5- **Juvenile osteochondrosis of tibia and fibula**
- M92.5Ø- **Unspecified leg**
  - **M92.5Ø1** **Right leg**
  - **M92.5Ø2** **Left leg**
  - **M92.5Ø3** **Bilateral**
  - **M92.5Ø9** **Unspecified leg**
- M92.51- **Right leg**
  - **M92.511** **Right leg**
  - **M92.512** **Left leg**
  - **M92.513** **Bilateral**
  - **M92.519** **Unspecified leg**
- M92.52- **Left leg**
  Including: Osgood-Schlatter disease
  - **M92.521** **Right leg**
  - **M92.522** **Left leg**
  - **M92.523** **Bilateral**
  - **M92.529** **Unspecified leg**
- M92.59- **Other juvenile osteochondrosis of tibia and fibula**
  - **M92.591** **Right leg**
  - **M92.592** **Left leg**
  - **M92.593** **Bilateral**
  - **M92.599** **Unspecified leg**

M92.6- **Juvenile osteochondrosis of tarsus**
Including: Calcaneum [Sever], os tibiale externum [Haglund], talus [Diaz], tarsal navicular [Köhler]
- **M92.6Ø** **Unspecified ankle**
- **M92.61** **Right ankle**
- **M92.62** **Left ankle**

M92.7- **Juvenile osteochondrosis of metatarsus**
Including: Fifth metatarsus [Iselin], second metatarsus [Freiberg]
- **M92.7Ø** **Unspecified foot**
- **M92.71** **Right foot**
- **M92.72** **Left foot**

M92.8 **Other specified**
Including: Calcaneal apophysitis

M92.9 **Unspecified**
Including: Apophysitis NOS, epiphysitis NOS, osteochondritis NOS, osteochondrosis NOS

M93- OTHER OSTEOCHONDROPATHIES

Excludes2:
osteochondrosis of spine (M42.-)

M93.Ø- **Slipped upper femoral epiphysis (nontraumatic)**
Including: capital (SCFE), upper (SUFE)
Use additional code for associated chondrolysis (M94.3)

Ch5

5. The Tabular List

M93.ØØ- **Unspecified**
- **M93.ØØ1** **Right hip** — *Indicator(s): HHSØ5: 62 | HHSØ7: 62*
- **M93.ØØ2** **Left hip** — *Indicator(s): HHSØ5: 62 | HHSØ7: 62*
- **M93.ØØ3** **Unspecified hip** — *Indicator(s): HHSØ5: 62 | HHSØ7: 62*
- N **M93.ØØ4** **Bilateral hips**

M93.Ø1- **Acute, stable**
- R **M93.Ø11** **Right hip** — *Indicator(s): HHSØ5: 62 | HHSØ7: 62*
- R **M93.Ø12** **Left hip** — *Indicator(s): HHSØ5: 62 | HHSØ7: 62*
- R **M93.Ø13** **Unspecified hip** — *Indicator(s): HHSØ5: 62 | HHSØ7: 62*
- N **M93.Ø14** **Bilateral hips**

M93.Ø2- **Chronic, stable**
- R **M93.Ø21** **Right hip** — *Indicator(s): HHSØ5: 62 | HHSØ7: 62*
- R **M93.Ø22** **Left hip** — *Indicator(s): HHSØ5: 62 | HHSØ7: 62*
- R **M93.Ø23** **Unspecified hip** — *Indicator(s): HHSØ5: 62 | HHSØ7: 62*
- N **M93.Ø24** **Bilateral hips**

M93.Ø3- **Acute on chronic, stable**
- R **M93.Ø31** **Right hip** — *Indicator(s): HHSØ5: 62 | HHSØ7: 62*
- R **M93.Ø32** **Left hip** — *Indicator(s): HHSØ5: 62 | HHSØ7: 62*
- R **M93.Ø33** **Unspecified hip** — *Indicator(s): HHSØ5: 62 | HHSØ7: 62*
- N **M93.Ø34** **Bilateral hips**

M93.Ø4- **Acute, unstable**
- N **M93.Ø41** **Right hip**
- N **M93.Ø42** **Left hip**
- N **M93.Ø43** **Unspecified hip**
- N **M93.Ø44** **Bilateral hips**

M93.Ø5- **Acute on chronic, unstable**
- N **M93.Ø51** **Right hip**
- N **M93.Ø52** **Left hip**
- N **M93.Ø53** **Unspecified hip**
- N **M93.Ø54** **Bilateral hips**

M93.Ø6- **Acute, uspecified stability**
- N **M93.Ø61** **Right hip**
- N **M93.Ø62** **Left hip**
- N **M93.Ø63** **Unspecified hip**
- N **M93.Ø64** **Bilateral hips**

M93.Ø7- **Acute on chronic, unspecified stability**
- N **M93.Ø71** **Right hip**
- N **M93.Ø72** **Left hip**
- N **M93.Ø73** **Unspecified hip**
- N **M93.Ø74** **Bilateral hips**

M93.1 **Kienböck's disease of adults**
Including: Adult osteochondrosis of carpal lunates
Indicator(s): Adult

M93.2- **Osteochondritis dissecans**
- **M93.2Ø** **Unspecified site**
- M93.21- **Shoulder**
  - **M93.211** **Right**
  - **M93.212** **Left**
  - **M93.219** **Unspecified**
- M93.22- **Elbow**
  - **M93.221** **Right**
  - **M93.222** **Left**
  - **M93.229** **Unspecified**
- M93.23- **Wrist**
  - **M93.231** **Right**
  - **M93.232** **Left**
  - **M93.239** **Unspecified**
- M93.24- **Joints of hand**
  - **M93.241** **Right**
  - **M93.242** **Left**
  - **M93.249** **Unspecified**
- M93.25- **Hip**
  - **M93.251** **Right**
  - **M93.252** **Left**
  - **M93.259** **Unspecified**
- M93.26- **Knee**
  - **M93.261** **Right**
  - **M93.262** **Left**
  - **M93.269** **Unspecified**
- M93.27- **Ankle and joints of foot**
  - **M93.271** **Right**
  - **M93.272** **Left**
  - **M93.279** **Unspecified**
- **M93.28** **Other site**
- **M93.29** **Multiple sites**

M93.8- **Other specified osteochondropathies**
- **M93.8Ø** **Unspecified site**
- M93.81- **Shoulder**
  - **M93.811** **Right**
  - **M93.812** **Left**
  - **M93.819** **Unspecified**
- M93.82- **Upper arm**
  - **M93.821** **Right**
  - **M93.822** **Left**
  - **M93.829** **Unspecified**
- M93.83- **Forearm**
  - **M93.831** **Right**
  - **M93.832** **Left**
  - **M93.839** **Unspecified**
- M93.84- **Hand**
  - **M93.841** **Right**
  - **M93.842** **Left**
  - **M93.849** **Unspecified**

Ch5
5. The Tabular List

M93.85- **Thigh**
M93.851 **Right**
M93.852 **Left**
M93.859 **Unspecified**
M93.86- **Lower leg**
M93.861 **Right**
M93.862 **Left**
M93.869 **Unspecified**
M93.87- **Ankle and foot**
M93.871 **Right**
M93.872 **Left**
M93.879 **Unspecified**
M93.88 **Other specified**
M93.89 **Multiple sites**

M93.9- **Osteochondropathy, unspecified**
Including: Apophysitis NOS, Epiphysitis NOS, Osteochondritis NOS, Osteochondrosis NOS
M93.9Ø **Unspecified site**
M93.91- **Shoulder**
M93.911 **Right**
M93.912 **Left**
M93.919 **Unspecified**
M93.92- **Upper arm**
M93.921 **Right**
M93.922 **Left**
M93.929 **Unspecified**
M93.93- **Forearm**
M93.931 **Right**
M93.932 **Left**
M93.939 **Unspecified**
M93.94- **Hand**
M93.941 **Right**
M93.942 **Left**
M93.949 **Unspecified**
M93.95- **Thigh**
M93.951 **Right**
M93.952 **Left**
M93.959 **Unspecified**
M93.96- **Lower leg**
M93.961 **Right**
M93.962 **Left**
M93.969 **Unspecified**
M93.97- **Ankle and foot**
M93.971 **Right**
M93.972 **Left**
M93.979 **Unspecified**
M93.98 **Other**
M93.99 **Multiple sites**

M94- OTHER DISORDERS OF CARTILAGE

M94.Ø **Chondrocostal junction syndrome [Tietze]**
Including: Costochondritis

M94.1 **Relapsing polychondritis**

M94.2- **Chondromalacia**
Excludes1:
chondromalacia patellae (M22.4)
M94.2Ø **Unspecified site**
M94.21- **Shoulder**
M94.211 **Right**
M94.212 **Left**
M94.219 **Unspecified**
M94.22- **Elbow**
M94.221 **Right**
M94.222 **Left**
M94.229 **Unspecified**
M94.23- **Wrist**
M94.231 **Right**
M94.232 **Left**
M94.239 **Unspecified**
M94.24- **Joints of hand**
M94.241 **Right**
M94.242 **Left**
M94.249 **Unspecified**
M94.25- **Hip**
M94.251 **Right**
M94.252 **Left**
M94.259 **Unspecified**
M94.26- **Knee**
M94.261 **Right**
M94.262 **Left**
M94.269 **Unspecified**
M94.27- **Ankle and joints of foot**
M94.271 **Right**
M94.272 **Left**
M94.279 **Unspecified**
M94.28 **Other site**
M94.29 **Multiple sites**

M94.3- **Chondrolysis**
Code First:
any associated slipped upper femoral epiphysis (nontraumatic) (M93.Ø-)
M94.35- **Chondrolysis, hip**
M94.351 **Right**
M94.352 **Left**
M94.359 **Unspecified**

M94.8- **Other specified disorders of cartilage**
M94.8xØ **Multiple sites**
M94.8x1 **Shoulder**
M94.8x2 **Upper arm**
M94.8x3 **Forearm**
M94.8x4 **Hand**
M94.8x5 **Thigh**
M94.8x6 **Lower leg**
M94.8x7 **Ankle and foot**
M94.8x8 **Other site**
M94.8x9 **Unspecified sites**

M94.9 **Disorder of cartilage, unspecified**

M95 OTHER DISORDERS OF THE MUSCULOSKELETAL SYSTEM AND CONNECTIVE TISSUE (M95) (M95-M95)

M95- OTHER ACQUIRED DEFORMITIES OF MUSCULOSKELETAL SYSTEM AND CONNECTIVE TISSUE

Excludes2:
acquired absence of limbs and organs (Z89-Z9Ø)
acquired deformities of limbs (M2Ø-M21)
congenital malformations and deformations of the musculoskeletal system (Q65-Q79)
deforming dorsopathies (M4Ø-M43)
dentofacial anomalies [including malocclusion] (M26.-)
postprocedural musculoskeletal disorders (M96.-)

M95.Ø **Nose**
Excludes2:
deviated nasal septum (J34.2)

M95.1- **Cauliflower ear**
Excludes2:
other acquired deformities of ear (H61.1)

M95.1Ø **Unspecified**
M95.11 **Right**
M95.12 **Left**

M95.2 **Head**
M95.3 **Neck**
M95.4 **Chest and rib**
M95.5 **Pelvis**
Excludes1:
maternal care for known or suspected disproportion (O33.-)

M95.8 **Other specified**
M95.9 **Unspecified**

M96 INTRAOPERATIVE AND POSTPROCEDURAL COMPLICATIONS AND DISORDERS OF MUSCULOSKELETAL SYSTEM, NOT ELSEWHERE CLASSIFIED (M96) (M96-M96)

M96- INTRAOPERATIVE AND POSTPROCEDURAL COMPLICATIONS AND DISORDERS OF MUSCULOSKELETAL SYSTEM, NOT ELSEWHERE CLASSIFIED

Excludes2:
arthropathy following intestinal bypass (MØ2.Ø-)
complications of internal orthopedic prosthetic devices, implants and grafts (T84.-)
disorders associated with osteoporosis (M8Ø)
periprosthetic fracture around internal prosthetic joint (M97.-)
presence of functional implants and other devices (Z96-Z97)

M96.Ø **Pseudarthrosis after fusion or arthrodesis**
Indicator(s): *CC*

M96.1 **Postlaminectomy syndrome, NEC**
M96.2 **Postradiation kyphosis**
M96.3 **Postlaminectomy kyphosis**
M96.4 **Postsurgical lordosis**
M96.5 **Postradiation scoliosis**

M99 BIOMECHANICAL LESIONS, NOT ELSEWHERE CLASSIFIED (M99) (M99-M99)

M99- BIOMECHANICAL LESIONS, NOT ELSEWHERE CLASSIFIED

Notes:
This category should not be used if the condition can be classified elsewhere.

M99.Ø- **Segmental and somatic dysfunction**

M99.ØØ **Head region**
M99.Ø1 **Cervical region**
M99.Ø2 **Thoracic region**
M99.Ø3 **Lumbar region**
M99.Ø4 **Sacral region**
M99.Ø5 **Pelvic region**
M99.Ø6 **Lower extremity**
M99.Ø7 **Upper extremity**
M99.Ø8 **Rib cage region**
M99.Ø9 **Abdomen and other regions**

M99.1- **Subluxation complex (vertebral)**

M99.1Ø **Head region**
Indicator(s): *CC | HAC: Ø5*
M99.11 **Cervical region**
Indicator(s): *CC | HAC: Ø5*
M99.12 **Thoracic region**
M99.13 **Lumbar region**
M99.14 **Sacral region**
M99.15 **Pelvic region**
M99.16 **Lower extremity**
M99.17 **Upper extremity**
M99.18 **Rib cage region**
Indicator(s): *CC | HAC: Ø5*
M99.19 **Abdomen and other regions**

M99.2- **Subluxation stenosis of neural canal**

M99.2Ø **Head region**
M99.21 **Cervical region**
M99.22 **Thoracic region**
M99.23 **Lumbar region**
M99.24 **Sacral region**
M99.25 **Pelvic region**
M99.26 **Lower extremity**
M99.27 **Upper extremity**
M99.28 **Rib cage region**
M99.29 **Abdomen and other regions**

M99.3- **Osseous stenosis of neural canal**

M99.3Ø **Head region**
M99.31 **Cervical region**
M99.32 **Thoracic region**
M99.33 **Lumbar region**
M99.34 **Sacral region**
M99.35 **Pelvic region**
M99.36 **Lower extremity**
M99.37 **Upper extremity**
M99.38 **Rib cage region**
M99.39 **Abdomen and other regions**

M99.4- **Connective tissue stenosis of neural canal**
- **M99.4Ø** **Head region**
- **M99.41** **Cervical region**
- **M99.42** **Thoracic region**
- **M99.43** **Lumbar region**
- **M99.44** **Sacral region**
- **M99.45** **Pelvic region**
- **M99.46** **Lower extremity**
- **M99.47** **Upper extremity**
- **M99.48** **Rib cage region**
- **M99.49** **Abdomen and other regions**

M99.5- **Intervertebral disc stenosis of neural canal**
- **M99.5Ø** **Head region**
- **M99.51** **Cervical region**
- **M99.52** **Thoracic region**
- **M99.53** **Lumbar region**
- **M99.54** **Sacral region**
- **M99.55** **Pelvic region**
- **M99.56** **Lower extremity**
- **M99.57** **Upper extremity**
- **M99.58** **Rib cage region**
- **M99.59** **Abdomen and other regions**

M99.6- **Osseous and subluxation stenosis of intervertebral foramina**
- **M99.6Ø** **Head region**
- **M99.61** **Cervical region**
- **M99.62** **Thoracic region**
- **M99.63** **Lumbar region**
- **M99.64** **Sacral region**
- **M99.65** **Pelvic region**
- **M99.66** **Lower extremity**
- **M99.67** **Upper extremity**
- **M99.68** **Rib cage region**
- **M99.69** **Abdomen and other regions**

M99.7- **Connective tissue and disc stenosis of intervertebral foramina**
- **M99.7Ø** **Head region**
- **M99.71** **Cervical region**
- **M99.72** **Thoracic region**
- **M99.73** **Lumbar region**
- **M99.74** **Sacral region**
- **M99.75** **Pelvic region**
- **M99.76** **Lower extremity**
- **M99.77** **Upper extremity**
- **M99.78** **Rib cage region**
- **M99.79** **Abdomen and other regions**

M99.8- **Other biomechanical lesions**
- **M99.8Ø** **Head region**
- **M99.81** **Cervical region**
- **M99.82** **Thoracic region**
- **M99.83** **Lumbar region**
- **M99.84** **Sacral region**
- **M99.85** **Pelvic region**
- **M99.86** **Lower extremity**
- **M99.87** **Upper extremity**
- **M99.88** **Rib cage region**
- **M99.89** **Abdomen and other regions**

M99.9 **Biomechanical lesion, unspecified**

See Appendix A — Coding Reference Tables for lists of the ICD-10-CM Tabular indicators, HAC categories, and HCC codes.

14. Diseases of the genitourinary system (NØØ-N99)

Excludes2:
certain conditions originating in the perinatal period (PØ4-P96)
certain infectious and parasitic diseases (AØØ-B99)
complications of pregnancy, childbirth and the puerperium (OØØ-O9A)
congenital malformations, deformations and chromosomal abnormalities (QØØ-Q99)
endocrine, nutritional and metabolic diseases (EØØ-E88)
injury, poisoning and certain other consequences of external causes (SØØ-T88)
neoplasms (CØØ-D49)
symptoms, signs and abnormal clinical and laboratory findings, not elsewhere classified (RØØ-R94)
See Guidelines: *1;C.2Ø.a.1*

OTHER DISEASES OF THE URINARY SYSTEM (N3Ø-N39)

Excludes2:
urinary infection (complicating):
abortion or ectopic or molar pregnancy (OØØ-OØ7, OØ8.8)
pregnancy, childbirth and the puerperium (O23.-, O75.3, O86.2-)

N3Ø- CYSTITIS
Use additional code to identify infectious agent (B95-B97)
Excludes1:
prostatocystitis (N41.3)

N3Ø.Ø- **Acute cystitis**
Excludes1:
irradiation cystitis (N3Ø.4-)
trigonitis (N3Ø.3-)
Indicator(s): *CC | HAC: Ø6*

N3Ø.ØØ Without hematuria
N3Ø.Ø1 With hematuria

N3Ø.1- **Interstitial cystitis (chronic)**

N3Ø.1Ø Without hematuria
N3Ø.11 With hematuria

N3Ø.2- **Other chronic cystitis**

N3Ø.2Ø Without hematuria
N3Ø.21 With hematuria

N3Ø.3- **Trigonitis**
Including: Urethrotrigonitis

N3Ø.3Ø Without hematuria
N3Ø.31 With hematuria

N3Ø.4- **Irradiation cystitis**
Indicator(s): *CC*

N3Ø.4Ø Without hematuria
N3Ø.41 With hematuria

N3Ø.8- **Other cystitis**
Including: Abscess of bladder

N3Ø.8Ø Without hematuria
N3Ø.81 With hematuria

N3Ø.9- **Cystitis, unspecified**

N3Ø.9Ø Without hematuria
N3Ø.91 With hematuria

N39- OTHER DISORDERS OF URINARY SYSTEM
Excludes2:
hematuria NOS (R31.-)
recurrent or persistent hematuria (NØ2.-)
recurrent or persistent hematuria with specified morphological lesion (NØ2.-)
proteinuria NOS (R8Ø.-)

N39.Ø Urinary tract infection, site not specified
Use additional code (B95-B97), to identify infectious agent.
Excludes1:
candidiasis of urinary tract (B37.4-)
neonatal urinary tract infection (P39.3)
pyuria (R82.81)
urinary tract infection of specified site, such as:
cystitis (N3Ø.-)
urethritis (N34.-)
Indicator(s): *CC | HAC: Ø6*

DISEASES OF MALE GENITAL ORGANS (N4Ø-N53)

N4Ø- BENIGN PROSTATIC HYPERPLASIA
Includes:
adenofibromatous hypertrophy of prostate
benign hypertrophy of the prostate
benign prostatic hypertrophy
BPH
enlarged prostate
nodular prostate
polyp of prostate
Excludes1:
benign neoplasms of prostate (adenoma, benign) (fibroadenoma) (fibroma) (myoma) (D29.1)
Excludes2:
malignant neoplasm of prostate (C61)

N4Ø.Ø Without lower urinary tract symptoms
Including: Enlarged prostate without LUTS, Enlarged prostate NOS

N4Ø.1 With lower urinary tract symptoms
Including: Enlarged prostate with LUTS
Use additional code for associated symptoms, when specified:
incomplete bladder emptying (R39.14)
nocturia (R35.1)
straining on urination (R39.16)
urinary frequency (R35.Ø)
urinary hesitancy (R39.11)
urinary incontinence (N39.4-)
urinary obstruction (N13.8)
urinary retention (R33.8)
urinary urgency (R39.15)
weak urinary stream (R39.12)

N4Ø.2 Nodular prostate without lower urinary tract symptoms
Including: Nodular prostate without LUTS

N4Ø.3 Nodular prostate with lower urinary tract symptoms
Use additional code for associated symptoms, when specified:
incomplete bladder emptying (R39.14)
nocturia (R35.1)
straining on urination (R39.16)
urinary frequency (R35.Ø)
urinary hesitancy (R39.11)
urinary incontinence (N39.4-)
urinary obstruction (N13.8)
urinary retention (R33.8)
urinary urgency (R39.15)
weak urinary stream (R39.12)

DISORDERS OF BREAST (N6Ø-N65)

Excludes1:
disorders of breast associated with childbirth (O91-O92)

N63- UNSPECIFIED LUMP

Including: Nodule(s) NOS

N63.Ø **Unspecified breast**

N63.1- **Right breast**

N63.1Ø **Unspecified quadrant**
N63.11 **Upper outer quadrant**
N63.12 **Upper inner quadrant**
N63.13 **Lower outer quadrant**
N63.14 **Lower inner quadrant**
N63.15 **Overlapping quadrants**

N63.2- **Left breast**

N63.2Ø **Unspecified quadrant**
N63.21 **Upper outer quadrant**
N63.22 **Upper inner quadrant**
N63.23 **Lower outer quadrant**
N63.24 **Lower inner quadrant**
N63.25 **Overlapping quadrants**

N63.3- **Axillary tail**

N63.31 **Right breast**
N63.32 **Left breast**

N63.4- **Subareolar**

N63.41 **Right breast**
N63.42 **Left breast**

NONINFLAMMATORY DISORDERS OF FEMALE GENITAL TRACT (N8Ø-N98)

N94- PAIN AND OTHER CONDITIONS ASSOCIATED WITH FEMALE GENITAL ORGANS AND MENSTRUAL CYCLE

N94.3 **Premenstrual tension syndrome**

Indicator(s): Female

N95- MENOPAUSAL AND OTHER PERIMENOPAUSAL DISORDERS

Including: Menopausal and other perimenopausal disorders due to naturally occurring (age-related) menopause and perimenopause

Excludes1:
excessive bleeding in the premenopausal period (N92.4)
menopausal and perimenopausal disorders due to artificial or premature menopause (E89.4-, E28.31-)
premature menopause (E28.31-)

Excludes2:
postmenopausal osteoporosis (M81.Ø-)
postmenopausal osteoporosis with current pathological fracture (M8Ø.Ø-)
postmenopausal urethritis (N34.2)

N95.1 **Menopausal and female climacteric states**

Including: Symptoms such as flushing, sleeplessness, headache, lack of concentration, associated with natural (age-related) menopause

Use additional code for associated symptoms

Excludes1:
asymptomatic menopausal state (Z78.Ø)
symptoms associated with artificial menopause (E89.41)
symptoms associated with premature menopause (E28.31Ø)

Indicator(s): Female

15. Pregnancy, childbirth and the puerperium (OØØ-O9A)

Notes:

CODES FROM THIS CHAPTER ARE FOR USE ONLY ON MATERNAL RECORDS, NEVER ON NEWBORN RECORDS

Codes from this chapter are for use for conditions related to or aggravated by the pregnancy, childbirth, or by the puerperium (maternal causes or obstetric causes)

Trimesters are counted from the first day of the last menstrual period. They are defined as follows:

1st trimester- less than 14 weeks Ø days

2nd trimester- 14 weeks Ø days to less than 28 weeks Ø days

3rd trimester- 28 weeks Ø days until delivery

Use additional code from category Z3A, Weeks of gestation, to identify the specific week of the pregnancy, if known.

Excludes1:

supervision of normal pregnancy (Z34.-)

Excludes2:

mental and behavioral disorders associated with the puerperium (F53.-)

obstetrical tetanus (A34)

postpartum necrosis of pituitary gland (E23.Ø)

puerperal osteomalacia (M83.Ø)

See Guidelines: 1;C.15.o | 1;C.15.a.1-5 | 1;C.15.b-c | 1;C.15.j-k | 1;C.15.o.1-4 | 1;C.15.q.3 | 1;C.2Ø.a.1

EDEMA, PROTEINURIA AND HYPERTENSIVE DISORDERS IN PREGNANCY, CHILDBIRTH AND THE PUERPERIUM (O1Ø-O16)

O1Ø- PRE-EXISTING HYPERTENSION COMPLICATING PREGNANCY, CHILDBIRTH AND THE PUERPERIUM

Includes:

pre-existing hypertension with pre-existing proteinuria complicating pregnancy, childbirth and the puerperium

Excludes2:

pre-existing hypertension with superimposed pre-eclampsia complicating pregnancy, childbirth and the puerperium (O11.-)

See Guidelines: 1;C.15.d

O1Ø.Ø- **Pre-existing essential hypertension complicating pregnancy, childbirth and the puerperium**

Including: Any condition in I1Ø specified as a reason for obstetric care during pregnancy, childbirth or the puerperium

O1Ø.Ø1- **Complicating pregnancy**
Indicator(s): HHSØ7: 211

O1Ø.Ø11 **First trimester**
Indicator(s): Female | CC

O1Ø.Ø12 **Second trimester**
Indicator(s): Female | CC

O1Ø.Ø13 **Third trimester**
Indicator(s): Female | CC

O1Ø.Ø19 **Unspecified trimester**
Indicator(s): Female

O1Ø.Ø3 **Complicating the puerperium**
Indicator(s): Female | HHSØ5: 2Ø8 | HHSØ7: 2Ø8

O12- GESTATIONAL [PREGNANCY-INDUCED] EDEMA AND PROTEINURIA WITHOUT HYPERTENSION

O12.Ø- **Gestational edema**

O12.ØØ **Unspecified trimester**
Indicator(s): Female | HHSØ7: 212

O12.Ø1 **First trimester**
Indicator(s): Female | HHSØ7: 212

O12.Ø2 **Second trimester**
Indicator(s): Female | HHSØ7: 212

O12.Ø3 **Third trimester**
Indicator(s): Female | HHSØ7: 212

O12.Ø4 **Complicating childbirth**
Indicator(s): Female | HHSØ5: 2Ø9 | HHSØ7: 2Ø9

O12.Ø5 **Complicating the puerperium**
Indicator(s): Female | HHSØ5: 2Ø9 | HHSØ7: 2Ø9

O12.1- **Gestational proteinuria**

O12.1Ø **Unspecified trimester**
Indicator(s): Female | HHSØ7: 211

O12.11 **First trimester**
Indicator(s): Female | CC | HHSØ7: 211

O12.12 **Second trimester**
Indicator(s): Female | CC | HHSØ7: 211

O12.13 **Third trimester**
Indicator(s): Female | CC | HHSØ7: 211

O12.14 **Complicating childbirth**
Indicator(s): Female | HHSØ5: 2Ø9 | HHSØ7: 2Ø9

O12.15 **Complicating the puerperium**
Indicator(s): Female | HHSØ5: 2Ø9 | HHSØ7: 2Ø9

O12.2- **Gestational edema with proteinuria**

O12.2Ø **Unspecified trimester**
Indicator(s): Female | HHSØ7: 211

O12.21 **First trimester**
Indicator(s): Female | CC | HHSØ7: 211

O12.22 **Second trimester**
Indicator(s): Female | CC | HHSØ7: 211

O12.23 **Third trimester**
Indicator(s): Female | CC | HHSØ7: 211

O12.24 **Complicating childbirth**
Indicator(s): Female | HHSØ5: 2Ø9 | HHSØ7: 2Ø9

O12.25 **Complicating the puerperium**
Indicator(s): Female | HHSØ5: 2Ø9 | HHSØ7: 2Ø9

O13- GESTATIONAL [PREGNANCY-INDUCED] HYPERTENSION WITHOUT SIGNIFICANT PROTEINURIA

Includes:

gestational hypertension NOS

transient hypertension of pregnancy

See Guidelines: 1;C.9.a.7

O13.1 **First trimester**
Indicator(s): Female | HHSØ7: 211

O13.2 **Second trimester**
Indicator(s): Female | HHSØ7: 211

O13.3 **Third trimester**
Indicator(s): Female | HHSØ7: 211

O13.5 **Complicating the puerperium**
Indicator(s): Female | HHSØ5: 2Ø8 | HHSØ7: 2Ø8

O13.9 **Unspecified trimester**
Indicator(s): Female | HHSØ7: 211

OTHER MATERNAL DISORDERS PREDOMINANTLY RELATED TO PREGNANCY (O2Ø-O29)

Excludes2:
maternal care related to the fetus and amniotic cavity and possible delivery problems (O3Ø-O48)
maternal diseases classifiable elsewhere but complicating pregnancy, labor and delivery, and the puerperium (O98-O99)

O21- EXCESSIVE VOMITING IN PREGNANCY
Indicator(s): HHSØ7: 212

O21.2 **Late**
Including: Excessive vomiting starting after 2Ø completed weeks of gestation
Indicator(s): Female

O21.8 **Other**
Including: Vomiting due to diseases classified elsewhere, complicating pregnancy
Use additional code, to identify cause.
Indicator(s): Female

O21.9 **Unspecified**
Indicator(s): Female

O23- INFECTIONS OF GENITOURINARY TRACT IN PREGNANCY
Use additional code to identify organism (B95.-, B96.-)
Excludes2:
gonococcal infections complicating pregnancy, childbirth and the puerperium (O98.2)
infections with a predominantly sexual mode of transmission NOS complicating pregnancy, childbirth and the puerperium (O98.3)
syphilis complicating pregnancy, childbirth and the puerperium (O98.1)
tuberculosis of genitourinary system complicating pregnancy, childbirth and the puerperium (O98.Ø)
venereal disease NOS complicating pregnancy, childbirth and the puerperium (O98.3)
Indicator(s): HHSØ7: 212

O23.4- **Unspecified infection of urinary tract in pregnancy**

O23.4Ø **Unspecified trimester**
Indicator(s): Female

O23.41 **First trimester**
Indicator(s): Female | CC

O23.42 **Second trimester**
Indicator(s): Female | CC

O23.43 **Third trimester**
Indicator(s): Female | CC

O24- DIABETES MELLITUS IN PREGNANCY, CHILDBIRTH, AND THE PUERPERIUM
See Guidelines: 1;C.15.g | 1;C.15.g-i | 1;C.15.h-i

O24.Ø- **Pre-existing type 1 diabetes mellitus, in pregnancy, childbirth and the puerperium**
Including: Juvenile onset diabetes mellitus; Ketosis-prone diabetes mellitus
Use additional code from category E1Ø to further identify any manifestations

O24.Ø1- **In pregnancy**
Indicator(s): CC | HHSØ7: 211

O24.Ø11 **First trimester**
Indicator(s): Female

O24.Ø12 **Second trimester**
Indicator(s): Female

O24.Ø13 **Third trimester**
Indicator(s): Female

O24.Ø19 **Unspecified trimester**
Indicator(s): Female

O24.Ø2 **In childbirth**
Indicator(s): Female | MCC | HHSØ5: 2Ø8 | HHSØ7: 2Ø8

O24.Ø3 **In the puerperium**
Indicator(s): Female | CC | HHSØ5: 2Ø8 | HHSØ7: 2Ø8

O24.1- **Pre-existing type 2 diabetes mellitus**
Including: Insulin-resistant diabetes mellitus
Use additional code (for):
from category E11 to further identify any manifestations
long-term (current) use of insulin (Z79.4)

O24.11- **Pre-existing type 2 diabetes mellitus, in pregnancy**
Indicator(s): CC | HHSØ7: 211

O24.111 **First trimester**
Indicator(s): Female

O24.112 **Second trimester**
Indicator(s): Female

O24.113 **Third trimester**
Indicator(s): Female

O24.119 **Unspecified trimester**
Indicator(s): Female

O24.12 **In childbirth**
Indicator(s): Female | MCC | HHSØ5: 2Ø8 | HHSØ7: 2Ø8

O24.13 **In the puerperium**
Indicator(s): Female | CC | HHSØ5: 2Ø8 | HHSØ7: 2Ø8

O24.3- **Unspecified pre-existing diabetes mellitus in pregnancy, childbirth and the puerperium**
Use additional code (for):
from category E11 to further identify any manifestation
long-term (current) use of insulin (Z79.4)

O24.31- **In pregnancy**
Indicator(s): CC | HHSØ7: 211

O24.311 **First trimester**
Indicator(s): Female

O24.312 **Second trimester**
Indicator(s): Female

O24.313 **Third trimester**
Indicator(s): Female

O24.319 **Unspecified trimester**
Indicator(s): Female

O24.32 **In childbirth**
Indicator(s): Female | MCC | HHSØ5: 2Ø8 | HHSØ7: 2Ø8

O24.33 **In the puerperium**
Indicator(s): Female | CC | HHSØ5: 2Ø8 | HHSØ7: 2Ø8

O24.4- **Gestational diabetes mellitus**
Including: Diabetes mellitus arising in pregnancy, Gestational diabetes mellitus NOS
See Guidelines: 1;C.15.h-i | 1;C.15.i

O24.41- **In pregnancy**
Indicator(s): HHSØ7: 212

O24.41Ø **Diet controlled**
Indicator(s): Female

O24.414 **Insulin controlled**
Indicator(s): Female

O24.415 **Controlled by oral hypoglycemic drugs**
Including: Antidiabetic drugs
Indicator(s): Female

O24.419 **Unspecified control**
Indicator(s): Female

O24.42- **In childbirth**
Indicator(s): HHSØ5: 2Ø9 | HHSØ7: 2Ø9

O24.42Ø **Diet controlled**
Indicator(s): Female

O24.424 **Insulin controlled**
Indicator(s): Female

O24.425 **Controlled by oral hypoglycemic drugs**
Including: Antidiabetic drugs
Indicator(s): Female

O24.429 **Unspecified control**
Indicator(s): Female

O24.43- **In the puerperium**
Indicator(s): HHSØ5: 2Ø9 | HHSØ7: 2Ø9

O24.43Ø **Diet controlled**
Indicator(s): Female

O24.434 **Insulin controlled**
Indicator(s): Female

O24.435 **Controlled by oral hypoglycemic drugs**
Including: Antidiabetic drugs
Indicator(s): Female

O24.439 **Unspecified control**
Indicator(s): Female

O24.8- **Other pre-existing diabetes mellitus in pregnancy, childbirth, and the puerperium**
Use additional code (for):
from categories EØ8, EØ9 and E13 to further identify any manifestation
long-term (current) use of insulin (Z79.4)

O24.81- **In pregnancy**
Indicator(s): CC | HHSØ7: 211

O24.811 **First trimester**
Indicator(s): Female

O24.812 **Second trimester**
Indicator(s): Female

O24.813 **Third trimester**
Indicator(s): Female

O24.819 **Unspecified trimester**
Indicator(s): Female

O24.82 **In childbirth**
Indicator(s): Female | MCC | HHSØ5: 2Ø8 | HHSØ7: 2Ø8

O24.83 **In the puerperium**
Indicator(s): Female | CC | HHSØ5: 2Ø8 | HHSØ7: 2Ø8

O24.9- **Unspecified diabetes mellitus in pregnancy, childbirth and the puerperium**
Use additional code *for long-term (current) use of insulin (Z79.4)*

O24.91- **In pregnancy**
Indicator(s): CC | HHSØ7: 211

O24.911 **First trimester**
Indicator(s): Female

O24.912 **Second trimester**
Indicator(s): Female

O24.913 **Third trimester**
Indicator(s): Female

O24.919 **Unspecified trimester**
Indicator(s): Female

O24.92 **In childbirth**
Indicator(s): Female | HHSØ5: 2Ø8 | HHSØ7: 2Ø8

O24.93 **In the puerperium**
Indicator(s): Female | CC | HHSØ5: 2Ø8 | HHSØ7: 2Ø8

O26- MATERNAL CARE FOR OTHER CONDITIONS PREDOMINANTLY RELATED TO PREGNANCY

O26.5- **Maternal hypotension syndrome**
Including: Supine hypotensive syndrome
Indicator(s): HHSØ7: 211

O26.5Ø **Unspecified trimester**
Indicator(s): Female

O26.51 **First trimester**
Indicator(s): Female

O26.52 **Second trimester**
Indicator(s): Female

O26.53 **Third trimester**
Indicator(s): Female

O26.7- **Subluxation of symphysis (pubis) in pregnancy, childbirth and the puerperium**
Excludes1:
traumatic separation of symphysis (pubis) during childbirth (O71.6)

O26.71- **In pregnancy**
Indicator(s): HHSØ7: 212

O26.711 **First trimester**
Indicator(s): Female

O26.712 **Second trimester**
Indicator(s): Female

O26.713 **Third trimester**
Indicator(s): Female

O26.719 **Unspecified trimester**
Indicator(s): Female

O26.72 **In childbirth**
Indicator(s): Female | HHSØ5: 2Ø9 | HHSØ7: 2Ø9

O26.73 **In the puerperium**
Indicator(s): Female | HHSØ5: 2Ø9 | HHSØ7: 2Ø9

O26.8- **Other specified pregnancy related conditions**

O26.81- **Pregnancy related exhaustion and fatigue**
Indicator(s): HHSØ7: 212

O26.811 **First trimester**
Indicator(s): Female

O26.812 **Second trimester**
Indicator(s): Female

O26.813 **Third trimester**
Indicator(s): Female

O26.819 **Unspecified trimester**
Indicator(s): Female

O26.82- **Pregnancy related peripheral neuritis**
Indicator(s): HHSØ7: 212

O26.821 **First trimester**
Indicator(s): Female

O26.822 **Second trimester**
Indicator(s): Female

O26.823 **Third trimester**
Indicator(s): Female

O26.829 **Unspecified trimester**
Indicator(s): Female

O26.89- **Other specified pregnancy related conditions**
Indicator(s): HHSØ7: 212

O26.891 First trimester
Indicator(s): Female

O26.892 Second trimester
Indicator(s): Female

O26.893 Third trimester
Indicator(s): Female

O26.899 Unspecified trimester
Indicator(s): Female

O26.9- **Pregnancy related conditions, unspecified**
Indicator(s): HHSØ7: 212

O26.9Ø Unspecified trimester
Indicator(s): Female

O26.91 First trimester
Indicator(s): Female

O26.92 Second trimester
Indicator(s): Female

O26.93 Third trimester
Indicator(s): Female

MATERNAL CARE RELATED TO THE FETUS AND AMNIOTIC CAVITY AND POSSIBLE DELIVERY PROBLEMS (O3Ø-O48)

O32- MATERNAL CARE FOR MALPRESENTATION OF FETUS

Includes:
the listed conditions as a reason for observation, hospitalization or other obstetric care of the mother, or for cesarean delivery before onset of labor
Excludes1:
malpresentation of fetus with obstructed labor (O64.-)

One of the following 7th characters is to be assigned to each code under category O32. 7th character Ø is for single gestations and multiple gestations where the fetus is unspecified. 7th characters 1 through 9 are for cases of multiple gestations to identify the fetus for which the code applies. The appropriate code from category O3Ø, Multiple gestation, must also be assigned when assigning a code from category O32 that has a 7th character of 1 through 9.

Ø - not applicable or unspecified
1 - fetus 1
2 - fetus 2
3 - fetus 3
4 - fetus 4
5 - fetus 5
9 - other fetus

See Guidelines: 1;C.15.a.6
Indicator(s): HHSØ7: 21Ø (7th 1/2/3/4/5/9), 211 (7th Ø)

O32.1xx_ Breech
Including: Maternal care for buttocks presentation, complete breech, or frank breech
Excludes1:
footling presentation (O32.8)
incomplete breech (O32.8)

O47- FALSE LABOR

Includes:
Braxton Hicks contractions
threatened labor
Excludes1:
preterm labor (O6Ø.-)
Indicator(s): HHSØ7: 212

O47.9 Unspecified
Indicator(s): Female

O48- LATE PREGNANCY

Indicator(s): HHSØ7: 212

O48.Ø Post-term pregnancy
Including: Pregnancy over 4Ø completed weeks to 42 completed weeks gestation
Indicator(s): Female

O48.1 Prolonged pregnancy
Including: Pregnancy which has advanced beyond 42 completed weeks gestation
Indicator(s): Female

16. Certain conditions originating in the perinatal period (PØØ-P96)

This Chapter was not included in this common codes list. For a complete listing of ICD-10-CM codes see FindACode.com

17. Congenital malformations, deformations and chromosomal abnormalities (QØØ-Q99)

Notes:
Codes from this chapter are not for use on maternal records
Excludes2:
inborn errors of metabolism (E7Ø-E88)
See Guidelines: *1;C.17 | 1;C.2Ø.a.1*
Indicator(s): *POAEx*

CONGENITAL MALFORMATIONS OF THE NERVOUS SYSTEM (QØØ-QØ7)

Indicator(s): *CMS22: 72 | CMS24: 72 | RxØ5: 157 | ESRD21: 72*

QØ5- SPINA BIFIDA
Includes:
hydromeningocele (spinal)
meningocele (spinal)
meningomyelocele
myelocele
myelomeningocele
rachischisis
spina bifida (aperta)(cystica)
syringomyelocele
Use additional code for any associated paraplegia (paraparesis) (G82.2-)
Excludes1:
Arnold-Chiari syndrome, type II (QØ7.Ø-)
spina bifida occulta (Q76.Ø)

QØ5.Ø **Cervical, with hydrocephalus**
Indicator(s): *CC*
QØ5.1 **Thoracic, with hydrocephalus**
Including: Dorsal, Thoracolumbar
Indicator(s): *CC*
QØ5.2 **Lumbar, with hydrocephalus**
Including: Lumbosacral
Indicator(s): *CC*
QØ5.3 **Sacral, with hydrocephalus**
Indicator(s): *CC*
QØ5.4 **Unspecified, with hydrocephalus**
Indicator(s): *CC*
QØ5.5 **Cervical, without hydrocephalus**
QØ5.6 **Thoracic, without hydrocephalus**
Including: Dorsal NOS, Thoracolumbar NOS
QØ5.7 **Lumbar, without hydrocephalus**
Including: Lumbosacral NOS
QØ5.8 **Sacral, without hydrocephalus**
QØ5.9 **Unspecified**

QØ7- OTHER CONGENITAL MALFORMATIONS OF NERVOUS SYSTEM
Excludes2:
congenital central alveolar hypoventilation syndrome (G47.35)
familial dysautonomia [Riley-Day] (G9Ø.1)
neurofibromatosis (nonmalignant) (Q85.Ø-)

QØ7.Ø- **Arnold-Chiari syndrome**
Including: Arnold-Chiari syndrome, type II
Excludes1:
Arnold-Chiari syndrome, type III (QØ1.-)
Arnold-Chiari syndrome, type IV (QØ4.8)
QØ7.ØØ **Without spina bifida or hydrocephalus**
QØ7.Ø1 **With spina bifida**
QØ7.Ø2 **With hydrocephalus**
Indicator(s): *CC*
QØ7.Ø3 **With spina bifida and hydrocephalus**
Indicator(s): *CC*

QØ7.9 **Unspecified**
Including: Anomaly, deformity, disease or lesion

CONGENITAL MALFORMATIONS OF EYE, EAR, FACE AND NECK (Q1Ø-Q18)

Excludes2:
cleft lip and cleft palate (Q35-Q37)
congenital malformation of cervical spine (QØ5.Ø, QØ5.5, Q67.5, Q76.Ø-Q76.4)
congenital malformation of larynx (Q31.-)
congenital malformation of lip NEC (Q38.Ø)
congenital malformation of nose (Q3Ø.-)
congenital malformation of parathyroid gland (Q89.2)
congenital malformation of thyroid gland (Q89.2)

Q18- OTHER CONGENITAL MALFORMATIONS OF FACE AND NECK
Excludes1:
cleft lip and cleft palate (Q35-Q37)
conditions classified to Q67.Ø-Q67.4
congenital malformations of skull and face bones (Q75.-)
cyclopia (Q87.Ø)
dentofacial anomalies [including malocclusion] (M26.-)
malformation syndromes affecting facial appearance (Q87.Ø)
persistent thyroglossal duct (Q89.2)

Q18.3 **Webbing of neck**
Including: Pterygium colli
Q18.4 **Macrostomia**
Q18.5 **Microstomia**
Q18.6 **Macrocheilia**
Including: Hypertrophy of lip, congenital
Q18.7 **Microcheilia**
Q18.8 **Other specified**
Including: Medial cyst, Medial fistula, Medial sinus
Q18.9 **Unspecified**
Including: Anomaly NOS

CONGENITAL MALFORMATIONS AND DEFORMATIONS OF THE MUSCULOSKELETAL SYSTEM (Q65-Q79)

Q65- CONGENITAL DEFORMITIES OF HIP
Excludes1:
clicking hip (R29.4)
Indicator(s): *HHSØ5: 62 | HHSØ7: 62*

Q65.Ø- **Congenital dislocation of hip, unilateral**
Q65.ØØ **Unspecified**
Q65.Ø1 **Right**
Q65.Ø2 **Left**
Q65.1 **Dislocation of hip, bilateral**
Q65.2 **Dislocation of hip, unspecified**
Q65.3- **Congenital partial dislocation of hip, unilateral**
Q65.3Ø **Unspecified**
Q65.31 **Right**
Q65.32 **Left**
Q65.4 **Partial dislocation of hip, bilateral**
Q65.5 **Partial dislocation of hip, unspecified**
Q65.6 **Unstable hip**
Including: Dislocatable hip

 See Appendix A — Coding Reference Tables for lists of the ICD-10-CM Tabular indicators, HAC categories, and HCC codes.

Q65.8- **Other congenital deformities of hip**

Q65.81 **Coxa valga**

Q65.82 **Coxa vara**

Q65.89 **Other specified**
Including: Anteversion of femoral neck, Congenital acetabular dysplasia

Q65.9 **Unspecified**

Q66- CONGENITAL DEFORMITIES OF FEET
Excludes1:
reduction defects of feet (Q72.-)
valgus deformities (acquired) (M21.Ø-)
varus deformities (acquired) (M21.1-)

Q66.5- **Congenital pes planus**
Including: Flat foot, rigid flat foot, spastic (everted) flat foot
Excludes1:
pes planus, acquired (M21.4)

Q66.5Ø **Unspecified**

Q66.51 **Right**

Q66.52 **Left**

Q66.6 **Other valgus deformities**
Including: Metatarsus valgus

Q66.8- **Other congenital deformities of feet**

Q66.8Ø **Vertical talus deformity, unspecified**

Q66.81 **Vertical talus deformity, right**

Q66.82 **Vertical talus deformity, left**

Q66.89 **Other specified**
Including: Asymmetric talipes, clubfoot NOS, talipes NOS, tarsal coalition, Hammer toe

Q67- CONGENITAL MUSCULOSKELETAL DEFORMITIES OF HEAD, FACE, SPINE AND CHEST
Excludes1:
congenital malformation syndromes classified to Q87.-
Potter's syndrome (Q6Ø.6)

Q67.Ø **Facial asymmetry**

Q67.1 **Compression facies**

Q67.2 **Dolichocephaly**

Q67.3 **Plagiocephaly**

Q67.4 **Other deformities of skull, face and jaw**
Including: Depressions in skull, Hemifacial atrophy or hypertrophy, Deviation of nasal septum, Squashed or bent nose
Excludes1:
dentofacial anomalies [including malocclusion] (M26.-)
syphilitic saddle nose (A5Ø.5)

Q67.5 **Deformity of spine**
Including: Postural scoliosis, scoliosis NOS
Excludes1:
infantile idiopathic scoliosis (M41.Ø)
scoliosis due to congenital bony malformation (Q76.3)
Indicator(s): CC

Q67.6 **Pectus excavatum**
Including: Congenital funnel chest

Q67.7 **Pectus carinatum**
Including: Congenital pigeon chest

Q67.8 **Other deformities of chest**
Including: Deformity of chest wall NOS
Indicator(s): CC

Q68- OTHER CONGENITAL MUSCULOSKELETAL DEFORMITIES
Excludes1:
reduction defects of limb(s) (Q71-Q73)
Excludes2:
congenital myotonic chondrodystrophy (G71.13)

Q68.Ø **Deformity of sternocleidomastoid muscle**
Including: Contracture of sternocleidomastoid (muscle), (Sternomastoid) torticollis, Sternomastoid tumor

Q68.2 **Deformity of knee**
Including: Dislocation, genu recurvatum

Q68.3 **Bowing of femur**
Excludes1:
anteversion of femur (neck) (Q65.89)

Q68.4 **Bowing of tibia and fibula**

Q68.5 **Bowing of long bones of leg, unspecified**

Q68.8 **Other specified**
Including: Deformity of clavicle, elbow, forearm, scapula, and wrist; dislocation of elbow, shoulder, and wrist

Q71- REDUCTION DEFECTS OF UPPER LIMB

Q71.Ø- **Congenital complete absence of upper limb**

Q71.ØØ **Unspecified limb**

Q71.Ø1 **Right**

Q71.Ø2 **Left**

Q71.Ø3 **Bilateral**

Q71.1- **Congenital absence of upper arm and forearm with hand present**

Q71.1Ø **Unspecified arm**

Q71.11 **Right**

Q71.12 **Left**

Q71.13 **Bilateral**

Q71.2- **Congenital absence of both forearm and hand**

Q71.2Ø **Unspecified limb**

Q71.21 **Right**

Q71.22 **Left**

Q71.23 **Bilateral**

Q71.3- **Congenital absence of hand and finger**

Q71.3Ø **Unspecified hand and finger**

Q71.31 **Right**

Q71.32 **Left**

Q71.33 **Bilateral**

Q71.4- **Longitudinal reduction defect of radius**
Including: Clubhand (congenital), Radial clubhand

Q71.4Ø **Unspecified radius**

Q71.41 **Right**

Q71.42 **Left**

Q71.43 **Bilateral**

Q71.5- **Longitudinal reduction defect of ulna**

Q71.5Ø **Unspecified ulna**

Q71.51 **Right**

Q71.52 **Left**

Q71.53 **Bilateral**

Q71.6- **Lobster-claw hand**

Q71.6Ø **Unspecified hand**

Q71.61 **Right**

Q71.62 **Left**

Q71.63 **Bilateral**

Q71.8- **Other reduction defects of upper limb**
Q71.81- **Congenital shortening of upper limb**
Q71.811 **Right**
Q71.812 **Left**
Q71.813 **Bilateral**
Q71.819 **Unspecified limb**
Q71.89- **Other reduction defects of upper limb**
Q71.891 **Right**
Q71.892 **Left**
Q71.893 **Bilateral**
Q71.899 **Unspecified limb**
Q71.9- **Unspecified reduction defect of upper limb**
Q71.90 **Unspecified limb**
Q71.91 **Right**
Q71.92 **Left**
Q71.93 **Bilateral**

Q72- REDUCTION DEFECTS OF LOWER LIMB
Q72.0- **Congenital complete absence of lower limb**
Q72.00 **Unspecified limb**
Q72.01 **Right**
Q72.02 **Left**
Q72.03 **Bilateral**
Q72.1- **Congenital absence of thigh and lower leg with foot present**
Q72.10 **Unspecified thigh**
Q72.11 **Right**
Q72.12 **Left**
Q72.13 **Bilateral**
Q72.2- **Congenital absence of both lower leg and foot**
Q72.20 **Unspecified limb**
Q72.21 **Right**
Q72.22 **Left**
Q72.23 **Bilateral**
Q72.3- **Congenital absence of foot and toe(s)**
Q72.30 **Unspecified foot and toe(s)**
Q72.31 **Right**
Q72.32 **Left**
Q72.33 **Bilateral**
Q72.4- **Longitudinal reduction defect of femur**
Including: Proximal femoral focal deficiency
Q72.40 **Unspecified femur**
Q72.41 **Right**
Q72.42 **Left**
Q72.43 **Bilateral**
Q72.5- **Longitudinal reduction defect of tibia**
Q72.50 **Unspecified tibia**
Q72.51 **Right**
Q72.52 **Left**
Q72.53 **Bilateral**
Q72.6- **Longitudinal reduction defect of fibula**
Q72.60 **Unspecified fibula**
Q72.61 **Right**
Q72.62 **Left**
Q72.63 **Bilateral**
Q72.7- **Split foot**
Q72.70 **Unspecified lower limb**
Q72.71 **Right**
Q72.72 **Left**
Q72.73 **Bilateral**
Q72.8- **Other reduction defects of lower limb**
Q72.81- **Congenital shortening**
Q72.811 **Right**
Q72.812 **Left**
Q72.813 **Bilateral**
Q72.819 **Unspecified limb**
Q72.89- **Other reduction defects**
Q72.891 **Right**
Q72.892 **Left**
Q72.893 **Bilateral**
Q72.899 **Unspecified limb**
Q72.9- **Unspecified reduction defect of lower limb**
Q72.90 **Unspecified limb**
Q72.91 **Right**
Q72.92 **Left**
Q72.93 **Bilateral**

Q73- REDUCTION DEFECTS OF UNSPECIFIED LIMB
Q73.0 **Absence**
Including: Amelia NOS
Q73.1 **Phocomelia**
Including: Phocomelia NOS
Q73.8 **Other reduction defects**
Including: Longitudinal reduction deformity, Ectromelia NOS, Hemimelia NOS, defect NOS

Q74- OTHER CONGENITAL MALFORMATIONS OF LIMB(S)
Excludes1:
polydactyly (Q69.-)
reduction defect of limb (Q71-Q73)
syndactyly (Q70.-)
Q74.0 **Upper limb(s), including shoulder girdle**
Including: Accessory carpal bones, Cleidocranial dysostosis, Pseudarthrosis of clavicle, Macrodactylia (fingers), Madelung's deformity, Radioulnar synostosis, Sprengel's deformity, Triphalangeal thumb
Q74.1 **Knee**
Including: Absence of patella, dislocation of patella, genu valgum, genu varum, Rudimentary patella
Excludes1:
congenital dislocation of knee (Q68.2)
congenital genu recurvatum (Q68.2)
nail patella syndrome (Q87.2)
Q74.2 **Lower limb(s), including pelvic girdle**
Including: Fusion of sacroiliac joint, malformation of ankle joint, malformation of sacroiliac joint
Excludes1:
anteversion of femur (neck) (Q65.89)
Q74.3 **Arthrogryposis multiplex congenita**
Indicator(s): CC
Q74.8 **Other specified**
Q74.9 **Unspecified**
Including: Anomaly NOS

Q75- OTHER CONGENITAL MALFORMATIONS OF SKULL AND FACE BONES

Excludes1:

congenital malformation of face NOS (Q18.-)

congenital malformation syndromes classified to Q87.-

dentofacial anomalies [including malocclusion] (M26.-)

musculoskeletal deformities of head and face (Q67.Ø-Q67.4)

skull defects associated with congenital anomalies of brain such as:

anencephaly (QØØ.Ø)

encephalocele (QØ1.-)

hydrocephalus (QØ3.-)

microcephaly (QØ2)

Q75.Ø Craniosynostosis

Including: Acrocephaly, Imperfect fusion of skull, Oxycephaly, Trigonocephaly

Q75.1 Craniofacial dysostosis

Including: Crouzon's disease

Q75.2 Hypertelorism

Q75.3 Macrocephaly

Q75.4 Mandibulofacial dysostosis

Including: Franceschetti syndrome, Treacher Collins syndrome

Q75.5 Oculomandibular dysostosis

Q75.8 Other specified

Including: Absence of skull bone, deformity of forehead, Platybasia

Q75.9 Unspecified

Including: Anomaly of face bones NOS, anomaly of skull NOS

Q76- CONGENITAL MALFORMATIONS OF SPINE AND BONY THORAX

Excludes1:

congenital musculoskeletal deformities of spine and chest (Q67.5-Q67.8)

Q76.Ø Spina bifida occulta

Excludes1:

meningocele (spinal) (QØ5.-)

spina bifida (aperta) (cystica) (QØ5.-)

Q76.1 Klippel-Feil syndrome

Including: Cervical fusion syndrome

Q76.2 Spondylolisthesis

Including: Spondylolysis

Excludes1:

spondylolisthesis (acquired) (M43.1-)

spondylolysis (acquired) (M43.Ø-)

Q76.3 Scoliosis due to congenital bony malformation

Including: Hemivertebra fusion or failure of segmentation with scoliosis

Indicator(s): CC

Q76.4- **Other congenital malformations of spine, not associated with scoliosis**

Indicator(s): POAEx

Q76.41- **Congenital kyphosis**

Q76.411 Occipito-atlanto-axial region

Q76.412 Cervical region

Q76.413 Cervicothoracic region

Q76.414 Thoracic region

Q76.415 Thoracolumbar region

Q76.419 Unspecified region

Q76.42- **Congenital lordosis**

Indicator(s): CC

Q76.425 Thoracolumbar region

Q76.426 Lumbar region

Q76.427 Lumbosacral region

Q76.428 Sacral and sacrococcygeal region

Q76.429 Unspecified region

Q76.49 Other

Including: Absence of vertebra NOS, fusion of spine NOS, malformation of lumbosacral (joint) (region) NOS, malformation of spine NOS, Hemivertebra NOS, Malformation of spine NOS, Platyspondylisis NOS, Supernumerary vertebra NOS

Q76.5 Cervical rib

Including: Supernumerary rib in cervical region

Q76.6 Other malformations of ribs

Including: Accessory rib, absence, fusion, malformation NOS

Excludes1:

short rib syndrome (Q77.2)

Indicator(s): CC

Q76.7 Malformation of sternum

Including: Absence, Sternum bifidum

Indicator(s): CC

Q76.8 Other malformations of bony thorax

Indicator(s): CC

Q76.9 Unspecified

Indicator(s): CC

Q77- OSTEOCHONDRODYSPLASIA WITH DEFECTS OF GROWTH OF TUBULAR BONES AND SPINE

Excludes1:

mucopolysaccharidosis (E76.Ø-E76.3)

Excludes2:

congenital myotonic chondrodystrophy (G71.13)

Q77.Ø Achondrogenesis

Including: Hypochondrogenesis

Indicator(s): HHSØ5: 62 | HHSØ7: 62

Q77.1 Thanatophoric short stature

Indicator(s): HHSØ5: 62 | HHSØ7: 62

Q77.2 Short rib syndrome

Including: Asphyxiating thoracic dysplasia [Jeune]

Indicator(s): CC | HHSØ5: 62 | HHSØ7: 62

Q77.3 Chondrodysplasia punctata

Excludes1:

Rhizomelic chondrodysplasia punctata (E71.43)

Indicator(s): HHSØ5: 61 | HHSØ7: 61

Q77.4 Achondroplasia

Including: Hypochondroplasia, Osteosclerosis congenita

Indicator(s): HHSØ5: 62 | HHSØ7: 62

Q77.5 Diastrophic dysplasia

Indicator(s): HHSØ5: 62 | HHSØ7: 62

Q77.6 Chondroectodermal dysplasia

Including: Ellis-van Creveld syndrome

Indicator(s): HHSØ5: 61 | HHSØ7: 61

Q77.7 Spondyloepiphyseal dysplasia

Indicator(s): HHSØ5: 62 | HHSØ7: 62

Q77.8 Other

Indicator(s): HHSØ5: 62 | HHSØ7: 62

Q77.9 Unspecified

Indicator(s): HHSØ5: 62 | HHSØ7: 62

Q78- OTHER OSTEOCHONDRODYSPLASIAS

Excludes2:
congenital myotonic chondrodystrophy (G71.13)

Q78.Ø Osteogenesis imperfecta
Including: Fragilitas ossium, Osteopsathyrosis
Indicator(s): CC | HHSØ5: 61 | HHSØ7: 61

Q78.1 Polyostotic fibrous dysplasia
Including: Albright (-McCune) (-Sternberg) syndrome
Indicator(s): HHSØ5: 61 | HHSØ7: 61

Q78.2 Osteopetrosis
Including: Albers-Schönberg syndrome, Osteosclerosis NOS
Indicator(s): CC | HHSØ5: 61 | HHSØ7: 61

Q78.3 Progressive diaphyseal dysplasia
Including: Camurati-Engelmann syndrome
Indicator(s): HHSØ5: 61 | HHSØ7: 61

Q78.4 Enchondromatosis
Including: Maffucci's syndrome, Ollier's disease
Indicator(s): HHSØ5: 62 | HHSØ7: 62

Q78.5 Metaphyseal dysplasia
Including: Pyle's syndrome
Indicator(s): HHSØ5: 61 | HHSØ7: 61

Q78.6 Multiple congenital exostoses
Including: Diaphyseal aclasis
Indicator(s): HHSØ5: 61 | HHSØ7: 61

Q78.8 Other specified
Including: Osteopoikilosis
Indicator(s): HHSØ5: 61 | HHSØ7: 61

Q78.9 Unspecified
Including: Chondrodystrophy NOS, Osteodystrophy NOS
Indicator(s): HHSØ5: 61 | HHSØ7: 61

Q79- CONGENITAL MALFORMATIONS OF MUSCULOSKELETAL SYSTEM, NOT ELSEWHERE CLASSIFIED

Excludes2:
congenital (sternomastoid) torticollis (Q68.Ø)

Q79.Ø Diaphragmatic hernia
Excludes1:
congenital hiatus hernia (Q4Ø.1)
Indicator(s): MCC | HHSØ5: 64 | HHSØ7: 64

Q79.1 Other malformations of diaphragm
Including: Absence, malformation NOS, Eventration
Indicator(s): MCC | HHSØ5: 64 | HHSØ7: 64

Q79.2 Exomphalos
Including: Omphalocele
Excludes1:
umbilical hernia (K42.-)
Indicator(s): MCC | HHSØ5: 64 | HHSØ7: 64

Q79.3 Gastroschisis
Indicator(s): MCC | HHSØ5: 64 | HHSØ7: 64

Q79.4 Prune belly syndrome
Including: Congenital prolapse of bladder mucosa, Eagle-Barrett syndrome
Indicator(s): MCC | HHSØ5: 64 | HHSØ7: 64

Q79.5- **Other congenital malformations of abdominal wall**
Excludes1:
umbilical hernia (K42.-)
Indicator(s): MCC

Q79.51 Hernia of bladder
Indicator(s): HHSØ5: 64 | HHSØ7: 64

Q79.59 Other

Q79.8 Other malformations of musculoskeletal system
Including: Absence of muscle, Absence of tendon, Accessory muscle, Amyotrophia congenita, constricting bands, shortening of tendon, Poland syndrome

Q79.9 Unspecified
Including: Anomaly NOS, deformity NOS

OTHER CONGENITAL MALFORMATIONS (Q8Ø-Q89)

Q87- OTHER SPECIFIED CONGENITAL MALFORMATION SYNDROMES AFFECTING MULTIPLE SYSTEMS

Use additional code(s) to identify all associated manifestations

Q87.4- **Marfan's syndrome**
Indicator(s): CC | RxØ5: 84 | HHSØ5: 62 | HHSØ7: 62

Q87.4Ø Unspecified

Q89- OTHER CONGENITAL MALFORMATIONS, NOT ELSEWHERE CLASSIFIED

Q89.9 Unspecified
Including: Anomaly NOS, deformity NOS

CHROMOSOMAL ABNORMALITIES, NOT ELSEWHERE CLASSIFIED (Q9Ø-Q99)

Excludes2:
mitochondrial metabolic disorders (E88.4-)

Q9Ø- DOWN SYNDROME

Use additional code(s) to identify any associated physical conditions and degree of intellectual disabilities (F7Ø-F79)
Indicator(s): HHSØ5: 97 | HHSØ7: 97

Q9Ø.9 Unspecified
Including: Trisomy 21 NOS

Q91- TRISOMY 18 AND TRISOMY 13

Indicator(s): CC | RxØ5: 148 | HHSØ5: 96 | HHSØ7: 96

Q91.7 13, unspecified

Q96- TURNER'S SYNDROME

Excludes1:
Noonan syndrome (Q87.19)
Indicator(s): HHSØ5: 97 | HHSØ7: 97

Q96.9 Unspecified
Indicator(s): Female

Q99- OTHER CHROMOSOME ABNORMALITIES, NOT ELSEWHERE CLASSIFIED

Indicator(s): HHSØ5: 97 | HHSØ7: 97

Q99.9 Unspecified

Ch5

5. The Tabular List

See Appendix A — Coding Reference Tables for lists of the ICD-10-CM Tabular indicators, HAC categories, and HCC codes.

18. Symptoms, signs and abnormal clinical and laboratory findings, not elsewhere classified (RØØ-R99)

Notes:

This chapter includes symptoms, signs, abnormal results of clinical or other investigative procedures, and ill-defined conditions regarding which no diagnosis classifiable elsewhere is recorded.

Signs and symptoms that point rather definitely to a given diagnosis have been assigned to a category in other chapters of the classification. In general, categories in this chapter include the less well-defined conditions and symptoms that, without the necessary study of the case to establish a final diagnosis, point perhaps equally to two or more diseases or to two or more systems of the body. Practically all categories in the chapter could be designated 'not otherwise specified', 'unknown etiology' or 'transient'. The Alphabetical Index should be consulted to determine which symptoms and signs are to be allocated here and which to other chapters. The residual subcategories, numbered .8, are generally provided for other relevant symptoms that cannot be allocated elsewhere in the classification.

The conditions and signs or symptoms included in categories RØØ-R94 consist of:

(a) cases for which no more specific diagnosis can be made even after all the facts bearing on the case have been investigated;

(b) signs or symptoms existing at the time of initial encounter that proved to be transient and whose causes could not be determined;

(c) provisional diagnosis in a patient who failed to return for further investigation or care;

(d) cases referred elsewhere for investigation or treatment before the diagnosis was made;

(e) cases in which a more precise diagnosis was not available for any other reason;

(f) certain symptoms, for which supplementary information is provided, that represent important problems in medical care in their own right.

Excludes2:

abnormal findings on antenatal screening of mother (O28.-)

certain conditions originating in the perinatal period (PØ4-P96)

signs and symptoms classified in the body system chapters

signs and symptoms of breast (N63, N64.5)

See Guidelines: *1;C.18.a-c | 1;C.2Ø.a.1 | 4;D*

SYMPTOMS AND SIGNS INVOLVING THE CIRCULATORY AND RESPIRATORY SYSTEMS (RØØ-RØ9)

RØØ- ABNORMALITIES OF HEART BEAT

Excludes1:

abnormalities originating in the perinatal period (P29.1-)

Excludes2:

specified arrhythmias (I47-I49)

RØØ.Ø **Tachycardia, unspecified**

Including: Rapid heart beat, Sinoauricular tachycardia NOS, Sinus [sinusal] tachycardia NOS

Excludes1:

neonatal tachycardia (P29.11)

paroxysmal tachycardia (I47.-)

RØØ.1 **Bradycardia, unspecified**

Including: Sinoatrial, Sinus, Vagal bradycardia; Slow heart beat

Use additional *code for adverse effect, if applicable, to identify drug (T36-T5Ø with fifth or sixth character 5)*

Excludes1:

neonatal bradycardia (P29.12)

RØØ.2 **Palpitations**

Including: Awareness of heart beat

RØØ.8 **Other**

RØØ.9 **Unspecified**

RØ1- CARDIAC MURMURS AND OTHER CARDIAC SOUNDS

Excludes1:

cardiac murmurs and sounds originating in the perinatal period (P29.8)

RØ1.Ø **Benign and innocent cardiac murmurs**

Including: Functional cardiac murmur

RØ1.1 **Cardiac murmur, unspecified**

Including: Cardiac bruit NOS, Heart murmur NOS, Systolic murmur NOS

RØ1.2 **Other cardiac sounds**

Including: Cardiac dullness (increased or decreased), Precordial friction

RØ3- ABNORMAL BLOOD-PRESSURE READING, WITHOUT DIAGNOSIS

RØ3.Ø **Elevated reading, without diagnosis of hypertension**

Notes:

This category is to be used to record an episode of elevated blood pressure in a patient in whom no formal diagnosis of hypertension has been made, or as an isolated incidental finding.

See Guidelines: *1;C.9.a.7*

Indicator(s): *QAdmit*

RØ3.1 **Nonspecific low reading**

Excludes1:

hypotension (I95.-)

maternal hypotension syndrome (O26.5-)

neurogenic orthostatic hypotension (G9Ø.3)

RØ4- HEMORRHAGE FROM RESPIRATORY PASSAGES

RØ4.Ø **Epistaxis**

Including: Hemorrhage from nose, Nosebleed

RØ4.1 **Hemorrhage from throat**

Excludes2:

hemoptysis (RØ4.2)

RØ4.2 **Hemoptysis**

Including: Blood-stained sputum, Cough with hemorrhage

Indicator(s): *CC*

RØ4.8- **Other sites**

Indicator(s): *CC*

R **RØ4.81** **Acute idiopathic hemorrhage in infants**

Including: in infants over 28 days old; AIPHI

Excludes1:

perinatal pulmonary hemorrhage (P26.-)

von Willebrand disease (D68.Ø-)

Indicator(s): *Pediatric*

RØ4.89 **Other**

Including: Pulmonary hemorrhage NOS

RØ4.9 **Unspecified**

Indicator(s): *CC*

RØ6- ABNORMALITIES OF BREATHING

Excludes1:
acute respiratory distress syndrome (J8Ø)
respiratory arrest (RØ9.2)
respiratory arrest of newborn (P28.81)
respiratory distress syndrome of newborn (P22.-)
respiratory failure (J96.-)
respiratory failure of newborn (P28.5)

RØ6.Ø- **Dyspnea**
Excludes1:
tachypnea NOS (RØ6.82)
transient tachypnea of newborn (P22.1)

RØ6.ØØ Unspecified

RØ6.Ø1 Orthopnea

RØ6.Ø2 Shortness of breath

RØ6.Ø9 Other

RØ6.1 Stridor
Excludes1:
congenital laryngeal stridor (P28.89)
laryngismus (stridulus) (J38.5)

RØ6.2 Wheezing
Excludes1:
Asthma (J45.-)

RØ6.3 Periodic breathing
Including: Cheyne-Stokes breathing
Indicator(s): CC | DSM-5

RØ6.4 Hyperventilation
Excludes1:
psychogenic hyperventilation (F45.8)

RØ6.5 Mouth breathing
Excludes2:
dry mouth NOS (R68.2)

RØ6.6 Hiccough
Excludes1:
psychogenic hiccough (F45.8)

RØ6.7 Sneezing

RØ6.8- **Other abnormalities**

R **RØ6.81 Apnea, NEC**
Including: Apnea NOS
Excludes1:
apnea (of) newborn (P28.4-)
sleep apnea (G47.3-)
sleep apnea of newborn (primary) (P28.3-)

RØ6.82 Tachypnea, NEC
Including: Tachypnea NOS
Excludes1:
transitory tachypnea of newborn (P22.1)

RØ6.83 Snoring

RØ6.89 Other
Including: Breath-holding (spells), Sighing

RØ6.9 Unspecified

RØ7- PAIN IN THROAT AND CHEST

Excludes1:
epidemic myalgia (B33.Ø)
Excludes2:
jaw pain R68.84
pain in breast (N64.4)

RØ7.Ø Pain in throat
Excludes1:
chronic sore throat (J31.2)
sore throat (acute) NOS (JØ2.9)
Excludes2:
dysphagia (R13.1-)
pain in neck (M54.2)

RØ7.1 Chest pain on breathing
Including: Painful respiration

RØ7.2 Precordial pain

RØ7.8- **Other chest pain**

RØ7.81 Pleurodynia
Including: Pleurodynia NOS
Excludes1:
epidemic pleurodynia (B33.Ø)

RØ7.82 Intercostal pain

RØ7.89 Other chest pain
Including: Anterior chest-wall pain NOS

RØ7.9 Chest pain, unspecified

RØ9- OTHER SYMPTOMS AND SIGNS INVOLVING THE CIRCULATORY AND RESPIRATORY SYSTEM

Excludes1:
acute respiratory distress syndrome (J8Ø)
respiratory arrest of newborn (P28.81)
respiratory distress syndrome of newborn (P22.Ø)
respiratory failure (J96.-)
respiratory failure of newborn (P28.5)

RØ9.Ø- **Asphyxia and hypoxemia**
Excludes1:
asphyxia due to carbon monoxide (T58.-)
asphyxia due to foreign body in respiratory tract (T17.-)
birth (intrauterine) asphyxia (P84)
hyperventilation (RØ6.4)
traumatic asphyxia (T71.-)
Excludes2:
hypercapnia (RØ6.89)

RØ9.Ø1 Asphyxia
Indicator(s): CC

RØ9.Ø2 Hypoxemia

RØ9.1 Pleurisy
Excludes1:
pleurisy with effusion (J9Ø)

RØ9.2 Respiratory arrest
Including: Cardiorespiratory failure
Excludes1:
cardiac arrest (I46.-)
respiratory arrest of newborn (P28.81)
respiratory distress of newborn (P22.Ø)
respiratory failure (J96.-)
respiratory failure of newborn (P28.5)
respiratory insufficiency (RØ6.89)
respiratory insufficiency of newborn (P28.5)
Indicator(s): MCC | CMS22: 83 | CMS24: 83 | ESRD21: 83 | HHSØ5: 126 | HHSØ7: 126

RØ9.3 Abnormal sputum
Including: Abnormal amount, color, odor of sputum; Excessive sputum
Excludes1:
blood-stained sputum (RØ4.2)

RØ9.8- **Other specified symptoms and signs**

RØ9.81 Nasal congestion

RØ9.82 Postnasal drip

RØ9.89 Other
Including: Bruit (arterial), Abnormal chest percussion, Feeling of foreign body in throat, Friction sounds in chest, Chest tympany, Choking sensation, Rales, Weak pulse
Excludes2:
foreign body in throat (T17.2-)
wheezing (RØ6.2)

SYMPTOMS AND SIGNS INVOLVING THE DIGESTIVE SYSTEM AND ABDOMEN (R1Ø-R19)

Excludes2:
congenital or infantile pylorospasm (Q4Ø.Ø)
gastrointestinal hemorrhage (K92.Ø-K92.2)
intestinal obstruction (K56.-)
newborn gastrointestinal hemorrhage (P54.Ø-P54.3)
newborn intestinal obstruction (P76.-)
pylorospasm (K31.3)
signs and symptoms involving the urinary system (R3Ø-R39)
symptoms referable to female genital organs (N94.-)
symptoms referable to male genital organs (N48-N5Ø)

R1Ø- ABDOMINAL AND PELVIC PAIN

Excludes1:
renal colic (N23)
Excludes2:
dorsalgia (M54.-)
flatulence and related conditions (R14.-)

R1Ø.Ø Acute abdomen
Including: Severe abdominal pain (generalized) (with abdominal rigidity)
Excludes1:
abdominal rigidity NOS (R19.3)
generalized abdominal pain NOS (R1Ø.84)
localized abdominal pain (R1Ø.1-R1Ø.3-)

R1Ø.1- **Pain localized to upper abdomen**

R1Ø.1Ø Unspecified

R1Ø.11 Right upper quadrant

R1Ø.12 Left upper quadrant

R1Ø.13 Epigastric
Including: Dyspepsia
Excludes1:
functional dyspepsia (K3Ø)

R1Ø.2 Pelvic and perineal
Excludes1:
vulvodynia (N94.81)

R1Ø.3- **Pain localized to other parts of lower abdomen**

R1Ø.3Ø Unspecified

R1Ø.31 Right lower quadrant

R1Ø.32 Left lower quadrant

R1Ø.33 Periumbilical

R1Ø.8- **Other abdominal pain**

R1Ø.81- **Abdominal tenderness**
Including: Abdominal tenderness NOS

R1Ø.811 Right upper quadrant

R1Ø.812 Left upper quadrant

R1Ø.813 Right lower quadrant

R1Ø.814 Left lower quadrant

R1Ø.815 Periumbilic

R1Ø.816 Epigastric

R1Ø.817 Generalized

R1Ø.819 Unspecified site

R1Ø.82- **Rebound abdominal tenderness**

R1Ø.821 Right upper quadrant

R1Ø.822 Left upper quadrant

R1Ø.823 Right lower quadrant

R1Ø.824 Left lower quadrant

R1Ø.825 Periumbilic

R1Ø.826 Epigastric

R1Ø.827 Generalized

R1Ø.829 Unspecified site

R1Ø.83 Colic
Including: Colic NOS, Infantile colic
Excludes1:
colic in adult and child over 12 months old (R1Ø.84)
Indicator(s): Pediatric

R1Ø.84 Generalized
Excludes1:
generalized abdominal pain associated with acute abdomen (R1Ø.Ø)

R1Ø.9 Unspecified abdominal pain

R11- NAUSEA AND VOMITING

Excludes1:
cyclical vomiting associated with migraine (G43.A-)
excessive vomiting in pregnancy (O21.-)
hematemesis (K92.Ø)
neonatal hematemesis (P54.Ø)
newborn vomiting (P92.Ø-)
psychogenic vomiting (F5Ø.89)
vomiting associated with bulimia nervosa (F5Ø.2)
vomiting following gastrointestinal surgery (K91.Ø)

R11.Ø Nausea
Including: Nausea NOS, Nausea without vomiting

R11.1- **Vomiting**

R11.1Ø Unspecified
Including: Vomiting NOS

R11.11 Vomiting without nausea

R11.12 Projectile vomiting

R11.13 Vomiting of fecal matter

R11.14 Bilious vomiting
Including: Bilious emesis

R11.15 Cyclical vomiting syndrome unrelated to migraine
Including: Cyclic vomiting syndrome NOS, Persistent vomiting
Excludes1:
cyclical vomiting in migraine (G43.A-)
Excludes2:
bulimia nervosa (F5Ø.2)
diabetes mellitus due to underlying condition (EØ8.-)

R11.2 Nausea with vomiting, unspecified
Including: Persistent nausea with vomiting NOS

Ch5

5. The Tabular List

Ch5

5. The Tabular List

R12 Heartburn
Excludes1:
dyspepsia NOS (R1Ø.13)
functional dyspepsia (K3Ø)

R13- APHAGIA AND DYSPHAGIA

R13.Ø Aphagia
Including: Inability to swallow
Excludes1:
psychogenic aphagia (F5Ø.9)

R13.1- **Dysphagia**
Code First:
if applicable, dysphagia following cerebrovascular disease (I69. with final characters -91)
Excludes1:
psychogenic dysphagia (F45.8)

R13.1Ø Unspecified
Including: Difficulty in swallowing NOS

R13.11 Oral phase

R13.12 Oropharyngeal phase

R13.13 Pharyngeal phase

R13.14 Pharyngoesophageal phase

R13.19 Other
Including: Cervical, Neurogenic dysphagia

R14- FLATULENCE AND RELATED CONDITIONS
Excludes1:
psychogenic aerophagy (F45.8)

R14.Ø Abdominal distension (gaseous)
Including: Bloating, Tympanites (abdominal) (intestinal)

R14.1 Gas pain

R14.2 Eructation

R14.3 Flatulence

R15- FECAL INCONTINENCE
Includes:
encopresis NOS
Excludes1:
fecal incontinence of nonorganic origin (F98.1)

R15.Ø Incomplete defecation
Excludes1:
constipation (K59.Ø-)
fecal impaction (K56.41)

R15.1 Fecal smearing
Including: Fecal soiling

R15.2 Fecal urgency

R15.9 Full incontinence of feces
Including: Fecal incontinence NOS
Indicator(s): DSM-5

R16- HEPATOMEGALY AND SPLENOMEGALY, NOT ELSEWHERE CLASSIFIED

R16.Ø Hepatomegaly
Including: Hepatomegaly NOS

R16.1 Splenomegaly
Including: Splenomegaly NOS

R16.2 Hepatomegaly with splenomegaly
Including: Hepatosplenomegaly NOS

R17 Unspecified jaundice
Excludes1:
neonatal jaundice (P55, P57-P59)
Indicator(s): CC

R18- ASCITES
Includes:
fluid in peritoneal cavity
Excludes1:
ascites in alcoholic cirrhosis (K7Ø.31)
ascites in alcoholic hepatitis (K7Ø.11)
ascites in toxic liver disease with chronic active hepatitis (K71.51)
Indicator(s): CC

R18.Ø Malignant
Code First:
malignancy, such as:
malignant neoplasm of ovary (C56.-)
secondary malignant neoplasm of retroperitoneum and peritoneum (C78.6)
Indicator(s): NoPDx/M

R18.8 Other
Including: Ascites NOS, Peritoneal effusion (chronic)

R19- OTHER SYMPTOMS AND SIGNS INVOLVING THE DIGESTIVE SYSTEM AND ABDOMEN
Excludes1:
acute abdomen (R1Ø.Ø)

R19.Ø- **Intra-abdominal and pelvic swelling, mass and lump**
Excludes1:
abdominal distension (gaseous) (R14.-)
ascites (R18.-)

R19.ØØ Unspecified site

R19.Ø1 Right upper quadrant

R19.Ø2 Left upper quadrant

R19.Ø3 Right lower quadrant

R19.Ø4 Left lower quadrant

R19.Ø5 Periumbilic
Including: Diffuse or generalized umbilical swelling or mass

R19.Ø6 Epigastric

R19.Ø7 Generalized
Including: Diffuse or generalized intra-abdominal or pelvic swelling or mass NOS

R19.Ø9 Other

R19.1- **Abnormal bowel sounds**

R19.11 Absent

R19.12 Hyperactive

R19.15 Other
Including: Abnormal bowel sounds NOS

R19.2 Visible peristalsis
Including: Hyperperistalsis

R19.3- **Abdominal rigidity**
Excludes1:
abdominal rigidity with severe abdominal pain (R1Ø.Ø)

R19.3Ø Unspecified site

R19.31 Right upper quadrant

R19.32 Left upper quadrant

R19.33 Right lower quadrant

R19.34 Left lower quadrant

R19.35 Periumbilic

R19.36 Epigastric

R19.37 Generalized

R19.4 **Change in bowel habit**
Excludes1:
constipation (K59.Ø-)
functional diarrhea (K59.1)

R19.5 **Other fecal abnormalities**
Including: Abnormal stool color, Bulky stools, Mucus in stools, Occult blood in feces, Occult blood in stools
Excludes1:
melena (K92.1)
neonatal melena (P54.1)

R19.6 **Halitosis**

R19.7 **Diarrhea, unspecified**
Including: Diarrhea NOS
Excludes1:
functional diarrhea (K59.1)
neonatal diarrhea (P78.3)
psychogenic diarrhea (F45.8)

R19.8 **Other specified symptoms and signs**

SYMPTOMS AND SIGNS INVOLVING THE SKIN AND SUBCUTANEOUS TISSUE (R2Ø-R23)

Excludes2:
symptoms relating to breast (N64.4-N64.5)

R2Ø- DISTURBANCES OF SKIN SENSATION

Excludes1:
dissociative anesthesia and sensory loss (F44.6)
psychogenic disturbances (F45.8)

R2Ø.Ø **Anesthesia**

R2Ø.1 **Hypoesthesia**

R2Ø.2 **Paresthesia**
Including: Formication, Pins and needles, Tingling
Excludes1:
acroparesthesia (I73.8)

R2Ø.3 **Hyperesthesia**

R2Ø.8 **Other**

R2Ø.9 **Unspecified**

R21 **Rash and other nonspecific skin eruption**
Includes:
rash NOS
Excludes1:
specified type of rash- code to condition
vesicular eruption (R23.8)

R22- LOCALIZED SWELLING, MASS AND LUMP OF SKIN AND SUBCUTANEOUS TISSUE

Includes:
subcutaneous nodules (localized)(superficial)
Excludes1:
abnormal findings on diagnostic imaging (R9Ø-R93)
edema (R6Ø.-)
enlarged lymph nodes (R59.-)
localized adiposity (E65)
swelling of joint (M25.4-)

R22.Ø **Head**

R22.1 **Neck**

R22.2 **Trunk**
Excludes1:
intra-abdominal or pelvic mass and lump (R19.Ø-)
intra-abdominal or pelvic swelling (R19.Ø-)
Excludes2:
breast mass and lump (N63)

R22.3- **Upper limb**

R22.3Ø **Unspecified limb**

R22.31 **Right**

R22.32 **Left**

R22.33 **Bilateral**

R22.4- **Lower limb**

R22.4Ø **Unspecified limb**

R22.41 **Right**

R22.42 **Left**

R22.43 **Bilateral**

R22.9 **Unspecified**

R23- OTHER SKIN CHANGES

R23.Ø **Cyanosis**
Excludes1:
acrocyanosis (I73.8)
cyanotic attacks of newborn (P28.2)

R23.1 **Pallor**
Including: Clammy skin

R23.2 **Flushing**
Including: Excessive blushing
Code First:
if applicable, menopausal and female climacteric states (N95.1)

R23.3 **Spontaneous ecchymoses**
Including: Petechiae
Excludes1:
ecchymoses of newborn (P54.5)
purpura (D69.-)

R23.4 **Changes in skin texture**
Including: Desquamation, Induration, Scaling
Excludes1:
epidermal thickening NOS (L85.9)

R23.8 **Other**

R23.9 **Unspecified**

SYMPTOMS AND SIGNS INVOLVING THE NERVOUS AND MUSCULOSKELETAL SYSTEMS (R25-R29)

R25- ABNORMAL INVOLUNTARY MOVEMENTS

Excludes1:
specific movement disorders (G2Ø-G26)
stereotyped movement disorders (F98.4)
tic disorders (F95.-)

R25.Ø **Abnormal head movements**

R25.1 **Tremor, unspecified**
Excludes1:
chorea NOS (G25.5)
essential tremor (G25.Ø)
hysterical tremor (F44.4)
intention tremor (G25.2)

R25.2 **Cramp and spasm**
Excludes2:
carpopedal spasm (R29.Ø)
charley-horse (M62.831)
infantile spasms (G4Ø.4-)
muscle spasm of back (M62.83Ø)
muscle spasm of calf (M62.831)

R25.3 **Fasciculation**
Including: Twitching NOS

R25.8 **Other**

R25.9 **Unspecified**

R26- ABNORMALITIES OF GAIT AND MOBILITY

Excludes1:
ataxia NOS (R27.Ø)
hereditary ataxia (G11.-)
locomotor (syphilitic) ataxia (A52.11)
immobility syndrome (paraplegic) (M62.3)

R26.Ø **Ataxic**
Including: Staggering gait

R26.1 **Paralytic**
Including: Spastic gait

R26.2 **Difficulty in walking, NEC**
Excludes1:
falling (R29.6)
unsteadiness on feet (R26.81)

R26.8- **Other abnormalities**

R26.81 **Unsteadiness on feet**

R26.89 **Other**

R26.9 **Unspecified**

R27- OTHER LACK OF COORDINATION

Excludes1:
ataxic gait (R26.Ø)
hereditary ataxia (G11.-)
vertigo NOS (R42)

R27.Ø **Ataxia, unspecified**
Excludes1:
ataxia following cerebrovascular disease (I69. with final characters -93)

R27.8 **Other**

R27.9 **Unspecified**

R29- OTHER SYMPTOMS AND SIGNS INVOLVING THE NERVOUS AND MUSCULOSKELETAL SYSTEMS

R29.Ø **Tetany**
Including: Carpopedal spasm
Excludes1:
hysterical tetany (F44.5)
neonatal tetany (P71.3)
parathyroid tetany (E2Ø.9)
post-thyroidectomy tetany (E89.2)
Indicator(s): CC

R29.1 **Meningismus**
Indicator(s): CC

R29.2 **Abnormal reflex**
Excludes2:
abnormal pupillary reflex (H57.Ø)
hyperactive gag reflex (J39.2)
vasovagal reaction or syncope (R55)

R29.3 **Abnormal posture**

R29.4 **Clicking hip**
Excludes1:
congenital deformities of hip (Q65.-)

R29.5 **Transient paralysis**
Code First:
any associated spinal cord injury (S14.Ø, S14.1-, S24.Ø, S24.1-, S34.Ø-, S34.1-)
Excludes1:
transient ischemic attack (G45.9)
Indicator(s): CC

R29.6 **Repeated falls**
Including: Falling, Tendency to fall
Excludes2:
at risk for falling (Z91.81)
history of falling (Z91.81)
See Guidelines: 1;C.18.d

R29.8- **Other symptoms and signs**

R29.81- **Involving the nervous system**

R29.81Ø **Facial weakness**
Including: Facial droop
Excludes1:
Bell's palsy (G51.Ø)
facial weakness following cerebrovascular disease (I69. with final characters -92)

R29.818 **Other**
Indicator(s): DSM-5

R29.89- **Involving the musculoskeletal system**
Excludes2:
pain in limb (M79.6-)

R29.89Ø **Loss of height**
Excludes1:
osteoporosis (M8Ø-M81)

R29.891 **Ocular torticollis**
Excludes1:
congenital (sternomastoid) torticollis Q68.Ø
psychogenic torticollis (F45.8)
spasmodic torticollis (G24.3)
torticollis due to birth injury (P15.8)
torticollis NOS M43.6

R29.898 **Other**

R29.9- **Unspecified symptoms and signs**

R29.9Ø **Nervous system**

R29.91 **Musculoskeletal system**

SYMPTOMS AND SIGNS INVOLVING THE GENITOURINARY SYSTEM (R3Ø-R39)

R3Ø- PAIN ASSOCIATED WITH MICTURITION

Excludes1:
psychogenic pain associated with micturition (F45.8)

R3Ø.Ø **Dysuria**
Including: Strangury

R3Ø.1 **Vesical tenesmus**

R3Ø.9 **Unspecified**
Including: Painful urination NOS

R31- HEMATURIA

Excludes1:
hematuria included with underlying conditions, such as:
acute cystitis with hematuria (N3Ø.Ø1)
recurrent and persistent hematuria in glomerular diseases (NØ2.-)

R31.Ø **Gross**

R31.1 **Benign essential microscopic**

R31.2- **Other microscopic hematuria**

R31.21 **Asymptomatic**
Including: AMH

R31.29 **Other**

R31.9 **Unspecified**

 See Appendix A — Coding Reference Tables for lists of the ICD-10-CM Tabular indicators, HAC categories, and HCC codes.

R32 **Unspecified urinary incontinence**
Including: Enuresis NOS
Excludes1:
functional urinary incontinence (R39.81)
nonorganic enuresis (F98.Ø)
stress incontinence and other specified urinary incontinence (N39.3-N39.4-)
urinary incontinence associated with cognitive impairment (R39.81)
Indicator(s): *DSM-5*

R33- RETENTION OF URINE
Excludes1:
psychogenic retention of urine (F45.8)

R33.Ø **Drug induced**
Use additional code for adverse effect, if applicable, to identify drug (T36-T5Ø with fifth or sixth character 5)

R33.8 **Other**
Code First:
if applicable, any causal condition, such as:
enlarged prostate (N4Ø.1)

R33.9 **Unspecified**

R34 **Anuria and oliguria**
Excludes1:
anuria and oliguria complicating abortion or ectopic or molar pregnancy (OØØ-OØ7, OØ8.4)
anuria and oliguria complicating pregnancy (O26.83-)
anuria and oliguria complicating the puerperium (O9Ø.4)

R35- POLYURIA
Code First:
if applicable, any causal condition, such as:
enlarged prostate (N4Ø.1)
Excludes1:
psychogenic polyuria (F45.8)

R35.Ø **Frequency of micturition**

R35.1 **Nocturia**

R36- URETHRAL DISCHARGE

R36.Ø **Without blood**

R36.1 **Hematospermia**
Indicator(s): *Male*

R36.9 **Unspecified**
Including: Penile discharge NOS, Urethrorrhea

R37 **Sexual dysfunction, unspecified**

R39- OTHER AND UNSPECIFIED SYMPTOMS AND SIGNS INVOLVING THE GENITOURINARY SYSTEM

R39.Ø **Extravasation of urine**
Indicator(s): *CC*

R39.1- **Other difficulties with micturition**
Code First:
if applicable, any causal condition, such as:
enlarged prostate (N4Ø.1)

R39.11 **Hesitancy**

R39.12 **Poor urinary stream**
Including: Weak urinary steam

R39.13 **Splitting of urinary stream**

R39.14 **Feeling of incomplete bladder emptying**

R39.15 **Urgency of urination**
Excludes1:
urge incontinence (N39.41, N39.46)

R39.16 **Straining to void**

R39.19- **Other difficulties with micturition**

R39.191 **Need to immediately re-void**

R39.192 **Position dependent**

R39.198 **Other**

R39.2 **Extrarenal uremia**
Including: Prerenal
Excludes1:
uremia NOS (N19)

R39.8- **Other**

R39.81 **Functional urinary incontinence**
Including: due to cognitive impairment, or severe physical disability or immobility
Excludes1:
stress incontinence and other specified urinary incontinence (N39.3-N39.4-)
urinary incontinence NOS (R32)

R39.82 **Chronic bladder pain**

R39.89 **Other**

R39.9 **Unspecified**

SYMPTOMS AND SIGNS INVOLVING COGNITION, PERCEPTION, EMOTIONAL STATE AND BEHAVIOR (R4Ø-R46)

Excludes2:
symptoms and signs constituting part of a pattern of mental disorder (FØ1-F99)

R4Ø- SOMNOLENCE, STUPOR AND COMA
Excludes1:
neonatal coma (P91.5)
somnolence, stupor and coma in diabetes (EØ8-E13)
somnolence, stupor and coma in hepatic failure (K72.-)
somnolence, stupor and coma in hypoglycemia (nondiabetic) (E15)

R4Ø.Ø **Somnolence**
Including: Drowsiness
Excludes1:
coma (R4Ø.2-)

R4Ø.1 **Stupor**
Including: Catatonic, Semicoma
Excludes1:
catatonic schizophrenia (F2Ø.2)
coma (R4Ø.2-)
depressive stupor (F31-F33)
dissociative stupor (F44.2)
manic stupor (F3Ø.2)

R4Ø.2- **Coma**
Code First:
any associated:
fracture of skull (SØ2.-)
intracranial injury (SØ6.-)
Notes:
One code from each subcategory, R4Ø.21-R4Ø.23, is required to complete the coma scale
See Guidelines: *1;C.18.e*

R4Ø.2Ø **Unspecified**
Including: Coma NOS, Unconsciousness NOS
Indicator(s): *MCC | CMS22: 8Ø | CMS24: 8Ø | ESRD21: 8Ø | HHSØ5: 122 | HHSØ7: 122*

R4Ø.21- **Coma scale, eyes open**

The following appropriate 7th character is to be added to subcategory R4Ø.21-:
Ø - unspecified time
1 - in the field [EMT or ambulance]
2 - at arrival to emergency department
3 - at hospital admission
4 - 24 hours or more after hospital admission

Indicator(s): NoPDx/M

R4Ø.211_ Never
Including: Eye opening score of 1

R4Ø.212_ To pain
Including: Eye opening score of 2

R4Ø.213_ To sound
Including: Eye opening score of 3

R4Ø.214_ Spontaneous
Including: Eye opening score of 4

R4Ø.22- **Coma scale, best verbal response**

The following appropriate 7th character is to be added to subcategory R4Ø.22-:
Ø - unspecified time
1 - in the field [EMT or ambulance]
2 - at arrival to emergency department
3 - at hospital admission
4 - 24 hours or more after hospital admission

Indicator(s): NoPDx/M

R4Ø.221_ None
Including: Verbal score of 1

R4Ø.222_ Incomprehensible words
Coma scale verbal score of 2
Incomprehensible sounds (2-5 years of age)
Moans/grunts to pain; restless ([2 years old)

R4Ø.223_ Inappropriate words
Including: Verbal score of 3; Inappropriate crying or screaming (less than 2 years of age); Screaming (2-5 years of age)

R4Ø.224_ Confused conversation
Including: Verbal score of 4; Inappropriate words (2-5 years of age); Irritable cries (less than 2 years of age)

R4Ø.225_ Oriented
Including: Verbal score of 5; Cooing or babbling or crying appropriately (less than 2 years of age); Uses appropriate words (2-5 years of age)

R4Ø.23- **Coma scale, best motor response**

The following appropriate 7th character is to be added to subcategory R4Ø.23-:
Ø - unspecified time
1 - in the field [EMT or ambulance]
2 - at arrival to emergency department
3 - at hospital admission
4 - 24 hours or more after hospital admission

Indicator(s): NoPDx/M

R4Ø.231_ None
Including: Motor score of 1

R4Ø.232_ Extension
Including: Abnormal extensor posturing to pain or noxious stimuli (less than 2 years of age); Motor score of 2; Extensor posturing to pain or noxious stimuli (2-5 years of age)

R4Ø.233_ Abnormal flexion
Including: Abnormal flexure posturing to pain or noxious stimuli (Ø-5 years of age); Motor score of 3; Flexion/decorticate posturing (less than 2 years of age)

R4Ø.234_ Flexion withdrawal
Including: Motor score of 4; Withdraws from pain or noxious stimuli (2-5 years of age)

R4Ø.235_ Localizes pain
Including: Motor score of 5; Localizes pain (2-5 years of age); Withdraws to touch (less than 2 years of age)

R4Ø.236_ Obeys commands
Including: Motor scale of 6; Normal or spontaneous movement (less than 2 years of age); Obeys commands (2-5 years of age)

R4Ø.3 Persistent vegetative state
Indicator(s): CC | CMS22: 8Ø | CMS24: 8Ø | ESRD21: 8Ø | HHSØ5: 122 | HHSØ7: 122

R4Ø.4 Transient alteration of awareness

R41- OTHER SYMPTOMS AND SIGNS INVOLVING COGNITIVE FUNCTIONS AND AWARENESS

Excludes1:
dissociative [conversion] disorders (F44.-)
mild cognitive impairment, so stated (G31.84)

R41.Ø Disorientation, unspecified
Including: Confusion NOS, Delirium NOS
Indicator(s): DSM-5

R41.1 Anterograde amnesia

R41.2 Retrograde amnesia

R41.3 Other amnesia
Including: Amnesia NOS, Memory loss NOS
Excludes1:
amnestic disorder due to known physiologic condition (FØ4)
amnestic syndrome due to psychoactive substance use (F1Ø-F19 with 5th character .6)
mild memory disturbance due to known physiological condition (FØ6.8)
transient global amnesia (G45.4)

R41.4 Neurologic neglect syndrome
Including: Asomatognosia, Hemi-akinesia, Hemi-inattention, Hemispatial neglect, Left-sided neglect, Sensory neglect, Visuospatial neglect
Excludes1:
visuospatial deficit (R41.842)
Indicator(s): CC

R41.8- **Other symptoms and signs**

R41.81 Age-related cognitive decline
Including: Senility NOS
Indicator(s): Adult

R41.82 Altered mental status, unspecified
Including: Change in mental status NOS
Excludes1:
altered level of consciousness (R4Ø.-)
altered mental status due to known condition - code to condition
delirium NOS (R41.Ø)

R41.83 Borderline intellectual functioning
Including: IQ level 71 to 84
Excludes1:
intellectual disabilities (F7Ø-F79)
Indicator(s): NoPDx/M | DSM-5

R41.84- **Other specified cognitive deficit**

<u>*Excludes1:*</u>

cognitive deficits as sequelae of cerebrovascular disease (I69.Ø1-, I69.11-, I69.21-, I69.31-, I69.81-, I69.91-)

R41.84Ø Attention and concentration

<u>*Excludes1:*</u>

attention-deficit hyperactivity disorders (F9Ø.-)

R41.841 Cognitive communication

R41.842 Visuospatial

R41.843 Psychomotor

R41.844 Frontal lobe and executive function

R41.89 Other

Including: Anosognosia

R41.9 Unspecified

Including: Unspecified neurocognitive disorder

<u>*Indicator(s):*</u> *DSM-5*

R42 Dizziness and giddiness

Including: Light-headedness, Vertigo NOS

<u>*Excludes1:*</u>

vertiginous syndromes (H81.-)

vertigo from infrasound (T75.23)

R43- DISTURBANCES OF SMELL AND TASTE

R43.Ø Anosmia

R43.1 Parosmia

R43.2 Parageusia

R43.8 Other

Including: Mixed disturbance

R43.9 Unspecified

R44- OTHER SYMPTOMS AND SIGNS INVOLVING GENERAL SENSATIONS AND PERCEPTIONS

<u>*Excludes1:*</u>

alcoholic hallucinations (F1Ø.151, F1Ø.251, F1Ø.951)

hallucinations in drug psychosis (F11-F19 with fifth to sixth characters 51)

hallucinations in mood disorders with psychotic symptoms (F3Ø.2, F31.5, F32.3, F33.3)

hallucinations in schizophrenia, schizotypal and delusional disorders (F2Ø-F29)

<u>*Excludes2:*</u>

disturbances of skin sensation (R2Ø.-)

R44.Ø Auditory hallucinations

<u>*Indicator(s):*</u> *CC*

R44.1 Visual hallucinations

R44.2 Other hallucinations

<u>*Indicator(s):*</u> *CC*

R44.3 Hallucinations, unspecified

<u>*Indicator(s):*</u> *CC*

R44.8 Other

R44.9 Unspecified

R45- SYMPTOMS AND SIGNS INVOLVING EMOTIONAL STATE

R45.Ø Nervousness

Including: Nervous tension

R45.1 Restlessness and agitation

R45.2 Unhappiness

R45.3 Demoralization and apathy

<u>*Excludes1:*</u>

anhedonia (R45.84)

R45.4 Irritability and anger

R45.5 Hostility

R45.6 Violent behavior

R45.7 State of emotional shock and stress, unspecified

R45.8- **Other symptoms and signs**

R45.81 Low self-esteem

R45.82 Worries

R45.83 Excessive crying of child, adolescent or adult

<u>*Excludes1:*</u>

excessive crying of infant (baby) R68.11

R45.84 Anhedonia

R45.85- **Homicidal and suicidal ideations**

<u>*Excludes1:*</u>

suicide attempt (T14.91)

R45.85Ø Homicidal

<u>*Indicator(s):*</u> *NoPDx/M*

R45.851 Suicidal

<u>*Indicator(s):*</u> *CC*

R45.86 Emotional lability

R45.87 Impulsiveness

R45.89 Other

R46- SYMPTOMS AND SIGNS INVOLVING APPEARANCE AND BEHAVIOR

<u>*Excludes1:*</u>

appearance and behavior in schizophrenia, schizotypal and delusional disorders (F2Ø-F29)

mental and behavioral disorders (FØ1-F99)

R46.Ø Very low level of personal hygiene

R46.1 Bizarre personal appearance

R46.2 Strange and inexplicable behavior

R46.3 Overactivity

R46.4 Slowness and poor responsiveness

<u>*Excludes1:*</u>

stupor (R4Ø.1)

R46.5 Suspiciousness and marked evasiveness

R46.6 Undue concern and preoccupation with stressful events

R46.7 Verbosity and circumstantial detail obscuring reason for contact

R46.8- **Other symptoms and signs**

<u>*Indicator(s):*</u> *NoPDx/M*

R46.81 Obsessive-compulsive behavior

<u>*Excludes1:*</u>

obsessive-compulsive disorder (F42.-)

R46.89 Other

SYMPTOMS AND SIGNS INVOLVING SPEECH AND VOICE (R47-R49)

R47- SPEECH DISTURBANCES, NOT ELSEWHERE CLASSIFIED

Excludes1:
autism (F84.Ø)
cluttering (F8Ø.81)
specific developmental disorders of speech and language (F8Ø.-)
stuttering (F8Ø.81)

R47.Ø- **Dysphasia and aphasia**

R47.Ø1 **Aphasia**
Excludes1:
aphasia following cerebrovascular disease (I69. with final characters -2Ø)
progressive isolated aphasia (G31.Ø1)
Indicator(s): *CC*

R47.Ø2 **Dysphasia**
Excludes1:
dysphasia following cerebrovascular disease (I69. with final characters -21)

R47.1 **Dysarthria and anarthria**
Excludes1:
dysarthria following cerebrovascular disease (I69. with final characters -22)

R47.8- **Other speech disturbances**
Excludes1:
dysarthria following cerebrovascular disease (I69. with final characters -28)

R47.81 **Slurred**

R47.82 **Fluency disorder in conditions classified elsewhere**
Including: Stuttering
Code First:
underlying disease or condition, such as:
Parkinson's disease (G2Ø)
Excludes1:
adult onset fluency disorder (F98.5)
childhood onset fluency disorder (F8Ø.81)
fluency disorder (stuttering) following cerebrovascular disease (I69. with final characters -23)
Indicator(s): *Manifestation*

R47.89 **Other**

R47.9 **Unspecified**

R48- DYSLEXIA AND OTHER SYMBOLIC DYSFUNCTIONS, NOT ELSEWHERE CLASSIFIED

Excludes1:
specific developmental disorders of scholastic skills (F81.-)

R48.Ø **Dyslexia and alexia**

R48.1 **Agnosia**
Including: Astereognosia (astereognosis), Autotopagnosia
Excludes1:
visual object agnosia (R48.3)

R48.2 **Apraxia**
Excludes1:
apraxia following cerebrovascular disease (I69. with final characters -9Ø)

R48.3 **Visual agnosia**
Including: Prosopagnosia, Simultanagnosia (asimultagnosia)

R48.8 **Other**
Including: Acalculia, Agraphia

R48.9 **Unspecified**

R49- VOICE AND RESONANCE DISORDERS

Excludes1:
psychogenic voice and resonance disorders (F44.4)

R49.Ø **Dysphonia**
Including: Hoarseness

R49.1 **Aphonia**
Including: Loss of voice

R49.2- **Hypernasality and hyponasality**

R49.21 **Hypernasality**

R49.22 **Hyponasality**

R49.8 **Other**

R49.9 **Unspecified**
Including: Change in voice NOS, Resonance disorder NOS

GENERAL SYMPTOMS AND SIGNS (R5Ø-R69)

R5Ø- FEVER OF OTHER AND UNKNOWN ORIGIN

Excludes1:
chills without fever (R68.83)
febrile convulsions (R56.Ø-)
fever of unknown origin during labor (O75.2)
fever of unknown origin in newborn (P81.9)
hypothermia due to illness (R68.Ø)
malignant hyperthermia due to anesthesia (T88.3)
puerperal pyrexia NOS (O86.4)

R5Ø.2 **Drug induced fever**
Use additional *code for adverse effect, if applicable, to identify drug (T36-T5Ø with fifth or sixth character 5)*
Excludes1:
postvaccination (postimmunization) fever (R5Ø.83)

R5Ø.8- **Other specified fever**

R5Ø.81 **Fever presenting with conditions classified elsewhere**
Code First:
underlying condition when associated fever is present, such as with:
leukemia (C91-C95)
neutropenia (D7Ø.-)
sickle-cell disease (D57.-)
Indicator(s): *Manifestation*

R5Ø.82 **Postprocedural fever**
Excludes1:
postprocedural infection (T81.4-)
posttransfusion fever (R5Ø.84)
postvaccination (postimmunization) fever (R5Ø.83)

R5Ø.83 **Postvaccination fever**
Including: Postimmunization fever

R5Ø.84 **Febrile nonhemolytic transfusion reaction**
Including: FNHTR, Posttransfusion fever

R5Ø.9 **Unspecified**
Including: Fever NOS, Fever of unknown origin [FUO], Fever with chills, Fever with rigors, Hyperpyrexia NOS, Persistent fever, Pyrexia NOS

R51- HEADACHE
Including: Facial pain NOS
Excludes1:
atypical face pain (G5Ø.1)
migraine and other headache syndromes (G43-G44)
trigeminal neuralgia (G5Ø.Ø)

R51.Ø With orthostatic component, not elsewhere classified
Including: positional

R51.9 Unspecified
Including: Facial pain NOS

R52 Pain, unspecified
Including: Acute NOS, Generalized NOS, Pain NOS
Excludes1:
acute and chronic pain, not elsewhere classified (G89.-)
localized pain, unspecified type - code to pain by site, such as:
abdomen pain (R1Ø.-)
back pain (M54.9)
breast pain (N64.4)
chest pain (RØ7.1-RØ7.9)
ear pain (H92.Ø-)
eye pain (H57.1)
headache (R51.9)
joint pain (M25.5-)
limb pain (M79.6-)
lumbar region pain (M54.5-)
pelvic and perineal pain (R1Ø.2)
shoulder pain (M25.51-)
spine pain (M54.-)
throat pain (RØ7.Ø)
tongue pain (K14.6)
tooth pain (KØ8.8)
renal colic (N23)
pain disorders exclusively related to psychological factors (F45.41)

R53- MALAISE AND FATIGUE

R53.Ø Neoplastic (malignant) related fatigue
Code First:
associated neoplasm

R53.1 Weakness
Including: Asthenia NOS
Excludes1:
age-related weakness (R54)
muscle weakness (generalized) (M62.81)
sarcopenia (M62.84)
senile asthenia (R54)

R53.2 Functional quadriplegia
Including: Complete immobility due to severe physical disability or frailty
Excludes1:
frailty NOS (R54)
hysterical paralysis (F44.4)
immobility syndrome (M62.3)
neurologic quadriplegia (G82.5-)
quadriplegia (G82.5Ø)
See Guidelines: *1;C.18.f*
Indicator(s): *MCC | CMS22: 7Ø | CMS24: 7Ø | ESRD21: 7Ø | HHSØ5: 1Ø7 | HHSØ7: 1Ø7*

R53.8- **Other malaise and fatigue**
Excludes1:
combat exhaustion and fatigue (F43.Ø)
congenital debility (P96.9)
exhaustion and fatigue due to excessive exertion (T73.3)
exhaustion and fatigue due to exposure (T73.2)
exhaustion and fatigue due to heat (T67.-)
exhaustion and fatigue due to pregnancy (O26.8-)
exhaustion and fatigue due to recurrent depressive episode (F33)
exhaustion and fatigue due to senile debility (R54)

R53.81 Other malaise
Including: Chronic debility, Debility NOS, General physical deterioration, Malaise NOS, Nervous debility
Excludes1:
age-related physical debility (R54)

R **R53.82 Chronic fatigue, unspecified**
Including: Chronic fatigue syndrome NOS

R53.83 Other fatigue
Including: Fatigue NOS, Lack of energy, Lethargy, Tiredness
Excludes2:
exhaustion and fatigue due to depressive episode (F32.-)

R54 Age-related physical debility
Including: Frailty, Old age, Senescence, Senile asthenia, Senile debility
Excludes1:
age-related cognitive decline (R41.81)
sarcopenia (M62.84)
senile psychosis (FØ3)
senility NOS (R41.81)
Indicator(s): *Adult*

R55 Syncope and collapse
Including: Blackout, Fainting, Vasovagal attack
Excludes1:
cardiogenic shock (R57.Ø)
carotid sinus syncope (G9Ø.Ø1)
heat syncope (T67.1)
neurocirculatory asthenia (F45.8)
neurogenic orthostatic hypotension (G9Ø.3)
orthostatic hypotension (I95.1)
postprocedural shock (T81.1-)
psychogenic syncope (F48.8)
shock NOS (R57.9)
shock complicating or following abortion or ectopic or molar pregnancy (OØØ-OØ7, OØ8.3)
shock complicating or following labor and delivery (O75.1)
Stokes-Adams attack (I45.9)
unconsciousness NOS (R4Ø.2-)

R56- CONVULSIONS, NOT ELSEWHERE CLASSIFIED
Excludes1:
dissociative convulsions and seizures (F44.5)
epileptic convulsions and seizures (G4Ø.-)
newborn convulsions and seizures (P9Ø)
Indicator(s): *CMS22: 79 | CMS24: 79 | RxØ5: 165 | ESRD21: 79 | HHSØ5: 12Ø | HHSØ7: 12Ø*

R56.Ø- **Febrile convulsions**
Indicator(s): *CC*

R56.ØØ Simple
Including: Febrile convulsion NOS, Febrile seizure NOS

R56.Ø1 Complex
Including: Atypical febrile seizure, Complex febrile seizure, Complicated febrile seizure
Excludes1:
status epilepticus (G4Ø.9Ø1)

Ch5

5. The Tabular List

R56.1 **Post traumatic seizures**
Excludes1:
post traumatic epilepsy (G4Ø.-)
Indicator(s): CC

R56.9 **Unspecified**
Including: Convulsion disorder, Fit NOS, Recurrent convulsions, Seizure(s) (convulsive) NOS

R57- SHOCK, NOT ELSEWHERE CLASSIFIED
Excludes1:
anaphylactic shock NOS (T78.2)
anaphylactic reaction or shock due to adverse food reaction (T78.Ø-)
anaphylactic shock due to adverse effect of correct drug or medicament properly administered (T88.6)
anaphylactic shock due to serum (T8Ø.5-)
electric shock (T75.4)
obstetric shock (O75.1)
postprocedural shock (T81.1-)
psychic shock (F43.Ø)
shock complicating or following ectopic or molar pregnancy (OØØ-OØ7, OØ8.3)
shock due to anesthesia (T88.2)
shock due to lightning (T75.Ø1)
traumatic shock (T79.4)
toxic shock syndrome (A48.3)

R57.Ø **Cardiogenic**
Excludes2:
septic shock (R65.21)
Indicator(s): MCC | CMS22: 84 | CMS24: 84 | ESRD21: 84 | HHSØ5: 127 | HHSØ7: 127

R57.1 **Hypovolemic**
Indicator(s): MCC | CMS22: 2 | CMS24: 2 | ESRD21: 2 | HHSØ5: 2 | HHSØ7: 2

R57.8 **Other**
Indicator(s): MCC | CMS22: 2 | CMS24: 2 | ESRD21: 2 | HHSØ5: 2 | HHSØ7: 2

R57.9 **Unspecified**
Including: Failure of peripheral circulation NOS
Indicator(s): CC | CMS22: 84 | CMS24: 84 | ESRD21: 84 | HHSØ5: 127 | HHSØ7: 127

R58 **Hemorrhage, not elsewhere classified**
Including: Hemorrhage NOS
Excludes1:
hemorrhage included with underlying conditions, such as:
acute duodenal ulcer with hemorrhage (K26.Ø)
acute gastritis with bleeding (K29.Ø1)
ulcerative enterocolitis with rectal bleeding (K51.Ø1)

R59- ENLARGED LYMPH NODES
Includes:
swollen glands
Excludes1:
lymphadenitis NOS (I88.9)
acute lymphadenitis (LØ4.-)
chronic lymphadenitis (I88.1)
mesenteric (acute) (chronic) lymphadenitis (I88.Ø)

R59.Ø **Localized**

R59.1 **Generalized**
Including: Lymphadenopathy NOS

R59.9 **Unspecified**

R6Ø- EDEMA, NOT ELSEWHERE CLASSIFIED
Excludes1:
angioneurotic edema (T78.3)
ascites (R18.-)
cerebral edema (G93.6)
cerebral edema due to birth injury (P11.Ø)
edema of larynx (J38.4)
edema of nasopharynx (J39.2)
edema of pharynx (J39.2)
gestational edema (O12.Ø-)
hereditary edema (Q82.Ø)
hydrops fetalis NOS (P83.2)
hydrothorax (J94.8)
newborn edema (P83.3)
pulmonary edema (J81.-)

R6Ø.Ø **Localized**

R6Ø.1 **Generalized**
Excludes2:
nutritional edema (E4Ø-E46)

R6Ø.9 **Unspecified**
Including: Fluid retention NOS

R61 **Generalized hyperhidrosis**
Including: Excessive sweating, Night sweats, Secondary hyperhidrosis
Code First:
if applicable, menopausal and female climacteric states (N95.1)
Excludes1:
focal (primary) (secondary) hyperhidrosis (L74.5-)
Frey's syndrome (L74.52)
localized (primary) (secondary) hyperhidrosis (L74.5-)

R62- LACK OF EXPECTED NORMAL PHYSIOLOGICAL DEVELOPMENT IN CHILDHOOD AND ADULTS
Excludes1:
delayed puberty (E3Ø.Ø)
gonadal dysgenesis (Q99.1)
hypopituitarism (E23.Ø)

R62.Ø **Delayed milestone in childhood**
Including: Delayed attainment of expected physiological developmental stage, Late talker, Late walker
Indicator(s): Pediatric

R62.5- **Other and unspecified**
Excludes1:
HIV disease resulting in failure to thrive (B2Ø)
physical retardation due to malnutrition (E45)

R62.5Ø **Unspecified**
Including: Infantilism NOS

R62.51 **Failure to thrive (child)**
Including: Failure to gain weight
Excludes1:
failure to thrive in child under 28 days old (P92.6)
Indicator(s): Pediatric

R **R62.52** **Short stature (child)**
Including: Lack of growth, Physical retardation, Short stature NOS
Excludes1:
short stature due to endocrine disorder (E34.3-)

R62.59 **Other**

R62.7 **Adult failure to thrive**
Indicator(s): Adult

Ch5

5. The Tabular List

R63- SYMPTOMS AND SIGNS CONCERNING FOOD AND FLUID INTAKE

Excludes1:
bulimia NOS (F5Ø.2)

R63.Ø Anorexia
Including: Loss of appetite
Excludes1:
anorexia nervosa (F5Ø.Ø-)
loss of appetite of nonorganic origin (F5Ø.89)

R63.1 Polydipsia
Including: Excessive thirst

R63.2 Polyphagia
Including: Excessive eating, Hyperalimentation NOS

R63.4 Abnormal weight loss

R63.5 Abnormal weight gain
Excludes1:
excessive weight gain in pregnancy (O26.Ø-)
obesity (E66.-)

R63.6 Underweight
Use additional code to identify body mass index (BMI), if known (Z68.-)
Excludes1:
abnormal weight loss (R63.4)
anorexia nervosa (F5Ø.Ø-)
malnutrition (E4Ø-E46)

R63.8 Other

R64 Cachexia
Including: Wasting syndrome
Code First:
underlying condition, if known
Excludes1:
abnormal weight loss (R63.4)
nutritional marasmus (E41)
Indicator(s): CC | CMS22: 21 | CMS24: 21 | ESRD21: 21 | HHSØ5: 23 | HHSØ7: 23

R65- SYMPTOMS AND SIGNS SPECIFICALLY ASSOCIATED WITH SYSTEMIC INFLAMMATION AND INFECTION

See Guidelines: 1;C.1.d.6 | 1;C.1.d
Indicator(s): NoPDx/M | CMS22: 2 | CMS24: 2 | ESRD21: 2 | HHSØ5: 2 | HHSØ7: 2

R65.1- **Systemic inflammatory response syndrome (SIRS) of non-infectious origin**
Code First:
underlying condition, such as:
heatstroke (T67.Ø-)
injury and trauma (SØØ-T88)
Excludes1:
sepsis- code to infection
severe sepsis (R65.2)
See Guidelines: 1;C.1.d.6

R65.1Ø Without acute organ dysfunction
Including: Systemic inflammatory response syndrome (SIRS) NOS
See Guidelines: 1;C.18.g
Indicator(s): CC

R65.11 With acute organ dysfunction
Use additional code to identify specific acute organ dysfunction, such as:
acute kidney failure (N17.-)
acute respiratory failure (J96.Ø-)
critical illness myopathy (G72.81)
critical illness polyneuropathy (G62.81)
disseminated intravascular coagulopathy [DIC] (D65)
encephalopathy (metabolic) (septic) (G93.41)
hepatic failure (K72.Ø-)
See Guidelines: 1;C.18.g
Indicator(s): MCC

R65.2- **Severe sepsis**
Including: Infection with associated acute organ dysfunction, Sepsis with acute organ dysfunction, Sepsis with multiple organ dysfunction, Systemic inflammatory response syndrome due to infectious process with acute organ dysfunction
Code First:
underlying infection, such as:
infection following a procedure (T81.4-)
infections following infusion, transfusion and therapeutic injection (T8Ø.2-)
puerperal sepsis (O85)
sepsis following complete or unspecified spontaneous abortion (OØ3.87)
sepsis following ectopic and molar pregnancy (OØ8.82)
sepsis following incomplete spontaneous abortion (OØ3.37)
sepsis following (induced) termination of pregnancy (OØ4.87)
sepsis NOS (A41.9)
Use additional code to identify specific acute organ dysfunction, such as:
acute kidney failure (N17.-)
acute respiratory failure (J96.Ø-)
critical illness myopathy (G72.81)
critical illness polyneuropathy (G62.81)
disseminated intravascular coagulopathy [DIC] (D65)
encephalopathy (metabolic) (septic) (G93.41)
hepatic failure (K72.Ø-)
See Guidelines: 1;C.1.d.5.b-c | 1;C.1.d | 1;C.1.d.1.a-b | 1;C.1.d.3-4 | 1;C.1.d.5 | 1;C.1.d.6 | 1;C.15.j | 1;C.15.j-k | 1;C.16.f
Indicator(s): MCC

R65.2Ø Without septic shock
Including: Severe sepsis NOS
See Guidelines: 1;C.1.d.5.c

R65.21 With septic shock
See Guidelines: 1;C.1.d.2 | 1;C.1.d.2.a

R68- OTHER GENERAL SYMPTOMS AND SIGNS

R68.Ø Hypothermia, not associated with low environmental temperature
Excludes1:
hypothermia NOS (accidental) (T68)
hypothermia due to anesthesia (T88.51)
hypothermia due to low environmental temperature (T68)
newborn hypothermia (P8Ø.-)

R68.1- **Nonspecific symptoms peculiar to infancy**
Excludes1:
colic, infantile (R1Ø.83)
neonatal cerebral irritability (P91.3)
teething syndrome (KØØ.7)

R68.11 Excessive crying of infant (baby)
Excludes1:
excessive crying of child, adolescent, or adult (R45.83)
Indicator(s): Pediatric

R68.12 Fussy infant (baby)
Including: Irritable infant
Indicator(s): Pediatric

R68.13 **Apparent life threatening event in infant (ALTE)**
Including: Apparent life threatening event in newborn, Brief resolved unexplained event (BRUE)
Code First:
confirmed diagnosis, if known
Use additional code(s) for associated signs and symptoms if no confirmed diagnosis established, or if signs and symptoms are not associated routinely with confirmed diagnosis, or provide additional information for cause of ALTE
Indicator(s): Pediatric

R68.19 **Other**
Indicator(s): Pediatric

R68.2 **Dry mouth, unspecified**
Excludes1:
dry mouth due to dehydration (E86.Ø)
dry mouth due to Sjögren syndrome (M35.Ø-)
salivary gland hyposecretion (K11.7)

R68.3 **Clubbing of fingers**
Including: Clubbing of nails
Excludes1:
congenital clubfinger (Q68.1)

R68.8- **Other general symptoms and signs**

R68.81 **Early satiety**

R68.82 **Decreased libido**
Including: Decreased sexual desire
Indicator(s): Adult

R68.83 **Chills (without fever)**
Including: Chills NOS
Excludes1:
chills with fever (R5Ø.9)

R68.84 **Jaw pain**
Including: Mandibular, Maxilla pain
Excludes1:
temporomandibular joint arthralgia (M26.62-)

R68.89 **Other**

R69 **Illness, unspecified**
Including: Unknown and unspecified cases of morbidity

ABNORMAL FINDINGS ON EXAMINATION OF BLOOD, WITHOUT DIAGNOSIS (R7Ø-R79)

Excludes2:
abnormal findings on antenatal screening of mother (O28.-)
abnormalities of lipids (E78.-)
abnormalities of platelets and thrombocytes (D69.-)
abnormalities of white blood cells classified elsewhere (D7Ø-D72)
coagulation hemorrhagic disorders (D65-D68)
diagnostic abnormal findings classified elsewhere - see Alphabetical Index
hemorrhagic and hematological disorders of newborn (P5Ø-P61)

R73- ELEVATED BLOOD GLUCOSE LEVEL

Excludes1:
diabetes mellitus (EØ8-E13)
diabetes mellitus in pregnancy, childbirth and the puerperium (O24.-)
neonatal disorders (P7Ø.Ø-P7Ø.2)
postsurgical hypoinsulinemia (E89.1)

R73.9 **Hyperglycemia, unspecified**

ABNORMAL FINDINGS ON EXAMINATION OF URINE, WITHOUT DIAGNOSIS (R8Ø-R82)

Excludes1:
abnormal findings on antenatal screening of mother (O28.-)
diagnostic abnormal findings classified elsewhere - see Alphabetical Index
specific findings indicating disorder of amino-acid metabolism (E7Ø-E72)
specific findings indicating disorder of carbohydrate metabolism (E73-E74)

R8Ø- PROTEINURIA

Excludes1:
gestational proteinuria (O12.1-)

R8Ø.Ø **Isolated**
Including: Idiopathic proteinuria
Excludes1:
isolated proteinuria with specific morphological lesion (NØ6.-)

R8Ø.1 **Persistent proteinuria, unspecified**

R8Ø.2 **Orthostatic proteinuria, unspecified**
Including: Postural proteinuria

R8Ø.3 **Bence Jones**

R8Ø.8 **Other**

R8Ø.9 **Unspecified**
Including: Albuminuria NOS

R81 **Glycosuria**
Excludes1:
renal glycosuria (E74.818)

R82- OTHER AND UNSPECIFIED ABNORMAL FINDINGS IN URINE

Includes:
chromoabnormalities in urine
Use additional code to identify any retained foreign body, if applicable (Z18.-)
Excludes2:
hematuria (R31.-)

R82.Ø **Chyluria**
Excludes1:
filarial chyluria (B74.-)
Indicator(s): CC

R82.1 **Myoglobinuria**
Indicator(s): CC

R82.2 **Biliuria**

R82.3 **Hemoglobinuria**
Excludes1:
hemoglobinuria due to hemolysis from external causes NEC (D59.6)
hemoglobinuria due to paroxysmal nocturnal [Marchiafava-Micheli] (D59.5)

R82.4 **Acetonuria**
Including: Ketonuria

R82.5 **Elevated urine levels of drugs, medicaments and biological substances**
Including: Elevated urine levels of catecholamines, indoleacetic acid, 17-ketosteroids, or steroids

R82.6 **Abnormal levels of substances chiefly nonmedicinal as to source**
Including: Abnormal urine level of heavy metals

 See Appendix A — Coding Reference Tables for lists of the ICD-10-CM Tabular indicators, HAC categories, and HCC codes.

R82.7- **Abnormal findings on microbiological examination of urine**
Including: Positive culture findings of urine
Excludes1:
colonization status (Z22.-)

R82.71 Bacteriuria

R82.79 Other
Including: Positive culture findings

R82.9- **Other and unspecified**

R82.90 Unspecified

R82.91 Chromoabnormalities
Including: Chromoconversion (dipstick), Idiopathic dipstick converts positive for blood with no cellular forms in sediment
Excludes1:
hemoglobinuria (R82.3)
myoglobinuria (R82.1)

ABNORMAL FINDINGS ON DIAGNOSTIC IMAGING AND IN FUNCTION STUDIES, WITHOUT DIAGNOSIS (R90-R94)

Includes:
nonspecific abnormal findings on diagnostic imaging by computerized axial tomography [CAT scan]
nonspecific abnormal findings on diagnostic imaging by magnetic resonance imaging [MRI][NMR]
nonspecific abnormal findings on diagnostic imaging by positron emission tomography [PET scan]
nonspecific abnormal findings on diagnostic imaging by thermography
nonspecific abnormal findings on diagnostic imaging by ultrasound [echogram]
nonspecific abnormal findings on diagnostic imaging by X-ray examination
Excludes1:
abnormal findings on antenatal screening of mother (O28.-)
diagnostic abnormal findings classified elsewhere - see Alphabetical Index

R90- ABNORMAL FINDINGS ON DIAGNOSTIC IMAGING OF CENTRAL NERVOUS SYSTEM

R90.0 Intracranial space-occupying lesion found on diagnostic imaging

R90.8- **Other abnormal findings**

R90.89 Other
Including: Other cerebrovascular abnormality found

R91- ABNORMAL FINDINGS ON DIAGNOSTIC IMAGING OF LUNG

R91.1 Solitary pulmonary nodule
Including: Coin lesion lung; subsegmental branch of the bronchial tree

R91.8 Other nonspecific abnormal finding of lung field
Including: Lung mass NOS found on diagnostic imaging of lung; Pulmonary infiltrate NOS; Shadow, lung

R93- ABNORMAL FINDINGS ON DIAGNOSTIC IMAGING OF OTHER BODY STRUCTURES

R93.0 Skull and head, NEC
Excludes1:
intracranial space-occupying lesion found on diagnostic imaging (R90.0)

R93.6 Limbs
Excludes2:
abnormal finding in skin and subcutaneous tissue (R93.8-)

R93.7 Other parts of musculoskeletal system
Excludes2:
abnormal findings on diagnostic imaging of skull (R93.0)

R93.9 Diagnostic imaging inconclusive due to excess body fat of patient

R94- ABNORMAL RESULTS OF FUNCTION STUDIES
Includes:
abnormal results of radionuclide [radioisotope] uptake studies
abnormal results of scintigraphy

R94.1- **Peripheral nervous system and special senses**

R94.13- **Of peripheral nervous system**

R94.130 Response to nerve stimulation, unspecified

R94.131 Electromyogram [EMG]
Excludes1:
electromyogram of eye (R94.113)

R94.138 Other study

R94.2 Pulmonary study
Including: Reduced ventilatory capacity, vital capacity

R94.3- **Cardiovascular**

R94.31 Electrocardiogram [ECG] [EKG]
Excludes1:
long QT syndrome (I45.81)

R99 ILL-DEFINED AND UNKNOWN CAUSE OF MORTALITY (R99) (R99-R99)

R99 Ill-defined and unknown cause of mortality
Including: Death (unexplained) NOS, Unspecified cause of mortality
See Guidelines: 1;C.18.h

19. Injury, poisoning and certain other consequences of external causes (SØØ-T88)

Notes:
Use secondary code(s) from Chapter 2Ø, External causes of morbidity, to indicate cause of injury. Codes within the T section that include the external cause do not require an additional external cause code
Use additional code to identify any retained foreign body, if applicable (Z18.-)
Excludes1:
birth trauma (P1Ø-P15)
obstetric trauma (O7Ø-O71)
Notes:
The chapter uses the S-section for coding different types of injuries related to single body regions and the T-section to cover injuries to unspecified body regions as well as poisoning and certain other consequences of external causes.
See Guidelines: *1;C.15.m | 1;C.19.a-b | 1;C.2Ø.a.1*

INJURIES TO THE HEAD (SØØ-SØ9)

Includes:
injuries of ear
injuries of eye
injuries of face [any part]
injuries of gum
injuries of jaw
injuries of oral cavity
injuries of palate
injuries of periocular area
injuries of scalp
injuries of temporomandibular joint area
injuries of tongue
injuries of tooth
Code Also
for any associated infection
Excludes2:
burns and corrosions (T2Ø-T32)
effects of foreign body in ear (T16)
effects of foreign body in larynx (T17.3)
effects of foreign body in mouth NOS (T18.Ø)
effects of foreign body in nose (T17.Ø-T17.1)
effects of foreign body in pharynx (T17.2)
effects of foreign body on external eye (T15.-)
frostbite (T33-T34)
insect bite or sting, venomous (T63.4)
See Guidelines: *1;C.19.b*

SØØ- SUPERFICIAL INJURY OF HEAD

Excludes1:
diffuse cerebral contusion (SØ6.2-)
focal cerebral contusion (SØ6.3-)
injury of eye and orbit (SØ5.-)
open wound of head (SØ1.-)

The appropriate 7th character is to be added to each code from category SØØ
A - initial encounter
D - subsequent encounter
S - sequela

Indicator(s): *POAEx (7th D/S)*

SØØ.Ø- **Superficial injury of scalp**
SØØ.Ø3x_ Contusion
Including: Bruise, Hematoma

SØØ.1- **Contusion of eyelid and periocular area**
Including: Black eye
Excludes2:
contusion of eyeball and orbital tissues (SØ5.1-)
SØØ.1Øx_ Unspecified side
SØØ.11x_ Right side
SØØ.12x_ Left side

SØØ.3- **Superficial injury of nose**
SØØ.33x_ Contusion
Including: Bruise, Hematoma

SØØ.4- **Superficial injury of ear**
SØØ.43- **Contusion**
Including: Bruise, Hematoma
SØØ.431_ Right
SØØ.432_ Left

SØØ.5- **Superficial injury of lip and oral cavity**
SØØ.53- **Contusion**
SØØ.531_ Lip
Including: Bruise, Hematoma
SØØ.532_ Oral cavity
Including: Bruise, Hematoma

SØØ.8- **Superficial injury of other parts of head**
Including: Superficial injuries of face [any part]
SØØ.83x_ Contusion
Including: Bruise, Hematoma

SØØ.9- **Unspecified part of head**
SØØ.93x_ Contusion
Including: Bruise, Hematoma

SØ2- FRACTURE OF SKULL AND FACIAL BONES

Notes:
A fracture not indicated as open or closed should be coded to closed
Code Also
any associated intracranial injury (SØ6.-)

The appropriate 7th character is to be added to each code from category SØ2
A - initial encounter for closed fracture
B - initial encounter for open fracture
D - subsequent encounter for fracture with routine healing
G - subsequent encounter for fracture with delayed healing
K - subsequent encounter for fracture with nonunion
S - sequela

See Guidelines: *1;C.18.e | 1;C.19.c*

SØ2.Øxx_ Vault of skull
Including: Frontal bone, parietal bone

SØ2.1- **Fracture of base of skull**
Excludes2:
lateral orbital wall (SØ2.84-)
medial orbital wall (SØ2.83-)
orbital floor (SØ2.3-)
Indicator(s): *CC (7th A/K) | MCC (7th B) | CMS24: 167 (7th A/B/S)*

SØ2.1Ø- **Unspecified fracture**
Indicator(s): *POAEx (7th D/G/K/S) | HAC: Ø5 (7th A/B)*
SØ2.1Ø1_ Right side
SØ2.1Ø2_ Left side
SØ2.1Ø9_ Unspecified side

 See Appendix A — Coding Reference Tables for lists of the ICD-10-CM Tabular indicators, HAC categories, and HCC codes.

S02.11- **Fracture of occiput**
Indicator(s): HAC: 05 (7th A/B)

S02.110_ Type I occipital condyle
S02.111_ Type II occipital condyle
S02.112_ Type III occipital condyle
S02.113_ Unspecified occipital condyle
S02.118_ Other
S02.119_ Unspecified
S02.11A_ Type I occipital condyle fracture, right side
S02.11B_ Type I occipital condyle fracture, left side
S02.11C_ Type II occipital condyle fracture, right side
S02.11D_ Type II occipital condyle fracture, left side
S02.11E_ Type III occipital condyle fracture, right side
S02.11F_ Type III occipital condyle fracture, left side
S02.11G_ Other fracture of occiput, right side
S02.11H_ Other fracture of occiput, left side

S02.12- **Fracture of orbital roof**
Indicator(s): POAEx (7th D/G/K/S) | HAC: 05 (7th A/B/K)

S02.121_ Right side
S02.122_ Left side
S02.129_ Unspecified side

S02.19x_ Other fracture
Including: Anterior fossa, ethmoid sinus, frontal sinus, middle fossa, posterior fossa, sphenoid, temporal bone

S02.2xx_ Nasal bones

S02.3- **Fracture of orbital floor**
Including: Inferior orbital wall
Excludes1:
orbit NOS (S02.85)
Excludes2:
lateral orbital wall (S02.84-)
medial orbital wall (S02.83-)
orbital roof (S02.1-)
Indicator(s): CC (7th A/B/K) | POAEx (7th D/G/K/S) | HAC: 05 (7th A/B) | CMS22: 167 (7th A/B/S) | CMS24: 167 (7th A/B/S) | ESRD21: 167 (7th A/B/S)

S02.30x_ Unspecified side
S02.31x_ Right side
S02.32x_ Left side

S02.4- **Fracture of malar, maxillary and zygoma bones**
Including: Superior maxilla, upper jaw (bone), zygomatic process of temporal bone
Indicator(s): CC (7th A/B/K) | POAEx (7th D/G/K/S) | HAC: 05 (7th A/B) | CMS22: 167 (7th A/B/S) | CMS24: 167 (7th A/B/S)

S02.40- **Fracture of malar, maxillary and zygoma bones, unspecified**

S02.400_ Malar fracture unspecified
S02.401_ Maxillary fracture, unspecified
S02.402_ Zygomatic
S02.40A_ Malar fracture, right side
S02.40B_ Malar fracture, left side
S02.40C_ Maxillary fracture, right side
S02.40D_ Maxillary fracture, left side
S02.40E_ Zygomatic fracture, right side
S02.40F_ Zygomatic fracture, left side

S02.41- **LeFort fracture**

S02.411_ LeFort I fracture
S02.412_ LeFort II fracture
S02.413_ LeFort III fracture

S02.42x_ Fracture of alveolus of maxilla

S02.5xx_ Tooth (traumatic)
Including: Broken tooth
Excludes1:
cracked tooth (nontraumatic) (K03.81)

S02.6- **Fracture of mandible**
Including: Lower jaw (bone)
Indicator(s): CC (7th A/B/K) | POAEx (7th D/G/K/S) | HAC: 05 (7th A/B) | CMS22: 167 (7th A/B/S) | CMS24: 167 (7th A/B/S)

S02.60- **Fracture of mandible, unspecified**

S02.600_ Unspecified part of body of mandible
S02.601_ Fracture of unspecified part of body of right mandible
S02.602_ Unspecified part of body of left mandible
S02.609_ Unspecified

S02.61- **Condylar process**

S02.610_ Unspecified side
S02.611_ Right
S02.612_ Left

S02.62- **Subcondylar process**

S02.620_ Unspecified side
S02.621_ Right
S02.622_ Left

S02.63- **Coronoid process**

S02.630_ Unspecified side
S02.631_ Right
S02.632_ Left

S02.64- **Ramus**

S02.640_ Unspecified side
S02.641_ Right
S02.642_ Left

S02.65- **Angle**

S02.650_ Unspecified side
S02.651_ Right
S02.652_ Left

S02.66x_ Symphysis

S02.67- **Alveolus**

S02.670_ Unspecified side
S02.671_ Right
S02.672_ Left

S02.69x_ Other specified site

S02.8- **Fractures of other specified skull and facial bones**
Including: Palate
Excludes2:
fracture of orbital floor (S02.3-)
fracture of orbital roof (S02.12-)
Indicator(s): CC (7th A/B/K) | POAEx (7th D/G/K/S) | CMS24: 167 (7th A/B/S) | ESRD21: 167 (7th A/B/S)

S02.80x_ Unspecified side
S02.81x_ Other specified skull and facial bones, right side
S02.82x_ Other specified skull and facial bones, left side

SØ2.83- **Fracture of medial orbital wall**
Excludes2:
orbital floor (SØ2.3-)
orbital roof (SØ2.12-)
Indicator(s): HAC: Ø5 (7th A/B/K)

SØ2.831_ Right side
SØ2.832_ Left side
SØ2.839_ Unspecified side

SØ2.84- **Fracture of lateral orbital wall**
Excludes2:
orbital floor (SØ2.3-)
orbital roof (SØ2.12-)
Indicator(s): HAC: Ø5 (7th A/B/K)

SØ2.841_ Right side
SØ2.842_ Left side
SØ2.849_ Unspecified side

SØ2.85x_ Fracture of orbit, unspecified
Including: Fracture of orbit NOS, orbit wall NOS
Excludes1:
lateral orbital wall (SØ2.84-)
medial orbital wall (SØ2.83-)
orbital floor (SØ2.3-)
orbital roof (SØ2.12-)

SØ2.9- **Fracture of unspecified skull and facial bones**
Indicator(s): POAEx (7th D/G/K/S) | HAC: Ø5 (7th A/B) | CMS22: 167 (7th A/B/S) | CMS24: 167 (7th A/B/S) | ESRD21: 167 (7th A/B/S)

SØ2.91x_ Skull
SØ2.92x_ Facial bones

SØ3- DISLOCATION AND SPRAIN OF JOINTS AND LIGAMENTS OF HEAD

Includes:
avulsion of joint (capsule) or ligament of head
laceration of cartilage, joint (capsule) or ligament of head
sprain of cartilage, joint (capsule) or ligament of head
traumatic hemarthrosis of joint or ligament of head
traumatic rupture of joint or ligament of head
traumatic subluxation of joint or ligament of head
traumatic tear of joint or ligament of head
Code Also
any associated open wound
Excludes2:
Strain of muscle or tendon of head (SØ9.1)
The appropriate 7th character is to be added to each code from category SØ3
A - initial encounter
D - subsequent encounter
S - sequela
Indicator(s): POAEx (7th D/S)

SØ3.Ø- **Dislocation of jaw**
Including: Jaw (cartilage) (meniscus), mandible, temporomandibular (joint)

SØ3.ØØx_ Unspecified side
SØ3.Ø1x_ Right side
SØ3.Ø2x_ Left side
SØ3.Ø3x_ Bilateral

SØ3.1xx_ Dislocation of septal cartilage of nose
SØ3.2xx_ Dislocation of tooth

SØ3.4- **Sprain of jaw**
Including: Temporomandibular (joint) (ligament)

SØ3.4Øx_ Unspecified side
SØ3.41x_ Right side
SØ3.42x_ Left side
SØ3.43x_ Bilateral

SØ3.8xx_ Sprain of other parts of head
SØ3.9xx_ Sprain of unspecified parts of head

SØ4- INJURY OF CRANIAL NERVE

Including: The selection of side should be based on the side of the body being affected
Code First:
any associated intracranial injury (SØ6.-)
Code Also
any associated:
open wound of head (SØ1.-)
skull fracture (SØ2.-)
The appropriate 7th character is to be added to each code from category SØ4
A - initial encounter
D - subsequent encounter
S - sequela
See Guidelines: 1;C.19.b.2
Indicator(s): CC (7th A) | POAEx (7th D/S)

SØ4.Ø- **Optic nerve and pathways**
Use additional code to identify any visual field defect or blindness (H53.4-, H54.-)

SØ4.Ø1- **Optic nerve**
Including: 2nd cranial nerve

SØ4.Ø11_ Right eye
SØ4.Ø12_ Left eye
SØ4.Ø19_ Unspecified eye
Including: Optic nerve NOS

SØ4.Ø2x_ Optic chiasm

SØ4.Ø3- **Optic tract and pathways**
Including: Optic radiation

SØ4.Ø31_ Right side
SØ4.Ø32_ Left side
SØ4.Ø39_ Unspecified side
Including: Injury NOS

SØ4.Ø4- **Visual cortex**

SØ4.Ø41_ Right side
SØ4.Ø42_ Left side
SØ4.Ø49_ Unspecified side
Including: Injury NOS

SØ4.1- **Oculomotor nerve**
Including: 3rd cranial nerve

SØ4.1Øx_ Unspecified side
SØ4.11x_ Right side
SØ4.12x_ Left side

SØ4.2- **Trochlear nerve**
Including: 4th cranial nerve

SØ4.2Øx_ Unspecified side
SØ4.21x_ Right side
SØ4.22x_ Left side

SØ4.3- **Trigeminal nerve**
Including: 5th cranial nerve
SØ4.3Øx_ Unspecified side
SØ4.31x_ Right side
SØ4.32x_ Left side

SØ4.4- **Abducent nerve**
Including: 6th cranial nerve
SØ4.4Øx_ Unspecified side
SØ4.41x_ Right side
SØ4.42x_ Left side

SØ4.5- **Facial nerve**
Including: 7th cranial nerve
SØ4.5Øx_ Unspecified side
SØ4.51x_ Right side
SØ4.52x_ Left side

SØ4.6- **Acoustic nerve**
Including: Auditory nerve, 8th cranial nerve
SØ4.6Øx_ Unspecified side
SØ4.61x_ Right side
SØ4.62x_ Left side

SØ4.7- **Accessory nerve**
Including: 11th cranial nerve
SØ4.7Øx_ Unspecified side
SØ4.71x_ Right side
SØ4.72x_ Left side

SØ4.8- **Other**

SØ4.81- **Olfactory [1st] nerve**
SØ4.811_ Right side
SØ4.812_ Left side
SØ4.819_ Unspecified side

SØ4.89- **Other**
Including: Vagus [1Øth] nerve
SØ4.891_ Right side
SØ4.892_ Left side
SØ4.899_ Unspecified side

SØ4.9xx_ Unspecified cranial nerve

SØ6- INTRACRANIAL INJURY

Includes:
traumatic brain injury
Code Also
any associated:
open wound of head (SØ1.-)
skull fracture (SØ2.-)
Use additional *code, if applicable, to identify mild neurocognitive disorders due to known physiological condition (FØ6.7-)*
Excludes1:
head injury NOS (SØ9.9Ø)

The appropriate 7th character is to be added to each code from category SØ6
A - initial encounter
D - subsequent encounter
S - sequela

Notes:
7th characters D and S do not apply to codes in category SØ6 with 6th character 7 - death due to brain injury prior to regaining consciousness, or 8 - death due to other cause prior to regaining consciousness.
See Guidelines: *1;C.18.e*

SØ6.Ø- **Concussion**
Including: Commotio cerebri
Excludes1:
concussion with other intracranial injuries classified in subcategories SØ6.1- to SØ6.6-, and SØ6.81- to SØ6.89-, code to specified intracranial injury
Indicator(s): *POAEx (7th D/S)*
SØ6.ØxØ_ Without loss of consciousness
R **SØ6.Øx1_ With loss of consciousness of 3Ø minutes or less**
Including: brief loss of consciousness
N **SØ6.ØxA_ Concussion with loss of consciousness status unknown**
Including: Concussion NOS

SØ9- OTHER AND UNSPECIFIED INJURIES OF HEAD

The appropriate 7th character is to be added to each code from category SØ9
A - initial encounter
D - subsequent encounter
S - sequela

Indicator(s): *POAEx (7th D/S)*

SØ9.1- **Injury of muscle and tendon of head**
Code Also
any associated open wound (SØ1.-)
Excludes2:
sprain to joints and ligament of head (SØ3.9)
SØ9.11x_ Strain

INJURIES TO THE NECK (S1Ø-S19)

Includes:
injuries of nape
injuries of supraclavicular region
injuries of throat
Excludes2:
burns and corrosions (T2Ø-T32)
effects of foreign body in esophagus (T18.1)
effects of foreign body in larynx (T17.3)
effects of foreign body in pharynx (T17.2)
effects of foreign body in trachea (T17.4)
frostbite (T33-T34)
insect bite or sting, venomous (T63.4)
See Guidelines: *1;C.19.b*

S1Ø- SUPERFICIAL INJURY OF NECK

The appropriate 7th character is to be added to each code from category S1Ø
A - initial encounter
D - subsequent encounter
S - sequela

Indicator(s): *POAEx (7th D/S)*

S1Ø.Øxx_ Contusion of throat
Including: Cervical esophagus, larynx, pharynx, trachea

S1Ø.8- **Superficial injury of other specified parts of neck**
S1Ø.83x_ Contusion

S1Ø.9- **Superficial injury of unspecified part of neck**
S1Ø.93x_ Contusion

S12- FRACTURE OF CERVICAL VERTEBRA AND OTHER PARTS OF NECK

Notes:

A fracture not indicated as displaced or nondisplaced should be coded to displaced

A fracture not indicated as open or closed should be coded to closed

Includes:

fracture of cervical neural arch
fracture of cervical spine
fracture of cervical spinous process
fracture of cervical transverse process
fracture of cervical vertebral arch
fracture of neck

Code First:

any associated cervical spinal cord injury (S14.Ø, S14.1-)

The appropriate 7th character is to be added to all codes from subcategories S12.Ø-S12.6

A - initial encounter for closed fracture
B - initial encounter for open fracture
D - subsequent encounter for fracture with routine healing
G - subsequent encounter for fracture with delayed healing
K - subsequent encounter for fracture with nonunion
S - sequela

See Guidelines: *1;C.19.c*

S12.Ø- **Fracture of first cervical vertebra**
Including: Atlas
Indicator(s): CC (7th A/K) | MCC (7th B) | POAEx (7th D/G/K/S) | HAC: Ø5 (7th A/B) | CMS22: 169 (7th A/B) | CMS24: 169 (7th A/B) | ESRD21: 169 (7th A/B) | HHSØ7: 228 (7th A/B)

S12.ØØ- **Unspecified**
S12.ØØØ_ Displaced
S12.ØØ1_ Nondisplaced
S12.Ø1x_ Stable burst
S12.Ø2x_ Unstable burst
S12.Ø3- **Posterior arch**
S12.Ø3Ø_ Displaced
S12.Ø31_ Nondisplaced
S12.Ø4- **Lateral mass**
S12.Ø4Ø_ Displaced
S12.Ø41_ Nondisplaced
S12.Ø9- **Other**
S12.Ø9Ø_ Displaced
S12.Ø91_ Nondisplaced

S12.1- **Fracture of second cervical vertebra**
Including: Axis
Indicator(s): CC (7th A/K) | MCC (7th B) | POAEx (7th D/G/K/S) | HAC: Ø5 (7th A/B) | CMS22: 169 (7th A/B) | CMS24: 169 (7th A/B) | ESRD21: 169 (7th A/B) | HHSØ7: 228 (7th A/B)

S12.1Ø- **Unspecified**
S12.1ØØ_ Displaced
S12.1Ø1_ Nondisplaced
S12.11- **Type II dens fracture**
S12.11Ø_ Anterior displaced
S12.111_ Posterior displaced
S12.112_ Nondisplaced
S12.12- **Other dens fracture**
S12.12Ø_ Displaced
S12.121_ Nondisplaced
S12.13- **Unspecified traumatic spondylolisthesis**
S12.13Ø_ Displaced
S12.131_ Nondisplaced
S12.14x_ Type III traumatic spondylolisthesis
S12.15- **Other traumatic spondylolisthesis**
S12.15Ø_ Displaced
S12.151_ Nondisplaced
S12.19- **Other**
S12.19Ø_ Displaced
S12.191_ Nondisplaced

S12.2- **Fracture of third cervical vertebra**
Indicator(s): CC (7th A/K) | MCC (7th B) | POAEx (7th D/G/K/S) | HAC: Ø5 (7th A/B) | CMS22: 169 (7th A/B) | CMS24: 169 (7th A/B) | ESRD21: 169 (7th A/B) | HHSØ7: 228 (7th A/B)

S12.2Ø- **Unspecified**
S12.2ØØ_ Displaced
S12.2Ø1_ Nondisplaced
S12.23- **Unspecified traumatic spondylolisthesis**
S12.23Ø_ Displaced
S12.231_ Nondisplaced
S12.24x_ Type III traumatic spondylolisthesis
S12.25- **Other traumatic spondylolisthesis**
S12.25Ø_ Displaced
S12.251_ Nondisplaced
S12.29- **Other**
S12.29Ø_ Displaced
S12.291_ Nondisplaced

S12.3- **Fracture of fourth cervical vertebra**
Indicator(s): CC (7th A/K) | MCC (7th B) | POAEx (7th D/G/K/S) | HAC: Ø5 (7th A/B) | CMS22: 169 (7th A/B) | CMS24: 169 (7th A/B) | ESRD21: 169 (7th A/B) | HHSØ7: 228 (7th A/B)

S12.3Ø- **Unspecified**
S12.3ØØ_ Displaced
S12.3Ø1_ Nondisplaced
S12.33- **Unspecified traumatic spondylolisthesis**
S12.33Ø_ Displaced
S12.331_ Nondisplaced
S12.34x_ Type III traumatic spondylolisthesis
S12.35- **Other traumatic spondylolisthesis**
S12.35Ø_ Displaced
S12.351_ Nondisplaced
S12.39- **Other**
S12.39Ø_ Displaced
S12.391_ Nondisplaced

S12.4- **Fracture of fifth cervical vertebra**
Indicator(s): CC (7th A/K) | MCC (7th B) | POAEx (7th D/G/K/S) | HAC: Ø5 (7th A/B) | CMS22: 169 (7th A/B) | CMS24: 169 (7th A/B) | ESRD21: 169 (7th A/B) | HHSØ7: 228 (7th A/B)

S12.4Ø- **Unspecified**
S12.4ØØ_ Displaced
S12.4Ø1_ Nondisplaced

S12.43- **Unspecified traumatic spondylolisthesis**

S12.430_ Displaced

S12.431_ Nondisplaced

S12.44x_ Type III traumatic spondylolisthesis

S12.45- **Other traumatic spondylolisthesis**

S12.450_ Displaced

S12.451_ Nondisplaced

S12.49- **Other**

S12.490_ Displaced

S12.491_ Nondisplaced

S12.5- **Fracture of sixth cervical vertebra**

Indicator(s): CC (7th A/K) | MCC (7th B) | POAEx (7th D/G/K/S) | HAC: Ø5 (7th A/B) | CMS22: 169 (7th A/B) | CMS24: 169 (7th A/B) | ESRD21: 169 (7th A/B) | HHSØ7: 228 (7th A/B)

S12.5Ø- **Unspecified**

S12.500_ Displaced

S12.501_ Nondisplaced

S12.53- **Unspecified traumatic spondylolisthesis**

S12.530_ Displaced

S12.531_ Nondisplaced

S12.54x_ Type III traumatic spondylolisthesis

S12.55- **Other traumatic spondylolisthesis**

S12.550_ Displaced

S12.551_ Nondisplaced

S12.59- **Other**

S12.590_ Displaced

S12.591_ Nondisplaced

S12.6- **Fracture of seventh cervical vertebra**

Indicator(s): CC (7th A/K) | MCC (7th B) | POAEx (7th D/G/K/S) | HAC: Ø5 (7th A/B) | CMS22: 169 (7th A/B) | CMS24: 169 (7th A/B) | ESRD21: 169 (7th A/B) | HHSØ7: 228 (7th A/B)

S12.6Ø- **Unspecified**

S12.600_ Displaced

S12.601_ Nondisplaced

S12.63- **Unspecified traumatic spondylolisthesis**

S12.630_ Displaced

S12.631_ Nondisplaced

S12.64x_ Type III traumatic spondylolisthesis

S12.65- **Other traumatic spondylolisthesis**

S12.650_ Displaced

S12.651_ Nondisplaced

S12.69- **Other**

S12.690_ Displaced

S12.691_ Nondisplaced

S12.8xx_ Fracture of other parts of neck

Including: Hyoid bone, Larynx, Thyroid cartilage, Trachea

The appropriate 7th character is to be added to code S12.8

A - initial encounter

D - subsequent encounter

S - sequela

S12.9xx_ Fracture of neck, unspecified

Including: Neck NOS, cervical spine NOS, cervical vertebra NOS

The appropriate 7th character is to be added to code S12.9

A - initial encounter

D - subsequent encounter

S - sequela

S13- DISLOCATION AND SPRAIN OF JOINTS AND LIGAMENTS AT NECK LEVEL

Includes:

avulsion of joint or ligament at neck level

laceration of cartilage, joint or ligament at neck level

sprain of cartilage, joint or ligament at neck level

traumatic hemarthrosis of joint or ligament at neck level

traumatic rupture of joint or ligament at neck level

traumatic subluxation of joint or ligament at neck level

traumatic tear of joint or ligament at neck level

Code Also

any associated open wound

Excludes2:

strain of muscle or tendon at neck level (S16.1)

The appropriate 7th character is to be added to each code from category S13

A - initial encounter

D - subsequent encounter

S - sequela

Indicator(s): POAEx (7th D/S)

S13.Øxx_ Traumatic rupture of cervical intervertebral disc

Excludes1:

rupture or displacement (nontraumatic) of cervical intervertebral disc NOS (M5Ø.-)

S13.1- **Subluxation and dislocation of cervical vertebrae**

Code Also

any associated:

open wound of neck (S11.-)

spinal cord injury (S14.1-)

Excludes2:

fracture of cervical vertebrae (S12.Ø-S12.3-)

Indicator(s): CC (7th A) | HAC: Ø5 (7th A)

S13.1Ø- **Unspecified**

S13.100_ Subluxation of unspecified cervical vertebrae

S13.101_ Dislocation of unspecified cervical vertebrae

S13.11- **CØ/C1**

Including: Atlantooccipital joint, atloidooccipital joint, occipitoatloid joint

S13.110_ Subluxation of CØ/C1 cervical vertebrae

S13.111_ Dislocation of CØ/C1 cervical vertebrae

S13.12- **C1/C2**

Including: Atlantoaxial joint

S13.120_ Subluxation of C1/C2 cervical vertebrae

S13.121_ Dislocation of C1/C2 cervical vertebrae

S13.13- **C2/C3**

S13.130_ **Subluxation of C2/C3 cervical vertebrae**

S13.131_ **Dislocation of C2/C3 cervical vertebrae**

S13.14- **C3/C4**

S13.140_ **Subluxation of C3/C4 cervical vertebrae**

S13.141_ **Dislocation of C3/C4 cervical vertebrae**

S13.15- **C4/C5**

S13.150_ **Subluxation of C4/C5 cervical vertebrae**

S13.151_ **Dislocation of C4/C5 cervical vertebrae**

S13.16- **C5/C6**

S13.160_ **Subluxation of C5/C6 cervical vertebrae**

S13.161_ **Dislocation of C5/C6 cervical vertebrae**

S13.17- **C6/C7**

S13.170_ **Subluxation of C6/C7 cervical vertebrae**

S13.171_ **Dislocation of C6/C7 cervical vertebrae**

S13.18- **C7/T1**

S13.180_ **Subluxation of C7/T1 cervical vertebrae**

S13.181_ **Dislocation of C7/T1 cervical vertebrae**

S13.2- **Dislocation of other and unspecified parts**
Indicator(s): CC (7th A) | HAC: Ø5 (7th A)

S13.2Øx_ **Unspecified**

S13.29x_ **Other**

S13.4xx_ **Sprain of ligaments of cervical spine**
Including: Anterior longitudinal (ligament), cervical; atlanto-axial, atlanto-occipital joints; Whiplash injury

S13.5xx_ **Sprain of thyroid region**
Including: Cricoarytenoid, cricothyroid (joint) (ligament); thyroid cartilage

S13.8xx_ **Sprain of other parts**

S13.9xx_ **Sprain of unspecified parts**

S14- INJURY OF NERVES AND SPINAL CORD AT NECK LEVEL

Notes:
Code to highest level of cervical cord injury

Code Also
any associated:
fracture of cervical vertebra (S12.Ø--S12.6.-)
open wound of neck (S11.-)
transient paralysis (R29.5)

The appropriate 7th character is to be added to each code from category S14
A - initial encounter
D - subsequent encounter
S - sequela

Indicator(s): POAEx (7th D/S)

S14.Øxx_ **Concussion and edema of cervical spinal cord**

S14.1- **Other and unspecified cervical spinal cord**

S14.1Ø- **Unspecified**
Indicator(s): CMS22: 72 | CMS24: 72 | ESRD21: 72 | HHSØ5: 11Ø | HHSØ7: 11Ø

S14.1Ø1_ **At C1 level**
S14.1Ø2_ **At C2 level**
S14.1Ø3_ **At C3 level**
S14.1Ø4_ **At C4 level**
S14.1Ø5_ **At C5 level**
S14.1Ø6_ **At C6 level**
S14.1Ø7_ **At C7 level**
S14.1Ø8_ **At C8 level**
S14.1Ø9_ **At unspecified level**
Including: Injury of cervical spinal cord NOS

S14.11- **Complete lesion**
Indicator(s): CMS22: 7Ø | CMS24: 7Ø | ESRD21: 7Ø

S14.111_ **At C1 level**
S14.112_ **At C2 level**
S14.113_ **At C3 level**
S14.114_ **At C4 level**
S14.115_ **At C5 level**
S14.116_ **At C6 level**
S14.117_ **At C7 level**
S14.118_ **At C8 level**
S14.119_ **At unspecified level**

S14.12- **Central cord syndrome**
Indicator(s): CMS22: 72 | CMS24: 72 | ESRD21: 72 | HHSØ5: 11Ø | HHSØ7: 11Ø

S14.121_ **At C1 level**
S14.122_ **At C2 level**
S14.123_ **At C3 level**
S14.124_ **At C4 level**
S14.125_ **At C5 level**
S14.126_ **At C6 level**
S14.127_ **At C7 level**
S14.128_ **At C8 level**
S14.129_ **At unspecified level**

S14.13- **Anterior cord syndrome**
Indicator(s): CMS22: 72 | CMS24: 72 | ESRD21: 72 | HHSØ5: 11Ø | HHSØ7: 11Ø

S14.131_ **At C1 level**
S14.132_ **At C2 level**
S14.133_ **At C3 level**
S14.134_ **At C4 level**
S14.135_ **At C5 level**
S14.136_ **At C6 level**
S14.137_ **At C7 level**
S14.138_ **At C8 level**
S14.139_ **At unspecified level**

S14.14- **Brown-Séquard syndrome**
Indicator(s): CMS22: 72 | CMS24: 72 | ESRD21: 72 | HHSØ5: 11Ø | HHSØ7: 11Ø

S14.141_ At C1 level
S14.142_ At C2 level
S14.143_ At C3 level
S14.144_ At C4 level
S14.145_ At C5 level
S14.146_ At C6 level
S14.147_ At C7 level
S14.148_ At C8 level
S14.149_ At unspecified level

S14.15- **Incomplete lesions**
Including: Incomplete lesion NOS, Posterior cord syndrome
Indicator(s): CMS22: 72 | CMS24: 72 | ESRD21: 72 | HHSØ5: 11Ø | HHSØ7: 11Ø

S14.151_ Lesion at C1 level
S14.152_ Lesion at C2 level
S14.153_ Lesion at C3 level
S14.154_ Lesion at C4 level
S14.155_ Lesion at C5 level
S14.156_ Lesion at C6 level
S14.157_ Lesion at C7 level
S14.158_ Lesion at C8 level
S14.159_ Lesion at unspecified level

S14.2xx_ Nerve root of cervical spine
S14.3xx_ Brachial plexus
S14.4xx_ Peripheral nerves
S14.5xx_ Cervical sympathetic nerves
S14.8xx_ Other specified nerves
S14.9xx_ Unspecified nerves

S16- INJURY OF MUSCLE, FASCIA AND TENDON AT NECK LEVEL

Code Also
any associated open wound (S11.-)
Excludes2:
sprain of joint or ligament at neck level (S13.9)

The appropriate 7th character is to be added to each code from category S16
A - initial encounter
D - subsequent encounter
S - sequela

Indicator(s): POAEx (7th D/S)

S16.1xx_ Strain
S16.2xx_ Laceration
S16.8xx_ Other specified injury
S16.9xx_ Unspecified injury

INJURIES TO THE THORAX (S2Ø-S29)

Includes:
injuries of breast
injuries of chest (wall)
injuries of interscapular area
Excludes2:
burns and corrosions (T2Ø-T32)
effects of foreign body in bronchus (T17.5)
effects of foreign body in esophagus (T18.1)
effects of foreign body in lung (T17.8)
effects of foreign body in trachea (T17.4)
frostbite (T33-T34)
injuries of axilla
injuries of clavicle
injuries of scapular region
injuries of shoulder
insect bite or sting, venomous (T63.4)
See Guidelines: 1;C.19.b

S2Ø- SUPERFICIAL INJURY OF THORAX

The appropriate 7th character is to be added to each code from category S2Ø
A - initial encounter
D - subsequent encounter
S - sequela

Indicator(s): POAEx (7th D/S)

S2Ø.Ø- **Contusion of breast**

S2Ø.ØØx_ Unspecified breast
S2Ø.Ø1x_ Right breast
S2Ø.Ø2x_ Left breast

S2Ø.2- **Contusion of thorax**

S2Ø.2Øx_ Unspecified

S2Ø.21- **Front wall**

S2Ø.211_ Right
S2Ø.212_ Left
S2Ø.219_ Unspecified

S2Ø.22- **Back wall**

S2Ø.221_ Right
S2Ø.222_ Left
S2Ø.229_ Unspecified

S22- FRACTURE OF RIB(S), STERNUM AND THORACIC SPINE

Notes:
A fracture not indicated as displaced or nondisplaced should be coded to displaced
A fracture not indicated as open or closed should be coded to closed

Includes:
fracture of thoracic neural arch
fracture of thoracic spinous process
fracture of thoracic transverse process
fracture of thoracic vertebra
fracture of thoracic vertebral arch

Code First:
any associated:
injury of intrathoracic organ (S27.-)
spinal cord injury (S24.Ø-, S24.1-)

Excludes1:
transection of thorax (S28.1)

Excludes2:
fracture of clavicle (S42.Ø-)
fracture of scapula (S42.1-)

The appropriate 7th character is to be added to each code from category S22
A - initial encounter for closed fracture
B - initial encounter for open fracture
D - subsequent encounter for fracture with routine healing
G - subsequent encounter for fracture with delayed healing
K - subsequent encounter for fracture with nonunion
S - sequela

See Guidelines: 1;C.19.c

Indicator(s): *POAEx (7th D/G/K/S) | HAC: Ø5 (7th A/B)*

S22.Ø- **Thoracic vertebra**
Indicator(s): *CC (7th A/K) | MCC (7th B) | CMS22: 169 (7th A/B) | CMS24: 169 (7th A/B) | ESRD21: 169 (7th A/B) | HHSØ7: 228 (7th A/B)*

S22.ØØ- **Unspecified thoracic vertebra**
- **S22.ØØØ_ Wedge compression**
- **S22.ØØ1_ Stable burst**
- **S22.ØØ2_ Unstable burst**
- **S22.ØØ8_ Other**
- **S22.ØØ9_ Unspecified**

S22.Ø1- **First thoracic vertebra**
- **S22.Ø1Ø_ Wedge compression**
- **S22.Ø11_ Stable burst**
- **S22.Ø12_ Unstable burst**
- **S22.Ø18_ Other**
- **S22.Ø19_ Unspecified**

S22.Ø2- **Second thoracic vertebra**
- **S22.Ø2Ø_ Wedge compression**
- **S22.Ø21_ Stable burst**
- **S22.Ø22_ Unstable burst**
- **S22.Ø28_ Other**
- **S22.Ø29_ Unspecified**

S22.Ø3- **Third thoracic vertebra**
- **S22.Ø3Ø_ Wedge compression**
- **S22.Ø31_ Stable burst**
- **S22.Ø32_ Unstable burst**
- **S22.Ø38_ Other**
- **S22.Ø39_ Unspecified**

S22.Ø4- **Fourth thoracic vertebra**
- **S22.Ø4Ø_ Wedge compression**
- **S22.Ø41_ Stable burst**
- **S22.Ø42_ Unstable burst**
- **S22.Ø48_ Other**
- **S22.Ø49_ Unspecified**

S22.Ø5- **T5-T6**
- **S22.Ø5Ø_ Wedge compression**
- **S22.Ø51_ Stable burst**
- **S22.Ø52_ Unstable burst**
- **S22.Ø58_ Other**
- **S22.Ø59_ Unspecified**

S22.Ø6- **T7-T8**
- **S22.Ø6Ø_ Wedge compression**
- **S22.Ø61_ Stable burst**
- **S22.Ø62_ Unstable burst**
- **S22.Ø68_ Other**
- **S22.Ø69_ Unspecified**

S22.Ø7- **T9-T1Ø**
- **S22.Ø7Ø_ Wedge compression**
- **S22.Ø71_ Stable burst**
- **S22.Ø72_ Unstable burst**
- **S22.Ø78_ Other**
- **S22.Ø79_ Unspecified**

S22.Ø8- **T11-T12**
- **S22.Ø8Ø_ Wedge compression**
- **S22.Ø81_ Stable burst**
- **S22.Ø82_ Unstable burst**
- **S22.Ø88_ Other**
- **S22.Ø89_ Unspecified**

S22.2- **Sternum**
Indicator(s): *CC (7th A/K) | MCC (7th B)*
- **S22.2Øx_ Unspecified**
- **S22.21x_ Manubrium**
- **S22.22x_ Body of sternum**
- **S22.23x_ Sternal manubrial dissociation**
- **S22.24x_ Xiphoid process**

S22.3- **One rib**
Indicator(s): *CC (7th A/K) | MCC (7th B)*
- **S22.31x_ Right side**
- **S22.32x_ Left side**
- **S22.39x_ Unspecified side**

S22.4- **Multiple fractures of ribs**
Including: Fractures of two or more ribs
Excludes1:
flail chest (S22.5-)
Indicator(s): *CC (7th A/K) | MCC (7th B)*
- **S22.41x_ Right side**
- **S22.42x_ Left side**
- **S22.43x_ Bilateral**
- **S22.49x_ Unspecified side**

S22.5xx_ Flail chest

S22.9xx_ Bony thorax, part unspecified

S23- DISLOCATION AND SPRAIN OF JOINTS AND LIGAMENTS OF THORAX

Includes:
avulsion of joint or ligament of thorax
laceration of cartilage, joint or ligament of thorax
sprain of cartilage, joint or ligament of thorax
traumatic hemarthrosis of joint or ligament of thorax
traumatic rupture of joint or ligament of thorax
traumatic subluxation of joint or ligament of thorax
traumatic tear of joint or ligament of thorax

Code Also
any associated open wound

Excludes2:
dislocation, sprain of sternoclavicular joint (S43.2, S43.6)
strain of muscle or tendon of thorax (S29.Ø1-)

The appropriate 7th character is to be added to each code from category S23
A - initial encounter
D - subsequent encounter
S - sequela

Indicator(s): POAEx (7th D/S)

S23.Øxx_ Traumatic rupture of thoracic intervertebral disc

Excludes1:
rupture or displacement (nontraumatic) of thoracic intervertebral disc NOS (M51.- with fifth character 4)

S23.1- **Subluxation and dislocation of thoracic vertebra**

Code Also
any associated:
open wound of thorax (S21.-)
spinal cord injury (S24.Ø-, S24.1-)

Excludes2:
fracture of thoracic vertebrae (S22.Ø-)

S23.1Ø- **Unspecified**
S23.1ØØ_ Subluxation unspecified
S23.1Ø1_ Dislocation unspecified

S23.11- **T1/T2**
S23.11Ø_ Subluxation T1/T2
S23.111_ Dislocation T1/T2

S23.12- **T2/T3-T3/T4**
S23.12Ø_ Subluxation T2/T3
S23.121_ Dislocation T2/T3
S23.122_ Subluxation T3/T4
S23.123_ Dislocation T3/T4

S23.13- **T4/T5-T5/T6**
S23.13Ø_ Subluxation T4/T5
S23.131_ Dislocation T4/T5
S23.132_ Subluxation T5/T6
S23.133_ Dislocation T5/T6

S23.14- **T6/T7-T7/T8**
S23.14Ø_ Subluxation T6/T7
S23.141_ Dislocation T6/T7
S23.142_ Subluxation T7/T8
S23.143_ Dislocation T7/T8

S23.15- **T8/T9-T9/T1Ø**
S23.15Ø_ Subluxation T8/T9
S23.151_ Dislocation T8/T9
S23.152_ Subluxation T9/T1Ø
S23.153_ Dislocation T9/T1Ø

S23.16- **T1Ø/T11-T11/T12**
S23.16Ø_ Subluxation T1Ø/T11
S23.161_ Dislocation T1Ø/T11
S23.162_ Subluxation T11/T12
S23.163_ Dislocation T11/T12

S23.17- **T12/L1**
S23.17Ø_ Subluxation T12/L1
S23.171_ Dislocation T12/L1

S23.2- **Dislocation of other and unspecified parts**
S23.2Øx_ Unspecified
S23.29x_ Other

S23.3xx_ Sprain of ligaments of thoracic spine

S23.4- **Sprain of ribs and sternum**
S23.41x_ Ribs
S23.42- **Sternum**
S23.42Ø_ Sternoclavicular (joint) (ligament)
S23.421_ Chondrosternal joint
S23.428_ Other
S23.429_ Unspecified

S23.8xx_ Sprain of other specified parts
S23.9xx_ Sprain of unspecified parts

S24- INJURY OF NERVES AND SPINAL CORD AT THORAX LEVEL

Notes:
Code to highest level of thoracic spinal cord injury
Injuries to the spinal cord (S24.Ø and S24.1) refer to the cord level and not bone level injury, and can affect nerve roots at and below the level given.

Code Also
any associated:
fracture of thoracic vertebra (S22.Ø-)
open wound of thorax (S21.-)
transient paralysis (R29.5)

Excludes2:
injury of brachial plexus (S14.3)

The appropriate 7th character is to be added to each code from category S24
A - initial encounter
D - subsequent encounter
S - sequela

Indicator(s): POAEx (7th D/S)

S24.Øxx_ Concussion and edema of thoracic spinal cord

S24.1- **Other and unspecified injuries of thoracic spinal cord**

S24.1Ø- **Unspecified**
Indicator(s): *HAC: Ø5 (7th A) | CMS22: 72 | CMS24: 72 | ESRD21: 72 | HHSØ5: 11Ø | HHSØ7: 11Ø*
S24.1Ø1_ At T1 level
S24.1Ø2_ At T2-T6 level
S24.1Ø3_ At T7-T1Ø level
S24.1Ø4_ At T11-T12 level
S24.1Ø9_ At unspecified level
Including: Injury of thoracic spinal cord NOS

S24.11- **Complete lesion**
Indicator(s): *CMS22: 71 | CMS24: 71 | ESRD21: 71*
S24.119_ At unspecified level

S24.13- **Anterior cord syndrome**
Indicator(s): CMS22: 72 | CMS24: 72 | ESRD21: 72 | HHSØ5: 11Ø | HHSØ7: 11Ø

S24.139_ At unspecified level

S24.14- **Brown-Séquard syndrome**
Indicator(s): CMS22: 72 | CMS24: 72 | ESRD21: 72 | HHSØ5: 11Ø | HHSØ7: 11Ø

S24.149_ At unspecified level

S24.15- **Other incomplete lesions**
Including: Incomplete lesion NOS, Posterior cord syndrome
Indicator(s): CMS22: 72 | CMS24: 72 | ESRD21: 72 | HHSØ5: 11Ø | HHSØ7: 11Ø

S24.159_ Lesion at unspecified level

S24.2xx_ Nerve root of thoracic spine

S24.3xx_ Peripheral nerves

S24.4xx_ Thoracic sympathetic nervous system
Including: Cardiac plexus, esophageal plexus, pulmonary plexus, stellate ganglion, thoracic sympathetic ganglion

S24.8xx_ Other specified nerves

S24.9xx_ Unspecified nerve

S29- OTHER AND UNSPECIFIED INJURIES OF THORAX

Code Also
any associated open wound (S21.-)

The appropriate 7th character is to be added to each code from category S29
A - initial encounter
D - subsequent encounter
S - sequela

Indicator(s): POAEx (7th D/S)

S29.Ø- **Muscle and tendon at thorax level**

S29.ØØ- **Unspecified**

S29.ØØ1_ Front wall

S29.ØØ2_ Back wall

S29.ØØ9_ Unspecified wall

S29.Ø1- **Strain**

S29.Ø12_ Back wall

S29.Ø19_ Unspecified wall

S29.9xx_ Unspecified injury

INJURIES TO THE ABDOMEN, LOWER BACK, LUMBAR SPINE, PELVIS AND EXTERNAL GENITALS (S3Ø-S39)

Includes:
injuries to the abdominal wall
injuries to the anus
injuries to the buttock
injuries to the external genitalia
injuries to the flank
injuries to the groin

Excludes2:
burns and corrosions (T2Ø-T32)
effects of foreign body in anus and rectum (T18.5)
effects of foreign body in genitourinary tract (T19.-)
effects of foreign body in stomach, small intestine and colon (T18.2-T18.4)
frostbite (T33-T34)
insect bite or sting, venomous (T63.4)

See Guidelines: 1;C.19.b

S3Ø- SUPERFICIAL INJURY OF ABDOMEN, LOWER BACK, PELVIS AND EXTERNAL GENITALS

Excludes2:
superficial injury of hip (S7Ø.-)

The appropriate 7th character is to be added to each code from category S3Ø
A - initial encounter
D - subsequent encounter
S - sequela

Indicator(s): POAEx (7th D/S)

S3Ø.Øxx_ Contusion of lower back and pelvis
Including: Buttock

S3Ø.1xx_ Contusion of abdominal wall
Including: Flank, groin

S32- FRACTURE OF LUMBAR SPINE AND PELVIS

Notes:
A fracture not indicated as displaced or nondisplaced should be coded to displaced
A fracture not indicated as opened or closed should be coded to closed

Includes:
fracture of lumbosacral neural arch
fracture of lumbosacral spinous process
fracture of lumbosacral transverse process
fracture of lumbosacral vertebra
fracture of lumbosacral vertebral arch

Code First:
any associated spinal cord and spinal nerve injury (S34.-)

Excludes1:
transection of abdomen (S38.3)

Excludes2:
fracture of hip NOS (S72.Ø-)

The appropriate 7th character is to be added to each code from category S32
A - initial encounter for closed fracture
B - initial encounter for open fracture
D - subsequent encounter for fracture with routine healing
G - subsequent encounter for fracture with delayed healing
K - subsequent encounter for fracture with nonunion
S - sequela

See Guidelines: 1;C.19.c
Indicator(s): POAEx (7th D/G/K/S) | HAC: Ø5 (7th A/B)

S32.Ø- **Lumbar vertebra**
Including: Fracture of lumbar spine NOS
Indicator(s): CC (7th A/K) | MCC (7th B) | CMS22: 169 (7th A/B) | CMS24: 169 (7th A/B) | ESRD21: 169 (7th A/B) | HHSØ7: 228 (7th A/B)

S32.ØØ- **Unspecified**

S32.ØØØ_ Wedge compression

S32.ØØ1_ Stable burst

S32.ØØ2_ Unstable burst

S32.ØØ8_ Other

S32.ØØ9_ Unspecified

S32.Ø1- **First**

S32.Ø1Ø_ Wedge compression

S32.Ø11_ Stable burst

S32.Ø12_ Unstable burst

S32.Ø18_ Other

S32.Ø19_ Unspecified

S32.Ø2- **Second**

S32.Ø2Ø_ Wedge compression

S32.Ø21_ Stable burst

S32.Ø22_ Unstable burst

S32.Ø28_ Other

S32.Ø29_ Unspecified

S32.Ø3- **Third**

S32.Ø3Ø_ Wedge compression

S32.Ø31_ Stable burst

S32.Ø32_ Unstable burst

S32.Ø38_ Other

S32.Ø39_ Unspecified

S32.Ø4- **Fourth**

S32.Ø4Ø_ Wedge compression

S32.Ø41_ Stable burst

S32.Ø42_ Unstable burst

S32.Ø48_ Other

S32.Ø49_ Unspecified

S32.Ø5- **Fifth**

S32.Ø5Ø_ Wedge compression

S32.Ø51_ Stable burst

S32.Ø52_ Unstable burst

S32.Ø58_ Other

S32.Ø59_ Unspecified

S32.1- **Sacrum**

For vertical fractures, code to most medial fracture extension. Use two codes if both a vertical and transverse fracture are present.

Code Also

any associated fracture of pelvic ring (S32.8-)

Indicator(s): CC (7th A/K) | MCC (7th B) | CMS22: 169 (7th A/B) | CMS24: 169 (7th A/B) | ESRD21: 169 (7th A/B) | HHSØ7: 228 (7th A/B)

S32.1Øx_ Unspecified fracture

S32.11- **Zone I fracture**

Including: Vertical sacral ala

S32.11Ø_ Nondisplaced

S32.111_ Minimally displaced

S32.112_ Severely displaced

S32.119_ Unspecified

S32.12- **Zone II fracture**

Including: Vertical foraminal region

S32.12Ø_ Nondisplaced

S32.121_ Minimally displaced

S32.122_ Severely displaced

S32.129_ Unspecified

S32.13- **Zone III fracture**

Including: Vertical fracture into spinal canal region

S32.13Ø_ Nondisplaced

S32.131_ Minimally displaced

S32.132_ Severely displaced

S32.139_ Unspecified

S32.14x_ Type 1 fracture

Including: Transverse flexion fracture of sacrum without displacement

S32.15x_ Type 2 fracture

Including: Transverse flexion fracture of sacrum with posterior displacement

S32.16x_ Type 3 fracture

Including: Transverse extension fracture of sacrum with anterior displacement

S32.17x_ Type 4 fracture

Including: Transverse segmental comminution of upper sacrum

S32.19x_ Other fracture

S32.2xx_ Coccyx

S32.3- **Ilium**

Excludes1:

fracture of ilium with associated disruption of pelvic ring (S32.8-)

Indicator(s): CC (7th A/K) | MCC (7th B) | CMS22: 17Ø (7th A/B) | CMS24: 17Ø (7th A/B) | ESRD21: 17Ø (7th A/B) | HHSØ7: 226 (7th A/B)

S32.3Ø- **Unspecified**

S32.3Ø1_ Right

S32.3Ø2_ Left

S32.3Ø9_ Unspecified

S32.31- **Avulsion**

S32.311_ Displaced right

S32.312_ Displaced left

S32.313_ Displaced unspecified

S32.314_ Nondisplaced right

S32.315_ Nondisplaced left

S32.316_ Nondisplaced unspecified

S32.39- **Other**

S32.391_ Right

S32.392_ Left

S32.399_ Unspecified

S32.4- **Acetabulum**

Code Also

any associated fracture of pelvic ring (S32.8-)

Indicator(s): CC (7th K) | MCC (7th A/B) | CMS22: 17Ø (7th A/B) | CMS24: 17Ø (7th A/B) | ESRD21: 17Ø (7th A/B) | HHSØ7: 226 (7th A/B)

S32.4Ø- **Unspecified**

S32.4Ø1_ Right

S32.4Ø2_ Left

S32.4Ø9_ Unspecified

S32.41- **Anterior wall**

S32.411_ Displaced right

S32.412_ Displaced left

S32.413_ Displaced unspecified

S32.414_ Nondisplaced right

S32.415_ Nondisplaced left

S32.416_ Nondisplaced unspecified

S32.42- **Posterior wall**

S32.421_ Displaced right

S32.422_ Displaced left

S32.423_ Displaced unspecified

S32.424_ Nondisplaced right

S32.425_ Nondisplaced left

S32.426_ Nondisplaced unspecified

S32.43- **Anterior column [iliopubic]**
- **S32.431_** **Displaced right**
- **S32.432_** **Displaced left**
- **S32.433_** **Displaced unspecified**
- **S32.434_** **Nondisplaced right**
- **S32.435_** **Nondisplaced left**
- **S32.436_** **Nondisplaced unspecified**

S32.44- **Posterior column [ilioischial]**
- **S32.441_** **Displaced right**
- **S32.442_** **Displaced left**
- **S32.443_** **Displaced unspecified**
- **S32.444_** **Nondisplaced right**
- **S32.445_** **Nondisplaced left**
- **S32.446_** **Nondisplaced unspecified**

S32.45- **Transverse**
- **S32.451_** **Displaced right**
- **S32.452_** **Displaced left**
- **S32.453_** **Displaced unspecified**
- **S32.454_** **Nondisplaced right**
- **S32.455_** **Nondisplaced left**
- **S32.456_** **Nondisplaced unspecified**

S32.46- **Associated transverse-posterior**
- **S32.461_** **Displaced right**
- **S32.462_** **Displaced left**
- **S32.463_** **Displaced unspecified**
- **S32.464_** **Nondisplaced right**
- **S32.465_** **Nondisplaced left**
- **S32.466_** **Nondisplaced unspecified**

S32.47- **Medial wall**
- **S32.471_** **Displaced right**
- **S32.472_** **Displaced left**
- **S32.473_** **Displaced unspecified**
- **S32.474_** **Nondisplaced right**
- **S32.475_** **Nondisplaced left**
- **S32.476_** **Nondisplaced unspecified**

S32.48- **Dome**
- **S32.481_** **Displaced right**
- **S32.482_** **Displaced left**
- **S32.483_** **Displaced unspecified**
- **S32.484_** **Nondisplaced right**
- **S32.485_** **Nondisplaced left**
- **S32.486_** **Nondisplaced unspecified**

S32.49- **Other specified**
- **S32.491_** **Right**
- **S32.492_** **Left**
- **S32.499_** **Unspecified**

S32.5- **Pubis**

Excludes1:
fracture of pubis with associated disruption of pelvic ring (S32.8-)
Indicator(s): CC (7th A/K) | MCC (7th B) | CMS22: 170 (7th A/B) | CMS24: 170 (7th A/B) | ESRD21: 170 (7th A/B) | HHS07: 226 (7th A/B)

S32.50- **Unspecified fracture**
- **S32.501_** **Right**
- **S32.502_** **Left**
- **S32.509_** **Unspecified**

S32.51- **Superior rim**
- **S32.511_** **Right**
- **S32.512_** **Left**
- **S32.519_** **Unspecified**

S32.59- **Other specified fracture**
- **S32.591_** **Right**
- **S32.592_** **Left**
- **S32.599_** **Unspecified**

S32.6- **Ischium**

Excludes1:
fracture of ischium with associated disruption of pelvic ring (S32.8-)
Indicator(s): CC (7th A/K) | MCC (7th B) | CMS22: 170 (7th A/B) | CMS24: 170 (7th A/B) | ESRD21: 170 (7th A/B) | HHS07: 226 (7th A/B)

S32.60- **Unspecified fracture**
- **S32.601_** **Right**
- **S32.602_** **Left**
- **S32.609_** **Unspecified**

S32.61- **Avulsion fracture**
- **S32.611_** **Displaced right**
- **S32.612_** **Displaced left**
- **S32.613_** **Displaced unspecified**
- **S32.614_** **Nondisplaced right**
- **S32.615_** **Nondisplaced left**
- **S32.616_** **Nondisplaced unspecified**

S32.69- **Other specified**
- **S32.691_** **Right**
- **S32.692_** **Left**
- **S32.699_** **Unspecified**

S32.8- **Other parts of pelvis**

Code Also
any associated:
fracture of acetabulum (S32.4-)
sacral fracture (S32.1-)
Indicator(s): CC (7th A/K) | MCC (7th B) | CMS22: 170 (7th A/B) | CMS24: 170 (7th A/B) | ESRD21: 170 (7th A/B) | HHS07: 226 (7th A/B)

S32.81- **Multiple fractures with disruption of pelvic ring**
Including: Multiple pelvic fractures with disruption of pelvic circle
- **S32.810_** **Stable**
- **S32.811_** **Unstable**

S32.82x_ **Multiple without disruption of pelvic ring**
Including: Without disruption of pelvic circle

S32.89x_ **Fracture of other parts of pelvis**

S32.9xx_ **Unspecified parts of lumbosacral spine and pelvis**
Including: Lumbosacral spine NOS, pelvis NOS

See Appendix A — Coding Reference Tables for lists of the ICD-10-CM Tabular indicators, HAC categories, and HCC codes.

S33- DISLOCATION AND SPRAIN OF JOINTS AND LIGAMENTS OF LUMBAR SPINE AND PELVIS

Includes:
avulsion of joint or ligament of lumbar spine and pelvis
laceration of cartilage, joint or ligament of lumbar spine and pelvis
sprain of cartilage, joint or ligament of lumbar spine and pelvis
traumatic hemarthrosis of joint or ligament of lumbar spine and pelvis
traumatic rupture of joint or ligament of lumbar spine and pelvis
traumatic subluxation of joint or ligament of lumbar spine and pelvis
traumatic tear of joint or ligament of lumbar spine and pelvis

Code Also
any associated open wound

Excludes1:
nontraumatic rupture or displacement of lumbar intervertebral disc NOS (M51.-)
obstetric damage to pelvic joints and ligaments (O71.6)

Excludes2:
dislocation and sprain of joints and ligaments of hip (S73.-)
strain of muscle of lower back and pelvis (S39.Ø1-)

The appropriate 7th character is to be added to each code from category S33
A - initial encounter
D - subsequent encounter
S - sequela

Indicator(s): POAEx (7th D/S)

S33.Øxx_ Traumatic rupture of lumbar intervertebral disc
Excludes1:
rupture or displacement (nontraumatic) of lumbar intervertebral disc NOS (M51.- with fifth character 6)

S33.1- **Subluxation and dislocation of lumbar vertebra**
Code Also
any associated:
open wound of abdomen, lower back and pelvis (S31)
spinal cord injury (S24.Ø, S24.1-, S34.Ø-, S34.1-)
Excludes2:
fracture of lumbar vertebrae (S32.Ø-)

S33.1Ø- **Unspecified lumbar vertebra**
S33.1ØØ_ Subluxation unspecified vertebra
S33.1Ø1_ Dislocation unspecified vertebra

S33.11- **L1/L2**
S33.11Ø_ Subluxation of L1/L2
S33.111_ Dislocation of L1/L2

S33.12- **L2/L3**
S33.12Ø_ Subluxation of L2/L3
S33.121_ Dislocation of L2/L3

S33.13- **L3/L4**
S33.13Ø_ Subluxation of L3/L4
S33.131_ Dislocation of L3/L4

S33.14- **L4/L5**
S33.14Ø_ Subluxation of L4/L5
S33.141_ Dislocation of L4/L5

S33.2xx_ Dislocation of sacroiliac and sacrococcygeal joint

S33.3- **Dislocation of other and unspecified parts**
S33.3Øx_ Unspecified parts
S33.39x_ Other parts

S33.4xx_ Traumatic rupture of symphysis pubis

S33.5xx_ Sprain of ligaments of lumbar spine

S33.6xx_ Sprain of sacroiliac joint

S33.8xx_ Sprain of other parts

S33.9xx_ Sprain of unspecified parts

S34- INJURY OF LUMBAR AND SACRAL SPINAL CORD AND NERVES AT ABDOMEN, LOWER BACK AND PELVIS LEVEL

Notes:
Code to highest level of lumbar cord injury
Injuries to the spinal cord (S34.Ø and S34.1) refer to the cord level and not bone level injury, and can affect nerve roots at and below the level given.

Code Also
any associated:
fracture of vertebra (S22.Ø-, S32.Ø-)
open wound of abdomen, lower back and pelvis (S31.-)
transient paralysis (R29.5)

The appropriate 7th character is to be added to each code from category S34
A - initial encounter
D - subsequent encounter
S - sequela

Indicator(s): POAEx (7th D/S)

S34.Ø- **Concussion and edema of lumbar and sacral spinal cord**
Indicator(s): *MCC (7th A) | CMS22: 72 | CMS24: 72 | ESRD21: 72 | HHSØ5: 11Ø | HHSØ7: 11Ø*

S34.Ø1x_ Lumbar spinal cord
S34.Ø2x_ Sacral spinal cord
Including: Conus medullaris

S34.1- **Other and unspecified injury of lumbar and sacral spinal cord**
Indicator(s): *MCC (7th A) | HAC: Ø5 (7th A) | CMS22: 72 | CMS24: 72 | ESRD21: 72 | HHSØ5: 11Ø | HHSØ7: 11Ø*

S34.1Ø- **Unspecified injury to lumbar spinal cord**
S34.1Ø1_ L1 level
Including: Level 1
S34.1Ø2_ L2 level
Including: Level 2
S34.1Ø3_ L3 level
Including: Level 3
S34.1Ø4_ L4 level
Including: Level 4
S34.1Ø5_ L5 level
Including: Level 5
S34.1Ø9_ Unspecified level

S34.11- **Complete lesion of lumbar spinal cord**
S34.111_ L1 level
Including: Level 1
S34.112_ L2 level
Including: Level 2
S34.113_ L3 level
Including: Level 3
S34.114_ L4 level
Including: Level 4
S34.115_ L5 level
Including: Level 5
S34.119_ Unspecified level

S34.12- **Incomplete lesion of lumbar spinal cord**

S34.121_ L1 level
Including: Level 1

S34.122_ L2 level
Including: Level 2

S34.123_ L3 level
Including: Level 3

S34.124_ L4 level
Including: Level 4

S34.125_ L5 level
Including: Level 5

S34.129_ Unspecified level

S34.13- **Sacral spinal cord**
Including: Other injury to conus medullaris

S34.131_ Complete lesion
Including: Conus medullaris

S34.132_ Incomplete lesion
Including: Conus medullaris

S34.139_ Unspecified
Including: Conus medullaris

S34.2- **Nerve root of lumbar and sacral spine**

S34.21x_ Lumbar spine

S34.22x_ Sacral spine

S34.3xx_ Cauda equina

S34.4xx_ Lumbosacral plexus

S34.5xx_ Lumbar, sacral and pelvic sympathetic nerves
Including: Celiac ganglion or plexus, hypogastric plexus, mesenteric plexus (inferior) (superior), splanchnic nerve

S34.6xx_ Peripheral nerve(s) at abdomen, lower back and pelvis level

S34.8xx_ Other nerves at abdomen, lower back and pelvis level

S34.9xx_ Unspecified nerves at abdomen, lower back and pelvis level

S39- OTHER AND UNSPECIFIED INJURIES OF ABDOMEN, LOWER BACK, PELVIS AND EXTERNAL GENITALS

Code Also
any associated open wound (S31.-)

Excludes2:
sprain of joints and ligaments of lumbar spine and pelvis (S33.-)

The appropriate 7th character is to be added to each code from category S39
A - initial encounter
D - subsequent encounter
S - sequela

Indicator(s): POAEx (7th D/S)

S39.Ø- **Muscle, fascia and tendon**

S39.ØØ- **Unspecified injury**

S39.ØØ1_ Unspecified

S39.ØØ2_ Unspecified

S39.ØØ3_ Unspecified

S39.Ø1- **Strain**

S39.Ø11_ Abdomen

S39.Ø12_ Lower back

S39.Ø13_ Pelvis

S39.Ø9- **Other injury**

S39.Ø91_ Abdomen

S39.Ø92_ Lower back

S39.Ø93_ Pelvis

S39.8- **Other specified injuries**

S39.81x_ Abdomen

S39.82x_ Lower back

S39.83x_ Pelvis

INJURIES TO THE SHOULDER AND UPPER ARM (S4Ø-S49)

Includes:
injuries of axilla
injuries of scapular region

Excludes2:
burns and corrosions (T2Ø-T32)
frostbite (T33-T34)
injuries of elbow (S5Ø-S59)
insect bite or sting, venomous (T63.4)

See Guidelines: 1;C.19.b

S4Ø- SUPERFICIAL INJURY OF SHOULDER AND UPPER ARM

The appropriate 7th character is to be added to each code from category S4Ø
A - initial encounter
D - subsequent encounter
S - sequela

Indicator(s): POAEx (7th D/S)

S4Ø.Ø- **Contusion of shoulder and upper arm**

S4Ø.Ø1- **Shoulder**

S4Ø.Ø11_ Right

S4Ø.Ø12_ Left

S4Ø.Ø19_ Unspecified

S4Ø.Ø2- **Upper arm**

S4Ø.Ø21_ Right

S4Ø.Ø22_ Left

S4Ø.Ø29_ Unspecified

S43- DISLOCATION AND SPRAIN OF JOINTS AND LIGAMENTS OF SHOULDER GIRDLE

Includes:
avulsion of joint or ligament of shoulder girdle
laceration of cartilage, joint or ligament of shoulder girdle
sprain of cartilage, joint or ligament of shoulder girdle
traumatic hemarthrosis of joint or ligament of shoulder girdle
traumatic rupture of joint or ligament of shoulder girdle
traumatic subluxation of joint or ligament of shoulder girdle
traumatic tear of joint or ligament of shoulder girdle

Code Also
any associated open wound

Excludes2:
strain of muscle, fascia and tendon of shoulder and upper arm (S46.-)

The appropriate 7th character is to be added to each code from category S43
A - initial encounter
D - subsequent encounter
S - sequela

Indicator(s): POAEx (7th D/S)

S43.Ø- **Subluxation and dislocation of shoulder joint**
Including: Glenohumeral joint

S43.ØØ- **Unspecified subluxation and dislocation of shoulder joint**
Including: Humerus NOS

S43.ØØ1_ Right

S43.ØØ2_ Left

S43.ØØ3_ Unspecified

S43.ØØ4_ **Right**
S43.ØØ5_ **Left**
S43.ØØ6_ **Unspecified**

S43.Ø1- **Anterior subluxation and dislocation of humerus**
S43.Ø11_ **Right**
S43.Ø12_ **Left**
S43.Ø13_ **Unspecified**
S43.Ø14_ **Right**
S43.Ø15_ **Left**
S43.Ø16_ **Unspecified**

S43.Ø2- **Posterior subluxation and dislocation of humerus**
S43.Ø21_ **Right**
S43.Ø22_ **Left**
S43.Ø23_ **Unspecified**
S43.Ø24_ **Right**
S43.Ø25_ **Left**
S43.Ø26_ **Unspecified**

S43.Ø3- **Inferior subluxation and dislocation of humerus**
S43.Ø31_ **Right**
S43.Ø32_ **Left**
S43.Ø33_ **Unspecified**
S43.Ø34_ **Right**
S43.Ø35_ **Left**
S43.Ø36_ **Unspecified**

S43.Ø8- **Other subluxation and dislocation**
S43.Ø81_ **Right**
S43.Ø82_ **Left**
S43.Ø83_ **Unspecified**
S43.Ø84_ **Right**
S43.Ø85_ **Left**
S43.Ø86_ **Unspecified**

S43.1- **Subluxation and dislocation of acromioclavicular joint**

S43.1Ø- **Unspecified dislocation of acromioclavicular joint**
S43.1Ø1_ **Right**
S43.1Ø2_ **Left**
S43.1Ø9_ **Unspecified**

S43.11- **Subluxation**
S43.111_ **Right**
S43.112_ **Left**
S43.119_ **Unspecified**

S43.12- **Dislocation 1ØØ%-2ØØ% displacement**
S43.121_ **Right**
S43.122_ **Left**
S43.129_ **Unspecified**

S43.13- **Dislocation greater than 2ØØ% displacement**
S43.131_ **Right**
S43.132_ **Left**
S43.139_ **Unspecified**

S43.14- **Inferior dislocation**
S43.141_ **Right**
S43.142_ **Left**
S43.149_ **Unspecified**

S43.15- **Posterior dislocation**
S43.151_ **Right**
S43.152_ **Left**
S43.159_ **Unspecified**

S43.2- **Subluxation and dislocation of sternoclavicular joint**
Indicator(s): CC (7th A) | HAC: Ø5 (7th A)

S43.2Ø- **Unspecified subluxation and dislocation**
S43.2Ø1_ **Subluxation right**
S43.2Ø2_ **Subluxation left**
S43.2Ø3_ **Subluxation unspecified**
S43.2Ø4_ **Disloaction right**
S43.2Ø5_ **Dislocation left**
S43.2Ø6_ **Dislocation unspecified**

S43.21- **Anterior subluxation and dislocation**
S43.211_ **Subluxation right**
S43.212_ **Subluxation left**
S43.213_ **Subluxation unspecified**
S43.214_ **Dislocation right**
S43.215_ **Dislocation left**
S43.216_ **Dislocation unspecified**

S43.22- **Posterior subluxation and dislocation**
S43.221_ **Subluxation right**
S43.222_ **Subluxation left**
S43.223_ **Subluxation unspecified**
S43.224_ **Dislocation right**
S43.225_ **Dislocation left**
S43.226_ **Dislocation unspecified**

S43.3- **Subluxation and dislocation of other and unspecified parts of shoulder girdle**

S43.3Ø- **Unspecified parts of shoulder girdle**
Including: Shoulder girdle NOS
S43.3Ø1_ **Right**
S43.3Ø2_ **Left**
S43.3Ø3_ **Unspecified**
S43.3Ø4_ **Right**
S43.3Ø5_ **Left**
S43.3Ø6_ **Unspecified**

S43.31- **Scapula**
S43.311_ **Right**
S43.312_ **Left**
S43.313_ **Unspecified**
S43.314_ **Right**
S43.315_ **Left**
S43.316_ **Unspecified**

S43.39- **Other parts of shoulder girdle**
S43.391_ **Right**
S43.392_ **Left**
S43.393_ **Unspecified**
S43.394_ **Right**
S43.395_ **Left**
S43.396_ **Unspecified**

S43.4- **Sprain of shoulder joint**

S43.40- **Unspecified**

S43.401_ Right

S43.402_ Left

S43.409_ Unspecified

S43.41- **Sprain of coracohumeral (ligament)**

S43.411_ Right

S43.412_ Left

S43.419_ Unspecified

S43.42- **Sprain of rotator cuff capsule**

Excludes1:

rotator cuff syndrome (complete) (incomplete), not specified as traumatic (M75.1-)

Excludes2:

injury of tendon of rotator cuff (S46.0-)

S43.421_ Right

S43.422_ Left

S43.429_ Unspecified

S43.43- **Superior glenoid labrum lesion**

Including: SLAP lesion

S43.431_ Right shoulder

S43.432_ Left shoulder

S43.439_ Unspecified shoulder

S43.49- **Other**

S43.491_ Right

S43.492_ Left

S43.499_ Unspecified

S43.5- **Sprain of acromioclavicular joint**

Including: Acromioclavicular ligament

S43.50x_ Unspecified joint

S43.51x_ Right joint

S43.52x_ Left joint

S43.6- **Sprain of sternoclavicular joint**

S43.60x_ Unspecified joint

S43.61x_ Right joint

S43.62x_ Left joint

S43.8- **Sprain of other specified parts of shoulder girdle**

S43.80x_ Unspecified shoulder girdle

S43.81x_ Right shoulder girdle

S43.82x_ Left shoulder girdle

S43.9- **Sprain of unspecified parts of shoulder girdle**

S43.90x_ Unspecified shoulder girdle

Including: Sprain NOS

S43.91x_ Right shoulder girdle

S43.92x_ Left shoulder girdle

S44- INJURY OF NERVES AT SHOULDER AND UPPER ARM LEVEL

Code Also

any associated open wound (S41.-)

Excludes2:

injury of brachial plexus (S14.3-)

The appropriate 7th character is to be added to each code from category S44

A - initial encounter

D - subsequent encounter

S - sequela

Indicator(s): *POAEx (7th D/S)*

S44.0- **Ulnar nerve at upper arm level**

Excludes1:

ulnar nerve NOS (S54.0)

S44.00x_ Unspecified arm

S44.01x_ Right arm

S44.02x_ Left arm

S44.1- **Median nerve at upper arm level**

Excludes1:

median nerve NOS (S54.1)

S44.10x_ Unspecified arm

S44.11x_ Right arm

S44.12x_ Left arm

S44.2- **Radial nerve at upper arm level**

Excludes1:

radial nerve NOS (S54.2)

S44.20x_ Unspecified arm

S44.21x_ Right arm

S44.22x_ Left arm

S44.3- **Axillary nerve**

S44.30x_ Unspecified arm

S44.31x_ Right arm

S44.32x_ Left arm

S44.4- **Musculocutaneous nerve**

S44.40x_ Unspecified arm

S44.41x_ Right arm

S44.42x_ Left arm

S44.5- **Cutaneous sensory nerve**

S44.50x_ Unspecified arm

S44.51x_ Right arm

S44.52x_ Left arm

S44.8- **Injury of other nerves at shoulder and upper arm level**

S44.8X- **Other nerves**

S44.8x1_ Right

S44.8x2_ Left

S44.8x9_ Unspecified

S44.9- **Unspecified nerve**

S44.90x_ Unspecified arm

S44.91x_ Right arm

S44.92x_ Left arm

S46- INJURY OF MUSCLE, FASCIA AND TENDON AT SHOULDER AND UPPER ARM LEVEL

Code Also

any associated open wound (S41.-)

Excludes2:

injury of muscle, fascia and tendon at elbow (S56.-)

sprain of joints and ligaments of shoulder girdle (S43.9)

The appropriate 7th character is to be added to each code from category S46

A - initial encounter

D - subsequent encounter

S - sequela

Indicator(s): *POAEx (7th D/S)*

S46.0- **Muscle(s) and tendon(s) of the rotator cuff of shoulder**

S46.00- **Unspecified injury**

S46.001_ Right

S46.002_ Left

S46.009_ Unspecified shoulder

S46.Ø1- **Strain**

S46.Ø11_ **Right**

S46.Ø12_ **Left**

S46.Ø19_ **Unspecified**

S46.Ø2- **Laceration**

Indicator(s): CC (7th A)

S46.Ø21_ **Right**

S46.Ø22_ **Left**

S46.Ø29_ **Unspecified**

S46.Ø9- **Other injury**

S46.Ø91_ **Right**

S46.Ø92_ **Left**

S46.Ø99_ **Unspecified**

S46.1- **Muscle, fascia and tendon of long head of biceps**

S46.1Ø- **Unspecified injury**

S46.1Ø1_ **Right arm**

S46.1Ø2_ **Left arm**

S46.1Ø9_ **Unspecified arm**

S46.11- **Strain**

S46.111_ **Right arm**

S46.112_ **Left arm**

S46.119_ **Unspecified arm**

S46.12- **Laceration**

Indicator(s): CC (7th A)

S46.121_ **Right arm**

S46.122_ **Left arm**

S46.129_ **Unspecified arm**

S46.19- **Other injury**

S46.191_ **Right arm**

S46.192_ **Left arm**

S46.199_ **Unspecified arm**

S46.2- **Muscle, fascia and tendon of other parts of biceps**

S46.2Ø- **Unspecified injury**

S46.2Ø1_ **Right arm**

S46.2Ø2_ **Left arm**

S46.2Ø9_ **Unspecified arm**

S46.21- **Strain**

S46.211_ **Right arm**

S46.212_ **Left arm**

S46.219_ **Unspecified arm**

S46.22- **Laceration**

Indicator(s): CC (7th A)

S46.221_ **Right arm**

S46.222_ **Left arm**

S46.229_ **Unspecified arm**

S46.29- **Other injury**

S46.291_ **Right arm**

S46.292_ **Left arm**

S46.299_ **Unspecified arm**

S46.3- **Muscle, fascia and tendon of triceps**

S46.3Ø- **Unspecified injury**

S46.3Ø1_ **Right arm**

S46.3Ø2_ **Left arm**

S46.3Ø9_ **Unspecified arm**

S46.31- **Strain**

S46.311_ **Right arm**

S46.312_ **Left arm**

S46.319_ **Unspecified arm**

S46.32- **Laceration**

Indicator(s): CC (7th A)

S46.321_ **Right arm**

S46.322_ **Left arm**

S46.329_ **Unspecified arm**

S46.39- **Other injury**

S46.391_ **Right arm**

S46.392_ **Left arm**

S46.399_ **Unspecified arm**

S46.8- **Other muscles, fascia and tendons**

S46.8Ø- **Unspecified injury**

S46.8Ø1_ **Right**

S46.8Ø2_ **Left**

S46.8Ø9_ **Unspecified arm**

S46.81- **Strain**

S46.811_ **Right**

S46.812_ **Left**

S46.819_ **Unspecified**

S46.82- **Laceration**

Indicator(s): CC (7th A)

S46.821_ **Right**

S46.822_ **Left**

S46.829_ **Unspecified**

S46.89- **Other injury**

S46.891_ **Right**

S46.892_ **Left**

S46.899_ **Unspecified**

S46.9- **Unspecified muscle, fascia and tendon**

S46.9Ø- **Unspecified injury**

S46.9Ø1_ **Right**

S46.9Ø2_ **Left**

S46.9Ø9_ **Unspecified arm**

S46.91- **Strain**

S46.911_ **Right**

S46.912_ **Left**

S46.919_ **Unspecified arm**

S46.92- **Laceration**

Indicator(s): CC (7th A)

S46.921_ **Right**

S46.922_ **Left**

S46.929_ **Unspecified arm**

S46.99- **Other injury**

S46.991_ **Right**

S46.992_ **Left**

S46.999_ **Unspecified arm**

S49- OTHER AND UNSPECIFIED INJURIES OF SHOULDER AND UPPER ARM

The appropriate 7th character is to be added to each code from subcategories S49.Ø and S49.1
- *A - initial encounter for closed fracture*
- *D - subsequent encounter for fracture with routine healing*
- *G - subsequent encounter for fracture with delayed healing*
- *K - subsequent encounter for fracture with nonunion*
- *P - subsequent encounter for fracture with malunion*
- *S - sequela*

See Guidelines: 1;C.19.c

S49.8- **Other specified injuries**

The appropriate 7th character is to be added to each code in subcategory S49.8
- *A - initial encounter*
- *D - subsequent encounter*
- *S - sequela*

Indicator(s): POAEx (7th D/S)

S49.8Øx_ Unspecified arm
S49.81x_ Right arm
S49.82x_ Left arm

S49.9- **Unspecified injury**

The appropriate 7th character is to be added to each code in subcategory S49.9
- *A - initial encounter*
- *D - subsequent encounter*
- *S - sequela*

Indicator(s): POAEx (7th D/S)

S49.9Øx_ Unspecified arm
S49.91x_ Right arm
S49.92x_ Left arm

INJURIES TO THE ELBOW AND FOREARM (S5Ø-S59)

Excludes2:
- *burns and corrosions (T2Ø-T32)*
- *frostbite (T33-T34)*
- *injuries of wrist and hand (S6Ø-S69)*
- *insect bite or sting, venomous (T63.4)*

See Guidelines: 1;C.19.b

S5Ø- SUPERFICIAL INJURY OF ELBOW AND FOREARM

Excludes2:
- *superficial injury of wrist and hand (S6Ø.-)*

The appropriate 7th character is to be added to each code from category S5Ø
- *A - initial encounter*
- *D - subsequent encounter*
- *S - sequela*

Indicator(s): POAEx (7th D/S)

S5Ø.Ø- **Contusion of elbow**

S5Ø.ØØx_ Unspecified elbow
S5Ø.Ø1x_ Right elbow
S5Ø.Ø2x_ Left elbow

S5Ø.1- **Contusion of forearm**

S5Ø.1Øx_ Unspecified forearm
S5Ø.11x_ Right forearm
S5Ø.12x_ Left forearm

S53- DISLOCATION AND SPRAIN OF JOINTS AND LIGAMENTS OF ELBOW

Includes:
- *avulsion of joint or ligament of elbow*
- *laceration of cartilage, joint or ligament of elbow*
- *sprain of cartilage, joint or ligament of elbow*
- *traumatic hemarthrosis of joint or ligament of elbow*
- *traumatic rupture of joint or ligament of elbow*
- *traumatic subluxation of joint or ligament of elbow*
- *traumatic tear of joint or ligament of elbow*

Code Also
- *any associated open wound*

Excludes2:
- *strain of muscle, fascia and tendon at forearm level (S56.-)*

The appropriate 7th character is to be added to each code from category S53
- *A - initial encounter*
- *D - subsequent encounter*
- *S - sequela*

Indicator(s): POAEx (7th D/S)

S53.Ø- **Subluxation and dislocation of radial head**
Including: Radiohumeral joint

Excludes1:
- *Monteggia's fracture-dislocation (S52.27-)*

S53.ØØ- **Unspecified**

S53.ØØ1_ Right
S53.ØØ2_ Left
S53.ØØ3_ Unspecified radial head
S53.ØØ4_ Right
S53.ØØ5_ Left
S53.ØØ6_ Unspecified radial head

S53.Ø1- **Anterior**
Including: Anteriomedial

S53.Ø11_ Right
S53.Ø12_ Left
S53.Ø13_ Unspecified
S53.Ø14_ Right
S53.Ø15_ Left
S53.Ø16_ Unspecified

S53.Ø2- **Posterior**
Including: Posteriolateral

S53.Ø21_ Right
S53.Ø22_ Left
S53.Ø23_ Unspecified
S53.Ø24_ Right
S53.Ø25_ Left
S53.Ø26_ Unspecified

S53.Ø3- **Nursemaid's elbow**

S53.Ø31_ Right
S53.Ø32_ Left
S53.Ø33_ Unspecified

S53.Ø9- **Other**

S53.Ø91_ Right
S53.Ø92_ Left
S53.Ø93_ Unspecified
S53.Ø94_ Right
S53.Ø95_ Left
S53.Ø96_ Unspecified

S53.1- **Subluxation and dislocation of ulnohumeral joint**
Including: Subluxation and dislocation of elbow NOS
Excludes1:
dislocation of radial head alone (S53.Ø-)

S53.1Ø- **Unspecified**
S53.1Ø1_ Right
S53.1Ø2_ Left
S53.1Ø3_ Unspecified ulnohumeral joint
S53.1Ø4_ Right
S53.1Ø5_ Left
S53.1Ø6_ Unspecified ulnohumeral joint

S53.11- **Anterior**
S53.111_ Right
S53.112_ Left
S53.113_ Unspecified
S53.114_ Right
S53.115_ Left
S53.116_ Unspecified

S53.12- **Posterior**
S53.121_ Right
S53.122_ Left
S53.123_ Unspecified
S53.124_ Right
S53.125_ Left
S53.126_ Unspecified

S53.13- **Medial**
S53.131_ Right
S53.132_ Left
S53.133_ Unspecified
S53.134_ Right
S53.135_ Left
S53.136_ Unspecified

S53.14- **Lateral**
S53.141_ Right
S53.142_ Left
S53.143_ Unspecified
S53.144_ Right
S53.145_ Left
S53.146_ Unspecified

S53.19- **Other**
S53.191_ Right
S53.192_ Left
S53.193_ Unspecified
S53.194_ Right
S53.195_ Left
S53.196_ Unspecified

S53.2- **Traumatic rupture of radial collateral ligament**
Excludes1:
sprain of radial collateral ligament NOS (S53.43-)
S53.2Øx_ Unspecified radial collateral ligament
S53.21x_ Right radial collateral ligament
S53.22x_ Left radial collateral ligament

S53.3- **Traumatic rupture of ulnar collateral ligament**
Excludes1:
sprain of ulnar collateral ligament (S53.44-)
S53.3Øx_ Unspecified ulnar collateral ligament
S53.31x_ Right ulnar collateral ligament
S53.32x_ Left ulnar collateral ligament

S53.4- **Sprain**
Excludes2:
traumatic rupture of radial collateral ligament (S53.2-)
traumatic rupture of ulnar collateral ligament (S53.3-)

S53.4Ø- **Unspecified**
S53.4Ø1_ Right
S53.4Ø2_ Left
S53.4Ø9_ Unspecified elbow
Including: Sprain of elbow NOS

S53.41- **Radiohumeral (joint) sprain**
S53.411_ Right elbow
S53.412_ Left elbow
S53.419_ Unspecified elbow

S53.42- **Ulnohumeral (joint) sprain**
S53.421_ Right elbow
S53.422_ Left elbow
S53.429_ Unspecified elbow

S53.43- **Radial collateral ligament sprain**
S53.431_ Right elbow
S53.432_ Left elbow
S53.439_ Unspecified elbow

S53.44- **Ulnar collateral ligament sprain**
S53.441_ Right elbow
S53.442_ Left elbow
S53.449_ Unspecified elbow

S53.49- **Other sprain of elbow**
S53.491_ Right
S53.492_ Left
S53.499_ Unspecified

S54- INJURY OF NERVES AT FOREARM LEVEL
Code Also
any associated open wound (S51.-)
Excludes2:
injury of nerves at wrist and hand level (S64.-)

The appropriate 7th character is to be added to each code from category S54
A - initial encounter
D - subsequent encounter
S - sequela

Indicator(s): *POAEx (7th D/S)*

S54.Ø- **Injury of ulnar nerve**
Including: Injury of ulnar nerve NOS
S54.ØØx_ Unspecified arm
S54.Ø1x_ Right arm
S54.Ø2x_ Left arm

S54.1- **Injury of median nerve**
Including: Injury of median nerve NOS
S54.1Øx_ Unspecified arm
S54.11x_ Right arm
S54.12x_ Left arm

S54.2- **Injury of radial nerve**
Including: Injury of radial nerve NOS
S54.2Øx_ Unspecified arm
S54.21x_ Right arm
S54.22x_ Left arm

S54.3- **Injury of cutaneous sensory nerve**
S54.3Øx_ Unspecified arm
S54.31x_ Right arm
S54.32x_ Left arm

S54.8- **Injury of other nerves at forearm level**
S54.8x1_ Right arm
S54.8x2_ Left arm
S54.8x9_ Unspecified arm

S54.9- **Unspecified nerve**
S54.9Øx_ Unspecified arm
S54.91x_ Right arm
S54.92x_ Left arm

S56- INJURY OF MUSCLE, FASCIA AND TENDON AT FOREARM LEVEL

Code Also
any associated open wound (S51.-)
Excludes2:
injury of muscle, fascia and tendon at or below wrist (S66.-)
sprain of joints and ligaments of elbow (S53.4-)

The appropriate 7th character is to be added to each code from category S56
A - initial encounter
D - subsequent encounter
S - sequela

Indicator(s): *POAEx (7th D/S)*

S56.Ø- **Flexor muscle, fascia and tendon of thumb**
S56.ØØ- **Unspecified injury**
S56.ØØ1_ Right
S56.ØØ2_ Left
S56.ØØ9_ Unspecified thumb
S56.Ø1- **Strain**
S56.Ø11_ Right
S56.Ø12_ Left
S56.Ø19_ Unspecified
S56.Ø9- **Other injury**
S56.Ø91_ Right
S56.Ø92_ Left
S56.Ø99_ Unspecified

S56.1- **Flexor muscle, fascia and tendon of other and unspecified finger**
S56.1Ø- **Unspecified injury**
S56.1Ø1_ Right index
S56.1Ø2_ Left index
S56.1Ø3_ Right middle
S56.1Ø4_ Left middle
S56.1Ø5_ Right ring
S56.1Ø6_ Left ring
S56.1Ø7_ Right little
S56.1Ø8_ Left little
S56.1Ø9_ Unspecified finger
S56.11- **Strain**
S56.111_ Right index
S56.112_ Left index
S56.113_ Right middle
S56.114_ Left middle
S56.115_ Right ring
S56.116_ Left ring
S56.117_ Right little
S56.118_ Left little
S56.119_ Unspecified finger
S56.19- **Other injury**
S56.191_ Right index
S56.192_ Left index
S56.193_ Right middle
S56.194_ Left middle
S56.195_ Right ring
S56.196_ Left ring
S56.197_ Right little
S56.198_ Left little
S56.199_ Unspecified finger

S56.2- **Other flexor muscle, fascia and tendon**
S56.2Ø- **Unspecified injury**
S56.2Ø1_ Right arm
S56.2Ø2_ Left arm
S56.2Ø9_ Unspecified arm
S56.21- **Strain**
S56.211_ Right arm
S56.212_ Left arm
S56.219_ Unspecified arm
S56.29- **Other injury**
S56.291_ Right arm
S56.292_ Left arm
S56.299_ Unspecified arm

S56.3- **Injury of extensor or abductor muscles, fascia and tendons of thumb**
S56.3Ø- **Unspecified injury**
S56.3Ø1_ Right
S56.3Ø2_ Left
S56.3Ø9_ Unspecified thumb
S56.31- **Strain**
S56.311_ Right
S56.312_ Left
S56.319_ Unspecified
S56.39- **Other injury**
S56.391_ Right
S56.392_ Left
S56.399_ Unspecified

S56.4- **Injury of extensor muscle, fascia and tendon of other and unspecified finger**
S56.4Ø- **Unspecified injury**
S56.4Ø1_ Right index
S56.4Ø2_ Left index
S56.4Ø3_ Right middle
S56.4Ø4_ Left middle
S56.4Ø5_ Right ring

S56.406_ **Left ring**
S56.407_ **Right little**
S56.408_ **Left little**
S56.409_ **Unspecified finger**
S56.41- **Strain**
S56.411_ **Right index**
S56.412_ **Left index**
S56.413_ **Right middle**
S56.414_ **Left middle**
S56.415_ **Right ring**
S56.416_ **Left ring**
S56.417_ **Right little**
S56.418_ **Left little**
S56.419_ **Unspecified finger**
S56.49- **Other injury**
S56.491_ **Right index**
S56.492_ **Left index**
S56.493_ **Right middle**
S56.494_ **Left middle**
S56.495_ **Right ring**
S56.496_ **Left ring**
S56.497_ **Right little**
S56.498_ **Left little**
S56.499_ **Unspecified finger**
S56.5- **Other extensor muscle, fascia and tendon**
S56.5Ø- **Unspecified injury**
S56.5Ø1_ **Right arm**
S56.5Ø2_ **Left arm**
S56.5Ø9_ **Unspecified arm**
S56.51- **Strain**
S56.511_ **Right arm**
S56.512_ **Left arm**
S56.519_ **Unspecified arm**
S56.59- **Other injury**
S56.591_ **Right arm**
S56.592_ **Left arm**
S56.599_ **Unspecified arm**
S56.8- **Injury of other muscles, fascia and tendons**
S56.8Ø- **Unspecified injury**
S56.8Ø1_ **Right arm**
S56.8Ø2_ **Left arm**
S56.8Ø9_ **Unspecified arm**
S56.81- **Strain**
S56.811_ **Right arm**
S56.812_ **Left arm**
S56.819_ **Unspecified arm**
S56.89- **Other injury**
S56.891_ **Right arm**
S56.892_ **Left arm**
S56.899_ **Unspecified arm**
S56.9- **Injury of unspecified muscles, fascia and tendons**
S56.9Ø- **Unspecified injury**
S56.9Ø1_ **Right arm**
S56.9Ø2_ **Left arm**
S56.9Ø9_ **Unspecified arm**
S56.91- **Strain**
S56.911_ **Right arm**
S56.912_ **Left arm**
S56.919_ **Unspecified arm**
S56.99- **Other injury**
S56.991_ **Right arm**
S56.992_ **Left arm**
S56.999_ **Unspecified arm**

S59- OTHER AND UNSPECIFIED INJURIES OF ELBOW AND FOREARM

Excludes2:
other and unspecified injuries of wrist and hand (S69.-)

The appropriate 7th character is to be added to each code from subcategories S59.Ø, S59.1, and S59.2
A - initial encounter for closed fracture
D - subsequent encounter for fracture with routine healing
G - subsequent encounter for fracture with delayed healing
K - subsequent encounter for fracture with nonunion
P - subsequent encounter for fracture with malunion
S - sequela

See Guidelines: 1;C.19.c

S59.8- **Other specified injuries**

The appropriate 7th character is to be added to each code in subcategory S59.8
A - initial encounter
D - subsequent encounter
S - sequela

Indicator(s): POAEx (7th D/S)

S59.8Ø- **Elbow**
S59.8Ø1_ **Right**
S59.8Ø2_ **Left**
S59.8Ø9_ **Unspecified**
S59.81- **Forearm**
S59.811_ **Right**
S59.812_ **Left**
S59.819_ **Unspecified**
S59.9- **Unspecified injury**

The appropriate 7th character is to be added to each code in subcategory S59.9
A - initial encounter
D - subsequent encounter
S - sequela

Indicator(s): POAEx (7th D/S)

S59.9Ø- **Elbow**
S59.9Ø1_ **Right**
S59.9Ø2_ **Left**
S59.9Ø9_ **Unspecified elbow**
S59.91- **Forearm**
S59.911_ **Right**
S59.912_ **Left**
S59.919_ **Unspecified forearm**

INJURIES TO THE WRIST, HAND AND FINGERS (S6Ø-S69)

Excludes2:
burns and corrosions (T2Ø-T32)
frostbite (T33-T34)
insect bite or sting, venomous (T63.4)
See Guidelines: 1;C.19.b

S6Ø- SUPERFICIAL INJURY OF WRIST, HAND AND FINGERS

The appropriate 7th character is to be added to each code from category S6Ø
A - initial encounter
D - subsequent encounter
S - sequela

Indicator(s): POAEx (7th D/S)

S6Ø.Ø- **Contusion of finger without damage to nail**
Excludes1:
contusion involving nail (matrix) (S6Ø.1)

S6Ø.Ø1- **Thumb**
S6Ø.Ø11_ Right
S6Ø.Ø12_ Left
S6Ø.Ø19_ Unspecified

S6Ø.Ø2- **Index finger**
S6Ø.Ø21_ Right
S6Ø.Ø22_ Left
S6Ø.Ø29_ Unspecified

S6Ø.Ø3- **Middle finger**
S6Ø.Ø31_ Right
S6Ø.Ø32_ Left
S6Ø.Ø39_ Unspecified

S6Ø.Ø4- **Ring finger**
S6Ø.Ø41_ Right
S6Ø.Ø42_ Left
S6Ø.Ø49_ Unspecified

S6Ø.Ø5- **Little finger**
S6Ø.Ø51_ Right
S6Ø.Ø52_ Left
S6Ø.Ø59_ Unspecified

S6Ø.1- **Contusion of finger with damage to nail**
S6Ø.1Øx_ Unspecified finger

S6Ø.11- **Thumb**
S6Ø.111_ Right
S6Ø.112_ Left
S6Ø.119_ Unspecified

S6Ø.12- **Index finger**
S6Ø.121_ Right
S6Ø.122_ Left
S6Ø.129_ Unspecified

S6Ø.13- **Middle finger**
S6Ø.131_ Right
S6Ø.132_ Left
S6Ø.139_ Unspecified

S6Ø.14- **Ring finger**
S6Ø.141_ Right
S6Ø.142_ Left
S6Ø.149_ Unspecified

S6Ø.15- **Little finger**
S6Ø.151_ Right
S6Ø.152_ Left
S6Ø.159_ Unspecified

S6Ø.2- **Contusion of wrist and hand**
Excludes2:
contusion of fingers (S6Ø.Ø-, S6Ø.1-)

S6Ø.21- **Wrist**
S6Ø.211_ Right
S6Ø.212_ Left
S6Ø.219_ Unspecified

S6Ø.22- **Hand**
S6Ø.221_ Right
S6Ø.222_ Left
S6Ø.229_ Unspecified

S63- DISLOCATION AND SPRAIN OF JOINTS AND LIGAMENTS AT WRIST AND HAND LEVEL

Includes:
avulsion of joint or ligament at wrist and hand level
laceration of cartilage, joint or ligament at wrist and hand level
sprain of cartilage, joint or ligament at wrist and hand level
traumatic hemarthrosis of joint or ligament at wrist and hand level
traumatic rupture of joint or ligament at wrist and hand level
traumatic subluxation of joint or ligament at wrist and hand level
traumatic tear of joint or ligament at wrist and hand level
Code Also
any associated open wound
Excludes2:
strain of muscle, fascia and tendon of wrist and hand (S66.-)

The appropriate 7th character is to be added to each code from category S63
A - initial encounter
D - subsequent encounter
S - sequela

Indicator(s): POAEx (7th D/S)

S63.Ø- **Subluxation and dislocation of wrist and hand joints**

S63.ØØ- **Unspecified**
Including: Carpal bone NOS, radius NOS
S63.ØØ1_ Right
S63.ØØ2_ Left
S63.ØØ3_ Subluxation unspecified wrist and hand
S63.ØØ4_ Right
S63.ØØ5_ Left
S63.ØØ6_ Dislocation unspecified wrist and hand

S63.Ø1- **Distal radioulnar joint**
S63.Ø11_ Right wrist
S63.Ø12_ Left wrist
S63.Ø13_ Unspecified wrist
S63.Ø14_ Right wrist
S63.Ø15_ Left wrist
S63.Ø16_ Unspecified wrist

S63.Ø2- **Radiocarpal joint**

- **S63.Ø21_** **Right wrist**
- **S63.Ø22_** **Left wrist**
- **S63.Ø23_** **Unspecified wrist**
- **S63.Ø24_** **Right wrist**
- **S63.Ø25_** **Left wrist**
- **S63.Ø26_** **Unspecified wrist**

S63.Ø3- **Midcarpal joint**

- **S63.Ø31_** **Right wrist**
- **S63.Ø32_** **Left wrist**
- **S63.Ø33_** **Unspecified wrist**
- **S63.Ø34_** **Right wrist**
- **S63.Ø35_** **Left wrist**
- **S63.Ø36_** **Unspecified wrist**

S63.Ø4- **Carpometacarpal joint of thumb**

Excludes2:
interphalangeal subluxation and dislocation of thumb (S63.1-)

- **S63.Ø41_** **Right**
- **S63.Ø42_** **Left**
- **S63.Ø43_** **Unspecified**
- **S63.Ø44_** **Right**
- **S63.Ø45_** **Left**
- **S63.Ø46_** **Unspecified**

S63.Ø5- **Other carpometacarpal joint**

Excludes2:
subluxation and dislocation of carpometacarpal joint of thumb (S63.Ø4-)

- **S63.Ø51_** **Right hand**
- **S63.Ø52_** **Left hand**
- **S63.Ø53_** **Unspecified hand**
- **S63.Ø54_** **Right hand**
- **S63.Ø55_** **Left hand**
- **S63.Ø56_** **Unspecified hand**

S63.Ø6- **Metacarpal (bone), proximal end**

- **S63.Ø61_** **Right hand**
- **S63.Ø62_** **Left hand**
- **S63.Ø63_** **Unspecified hand**
- **S63.Ø64_** **Right hand**
- **S63.Ø65_** **Left hand**
- **S63.Ø66_** **Unspecified hand**

S63.Ø7- **Distal end of ulna**

- **S63.Ø71_** **Right**
- **S63.Ø72_** **Left**
- **S63.Ø73_** **Unspecified**
- **S63.Ø74_** **Right**
- **S63.Ø75_** **Left**
- **S63.Ø76_** **Unspecified**

S63.Ø9- **Other**

- **S63.Ø91_** **Right**
- **S63.Ø92_** **Left**
- **S63.Ø93_** **Unspecified**
- **S63.Ø94_** **Right**
- **S63.Ø95_** **Left**
- **S63.Ø96_** **Unspecified**

S63.1- **Subluxation and dislocation of thumb**

S63.1Ø- **Unspecified**

- **S63.1Ø1_** **Right**
- **S63.1Ø2_** **Left**
- **S63.1Ø3_** **Subluxation unspecified thumb**
- **S63.1Ø4_** **Right**
- **S63.1Ø5_** **Left**
- **S63.1Ø6_** **Dislocation unspecified thumb**

S63.11- **Metacarpophalangeal joint**

- **S63.111_** **Right**
- **S63.112_** **Left**
- **S63.113_** **Unspecified**
- **S63.114_** **Right**
- **S63.115_** **Left**
- **S63.116_** **Unspecified**

S63.12- **Unspecified interphalangeal joint**

- **S63.121_** **Subluxation, right**
- **S63.122_** **Subluxation, left**
- **S63.123_** **Subluxation, unspecified**
- **S63.124_** **Dislocation, right**
- **S63.125_** **Dislocation, left**
- **S63.126_** **Dislocation unspecified**

S63.2- **Subluxation and dislocation of other finger(s)**

Excludes2:
subluxation and dislocation of thumb (S63.1-)

S63.2Ø- **Unspecified subluxation**

- **S63.2ØØ_** **Right index**
- **S63.2Ø1_** **Left index**
- **S63.2Ø2_** **Right middle**
- **S63.2Ø3_** **Left middle**
- **S63.2Ø4_** **Right ring**
- **S63.2Ø5_** **Left ring**
- **S63.2Ø6_** **Right little**
- **S63.2Ø7_** **Left little**
- **S63.2Ø8_** **Other finger**
  Including: Specified finger with unspecified laterality
- **S63.2Ø9_** **Unspecified finger**

S63.21- **Subluxation of metacarpophalangeal joint**

- **S63.21Ø_** **Right index**
- **S63.211_** **Left index**
- **S63.212_** **Right middle**
- **S63.213_** **Left middle**
- **S63.214_** **Right ring**
- **S63.215_** **Left ring**
- **S63.216_** **Right little**
- **S63.217_** **Left little**
- **S63.218_** **Other finger**
  Including: Specified finger with unspecified laterality
- **S63.219_** **Unspecified**

S63.22- **Subluxation of unspecified interphalangeal joint**
- **S63.22Ø_ Right index**
- **S63.221_ Left index**
- **S63.222_ Right middle**
- **S63.223_ Left middle**
- **S63.224_ Right ring**
- **S63.225_ Left ring**
- **S63.226_ Right little**
- **S63.227_ Left little**
- **S63.228_ Other finger**
  Including: Specified finger with unspecified laterality
- **S63.229_ Unspecified finger**

S63.23- **Subluxation of proximal interphalangeal joint**
- **S63.23Ø_ Right index**
- **S63.231_ Left index**
- **S63.232_ Right middle**
- **S63.233_ Left middle**
- **S63.234_ Right ring**
- **S63.235_ Left ring**
- **S63.236_ Right little**
- **S63.237_ Left little**
- **S63.238_ Other finger**
  Including: Specified finger with unspecified laterality
- **S63.239_ Unspecified**

S63.24- **Subluxation of distal interphalangeal joint**
- **S63.24Ø_ Right index**
- **S63.241_ Left index**
- **S63.242_ Right middle**
- **S63.243_ Left middle**
- **S63.244_ Right ring**
- **S63.245_ Left ring**
- **S63.246_ Right little**
- **S63.247_ Left little**
- **S63.248_ Other finger**
  Including: Specified finger with unspecified laterality
- **S63.249_ Unspecified**

S63.25- **Unspecified dislocation**
- **S63.25Ø_ Right index**
- **S63.251_ Left index**
- **S63.252_ Right middle**
- **S63.253_ Left middle**
- **S63.254_ Right ring**
- **S63.255_ Left ring**
- **S63.256_ Right little**
- **S63.257_ Left little**
- **S63.258_ Other finger**
  Including: Specified finger with unspecified laterality
- **S63.259_ Unspecified finger**
  Including: Unspecified finger with unspecified laterality

S63.26- **Dislocation of metacarpophalangeal joint**
- **S63.26Ø_ Right index**
- **S63.261_ Left index**
- **S63.262_ Right middle**
- **S63.263_ Left middle**
- **S63.264_ Right ring**
- **S63.265_ Left ring**
- **S63.266_ Right little**
- **S63.267_ Left little**
- **S63.268_ Other finger**
  Including: Specified finger with unspecified laterality
- **S63.269_ Unspecified**

S63.27- **Dislocation of unspecified interphalangeal joint**
- **S63.27Ø_ Right index**
- **S63.271_ Left index**
- **S63.272_ Right middle**
- **S63.273_ Left middle**
- **S63.274_ Right ring**
- **S63.275_ Left ring**
- **S63.276_ Right little**
- **S63.277_ Left little**
- **S63.278_ Other finger**
  Including: Specified finger with unspecified laterality
- **S63.279_ Unspecified finger**
  Including: Unspecified finger without specified laterality

S63.28- **Dislocation of proximal interphalangeal joint**
- **S63.28Ø_ Right index**
- **S63.281_ Left index**
- **S63.282_ Right middle**
- **S63.283_ Left middle**
- **S63.284_ Right ring**
- **S63.285_ Left ring**
- **S63.286_ Right little**
- **S63.287_ Left little**
- **S63.288_ Other finger**
  Including: Specified finger with unspecified laterality
- **S63.289_ Unspecified**

S63.29- **Dislocation of distal interphalangeal joint**
- **S63.29Ø_ Right index**
- **S63.291_ Left index**
- **S63.292_ Right middle**
- **S63.293_ Left middle**
- **S63.294_ Right ring**
- **S63.295_ Left ring**
- **S63.296_ Right little**
- **S63.297_ Left little**
- **S63.298_ Other finger**
  Including: Specified finger with unspecified laterality
- **S63.299_ Unspecified**

S63.3- **Traumatic rupture of ligament of wrist**

S63.3Ø- **Unspecified ligament**

S63.3Ø1_ Right

S63.3Ø2_ Left

S63.3Ø9_ Unspecified wrist

S63.31- **Collateral ligament**

S63.311_ Right

S63.312_ Left

S63.319_ Unspecified

S63.32- **Radiocarpal ligament**

S63.321_ Right

S63.322_ Left

S63.329_ Unspecified

S63.33- **Ulnocarpal (palmar) ligament**

S63.331_ Right

S63.332_ Left

S63.339_ Unspecified

S63.39- **Other ligament**

S63.391_ Right

S63.392_ Left

S63.399_ Unspecified

S63.4- **Traumatic rupture of ligament of finger at metacarpophalangeal and interphalangeal joint(s)**

S63.4Ø- **Unspecified ligament of finger**

S63.4ØØ_ Right index

S63.4Ø1_ Left index

S63.4Ø2_ Right middle

S63.4Ø3_ Left middle

S63.4Ø4_ Right ring

S63.4Ø5_ Left ring

S63.4Ø6_ Right little

S63.4Ø7_ Left little

S63.4Ø8_ Other finger
Including: Specified finger with unspecified laterality

S63.4Ø9_ Unspecified finger

S63.41- **Collateral ligament of finger**

S63.41Ø_ Right index

S63.411_ Left index

S63.412_ Right middle

S63.413_ Left middle

S63.414_ Right ring

S63.415_ Left ring

S63.416_ Right little

S63.417_ Left little

S63.418_ Other finger
Including: Specified finger with unspecified laterality

S63.419_ Unspecified

S63.42- **Palmar ligament of finger**

S63.42Ø_ Right index

S63.421_ Left index

S63.422_ Right middle

S63.423_ Left middle

S63.424_ Right ring

S63.425_ Left ring

S63.426_ Right little

S63.427_ Left little

S63.428_ Other finger
Including: Specified finger with unspecified laterality

S63.429_ Unspecified

S63.43- **Volar plate of finger**

S63.43Ø_ Right index

S63.431_ Left index

S63.432_ Right middle

S63.433_ Left middle

S63.434_ Right ring

S63.435_ Left ring

S63.436_ Right little

S63.437_ Left little

S63.438_ Other finger
Including: Specified finger with unspecified laterality

S63.439_ Unspecified

S63.49- **Other ligament of finger**

S63.49Ø_ Right index

S63.491_ Left index

S63.492_ Right middle

S63.493_ Left middle

S63.494_ Right ring

S63.495_ Left ring

S63.496_ Right little

S63.497_ Left little

S63.498_ Other finger
Including: Specified finger with unspecified laterality

S63.499_ Unspecified

S63.5- **Other and unspecified sprain of wrist**

S63.5Ø- **Unspecified**

S63.5Ø1_ Right

S63.5Ø2_ Left

S63.5Ø9_ Unspecified wrist

S63.51- **Sprain of carpal (joint)**

S63.511_ Right

S63.512_ Left

S63.519_ Unspecified

S63.52- **Sprain of radiocarpal joint**
Excludes1:
traumatic rupture of radiocarpal ligament (S63.32-)

S63.521_ Right wrist

S63.522_ Left wrist

S63.529_ Unspecified wrist

S63.59- **Other specified sprain of wrist**

S63.591_ Right

S63.592_ Left

S63.599_ Unspecified

S63.6- **Other and unspecified sprain of finger(s)**
Excludes1:
traumatic rupture of ligament of finger at metacarpophalangeal and interphalangeal joint(s) (S63.4-)

S63.6Ø- **Unspecified sprain of thumb**
S63.6Ø1_ Right
S63.6Ø2_ Left
S63.6Ø9_ Unspecified thumb

S63.61- **Unspecified sprain of other and unspecified finger(s)**
S63.61Ø_ Right index finger
S63.611_ Left index finger
S63.612_ Right middle finger
S63.613_ Left middle finger
S63.614_ Right ring finger
S63.615_ Left ring finger
S63.616_ Right little finger
S63.617_ Left little finger
S63.618_ Unspecified finger
Including: Specified finger with unspecified laterality
S63.619_ Unspecified finger

S63.62- **Sprain of interphalangeal joint of thumb**
S63.621_ Right
S63.622_ Left
S63.629_ Unspecified

S63.63- **Sprain of interphalangeal joint of other and unspecified finger(s)**
S63.63Ø_ Right index finger
S63.631_ Left index finger
S63.632_ Right middle finger
S63.633_ Left middle finger
S63.634_ Right ring finger
S63.635_ Left ring finger
S63.636_ Right little finger
S63.637_ Left little finger
S63.638_ Other
S63.639_ Unspecified

S63.64- **Sprain of metacarpophalangeal joint of thumb**
S63.641_ Right
S63.642_ Left
S63.649_ Unspecified

S63.65- **Sprain of metacarpophalangeal joint of other and unspecified finger(s)**
S63.65Ø_ Right index finger
S63.651_ Left index finger
S63.652_ Right middle finger
S63.653_ Left middle finger
S63.654_ Right ring finger
S63.655_ Left ring finger
S63.656_ Right little finger
S63.657_ Left little finger
S63.658_ Other
Including: Specified finger with unspecified laterality
S63.659_ Unspecified

S63.68- **Other sprain of thumb**
S63.681_ Right
S63.682_ Left
S63.689_ Unspecified

S63.69- **Other sprain of other and unspecified finger(s)**
S63.69Ø_ Right index finger
S63.691_ Left index finger
S63.692_ Right middle finger
S63.693_ Left middle finger
S63.694_ Right ring finger
S63.695_ Left ring finger
S63.696_ Right little finger
S63.697_ Left little finger
S63.698_ Other finger
Including: Specified finger with unspecified laterality
S63.699_ Unspecified

S63.8- **Sprain of other part of wrist and hand**
S63.8x1_ Right
S63.8x2_ Left
S63.8x9_ Unspecified

S63.9- **Sprain of unspecified part of wrist and hand**
S63.9Øx_ Unspecified wrist and hand
S63.91x_ Right wrist and hand
S63.92x_ Left wrist and hand

S64- INJURY OF NERVES AT WRIST AND HAND LEVEL
Code Also
any associated open wound (S61.-)

The appropriate 7th character is to be added to each code from category S64
A - initial encounter
D - subsequent encounter
S - sequela

Indicator(s): *POAEx (7th D/S)*

S64.Ø- **Injury of ulnar nerve**
S64.ØØx_ Unspecified arm
S64.Ø1x_ Right arm
S64.Ø2x_ Left arm

S64.1- **Injury of median nerve at wrist and hand level**
S64.1Øx_ Unspecified arm
S64.11x_ Right arm
S64.12x_ Left arm

S64.2- **Injury of radial nerve at wrist and hand level**
S64.2Øx_ Unspecified arm
S64.21x_ Right arm
S64.22x_ Left arm

S64.3- **Injury of digital nerve of thumb**
S64.3Øx_ Unspecified thumb
S64.31x_ Right thumb
S64.32x_ Left thumb

S64.4- **Injury of digital nerve of other and unspecified finger**
S64.4Øx_ Unspecified finger

S64.49- **Other finger**
S64.49Ø_ Right index
S64.491_ Left index
S64.492_ Right middle
S64.493_ Left middle

See Appendix A — Coding Reference Tables for lists of the ICD-10-CM Tabular indicators, HAC categories, and HCC codes.

S64.494_ **Right ring**
S64.495_ **Left ring**
S64.496_ **Right little**
S64.497_ **Left little**
S64.498_ **Other**
Including: Specified finger with unspecified laterality

S64.8- **Injury of other nerves at wrist and hand level**
S64.8x1_ **Right arm**
S64.8x2_ **Left arm**
S64.8x9_ **Unspecified arm**

S64.9- **Injury of unspecified nerve at wrist and hand level**
S64.9Øx_ **Unspecified arm**
S64.91x_ **Right arm**
S64.92x_ **Left arm**

S66- INJURY OF MUSCLE, FASCIA AND TENDON AT WRIST AND HAND LEVEL

Code Also
any associated open wound (S61.-)
Excludes2:
sprain of joints and ligaments of wrist and hand (S63.-)

The appropriate 7th character is to be added to each code from category S66
A - initial encounter
D - subsequent encounter
S - sequela

Indicator(s): POAEx (7th D/S)

S66.Ø- **Long flexor muscle, fascia and tendon of thumb**
S66.ØØ- **Unspecified injury**
S66.ØØ1_ **Right**
S66.ØØ2_ **Left**
S66.ØØ9_ **Unspecified thumb**
S66.Ø1- **Strain**
S66.Ø11_ **Right**
S66.Ø12_ **Left**
S66.Ø19_ **Unspecified**
S66.Ø9- **Other specified injury**
S66.Ø91_ **Right**
S66.Ø92_ **Left**
S66.Ø99_ **Unspecified**

S66.1- **Flexor muscle, fascia and tendon of other and unspecified finger**
Excludes2:
Injury of long flexor muscle, fascia and tendon of thumb at wrist and hand level (S66.Ø-)
S66.1Ø- **Unspecified injury**
S66.1ØØ_ **Right index**
S66.1Ø1_ **Left index**
S66.1Ø2_ **Right middle**
S66.1Ø3_ **Left middle**
S66.1Ø4_ **Right ring**
S66.1Ø5_ **Left ring**
S66.1Ø6_ **Right little**
S66.1Ø7_ **Left little**
S66.1Ø8_ **Other finger**
Including: Specified finger with unspecified laterality
S66.1Ø9_ **Unspecified finger**
S66.11- **Strain**
S66.11Ø_ **Right index**
S66.111_ **Left index**
S66.112_ **Right middle**
S66.113_ **Left middle**
S66.114_ **Right ring**
S66.115_ **Left ring**
S66.116_ **Right little**
S66.117_ **Left little**
S66.118_ **Other finger**
Including: Specified finger with unspecified laterality
S66.119_ **Unspecified finger**
S66.19- **Other injury**
S66.19Ø_ **Right index**
S66.191_ **Left index**
S66.192_ **Right middle**
S66.193_ **Left middle**
S66.194_ **Right ring**
S66.195_ **Left ring**
S66.196_ **Right little**
S66.197_ **Left little**
S66.198_ **Other finger**
Including: Specified finger with unspecified laterality
S66.199_ **Unspecified finger**

S66.2- **Extensor muscle, fascia and tendon of thumb**
S66.2Ø- **Unspecified injury**
S66.2Ø1_ **Right**
S66.2Ø2_ **Left**
S66.2Ø9_ **Unspecified thumb**
S66.21- **Strain**
S66.211_ **Right**
S66.212_ **Left**
S66.219_ **Unspecified**
S66.29- **Other specified injury**
S66.291_ **Right**
S66.292_ **Left**
S66.299_ **Unspecified**

S66.3- **Extensor muscle, fascia and tendon of other and unspecified finger**
Excludes2:
Injury of extensor muscle, fascia and tendon of thumb at wrist and hand level (S66.2-)
S66.3Ø- **Unspecified injury**
S66.3ØØ_ **Right index**
S66.3Ø1_ **Left index**
S66.3Ø2_ **Right middle**
S66.3Ø3_ **Left middle**
S66.3Ø4_ **Right ring**
S66.3Ø5_ **Left ring**
S66.3Ø6_ **Right little**
S66.3Ø7_ **Left little**
S66.3Ø8_ **Other finger**
Including: Specified finger with unspecified laterality
S66.3Ø9_ **Unspecified finger**

S66.31- **Strain**
- **S66.31Ø_** **Right index**
- **S66.311_** **Left index**
- **S66.312_** **Right middle**
- **S66.313_** **Left middle**
- **S66.314_** **Right ring**
- **S66.315_** **Left ring**
- **S66.316_** **Right little**
- **S66.317_** **Left little**
- **S66.318_** **Other finger**
  Including: Specified finger with unspecified laterality
- **S66.319_** **Unspecified finger**

S66.39- **Other injury**
- **S66.39Ø_** **Right index**
- **S66.391_** **Left index**
- **S66.392_** **Right middle**
- **S66.393_** **Left middle**
- **S66.394_** **Right ring**
- **S66.395_** **Left ring**
- **S66.396_** **Right little**
- **S66.397_** **Left little**
- **S66.398_** **Other finger**
  Including: Specified finger with unspecified laterality
- **S66.399_** **Unspecified finger**

S66.4- **Intrinsic muscle, fascia and tendon of thumb**

S66.4Ø- **Unspecified injury**
- **S66.4Ø1_** **Right**
- **S66.4Ø2_** **Left**
- **S66.4Ø9_** **Unspecified thumb**

S66.41- **Strain**
- **S66.411_** **Right**
- **S66.412_** **Left**
- **S66.419_** **Unspecified**

S66.49- **Other specified injury**
- **S66.491_** **Right**
- **S66.492_** **Left**
- **S66.499_** **Unspecified**

S66.5- **Intrinsic muscle, fascia and tendon of other and unspecified finger**

Excludes2:
injury of intrinsic muscle, fascia and tendon of thumb at wrist and hand level (S66.4-)

S66.5Ø- **Unspecified injury**
- **S66.5ØØ_** **Right index**
- **S66.5Ø1_** **Left index**
- **S66.5Ø2_** **Right middle**
- **S66.5Ø3_** **Left middle**
- **S66.5Ø4_** **Right ring**
- **S66.5Ø5_** **Left ring**
- **S66.5Ø6_** **Right little**
- **S66.5Ø7_** **Left little**
- **S66.5Ø8_** **Other finger**
  Including: Specified finger with unspecified laterality
- **S66.5Ø9_** **Unspecified finger**

S66.51- **Strain**
- **S66.51Ø_** **Right index**
- **S66.511_** **Left index**
- **S66.512_** **Right middle**
- **S66.513_** **Left middle**
- **S66.514_** **Right ring**
- **S66.515_** **Left ring**
- **S66.516_** **Right little**
- **S66.517_** **Left little**
- **S66.518_** **Other finger**
  Including: Specified finger with unspecified laterality
- **S66.519_** **Unspecified finger**

S66.59- **Other injury**
- **S66.59Ø_** **Right index**
- **S66.591_** **Left index**
- **S66.592_** **Right middle**
- **S66.593_** **Left middle**
- **S66.594_** **Right ring**
- **S66.595_** **Left ring**
- **S66.596_** **Right little**
- **S66.597_** **Left little**
- **S66.598_** **Other finger**
  Including: Specified finger with unspecified laterality
- **S66.599_** **Unspecified finger**

S66.8- **Other specified muscles, fascia and tendons**

S66.8Ø- **Unspecified injury**
- **S66.8Ø1_** **Right**
- **S66.8Ø2_** **Left**
- **S66.8Ø9_** **Unspecified hand**

S66.81- **Strain**
- **S66.811_** **Right**
- **S66.812_** **Left**
- **S66.819_** **Unspecified**

S66.89- **Other injury**
- **S66.891_** **Right**
- **S66.892_** **Left**
- **S66.899_** **Unspecified**

S66.9- **Unspecified muscle, fascia and tendon**

S66.9Ø- **Unspecified injury**
- **S66.9Ø1_** **Right**
- **S66.9Ø2_** **Left**
- **S66.9Ø9_** **Unspecified hand**

S66.91- **Strain**
- **S66.911_** **Right**
- **S66.912_** **Left**
- **S66.919_** **Unspecified hand**

S66.99- **Other injury**
- **S66.991_** **Right**
- **S66.992_** **Left**
- **S66.999_** **Unspecified hand**

S69- OTHER AND UNSPECIFIED INJURIES OF WRIST, HAND AND FINGER(S)

The appropriate 7th character is to be added to each code from category S69
A - initial encounter
D - subsequent encounter
S - sequela

Indicator(s): POAEx (7th D/S)

S69.8- **Other specified**

S69.80x_ **Unspecified wrist, hand and finger(s)**
S69.81x_ **Right wrist, hand and finger(s)**
S69.82x_ **Left wrist, hand and finger(s)**

S69.9- **Unspecified**

S69.90x_ **Unspecified wrist, hand and finger(s)**
S69.91x_ **Right wrist, hand and finger(s)**
S69.92x_ **Left wrist, hand and finger(s)**

INJURIES TO THE HIP AND THIGH (S70-S79)

Excludes2:
burns and corrosions (T20-T32)
frostbite (T33-T34)
snake bite (T63.0-)
venomous insect bite or sting (T63.4-)
See Guidelines: 1;C.19.b

S70- SUPERFICIAL INJURY OF HIP AND THIGH

The appropriate 7th character is to be added to each code from category S70
A - initial encounter
D - subsequent encounter
S - sequela

Indicator(s): POAEx (7th D/S)

S70.0- **Contusion of hip**

S70.00x_ **Unspecified hip**
S70.01x_ **Right hip**
S70.02x_ **Left hip**

S70.1- **Contusion of thigh**

S70.10x_ **Unspecified thigh**
S70.11x_ **Right thigh**
S70.12x_ **Left thigh**

S73- DISLOCATION AND SPRAIN OF JOINT AND LIGAMENTS OF HIP

Includes:
avulsion of joint or ligament of hip
laceration of cartilage, joint or ligament of hip
sprain of cartilage, joint or ligament of hip
traumatic hemarthrosis of joint or ligament of hip
traumatic rupture of joint or ligament of hip
traumatic subluxation of joint or ligament of hip
traumatic tear of joint or ligament of hip
Code Also
any associated open wound
Excludes2:
strain of muscle, fascia and tendon of hip and thigh (S76.-)

The appropriate 7th character is to be added to each code from category S73
A - initial encounter
D - subsequent encounter
S - sequela

Indicator(s): POAEx (7th D/S)

S73.0- **Subluxation and dislocation**

Excludes2:
dislocation and subluxation of hip prosthesis (T84.020, T84.021)
Indicator(s): CC (7th A) | HAC: 05 (7th A) | CMS22: 170 (7th A) | CMS24: 170 (7th A) | ESRD21: 170 (7th A)

S73.00- **Unspecified subluxation and dislocation**
Including: hip NOS

S73.001_ **Right**
S73.002_ **Left**
S73.003_ **Unspecified hip**
S73.004_ **Right**
S73.005_ **Left**
S73.006_ **Unspecified hip**

S73.01- **Posterior**

S73.011_ **Right**
S73.012_ **Left**
S73.013_ **Unspecified**
S73.014_ **Right**
S73.015_ **Left**
S73.016_ **Unspecified**

S73.02- **Obturator**

S73.021_ **Right**
S73.022_ **Left**
S73.023_ **Unspecified**
S73.024_ **Right**
S73.025_ **Left**
S73.026_ **Unspecified**

S73.03- **Other anterior dislocation**

S73.031_ **Subluxation right**
S73.032_ **Subluxation left**
S73.033_ **Subluxation unspecified**
S73.034_ **Right**
S73.035_ **Left**
S73.036_ **Unspecified**

S73.04- **Central dislocation**

S73.041_ **Subluxation right**
S73.042_ **Subluxation left**
S73.043_ **Subluxation unspecified**
S73.044_ **Right**
S73.045_ **Left**
S73.046_ **Unspecified**

S73.1- **Sprain of hip**

S73.10- **Unspecified sprain**

S73.101_ **Right**
S73.102_ **Left**
S73.109_ **Unspecified hip**

S73.11- **Iliofemoral ligament sprain**

S73.111_ **Right**
S73.112_ **Left**
S73.119_ **Unspecified**

S73.12- **Ischiocapsular (ligament) sprain**

S73.121_ **Right**
S73.122_ **Left**
S73.129_ **Unspecified**

S73.19- **Other sprain**
- **S73.191_ Right**
- **S73.192_ Left**
- **S73.199_ Unspecified**

S74- INJURY OF NERVES AT HIP AND THIGH LEVEL

Code Also
any associated open wound (S71.-)
Excludes2:
injury of nerves at ankle and foot level (S94.-)
injury of nerves at lower leg level (S84.-)

The appropriate 7th character is to be added to each code from category S74
A - initial encounter
D - subsequent encounter
S - sequela

Indicator(s): POAEx (7th D/S)

S74.Ø- **Sciatic nerve**
- **S74.ØØx_ Unspecified leg**
- **S74.Ø1x_ Right leg**
- **S74.Ø2x_ Left leg**

S74.1- **Femoral nerve**
- **S74.1Øx_ Unspecified leg**
- **S74.11x_ Right leg**
- **S74.12x_ Left leg**

S74.2- **Cutaneous sensory nerve**
- **S74.2Øx_ Unspecified leg**
- **S74.21x_ Right leg**
- **S74.22x_ Left leg**

S74.8- **Other nerves**
- **S74.8x1_ Right leg**
- **S74.8x2_ Left leg**
- **S74.8x9_ Unspecified leg**

S74.9- **Unspecified nerve**
- **S74.9Øx_ Unspecified leg**
- **S74.91x_ Right leg**
- **S74.92x_ Left leg**

S76- INJURY OF MUSCLE, FASCIA AND TENDON AT HIP AND THIGH LEVEL

Code Also
any associated open wound (S71.-)
Excludes2:
injury of muscle, fascia and tendon at lower leg level (S86)
sprain of joint and ligament of hip (S73.1)

The appropriate 7th character is to be added to each code from category S76
A - initial encounter
D - subsequent encounter
S - sequela

Indicator(s): POAEx (7th D/S)

S76.Ø- **Hip**

S76.ØØ- **Unspecified injury**
- **S76.ØØ1_ Right**
- **S76.ØØ2_ Left**
- **S76.ØØ9_ Unspecified hip**

S76.Ø1- **Strain**
- **S76.Ø11_ Right**
- **S76.Ø12_ Left**
- **S76.Ø19_ Unspecified**

S76.Ø2- **Laceration**
Indicator(s): CC (7th A)
- **S76.Ø21_ Right**
- **S76.Ø22_ Left**
- **S76.Ø29_ Unspecified**

S76.Ø9- **Other specified injury**
- **S76.Ø91_ Right**
- **S76.Ø92_ Left**
- **S76.Ø99_ Unspecified**

S76.1- **Quadriceps muscle, fascia and tendon**
Including: Injury of patellar ligament (tendon)

S76.1Ø- **Unspecified injury**
- **S76.1Ø1_ Right**
- **S76.1Ø2_ Left**
- **S76.1Ø9_ Unspecified part**

S76.11- **Strain**
- **S76.111_ Right**
- **S76.112_ Left**
- **S76.119_ Unspecified**

S76.12- **Laceration**
Indicator(s): CC (7th A)
- **S76.121_ Right**
- **S76.122_ Left**
- **S76.129_ Unspecified**

S76.19- **Other specified injury**
- **S76.191_ Right**
- **S76.192_ Left**
- **S76.199_ Unspecified**

S76.2- **Adductor muscle, fascia and tendon of thigh**

S76.2Ø- **Unspecified injury**
- **S76.2Ø1_ Right**
- **S76.2Ø2_ Left**
- **S76.2Ø9_ Unspecified thigh**

S76.21- **Strain**
- **S76.211_ Right**
- **S76.212_ Left**
- **S76.219_ Unspecified**

S76.22- **Laceration**
Indicator(s): CC (7th A)
- **S76.221_ Right**
- **S76.222_ Left**
- **S76.229_ Unspecified**

S76.29- **Other injury**
- **S76.291_ Right**
- **S76.292_ Left**
- **S76.299_ Unspecified**

S76.3- **The posterior muscle group at thigh level**

S76.3Ø- **Unspecified injury**

S76.3Ø1_ **Right**

S76.3Ø2_ **Left**

S76.3Ø9_ **Unspecified thigh**

S76.31- **Strain**

S76.311_ **Right**

S76.312_ **Left**

S76.319_ **Unspecified**

S76.32- **Laceration**

Indicator(s): CC (7th A)

S76.321_ **Right**

S76.322_ **Left**

S76.329_ **Unspecified**

S76.39- **Other specified injury**

S76.391_ **Right**

S76.392_ **Left**

S76.399_ **Unspecified**

S76.8- **Other specified muscles, fascia and tendons at thigh level**

S76.8Ø- **Unspecified injury**

S76.8Ø1_ **Right**

S76.8Ø2_ **Left**

S76.8Ø9_ **Unspecified thigh**

S76.81- **Strain**

S76.811_ **Right**

S76.812_ **Left**

S76.819_ **Unspecified**

S76.82- **Laceration**

Indicator(s): CC (7th A)

S76.821_ **Right**

S76.822_ **Left**

S76.829_ **Unspecified**

S76.89- **Other injury**

S76.891_ **Right**

S76.892_ **Left**

S76.899_ **Unspecified**

S76.9- **Unspecified muscles, fascia and tendons at thigh level**

S76.9Ø- **Unspecified injury**

S76.9Ø1_ **Right**

S76.9Ø2_ **Left**

S76.9Ø9_ **Unspecified thigh**

S76.91- **Strain**

S76.911_ **Right**

S76.912_ **Left**

S76.919_ **Unspecified thigh**

S76.92- **Laceration**

Indicator(s): CC (7th A)

S76.921_ **Right**

S76.922_ **Left**

S76.929_ **Unspecified thigh**

S76.99- **Other specified injury**

S76.991_ **Right**

S76.992_ **Left**

S76.999_ **Unspecified thigh**

S79- OTHER AND UNSPECIFIED INJURIES OF HIP AND THIGH

Notes:

A fracture not indicated as open or closed should be coded to closed

The appropriate 7th character is to be added to each code from subcategories S79.Ø and S79.1

A - initial encounter for closed fracture

D - subsequent encounter for fracture with routine healing

G - subsequent encounter for fracture with delayed healing

K - subsequent encounter for fracture with nonunion

P - subsequent encounter for fracture with malunion

S - sequela

See Guidelines: 1;C.19.c

S79.8- **Other specified injuries**

The appropriate 7th character is to be added to each code in subcategory S79.8

A - initial encounter

D - subsequent encounter

S - sequela

Indicator(s): POAEx (7th D/S)

S79.81- **Hip**

S79.811_ **Right**

S79.812_ **Left**

S79.819_ **Unspecified**

S79.82- **Thigh**

S79.821_ **Right**

S79.822_ **Left**

S79.829_ **Unspecified**

S79.9- **Unspecified injury**

The appropriate 7th character is to be added to each code in subcategory S79.9

A - initial encounter

D - subsequent encounter

S - sequela

Indicator(s): POAEx (7th D/S)

S79.91- **Hip**

S79.911_ **Right**

S79.912_ **Left**

S79.919_ **Unspecified hip**

S79.92- **Thigh**

S79.921_ **Right**

S79.922_ **Left**

S79.929_ **Unspecified thigh**

INJURIES TO THE KNEE AND LOWER LEG (S8Ø-S89)

Excludes2:
burns and corrosions (T2Ø-T32)
frostbite (T33-T34)
injuries of ankle and foot, except fracture of ankle and malleolus (S9Ø-S99)
insect bite or sting, venomous (T63.4)
See Guidelines: 1;C.19.b

S8Ø- SUPERFICIAL INJURY OF KNEE AND LOWER LEG
Excludes2:
superficial injury of ankle and foot (S9Ø.-)
The appropriate 7th character is to be added to each code from category S8Ø
A - initial encounter
D - subsequent encounter
S - sequela
Indicator(s): POAEx (7th D/S)

S8Ø.Ø- **Contusion of knee**
S8Ø.ØØx_ Unspecified knee
S8Ø.Ø1x_ Right knee
S8Ø.Ø2x_ Left knee

S8Ø.1- **Contusion of lower leg**
S8Ø.1Øx_ Unspecified leg
S8Ø.11x_ Right leg
S8Ø.12x_ Left leg

S83- DISLOCATION AND SPRAIN OF JOINTS AND LIGAMENTS OF KNEE
Includes:
avulsion of joint or ligament of knee
laceration of cartilage, joint or ligament of knee
sprain of cartilage, joint or ligament of knee
traumatic hemarthrosis of joint or ligament of knee
traumatic rupture of joint or ligament of knee
traumatic subluxation of joint or ligament of knee
traumatic tear of joint or ligament of knee
Code Also
any associated open wound
Excludes2:
derangement of patella (M22.Ø-M22.3)
injury of patellar ligament (tendon) (S76.1-)
internal derangement of knee (M23.-)
old dislocation of knee (M24.36)
pathological dislocation of knee (M24.36)
recurrent dislocation of knee (M22.Ø)
strain of muscle, fascia and tendon of lower leg (S86.-)
The appropriate 7th character is to be added to each code from category S83
A - initial encounter
D - subsequent encounter
S - sequela
Indicator(s): POAEx (7th D/S)

S83.Ø- **Subluxation and dislocation of patella**
S83.ØØ- **Unspecified**
S83.ØØ1_ Right
S83.ØØ2_ Left
S83.ØØ3_ Unspecified patella
S83.ØØ4_ Right
S83.ØØ5_ Left
S83.ØØ6_ Unspecified patella

S83.Ø1- **Lateral**
S83.Ø11_ Right
S83.Ø12_ Left
S83.Ø13_ Unspecified
S83.Ø14_ Right
S83.Ø15_ Left
S83.Ø16_ Unspecified

S83.Ø9- **Other**
S83.Ø91_ Right
S83.Ø92_ Left
S83.Ø93_ Unspecified
S83.Ø94_ Right
S83.Ø95_ Left
S83.Ø96_ Unspecified

S83.1- **Subluxation and dislocation of knee**
Excludes2:
instability of knee prosthesis (T84.Ø22, T84.Ø23)

S83.1Ø- **Unspecified**
S83.1Ø1_ Right
S83.1Ø2_ Left
S83.1Ø3_ Unspecified knee
S83.1Ø4_ Right
S83.1Ø5_ Left
S83.1Ø6_ Unspecified knee

S83.11- **Anterior subluxation and dislocation of proximal end of tibia**
Including: Posterior subluxation and dislocation of distal end of femur
S83.111_ Right knee
S83.112_ Left knee
S83.113_ Unspecified knee
S83.114_ Right knee
S83.115_ Left knee
S83.116_ Unspecified knee

S83.12- **Posterior subluxation and dislocation of proximal end of tibia**
Including: Anterior dislocation of distal end of femur
S83.121_ Right knee
S83.122_ Left knee
S83.123_ Unspecified knee
S83.124_ Right knee
S83.125_ Left knee
S83.126_ Unspecified knee

S83.13- **Medial subluxation and dislocation of proximal end of tibia**
S83.131_ Right knee
S83.132_ Left knee
S83.133_ Unspecified knee
S83.134_ Right knee
S83.135_ Left knee
S83.136_ Unspecified knee

S83.14- **Lateral subluxation and dislocation of proximal end of tibia**
- **S83.141_ Right knee**
- **S83.142_ Left knee**
- **S83.143_ Unspecified knee**
- **S83.144_ Right knee**
- **S83.145_ Left knee**
- **S83.146_ Unspecified knee**

S83.19- **Other**
- **S83.191_ Right**
- **S83.192_ Left**
- **S83.193_ Unspecified**
- **S83.194_ Right**
- **S83.195_ Left**
- **S83.196_ Unspecified**

S83.2- **Tear of meniscus, current injury**

Excludes1:
old bucket-handle tear (M23.2)

S83.2Ø- **Unspecified meniscus**
Including: Tear of meniscus of knee NOS
- **S83.2ØØ_ Bucket-handle tear right knee**
- **S83.2Ø1_ Bucket-handle tear left knee**
- **S83.2Ø2_ Bucket-handle tear unspecified knee**
- **S83.2Ø3_ Other tear right knee**
- **S83.2Ø4_ Other tear left knee**
- **S83.2Ø5_ Other tear unspecified knee**
- **S83.2Ø6_ Right knee**
- **S83.2Ø7_ Left knee**
- **S83.2Ø9_ Unspecified tear unspecified knee**

S83.21- **Bucket-handle tear of medial meniscus**
- **S83.211_ Right knee**
- **S83.212_ Left knee**
- **S83.219_ Unspecified knee**

S83.22- **Peripheral tear of medial meniscus**
- **S83.221_ Right knee**
- **S83.222_ Left knee**
- **S83.229_ Unspecified knee**

S83.23- **Complex tear of medial meniscus**
- **S83.231_ Right knee**
- **S83.232_ Left knee**
- **S83.239_ Unspecified knee**

S83.24- **Other tear of medial meniscus**
- **S83.241_ Right knee**
- **S83.242_ Left knee**
- **S83.249_ Unspecified knee**

S83.25- **Bucket-handle tear of lateral meniscus**
- **S83.251_ Right knee**
- **S83.252_ Left knee**
- **S83.259_ Unspecified knee**

S83.26- **Peripheral tear of lateral meniscus**
- **S83.261_ Right knee**
- **S83.262_ Left knee**
- **S83.269_ Unspecified knee**

S83.27- **Complex tear of lateral meniscus**
- **S83.271_ Right knee**
- **S83.272_ Left knee**
- **S83.279_ Unspecified knee**

S83.28- **Other tear of lateral meniscus**
- **S83.281_ Right knee**
- **S83.282_ Left knee**
- **S83.289_ Unspecified knee**

S83.3- **Tear of articular cartilage of knee, current**
- **S83.3Øx_ Unspecified knee**
- **S83.31x_ Right knee**
- **S83.32x_ Left knee**

S83.4- **Sprain of collateral ligament**

S83.4Ø- **Unspecified collateral ligament**
- **S83.4Ø1_ Right**
- **S83.4Ø2_ Left**
- **S83.4Ø9_ Unspecified knee**

S83.41- **Medial collateral ligament**
Including: Sprain of tibial collateral ligament
- **S83.411_ Right**
- **S83.412_ Left**
- **S83.419_ Unspecified**

S83.42- **Lateral collateral ligament**
Including: Sprain of fibular collateral ligament
- **S83.421_ Right**
- **S83.422_ Left**
- **S83.429_ Unspecified**

S83.5- **Sprain of cruciate ligament of knee**

S83.5Ø- **Unspecified cruciate ligament**
- **S83.5Ø1_ Right**
- **S83.5Ø2_ Left**
- **S83.5Ø9_ Unspecified knee**

S83.51- **Anterior cruciate ligament**
- **S83.511_ Right**
- **S83.512_ Left**
- **S83.519_ Unspecified**

S83.52- **Posterior cruciate ligament**
- **S83.521_ Right**
- **S83.522_ Left**
- **S83.529_ Unspecified**

S83.6- **Sprain of the superior tibiofibular joint and ligament**
- **S83.6Øx_ Unspecified knee**
- **S83.61x_ Right knee**
- **S83.62x_ Left knee**

S83.8- **Sprain of other specified parts of knee**

S83.8X- **Other specified parts**
- **S83.8x1_ Right**
- **S83.8x2_ Left**
- **S83.8x9_ Unspecified**

S83.9- **Sprain of unspecified site of knee**
- **S83.9Øx_ Unspecified knee**
- **S83.91x_ Right knee**
- **S83.92x_ Left knee**

S84- INJURY OF NERVES AT LOWER LEG LEVEL

<u>Code Also</u>

any associated open wound (S81.-)

<u>Excludes2:</u>

injury of nerves at ankle and foot level (S94.-)

The appropriate 7th character is to be added to each code from category S84

A - initial encounter

D - subsequent encounter

S - sequela

<u>Indicator(s):</u> POAEx (7th D/S)

S84.Ø- **Tibial nerve**

S84.ØØx_ Unspecified leg

S84.Ø1x_ Right leg

S84.Ø2x_ Left leg

S84.1- **Peroneal nerve**

S84.1Øx_ Unspecified leg

S84.11x_ Right leg

S84.12x_ Left leg

S84.2- **Cutaneous sensory nerve**

S84.2Øx_ Unspecified leg

S84.21x_ Right leg

S84.22x_ Left leg

S84.8- **Injury of other nerves at lower leg level**

S84.8Ø- **Other nerves**

S84.8Ø1_ Right

S84.8Ø2_ Left

S84.8Ø9_ Unspecified

S84.9- **Unspecified nerve**

S84.9Øx_ Unspecified leg

S84.91x_ Right leg

S84.92x_ Left leg

S86- INJURY OF MUSCLE, FASCIA AND TENDON AT LOWER LEG LEVEL

<u>Code Also</u>

any associated open wound (S81.-)

<u>Excludes2:</u>

injury of muscle, fascia and tendon at ankle (S96.-)

injury of patellar ligament (tendon) (S76.1-)

sprain of joints and ligaments of knee (S83.-)

The appropriate 7th character is to be added to each code from category S86

A - initial encounter

D - subsequent encounter

S - sequela

<u>Indicator(s):</u> POAEx (7th D/S)

S86.Ø- **Achilles tendon**

S86.ØØ- **Unspecified injury**

S86.ØØ1_ Right

S86.ØØ2_ Left

S86.ØØ9_ Unspecified leg

S86.Ø1- **Strain**

S86.Ø11_ Right

S86.Ø12_ Left

S86.Ø19_ Unspecified

S86.Ø2- **Laceration**

<u>Indicator(s):</u> CC (7th A)

S86.Ø21_ Right

S86.Ø22_ Left

S86.Ø29_ Unspecified

S86.Ø9- **Other specified injury**

S86.Ø91_ Right

S86.Ø92_ Left

S86.Ø99_ Unspecified

S86.1- **Other muscle(s) and tendon(s) of posterior muscle group**

S86.1Ø- **Unspecified injury**

S86.1Ø1_ Right

S86.1Ø2_ Left

S86.1Ø9_ Unspecified leg

S86.11- **Strain**

S86.111_ Right

S86.112_ Left

S86.119_ Unspecified

S86.12- **Laceration**

<u>Indicator(s):</u> CC (7th A)

S86.121_ Right

S86.122_ Left

S86.129_ Unspecified

S86.19- **Other injury**

S86.191_ Right

S86.192_ Left

S86.199_ Unspecified

S86.2- **Muscle(s) and tendon(s) of anterior muscle group**

S86.2Ø- **Unspecified injury**

S86.2Ø1_ Right

S86.2Ø2_ Left

S86.2Ø9_ Unspecified leg

S86.21- **Strain**

S86.211_ Right

S86.212_ Left

S86.219_ Unspecified

S86.22- **Laceration**

<u>Indicator(s):</u> CC (7th A)

S86.221_ Right

S86.222_ Left

S86.229_ Unspecified

S86.29- **Other injury**

S86.291_ Right

S86.292_ Left

S86.299_ Unspecified

S86.3- **Muscle(s) and tendon(s) of peroneal muscle group**

S86.3Ø- **Unspecified injury**

S86.3Ø1_ Right

S86.3Ø2_ Left

S86.3Ø9_ Unspecified leg

S86.31- **Strain**
S86.311_ Right
S86.312_ Left
S86.319_ Unspecified
S86.32- **Laceration**
Indicator(s): CC (7th A)
S86.321_ Right
S86.322_ Left
S86.329_ Unspecified
S86.39- **Other injury**
S86.391_ Right
S86.392_ Left
S86.399_ Unspecified
S86.8- **Other muscles and tendons**
S86.8Ø- **Unspecified injury**
S86.8Ø1_ Right
S86.8Ø2_ Left
S86.8Ø9_ Unspecified leg
S86.81- **Strain**
S86.811_ Right
S86.812_ Left
S86.819_ Unspecified
S86.82- **Laceration**
Indicator(s): CC (7th A)
S86.821_ Right
S86.822_ Left
S86.829_ Unspecified
S86.89- **Other injury**
S86.891_ Right
S86.892_ Left
S86.899_ Unspecified
S86.9- **Unspecified muscle and tendon**
S86.9Ø- **Unspecified injury**
S86.9Ø1_ Right
S86.9Ø2_ Left
S86.9Ø9_ Unspecified leg
S86.91- **Strain**
S86.911_ Right
S86.912_ Left
S86.919_ Unspecified
S86.92- **Laceration**
Indicator(s): CC (7th A)
S86.921_ Right
S86.922_ Left
S86.929_ Unspecified
S86.99- **Other injury**
S86.991_ Right
S86.992_ Left
S86.999_ Unspecified

S89- OTHER AND UNSPECIFIED INJURIES OF LOWER LEG

Notes:
A fracture not indicated as open or closed should be coded to closed
Excludes2:
other and unspecified injuries of ankle and foot (S99.-)

The appropriate 7th character is to be added to each code from subcategories S89.Ø, S89.1, S89.2, and S89.3
A - initial encounter for closed fracture
D - subsequent encounter for fracture with routine healing
G - subsequent encounter for fracture with delayed healing
K - subsequent encounter for fracture with nonunion
P - subsequent encounter for fracture with malunion
S - sequela

See Guidelines: 1;C.19.c

S89.8- **Other specified injuries**
The appropriate 7th character is to be added to each code in subcategory S89.8
A - initial encounter
D - subsequent encounter
S - sequela
Indicator(s): POAEx (7th D/S)
S89.8Øx_ Unspecified lower leg
S89.81x_ Right lower leg
S89.82x_ Left lower leg
S89.9- **Unspecified injury**
The appropriate 7th character is to be added to each code in subcategory S89.9
A - initial encounter
D - subsequent encounter
S - sequela
Indicator(s): POAEx (7th D/S)
S89.9Øx_ Unspecified lower leg
S89.91x_ Right lower leg
S89.92x_ Left lower leg

INJURIES TO THE ANKLE AND FOOT (S9Ø-S99)

Excludes2:
burns and corrosions (T2Ø-T32)
fracture of ankle and malleolus (S82.-)
frostbite (T33-T34)
insect bite or sting, venomous (T63.4)
See Guidelines: 1;C.19.b

S9Ø- SUPERFICIAL INJURY OF ANKLE, FOOT AND TOES

The appropriate 7th character is to be added to each code from category S9Ø
A - initial encounter
D - subsequent encounter
S - sequela
Indicator(s): POAEx (7th D/S)

S9Ø.Ø- **Contusion of ankle**
S9Ø.ØØx_ Unspecified ankle
S9Ø.Ø1x_ Right ankle
S9Ø.Ø2x_ Left ankle

S9Ø.1- **Contusion of toe without damage to nail**

S9Ø.11- **Great toe**

S9Ø.111_ **Right**

S9Ø.112_ **Left**

S9Ø.119_ **Unspecified**

S9Ø.12- **Lesser toe**

S9Ø.121_ **Right**

S9Ø.122_ **Left**

S9Ø.129_ **Unspecified**

Including: Contusion of toe NOS

S9Ø.2- **Contusion of toe with damage to nail**

S9Ø.21- **Great toe**

S9Ø.211_ **Right**

S9Ø.212_ **Left**

S9Ø.219_ **Unspecified**

S9Ø.22- **Lesser toe**

S9Ø.221_ **Right**

S9Ø.222_ **Left**

S9Ø.229_ **Unspecified**

S9Ø.3- **Contusion of foot**

Excludes2:

contusion of toes (S9Ø.1-, S9Ø.2-)

S9Ø.3Øx_ **Unspecified foot**

Including: Contusion of foot NOS

S9Ø.31x_ **Right foot**

S9Ø.32x_ **Left foot**

S93- DISLOCATION AND SPRAIN OF JOINTS AND LIGAMENTS AT ANKLE, FOOT AND TOE LEVEL

Includes:

avulsion of joint or ligament of ankle, foot and toe

laceration of cartilage, joint or ligament of ankle, foot and toe

sprain of cartilage, joint or ligament of ankle, foot and toe

traumatic hemarthrosis of joint or ligament of ankle, foot and toe

traumatic rupture of joint or ligament of ankle, foot and toe

traumatic subluxation of joint or ligament of ankle, foot and toe

traumatic tear of joint or ligament of ankle, foot and toe

Code Also

any associated open wound

Excludes2:

strain of muscle and tendon of ankle and foot (S96.-)

The appropriate 7th character is to be added to each code from category S93

A - initial encounter

D - subsequent encounter

S - sequela

Indicator(s): POAEx (7th D/S)

S93.Ø- **Subluxation and dislocation of ankle joint**

Including: Astragalus; fibula, lower end; talus; tibia, lower end

S93.Ø1x_ **Subluxation of right ankle joint**

S93.Ø2x_ **Subluxation of left ankle joint**

S93.Ø3x_ **Subluxation of unspecified ankle joint**

S93.Ø4x_ **Dislocation of right ankle joint**

S93.Ø5x_ **Dislocation of left ankle joint**

S93.Ø6x_ **Dislocation of unspecified ankle joint**

S93.1- **Subluxation and dislocation of toe**

S93.1Ø- **Unspecified**

Including: Toe NOS

S93.1Ø1_ **Right toe(s)**

S93.1Ø2_ **Left toe(s)**

S93.1Ø3_ **Subluxation unspecified toe(s)**

S93.1Ø4_ **Right toe(s)**

S93.1Ø5_ **Left toe(s)**

S93.1Ø6_ **Dislocation unspecified toe(s)**

S93.11- **Dislocation of interphalangeal joint**

S93.111_ **Right great toe**

S93.112_ **Left great toe**

S93.113_ **Unspecified great toe**

S93.114_ **Right lesser toe(s)**

S93.115_ **Left lesser toe(s)**

S93.116_ **Unspecified lesser toe(s)**

S93.119_ **Unspecified toe(s)**

S93.12- **Dislocation of metatarsophalangeal joint**

S93.121_ **Right great toe**

S93.122_ **Left great toe**

S93.123_ **Unspecified great toe**

S93.124_ **Right lesser toe(s)**

S93.125_ **Left lesser toe(s)**

S93.126_ **Unspecified lesser toe(s)**

S93.129_ **Unspecified toe(s)**

S93.13- **Subluxation of interphalangeal joint**

S93.131_ **Right great toe**

S93.132_ **Left great toe**

S93.133_ **Unspecified great toe**

S93.134_ **Right lesser toe(s)**

S93.135_ **Left lesser toe(s)**

S93.136_ **Unspecified lesser toe(s)**

S93.139_ **Unspecified toe(s)**

S93.14- **Subluxation of metatarsophalangeal joint**

S93.141_ **Right great toe**

S93.142_ **Left great toe**

S93.143_ **Unspecified great toe**

S93.144_ **Right lesser toe(s)**

S93.145_ **Left lesser toe(s)**

S93.146_ **Unspecified lesser toe(s)**

S93.149_ **Unspecified toe(s)**

S93.3- **Subluxation and dislocation of foot**

Excludes2:

dislocation of toe (S93.1-)

S93.3Ø- **Unspecified**

Including: Foot NOS

S93.3Ø1_ **Right**

S93.3Ø2_ **Left**

S93.3Ø3_ **Subluxation unspecified foot**

S93.3Ø4_ **Right**

S93.3Ø5_ **Left**

S93.3Ø6_ **Dislocation unspecified foot**

S93.31- **Tarsal joint**
S93.311_ Right foot
S93.312_ Left foot
S93.313_ Unspecified foot
S93.314_ Right foot
S93.315_ Left foot
S93.316_ Unspecified foot

S93.32- **Tarsometatarsal joint**
S93.321_ Right foot
S93.322_ Left foot
S93.323_ Unspecified foot
S93.324_ Right foot
S93.325_ Left foot
S93.326_ Unspecified foot

S93.33- **Other**
S93.331_ Right
S93.332_ Left
S93.333_ Unspecified
S93.334_ Right
S93.335_ Left
S93.336_ Unspecified

S93.4- **Sprain of ankle**
Excludes2:
injury of Achilles tendon (S86.Ø-)

S93.4Ø- **Sprain of unspecified ligament**
Including: Ankle NOS
S93.4Ø1_ Right
S93.4Ø2_ Left
S93.4Ø9_ Unspecified ankle

S93.41- **Sprain of calcaneofibular ligament**
S93.411_ Right ankle
S93.412_ Left ankle
S93.419_ Unspecified ankle

S93.42- **Sprain of deltoid ligament**
S93.421_ Right ankle
S93.422_ Left ankle
S93.429_ Unspecified ankle

S93.43- **Sprain of tibiofibular ligament**
S93.431_ Right ankle
S93.432_ Left ankle
S93.439_ Unspecified ankle

S93.49- **Sprain of other ligament**
Including: Internal collateral ligament, talofibular ligament
S93.491_ Right
S93.492_ Left
S93.499_ Unspecified

S93.5- **Sprain of toe**

S93.5Ø- **Unspecified sprain**
S93.5Ø1_ Right great
S93.5Ø2_ Left great
S93.5Ø3_ Unspecified great toe
S93.5Ø4_ Right lesser toe(s)
S93.5Ø5_ Left lesser toe(s)
S93.5Ø6_ Unspecified lesser toe(s)
S93.5Ø9_ Unspecified toe(s)

S93.51- **Sprain of interphalangeal joint**
S93.511_ Right great
S93.512_ Left great
S93.513_ Unspecified great
S93.514_ Right lesser toe(s)
S93.515_ Left lesser toe(s)
S93.516_ Unspecified lesser toe(s)
S93.519_ Unspecified toe(s)

S93.52- **Sprain of metatarsophalangeal joint**
S93.521_ Right great
S93.522_ Left great
S93.523_ Unspecified great
S93.524_ Right lesser toe(s)
S93.525_ Left lesser toe(s)
S93.526_ Unspecified lesser toe(s)
S93.529_ Unspecified toe(s)

S93.6- **Sprain of foot**
Excludes2:
sprain of metatarsophalangeal joint of toe (S93.52-)
sprain of toe (S93.5-)

S93.6Ø- **Unspecified sprain**
S93.6Ø1_ Right
S93.6Ø2_ Left
S93.6Ø9_ Unspecified foot

S93.61- **Sprain of tarsal ligament**
S93.611_ Right
S93.612_ Left
S93.619_ Unspecified

S93.62- **Sprain of tarsometatarsal ligament**
S93.621_ Right
S93.622_ Left
S93.629_ Unspecified

S93.69- **Other sprain**
S93.691_ Right
S93.692_ Left
S93.699_ Unspecified

S94- INJURY OF NERVES AT ANKLE AND FOOT LEVEL
Code Also
any associated open wound (S91.-)

The appropriate 7th character is to be added to each code from category S94
A - initial encounter
D - subsequent encounter
S - sequela

Indicator(s): POAEx (7th D/S)

S94.Ø- **Lateral plantar nerve**
S94.ØØx_ Unspecified leg
S94.Ø1x_ Right leg
S94.Ø2x_ Left leg

S94.1- **Medial plantar nerve**
S94.1Øx_ Unspecified leg
S94.11x_ Right leg
S94.12x_ Left leg

Ch5

5. The Tabular List

S94.2- **Deep peroneal nerve**
Including: Injury of terminal, lateral branch of deep peroneal nerve
S94.2Øx_ Unspecified leg
S94.21x_ Right leg
S94.22x_ Left leg

S94.3- **Cutaneous sensory nerve**
S94.3Øx_ Unspecified leg
S94.31x_ Right leg
S94.32x_ Left leg

S94.8- **Injury of other nerves at ankle and foot level**
S94.8X- **Other nerves**
S94.8x1_ Right leg
S94.8x2_ Left leg
S94.8x9_ Unspecified leg

S94.9- **Unspecified nerve**
S94.9Øx_ Unspecified leg
S94.91x_ Right leg
S94.92x_ Left leg

S96- INJURY OF MUSCLE AND TENDON AT ANKLE AND FOOT LEVEL

Code Also
any associated open wound (S91.-)
Excludes2:
injury of Achilles tendon (S86.Ø-)
sprain of joints and ligaments of ankle and foot (S93.-)

The appropriate 7th character is to be added to each code from category S96
A - initial encounter
D - subsequent encounter
S - sequela

Indicator(s): POAEx (7th D/S)

S96.Ø- **Long flexor muscle of toe**
S96.ØØ- **Unspecified injury**
S96.ØØ1_ Right
S96.ØØ2_ Left
S96.ØØ9_ Unspecified foot
S96.Ø1- **Strain**
S96.Ø11_ Right
S96.Ø12_ Left
S96.Ø19_ Unspecified
S96.Ø2- **Laceration**
Indicator(s): CC (7th A)
S96.Ø21_ Right
S96.Ø22_ Left
S96.Ø29_ Unspecified
S96.Ø9- **Other injury**
S96.Ø91_ Right
S96.Ø92_ Left
S96.Ø99_ Unspecified

S96.1- **Long extensor muscle of toe**
S96.1Ø- **Unspecified injury**
S96.1Ø1_ Right
S96.1Ø2_ Left
S96.1Ø9_ Unspecified foot
S96.11- **Strain**
S96.111_ Right
S96.112_ Left
S96.119_ Unspecified
S96.12- **Laceration**
Indicator(s): CC (7th A)
S96.121_ Right
S96.122_ Left
S96.129_ Unspecified
S96.19- **Other specified injury**
S96.191_ Right
S96.192_ Left
S96.199_ Unspecified

S96.2- **Intrinsic muscle and tendon**
S96.2Ø- **Unspecified injury**
S96.2Ø1_ Right
S96.2Ø2_ Left
S96.2Ø9_ Unspecified foot
S96.21- **Strain**
S96.211_ Right
S96.212_ Left
S96.219_ Unspecified
S96.22- **Laceration**
Indicator(s): CC (7th A)
S96.221_ Right
S96.222_ Left
S96.229_ Unspecified
S96.29- **Other specified injury**
S96.291_ Right
S96.292_ Left
S96.299_ Unspecified

S96.8- **Other specified muscles and tendons**
S96.8Ø- **Unspecified injury**
S96.8Ø1_ Right
S96.8Ø2_ Left
S96.8Ø9_ Unspecified foot
S96.81- **Strain**
S96.811_ Right
S96.812_ Left
S96.819_ Unspecified
S96.82- **Laceration**
Indicator(s): CC (7th A)
S96.821_ Right
S96.822_ Left
S96.829_ Unspecified
S96.89- **Other specified injury**
S96.891_ Right
S96.892_ Left
S96.899_ Unspecified

S96.9- **Unspecified muscle and tendon**
S96.9Ø- **Unspecified injury**
S96.9Ø1_ Right
S96.9Ø2_ Left
S96.9Ø9_ Unspecified foot

S96.91- **Strain**

S96.911_ Right

S96.912_ Left

S96.919_ Unspecified foot

S96.92- **Laceration**

Indicator(s): CC (7th A)

S96.921_ Right

S96.922_ Left

S96.929_ Unspecified foot

S96.99- **Other specified injury**

S96.991_ Right

S96.992_ Left

S96.999_ Unspecified foot

S99- OTHER AND UNSPECIFIED INJURIES OF ANKLE AND FOOT

S99.8- **Other specified injuries**

The appropriate 7th character is to be added to each code from subcategory S99.8

A - initial encounter

D - subsequent encounter

S - sequela

Indicator(s): POAEx (7th D/S)

S99.81- **Ankle**

S99.811_ Right

S99.812_ Left

S99.819_ Unspecified

S99.82- **Foot**

S99.821_ Right

S99.822_ Left

S99.829_ Unspecified

S99.9- **Unspecified injury**

The appropriate 7th character is to be added to each code from subcategory S99.9

A - initial encounter

D - subsequent encounter

S - sequela

Indicator(s): POAEx (7th D/S)

S99.91- **Ankle**

S99.911_ Right

S99.912_ Left

S99.919_ Unspecified ankle

S99.92- **Foot**

S99.921_ Right

S99.922_ Left

S99.929_ Unspecified foot

INJURY, POISONING AND CERTAIN OTHER CONSEQUENCES OF EXTERNAL CAUSES (TØ7-T88)

POISONING BY, ADVERSE EFFECTS OF AND UNDERDOSING OF DRUGS, MEDICAMENTS AND BIOLOGICAL SUBSTANCES (T36-T5Ø)

Includes:

adverse effect of correct substance properly administered

poisoning by overdose of substance

poisoning by wrong substance given or taken in error

underdosing by (inadvertently) (deliberately) taking less substance than prescribed or instructed

Code First:

for adverse effects, the nature of the adverse effect, such as:

adverse effect NOS (T88.7)

aspirin gastritis (K29.-)

blood disorders (D56-D76)

contact dermatitis (L23-L25)

dermatitis due to substances taken internally (L27.-)

nephropathy (N14.Ø-N14.2)

Notes:

The drug giving rise to the adverse effect should be identified by use of codes from categories T36-T5Ø with fifth or sixth character 5.

Use additional code(s) to specify:

manifestations of poisoning

underdosing or failure in dosage during medical and surgical care (Y63.6, Y63.8-Y63.9)

underdosing of medication regimen (Z91.12-, Z91.13-)

Excludes1:

toxic reaction to local anesthesia in pregnancy (O29.3-)

Excludes2:

abuse and dependence of psychoactive substances (F1Ø-F19)

abuse of non-dependence-producing substances (F55.-)

immunodeficiency due to drugs (D84.821)

drug reaction and poisoning affecting newborn (PØØ-P96)

pathological drug intoxication (inebriation) (F1Ø-F19)

See Guidelines: 1;C.19.e | 1;C.19.e.5 | 1;C.19.e.5.b

Indicator(s): POAEx (7th D/S)

T43- POISONING BY, ADVERSE EFFECT OF AND UNDERDOSING OF PSYCHOTROPIC DRUGS, NOT ELSEWHERE CLASSIFIED

Excludes1:

appetite depressants (T5Ø.5-)

barbiturates (T42.3-)

benzodiazepines (T42.4-)

methaqualone (T42.6-)

psychodysleptics [hallucinogens] (T4Ø.7-T4Ø.9-)

Excludes2:

drug dependence and related mental and behavioral disorders due to psychoactive substance use (F1Ø.- -F19.-)

The appropriate 7th character is to be added to each code from category T43

A - initial encounter

D - subsequent encounter

S - sequela

T43.6- **Poisoning by, adverse effect of and underdosing of psychostimulants**

Excludes1:

poisoning by, adverse effect of and underdosing of cocaine (T4Ø.5-)

T43.65- **Poisoning by, adverse effect of and underdosing of methamphetamines**

N **T43.651_ Poisoning by methamphetamines accidental (unintentional)**

Including: Poisoning by methamphetamines NOS

N **T43.652_ Poisoning by methamphetamines intentional self-harm**

N **T43.653_ Poisoning by methamphetamines, assault**

N **T43.654_ Poisoning by methamphetamines, undetermined**

N **T43.655_ Adverse effect of methamphetamines**

N **T43.656_ Underdosing of methamphetamines**

2Ø. External causes of morbidity (VØØ-Y99)

Notes:

This chapter permits the classification of environmental events and circumstances as the cause of injury, and other adverse effects. Where a code from this section is applicable, it is intended that it shall be used secondary to a code from another chapter of the Classification indicating the nature of the condition. Most often, the condition will be classifiable to Chapter 19, Injury, poisoning and certain other consequences of external causes (SØØ-T88). Other conditions that may be stated to be due to external causes are classified in Chapters I to XVIII. For these conditions, codes from Chapter 2Ø should be used to provide additional information as to the cause of the condition.

See Guidelines: *1;C.2Ø.a-i | 1;C.2Ø.k*

ACCIDENTS (VØØ-X58)

TRANSPORT ACCIDENTS (VØØ-V99)

Notes:

This section is structured in 12 groups. Those relating to land transport accidents (VØØ-V89) reflect the victim's mode of transport and are subdivided to identify the victim's 'counterpart' or the type of event. The vehicle of which the injured person is an occupant is identified in the first two characters since it is seen as the most important factor to identify for prevention purposes. A transport accident is one in which the vehicle involved must be moving or running or in use for transport purposes at the time of the accident.

Use additional code to identify:

Airbag injury (W22.1)

Type of street or road (Y92.4-)

Use of cellular telephone and other electronic equipment at the time of the transport accident (Y93.C-)

Excludes1:

agricultural vehicles in stationary use or maintenance (W31.-)

assault by crashing of motor vehicle (YØ3.-)

automobile or motor cycle in stationary use or maintenance-code to type of accident

crashing of motor vehicle, undetermined intent (Y32)

intentional self-harm by crashing of motor vehicle (X82)

Excludes2:

transport accidents due to cataclysm (X34-X38)

Notes:

Definitions related to transport accidents:

(a) A transport accident (VØØ-V99) is any accident involving a device designed primarily for, or used at the time primarily for, conveying persons or good from one place to another.

(b) A public highway [trafficway] or street is the entire width between property lines (or other boundary lines) of land open to the public as a matter of right or custom for purposes of moving persons or property from one place to another. A roadway is that part of the public highway designed, improved and customarily used for vehicular traffic.

(c) A traffic accident is any vehicle accident occurring on the public highway [i.e. originating on, terminating on, or involving a vehicle partially on the highway]. A vehicle accident is assumed to have occurred on the public highway unless another place is specified, except in the case of accidents involving only off-road motor vehicles, which are classified as nontraffic accidents unless the contrary is stated.

(d) A nontraffic accident is any vehicle accident that occurs entirely in any place other than a public highway.

(cont)

(e) A pedestrian is any person involved in an accident who was not at the time of the accident riding in or on a motor vehicle, railway train, streetcar or animal-drawn or other vehicle, or on a pedal cycle or animal. This includes, a person changing a tire, working on a parked car, or a person on foot. It also includes the user of a pedestrian conveyance such as a baby stroller, ice-skates, skis, sled, roller skates, a skateboard, nonmotorized or motorized wheelchair, motorized mobility scooter, or nonmotorized scooter.

(f) A driver is an occupant of a transport vehicle who is operating or intending to operate it.

(g) A passenger is any occupant of a transport vehicle other than the driver, except a person traveling on the outside of the vehicle.

(h) A person on the outside of a vehicle is any person being transported by a vehicle but not occupying the space normally reserved for the driver or passengers, or the space intended for the transport of property. This includes a person travelling on the bodywork, bumper, fender, roof, running board or step of a vehicle, as well as, hanging on the outside of the vehicle.

(i) A pedal cycle is any land transport vehicle operated solely by nonmotorized pedals including a bicycle or tricycle.

(j) A pedal cyclist is any person riding a pedal cycle or in a sidecar or trailer attached to a pedal cycle.

(k) A motorcycle is a two-wheeled motor vehicle with one or two riding saddles and sometimes with a third wheel for the support of a sidecar. The sidecar is considered part of the motorcycle. This includes a moped, motor scooter, or motorized bicycle.

(l) A motorcycle rider is any person riding a motorcycle or in a sidecar or trailer attached to the motorcycle.

(m) A three-wheeled motor vehicle is a motorized tricycle designed primarily for on-road use. This includes a motor-driven tricycle, a motorized rickshaw, or a three-wheeled motor car.

(n) A car [automobile] is a four-wheeled motor vehicle designed primarily for carrying up to 7 persons. A trailer being towed by the car is considered part of the car. It does not include a van or minivan - see definition (o)

(o) A pick-up truck or van is a four or six-wheeled motor vehicle designed for carrying passengers as well as property or cargo weighing less than the local limit for classification as a heavy goods vehicle, and not requiring a special driver's license. This includes a minivan and a sport-utility vehicle (SUV).

(p) A heavy transport vehicle is a motor vehicle designed primarily for carrying property, meeting local criteria for classification as a heavy goods vehicle in terms of weight and requiring a special driver's license.

(q) A bus (coach) is a motor vehicle designed or adapted primarily for carrying more than 1Ø passengers, and requiring a special driver's license.

(r) A railway train or railway vehicle is any device, with or without freight or passenger cars couple to it, designed for traffic on a railway track. This includes subterranean (subways) or elevated trains.

(s) A streetcar, is a device designed and used primarily for transporting passengers within a municipality, running on rails, usually subject to normal traffic control signals, and operated principally on a right-of-way that forms part of the roadway. This includes a tram or trolley that runs on rails. A trailer being towed by a streetcar is considered part of the streetcar.

(t) A special vehicle mainly used on industrial premises is a motor vehicle designed primarily for use within the buildings and premises of industrial or commercial establishments. This includes battery-powered airport passenger vehicles or baggage/mail trucks, forklifts, coal-cars in a coal mine, logging cars and trucks used in mines or quarries.

See Appendix A — Coding Reference Tables for lists of the ICD-10-CM Tabular indicators, HAC categories, and HCC codes.

(cont)

(u) A special vehicle mainly used in agriculture is a motor vehicle designed specifically for use in farming and agriculture (horticulture), to work the land, tend and harvest crops and transport materials on the farm. This includes harvesters, farm machinery and tractor and trailers.

(v) A special construction vehicle is a motor vehicle designed specifically for use on construction and demolition sites. This includes bulldozers, diggers, earth levellers, dump trucks. backhoes, front-end loaders, pavers, and mechanical shovels.

(w) A special all-terrain vehicle is a motor vehicle of special design to enable it to negotiate over rough or soft terrain, snow or sand. Examples of special design are high construction, special wheels and tires, tracks, and support on a cushion of air. This includes snow mobiles, All-terrain vehicles (ATV), and dune buggies. It does not include passenger vehicle designated as Sport Utility Vehicles. (SUV)

(x) A watercraft is any device designed for transporting passengers or goods on water. This includes motor or sail boats, ships, and hovercraft.

(y) An aircraft is any device for transporting passengers or goods in the air. This includes hot-air balloons, gliders, helicopters and airplanes.

(z) A military vehicle is any motorized vehicle operating on a public roadway owned by the military and being operated by a member of the military.

PEDESTRIAN INJURED IN TRANSPORT ACCIDENT (VØØ-VØ9)

Includes:
person changing tire on transport vehicle
person examining engine of vehicle broken down in (on side of) road
Excludes1:
fall due to non-transport collision with other person (WØ3)
pedestrian on foot falling (slipping) on ice and snow (WØØ.-)
struck or bumped by another person (W51)

VØØ- PEDESTRIAN CONVEYANCE ACCIDENT

Use additional place of occurrence and activity external cause codes, if known (Y92.-, Y93.-)
Excludes1:
collision with another person without fall (W51)
fall due to person on foot colliding with another person on foot (WØ3)
fall from non-moving wheelchair, nonmotorized scooter and motorized mobility scooter without collision (WØ5.-)
pedestrian (conveyance) collision with other land transport vehicle (VØ1-VØ9)
pedestrian on foot falling (slipping) on ice and snow (WØØ.-)

The appropriate 7th character is to be added to each code from category VØØ
A - initial encounter
D - subsequent encounter
S - sequela

VØØ.Ø- **Pedestrian on foot injured in collision with pedestrian conveyance**
Indicator(s): POAEx
VØØ.Ø1x_ Roller-skater
VØØ.Ø2x_ Skateboarder
VØØ.Ø3- **Standing micro-mobility pedestrian conveyance**
VØØ.Ø31_ Electric scooter
VØØ.Ø38_ Other
Including: hoverboard, segway
VØØ.Ø9x_ Other

VØØ.1- **Rolling-type pedestrian conveyance accident**
Excludes1:
accident with baby stroller (VØØ.82-)
accident with wheelchair (powered) (VØØ.81-)
accident with motorized mobility scooter (VØØ.83-)
Indicator(s): POAEx

VØØ.11- **In-line roller-skate accident**
VØØ.111_ Fall from
VØØ.112_ Colliding with stationary object
VØØ.118_ Other
Excludes1:
roller-skater collision with other land transport vehicle (VØ1-VØ9 with 5th character 1)

VØØ.12- **Non-in- line roller-skate accident**
VØØ.121_ Fall from
VØØ.122_ Colliding with stationary object
VØØ.128_ Other
Excludes1:
roller-skater collision with other land transport vehicle (VØ1-VØ9 with 5th character 1)

VØØ.13- **Skateboard accident**
VØØ.131_ Fall from
VØØ.132_ Colliding with stationary object
VØØ.138_ Other
Excludes1:
skateboarder collision with other land transport vehicle (VØ1-VØ9 with 5th character 2)

VØØ.14- **Scooter (nonmotorized) accident**
Excludes1:
motor scooter accident (V2Ø-V29)
VØØ.141_ Fall from
VØØ.142_ Colliding with stationary object
VØØ.148_ Other
Excludes1:
scooter (nonmotorized) collision with other land transport vehicle (VØ1-VØ9 with fifth character 9)

VØØ.15- **Heelies accident**
Including: Rolling shoe, Wheeled shoe, Wheelies
VØØ.151_ Fall from
VØØ.152_ Colliding with stationary object
VØØ.158_ Other

VØØ.18- **Accident on other rolling-type pedestrian conveyance**
VØØ.181_ Fall from
VØØ.182_ Colliding with stationary object
VØØ.188_ Other

VØØ.2- **Gliding-type pedestrian conveyance accident**
Indicator(s): POAEx

VØØ.21- **Ice-skates accident**
VØØ.211_ Fall from
VØØ.212_ Colliding with stationary object
VØØ.218_ Other
Excludes1:
ice-skater collision with other land transport vehicle (VØ1-VØ9 with 5th character 9)

VØØ.22- **Sled accident**

VØØ.221_ Fall from

VØØ.222_ Colliding with stationary object

VØØ.228_ Other

Excludes1:

sled collision with other land transport vehicle (VØ1-VØ9 with 5th character 9)

VØØ.28- **Other gliding-type pedestrian conveyance accident**

VØØ.281_ Fall from

VØØ.282_ Colliding with stationary object

VØØ.288_ Other

Excludes1:

gliding-type pedestrian conveyance collision with other land transport vehicle (VØ1-VØ9 with 5th character 9)

VØØ.3- **Flat-bottomed pedestrian conveyance accident**

Indicator(s): POAEx

VØØ.31- **Snowboard accident**

VØØ.311_ Fall from

VØØ.312_ Colliding with stationary object

VØØ.318_ Other

Excludes1:

snowboarder collision with other land transport vehicle (VØ1-VØ9 with 5th character 9)

VØØ.32- **Snow-ski accident**

VØØ.321_ Fall from

VØØ.322_ Colliding with stationary object

VØØ.328_ Other

Excludes1:

snow-skier collision with other land transport vehicle (VØ1-VØ9 with 5th character 9)

VØØ.38- **Other flat-bottomed pedestrian conveyance accident**

VØØ.381_ Fall from

VØØ.382_ Colliding with stationary object

VØØ.388_ Other

VØØ.8- **Accident on other pedestrian conveyance**

VØØ.81- **Accident with wheelchair (powered)**

VØØ.811_ Fall from moving

Excludes1:

fall from non-moving wheelchair (WØ5.Ø)

VØØ.812_ Colliding with stationary object

VØØ.818_ Other

VØØ.82- **Accident with baby stroller**

Indicator(s): POAEx

VØØ.821_ Fall from

VØØ.822_ Colliding with stationary object

VØØ.828_ Other

VØØ.83- **Accident with motorized mobility scooter**

VØØ.831_ Fall from

Excludes1:

fall from non-moving motorized mobility scooter (WØ5.2)

VØØ.832_ Colliding with stationary object

VØØ.838_ Other

VØØ.84- **Standing micro-mobility pedestrian conveyance**

Indicator(s): POAEx

VØØ.841_ Fall

VØØ.842_ Colliding with stationary object

VØØ.848_ Other accident

Including: hoverboard, segway

VØØ.89- **Accident on other pedestrian conveyance**

Indicator(s): POAEx

VØØ.891_ Fall from

VØØ.892_ Colliding with stationary object

VØØ.898_ Other

Excludes1:

other pedestrian (conveyance) collision with other land transport vehicle (VØ1-VØ9 with 5th character 9)

VØ1- PEDESTRIAN INJURED IN COLLISION WITH PEDAL CYCLE

The appropriate 7th character is to be added to each code from category VØ1

A - initial encounter

D - subsequent encounter

S - sequela

Indicator(s): POAEx

VØ1.Ø- **Pedestrian injured in collision with pedal cycle in nontraffic accident**

VØ1.ØØx_ Pedestrian on foot

Including: Pedestrian NOS

VØ1.Ø1x_ Pedestrian on roller-skates

VØ1.Ø2x_ Pedestrian on skateboard

VØ1.Ø3- **Pedestrian on standing micro-mobility pedestrian conveyance**

VØ1.Ø31_ Standing electric scooter

VØ1.Ø38_ Other standing micro-mobility pedestrian conveyance

Including: hoverboard, segway

VØ1.Ø9x_ Pedestrian with other conveyance

Including: Pedestrian with baby stroller, on ice-skates, on nonmotorized scooter, on sled, on snowboard, on snow-skis, in wheelchair (powered), in motorized mobility scooter

VØ1.1- **Pedestrian injured in collision with pedal cycle in traffic accident**

VØ1.1Øx_ Pedestrian on foot

Including: Pedestrian NOS

VØ1.11x_ Pedestrian on roller-skates

VØ1.12x_ Pedestrian on skateboard

VØ1.13- **Pedestrian on standing micro-mobility pedestrian conveyance**

VØ1.131_ Standing electric scooter

VØ1.138_ Other standing micro-mobility pedestrian conveyance

Including: hoverboard, segway

VØ1.19x_ Pedestrian with other conveyance

Including: Pedestrian with baby stroller, on ice-skates, on nonmotorized scooter, on sled, on snowboard, on snow-skis, in wheelchair (powered), in motorized mobility scooter

VØ1.9- **Pedestrian injured in collision with pedal cycle, unspecified whether traffic or nontraffic accident**

VØ1.9Øx_ Pedestrian on foot
Including: Pedestrian NOS

VØ1.91x_ Pedestrian on roller-skates

VØ1.92x_ Pedestrian on skateboard

VØ1.93- **Pedestrian on standing micro-mobility pedestrian conveyance**

VØ1.931_ Standing electric scooter

VØ1.938_ Other standing micro-mobility pedestrian conveyance
Including: hoverboard, segway

VØ1.99x_ Pedestrian with other conveyance
Including: Pedestrian with baby stroller, on ice-skates, on nonmotorized scooter, on sled, on snowboard, on snow-skis, in wheelchair (powered), in motorized mobility scooter

VØ2- PEDESTRIAN INJURED IN COLLISION WITH TWO- OR THREE-WHEELED MOTOR VEHICLE

The appropriate 7th character is to be added to each code from category VØ2
A - initial encounter
D - subsequent encounter
S - sequela

Indicator(s): POAEx

VØ2.Ø- **Pedestrian injured in collision with two- or three-wheeled motor vehicle in nontraffic accident**

VØ2.ØØx_ Pedestrian on foot
Including: Pedestrian NOS

VØ2.Ø1x_ Pedestrian on roller-skates

VØ2.Ø2x_ Pedestrian on skateboard

VØ2.Ø3- **Pedestrian on standing micro-mobility pedestrian conveyance injured in collision with two- or three-wheeled motor vehicle in nontraffic accident**

VØ2.Ø31_ Standing electric scooter

VØ2.Ø38_ Other standing micro-mobility pedestrian conveyance
Including: hoverboard, segway

VØ2.Ø9x_ Pedestrian with other conveyance
Including: Pedestrian with baby stroller, on ice-skates, on nonmotorized scooter, on sled, on snowboard, on snow-skis, in wheelchair (powered), in motorized mobility scooter

VØ2.1- **Pedestrian injured in collision with two- or three-wheeled motor vehicle in traffic accident**

VØ2.1Øx_ Pedestrian on foot
Including: Pedestrian NOS

VØ2.11x_ Pedestrian on roller-skates

VØ2.12x_ Pedestrian on skateboard

VØ2.13- **Pedestrian on standing micro-mobility pedestrian conveyance injured in collision with two- or three-wheeled motor vehicle in traffic accident**

VØ2.131_ Standing electric scooter

VØ2.138_ Other standing micro-mobility pedestrian conveyance
Including: hoverboard, segway

VØ2.19x_ Pedestrian with other conveyance
Including: Pedestrian with baby stroller, on ice-skates, on nonmotorized scooter, on sled, on snowboard, on snow-skis, in wheelchair (powered), in motorized mobility scooter

VØ2.9- **Pedestrian injured in collision with two- or three-wheeled motor vehicle, unspecified whether traffic or nontraffic accident**

VØ2.9Øx_ Pedestrian on foot
Including: Pedestrian NOS

VØ2.91x_ Pedestrian on roller-skates

VØ2.92x_ Pedestrian on skateboard

VØ2.93- **Pedestrian on standing micro-mobility pedestrian conveyance injured in collision with two- or three-wheeled motor vehicle, unspecified whether traffic or nontraffic accident**

VØ2.931_ Standing electric scooter

VØ2.938_ Other standing micro-mobility pedestrian conveyance
Including: hoverboard, segway

VØ2.99x_ Pedestrian with other conveyance
Including: Pedestrian with baby stroller, on ice-skates, on nonmotorized scooter, on sled, on snowboard, on snow-skis, in wheelchair (powered), in motorized mobility scooter

VØ3- PEDESTRIAN INJURED IN COLLISION WITH CAR, PICK-UP TRUCK OR VAN

The appropriate 7th character is to be added to each code from category VØ3
A - initial encounter
D - subsequent encounter
S - sequela

VØ3.Ø- **Pedestrian injured in collision with car, pick-up truck or van in nontraffic accident**
Indicator(s): POAEx

VØ3.ØØx_ Pedestrian on foot
Including: Pedestrian NOS

VØ3.Ø1x_ Pedestrian on roller-skates

VØ3.Ø2x_ Pedestrian on skateboard

VØ3.Ø3- **Pedestrian on standing micro-mobility pedestrian conveyance injured in collision with car, pick-up or van in nontraffic accident**

VØ3.Ø31_ Standing electric scooter

VØ3.Ø38_ Other standing micro-mobility pedestrian conveyance
Including: hoverboard, segway

VØ3.Ø9x_ Pedestrian with other conveyance
Including: Pedestrian with baby stroller, on ice-skates, on nonmotorized scooter, on sled, on snowboard, on snow-skis, in wheelchair (powered), in motorized mobility scooter

VØ3.1- **Pedestrian injured in collision with car, pick-up truck or van in traffic accident**

VØ3.1Øx_ Pedestrian on foot
Including: Pedestrian NOS

VØ3.11x_ Pedestrian on roller-skates

VØ3.12x_ Pedestrian on skateboard

VØ3.13- **Pedestrian on standing micro-mobility pedestrian conveyance injured in collision with car, pick-up or van in traffic accident**

VØ3.131_ Standing electric scooter

VØ3.138_ Other standing micro-mobility pedestrian conveyance
Including: hoverboard, segway

VØ3.19x_ Pedestrian with other conveyance
Including: Pedestrian with baby stroller, on ice-skates, on nonmotorized scooter, on sled, on snowboard, on snow-skis, in wheelchair (powered), in motorized mobility scooter

VØ3.9- **Pedestrian injured in collision with car, pick-up truck or van, unspecified whether traffic or nontraffic accident**
Indicator(s): POAEx

VØ3.9Øx_ Pedestrian on foot
Including: Pedestrian NOS

VØ3.91x_ Pedestrian on roller-skates

VØ3.92x_ Pedestrian on skateboard

VØ3.93- **Pedestrian on standing micro-mobility pedestrian conveyance injured in collision with car, pick-up or van, unspecified whether traffic or nontraffic accident**

VØ3.931_ Standing electric scooter

VØ3.938_ Other standing micro-mobility pedestrian conveyance
Including: hoverboard, segway

VØ3.99x_ Pedestrian with other conveyance
Including: Pedestrian with baby stroller, on ice-skates, on nonmotorized scooter, on sled, on snowboard, on snow-skis, in wheelchair (powered), in motorized mobility scooter

VØ4- PEDESTRIAN INJURED IN COLLISION WITH HEAVY TRANSPORT VEHICLE OR BUS

Excludes1:
pedestrian injured in collision with military vehicle (VØ9.Ø1, VØ9.21)

The appropriate 7th character is to be added to each code from category VØ4
A - initial encounter
D - subsequent encounter
S - sequela

Indicator(s): POAEx

VØ4.Ø- **Pedestrian injured in collision with heavy transport vehicle or bus in nontraffic accident**

VØ4.ØØx_ Pedestrian on foot
Including: Pedestrian NOS

VØ4.Ø1x_ Pedestrian on roller-skates

VØ4.Ø2x_ Pedestrian on skateboard

VØ4.Ø3- **Pedestrian on standing micro-mobility pedestrian conveyance injured in collision with heavy transport vehicle or bus in nontraffic accident**

VØ4.Ø31_ Standing electric scooter

VØ4.Ø38_ Other standing micro-mobility pedestrian conveyance
Including: hoverboard, segway

VØ4.Ø9x_ Pedestrian with other conveyance
Including: Pedestrian with baby stroller, on ice-skates, on nonmotorized scooter, on sled, on snowboard, on snow-skis, in wheelchair (powered), in motorized mobility scooter

VØ4.1- **Pedestrian injured in collision with heavy transport vehicle or bus in traffic accident**

VØ4.1Øx_ Pedestrian on foot
Including: Pedestrian NOS

VØ4.11x_ Pedestrian on roller-skates

VØ4.12x_ Pedestrian on skateboard

VØ4.13- **Pedestrian on standing micro-mobility pedestrian conveyance injured in collision with heavy transport vehicle or bus in traffic accident**

VØ4.131_ Standing electric scooter

VØ4.138_ Other standing micro-mobility pedestrian conveyance
Including: hoverboard, segway

VØ4.19x_ Pedestrian with other conveyance
Including: Pedestrian with baby stroller, on ice-skates, on nonmotorized scooter, on sled, on snowboard, on snow-skis, in wheelchair (powered), in motorized mobility scooter

VØ4.9- **Pedestrian injured in collision with heavy transport vehicle or bus, unspecified whether traffic or nontraffic accident**

VØ4.9Øx_ Pedestrian on foot
Including: Pedestrian NOS

VØ4.91x_ Pedestrian on roller-skates

VØ4.92x_ Pedestrian on skateboard

VØ4.93- **Pedestrian on standing micro-mobility pedestrian conveyance injured in collision with heavy transport vehicle or bus, unspecified whether traffic or nontraffic accident**

VØ4.931_ Standing electric scooter

VØ4.938_ Other standing micro-mobility pedestrian conveyance
Including: hoverboard, segway

VØ4.99x_ Pedestrian with other conveyance
Including: Pedestrian with baby stroller, on ice-skates, on nonmotorized scooter, on sled, on snowboard, on snow-skis, in wheelchair (powered), in motorized mobility scooter

VØ5- PEDESTRIAN INJURED IN COLLISION WITH RAILWAY TRAIN OR RAILWAY VEHICLE

The appropriate 7th character is to be added to each code from category VØ5
A - initial encounter
D - subsequent encounter
S - sequela

Indicator(s): POAEx

VØ5.Ø- **Pedestrian injured in collision with railway train or railway vehicle in nontraffic accident**

VØ5.ØØx_ Pedestrian on foot
Including: Pedestrian NOS

VØ5.Ø1x_ Pedestrian on roller-skates

VØ5.Ø2x_ Pedestrian on skateboard

See Appendix A — Coding Reference Tables for lists of the ICD-10-CM Tabular indicators, HAC categories, and HCC codes.

V05.03- **Pedestrian on standing micro-mobility pedestrian conveyance injured in collision with railway train or railway vehicle in nontraffic accident**

V05.031_ Standing electric scooter

V05.038_ Other standing micro-mobility pedestrian conveyance
Including: hoverboard, segway

V05.09x_ Pedestrian with other conveyance
Including: Pedestrian with baby stroller, on ice-skates, on nonmotorized scooter, on sled, on snowboard, on snow-skis, in wheelchair (powered), in motorized mobility scooter

V05.1- **Pedestrian injured in collision with railway train or railway vehicle in traffic accident**

V05.10x_ Pedestrian on foot
Including: Pedestrian NOS

V05.11x_ Pedestrian on roller-skates

V05.12x_ Pedestrian on skateboard

V05.13- **Pedestrian on standing micro-mobility pedestrian conveyance injured in collision with railway train or railway vehicle in traffic accident**

V05.131_ Standing electric scooter

V05.138_ Other standing micro-mobility pedestrian conveyance
Including: hoverboard, segway

V05.19x_ Pedestrian with other conveyance
Including: Pedestrian with baby stroller, on ice-skates, on nonmotorized scooter, on sled, on snowboard, on snow-skis, in wheelchair (powered), in motorized mobility scooter

V05.9- **Pedestrian injured in collision with railway train or railway vehicle, unspecified whether traffic or nontraffic accident**

V05.90x_ Pedestrian on foot
Including: Pedestrian NOS

V05.91x_ Pedestrian on roller-skates

V05.92x_ Pedestrian on skateboard

V05.93- **Pedestrian on standing micro-mobility pedestrian conveyance injured in collision with railway train or railway vehicle, unspecified whether traffic or nontraffic accident**

V05.931_ Standing electric scooter

V05.938_ Other standing micro-mobility pedestrian conveyance
Including: hoverboard, segway

V05.99x_ Pedestrian with other conveyance
Including: Pedestrian with baby stroller, on ice-skates, on nonmotorized scooter, on sled, on snowboard, on snow-skis, in wheelchair (powered), in motorized mobility scooter

V06- PEDESTRIAN INJURED IN COLLISION WITH OTHER NONMOTOR VEHICLE

Includes:
collision with animal-drawn vehicle, animal being ridden, nonpowered streetcar

Excludes1:
pedestrian injured in collision with pedestrian conveyance (V00.0-)

The appropriate 7th character is to be added to each code from category V06
A - initial encounter
D - subsequent encounter
S - sequela

Indicator(s): POAEx

V06.0- **Pedestrian injured in collision with other nonmotor vehicle in nontraffic accident**

V06.00x_ Pedestrian on foot
Including: Pedestrian NOS

V06.01x_ Pedestrian on roller-skates

V06.02x_ Pedestrian on skateboard

V06.03- **Pedestrian on standing micro-mobility pedestrian conveyance injured in collision with other nonmotor vehicle in nontraffic accident**

V06.031_ Standing electric scooter

V06.038_ Other standing micro-mobility pedestrian conveyance
Including: hoverboard, segway

V06.09x_ Pedestrian with other conveyance
Including: Pedestrian with baby stroller, on ice-skates, on nonmotorized scooter, on sled, on snowboard, on snow-skis, in wheelchair (powered), in motorized mobility scooter

V06.1- **Pedestrian injured in collision with other nonmotor vehicle in traffic accident**

V06.10x_ Pedestrian on foot
Including: Pedestrian NOS

V06.11x_ Pedestrian on roller-skates

V06.12x_ Pedestrian on skateboard

V06.13- **Pedestrian on standing micro-mobility pedestrian conveyance injured in collision with other nonmotor vehicle in traffic accident**

V06.131_ Standing electric scooter

V06.138_ Other standing micro-mobility pedestrian conveyance
Including: hoverboard, segway

V06.19x_ Pedestrian with other conveyance
Including: Pedestrian with baby stroller, on ice-skates, on nonmotorized scooter, on sled, on snowboard, on snow-skis, in wheelchair (powered), in motorized mobility scooter

V06.9- **Pedestrian injured in collision with other nonmotor vehicle, unspecified whether traffic or nontraffic accident**

V06.90x_ Pedestrian on foot
Including: Pedestrian NOS

V06.91x_ Pedestrian on roller-skates

V06.92x_ Pedestrian on skateboard

VØ6.93- **Pedestrian on standing micro-mobility pedestrian conveyance injured in collision with other nonmotor vehicle, unspecified whether traffic or nontraffic accident**

VØ6.931_ Standing electric scooter

VØ6.938_ Other standing micro-mobility pedestrian conveyance

Including: hoverboard, segway

VØ6.99x_ Pedestrian with other conveyance

Including: Pedestrian with baby stroller, on ice-skates, on nonmotorized scooter, on sled, on snowboard, on snow-skis, in wheelchair (powered), in motorized mobility scooter

VØ9- PEDESTRIAN INJURED IN OTHER AND UNSPECIFIED TRANSPORT ACCIDENTS

The appropriate 7th character is to be added to each code from category VØ9

A - initial encounter

D - subsequent encounter

S - sequela

Indicator(s): *POAEx*

VØ9.Ø- **Pedestrian injured in nontraffic accident involving other and unspecified motor vehicles**

VØ9.ØØx_ Unspecified motor vehicles

VØ9.Ø1x_ Military vehicle

VØ9.Ø9x_ Other motor vehicles

Including: Special vehicle

VØ9.1xx_ Unspecified nontraffic accident

VØ9.2- **Pedestrian injured in traffic accident involving other and unspecified motor vehicles**

VØ9.2Øx_ Unspecified motor vehicles

VØ9.21x_ Military vehicle

VØ9.29x_ Other motor vehicles

VØ9.3xx_ Unspecified traffic accident

VØ9.9xx_ Unspecified transport accident

PEDAL CYCLE RIDER INJURED IN TRANSPORT ACCIDENT (V1Ø-V19)

Includes:

any non-motorized vehicle, excluding an animal-drawn vehicle, or a sidecar or trailer attached to the pedal cycle

Excludes2:

rupture of pedal cycle tire (W37.Ø)

Indicator(s): *POAEx*

V1Ø- PEDAL CYCLE RIDER INJURED IN COLLISION WITH PEDESTRIAN OR ANIMAL

Excludes1:

pedal cycle rider collision with animal-drawn vehicle or animal being ridden (V16.-)

The appropriate 7th character is to be added to each code from category V1Ø

A - initial encounter

D - subsequent encounter

S - sequela

V1Ø.Øxx_ Driver in nontraffic accident

V1Ø.1xx_ Passenger in nontraffic accident

V1Ø.2xx_ Unspecified cyclist in nontraffic accident

V1Ø.3xx_ Person boarding or alighting a pedal cycle

V1Ø.4xx_ Driver in traffic accident

V1Ø.5xx_ Passenger in traffic accident

V1Ø.9xx_ Unspecified cyclist in traffic accident

V11- PEDAL CYCLE RIDER INJURED IN COLLISION WITH OTHER PEDAL CYCLE

The appropriate 7th character is to be added to each code from category V11

A - initial encounter

D - subsequent encounter

S - sequela

V11.Øxx_ Driver in nontraffic accident

V11.1xx_ Passenger in nontraffic accident

V11.2xx_ Unspecified cyclist in nontraffic accident

V11.3xx_ Person boarding or alighting a pedal cycle

V11.4xx_ Driver in traffic accident

V11.5xx_ Passenger in traffic accident

V11.9xx_ Unspecified cyclist in traffic accident

V12- PEDAL CYCLE RIDER INJURED IN COLLISION WITH TWO- OR THREE-WHEELED MOTOR VEHICLE

The appropriate 7th character is to be added to each code from category V12

A - initial encounter

D - subsequent encounter

S - sequela

V12.Øxx_ Driver in nontraffic accident

V12.1xx_ Passenger in nontraffic accident

V12.2xx_ Unspecified cyclist in nontraffic accident

V12.3xx_ Person boarding or alighting a pedal cycle

V12.4xx_ Driver in traffic accident

V12.5xx_ Passenger in traffic accident

V12.9xx_ Unspecified cyclist in traffic accident

V13- PEDAL CYCLE RIDER INJURED IN COLLISION WITH CAR, PICK-UP TRUCK OR VAN

The appropriate 7th character is to be added to each code from category V13

A - initial encounter

D - subsequent encounter

S - sequela

V13.Øxx_ Driver in nontraffic accident

V13.1xx_ Passenger in nontraffic accident

V13.2xx_ Unspecified cyclist in nontraffic accident

V13.3xx_ Person boarding or alighting a pedal cycle

V13.4xx_ Driver in traffic accident

V13.5xx_ Passenger in traffic accident

V13.9xx_ Unspecified cyclist in traffic accident

V14- PEDAL CYCLE RIDER INJURED IN COLLISION WITH HEAVY TRANSPORT VEHICLE OR BUS

Excludes1:

pedal cycle rider injured in collision with military vehicle (V19.81)

The appropriate 7th character is to be added to each code from category V14

A - initial encounter

D - subsequent encounter

S - sequela

V14.Øxx_ Driver in nontraffic accident

V14.1xx_ Passenger in nontraffic accident

V14.2xx_ Unspecified cyclist in nontraffic accident

V14.3xx_ Person boarding or alighting a pedal cycle

V14.4xx_ Driver in traffic accident

V14.5xx_ Passenger in traffic accident

V14.9xx_ Unspecified cyclist in traffic accident

See Appendix A — Coding Reference Tables for lists of the ICD-10-CM Tabular indicators, HAC categories, and HCC codes.

V15- PEDAL CYCLE RIDER INJURED IN COLLISION WITH RAILWAY TRAIN OR RAILWAY VEHICLE

The appropriate 7th character is to be added to each code from category V15
A - initial encounter
D - subsequent encounter
S - sequela

V15.Øxx_ Driver in nontraffic accident
V15.1xx_ Passenger in nontraffic accident
V15.2xx_ Unspecified cyclist in nontraffic accident
V15.3xx_ Person boarding or alighting a pedal cycle
V15.4xx_ Driver in traffic accident
V15.5xx_ Passenger in traffic accident
V15.9xx_ Unspecified cyclist in traffic accident

V16- PEDAL CYCLE RIDER INJURED IN COLLISION WITH OTHER NONMOTOR VEHICLE

Includes:
collision with animal-drawn vehicle, animal being ridden, streetcar

The appropriate 7th character is to be added to each code from category V16
A - initial encounter
D - subsequent encounter
S - sequela

V16.Øxx_ Driver in nontraffic accident
V16.1xx_ Passenger in nontraffic accident
V16.2xx_ Unspecified cyclist in nontraffic accident
V16.3xx_ Person boarding or alighting in nontraffic accident
V16.4xx_ Driver in traffic accident
V16.5xx_ Passenger in traffic accident
V16.9xx_ Unspecified cyclist in traffic accident

V17- PEDAL CYCLE RIDER INJURED IN COLLISION WITH FIXED OR STATIONARY OBJECT

The appropriate 7th character is to be added to each code from category V17
A - initial encounter
D - subsequent encounter
S - sequela

V17.Øxx_ Driver in nontraffic accident
V17.1xx_ Passenger in nontraffic accident
V17.2xx_ Unspecified cyclist in nontraffic accident
V17.3xx_ Person boarding or alighting a pedal cycle
V17.4xx_ Driver in traffic accident
V17.5xx_ Passenger in traffic accident
V17.9xx_ Unspecified cyclist in traffic accident

V18- PEDAL CYCLE RIDER INJURED IN NONCOLLISION TRANSPORT ACCIDENT

Includes:
fall or thrown from pedal cycle (without antecedent collision)
overturning pedal cycle NOS
overturning pedal cycle without collision

The appropriate 7th character is to be added to each code from category V18
A - initial encounter
D - subsequent encounter
S - sequela

V18.Øxx_ Driver in nontraffic accident
V18.1xx_ Passenger in nontraffic accident
V18.2xx_ Unspecified cyclist in nontraffic accident
V18.3xx_ Person boarding or alighting a pedal cycle
V18.4xx_ Driver in traffic accident
V18.5xx_ Passenger in traffic accident
V18.9xx_ Unspecified cyclist in traffic accident

V19- PEDAL CYCLE RIDER INJURED IN OTHER AND UNSPECIFIED TRANSPORT ACCIDENTS

The appropriate 7th character is to be added to each code from category V19
A - initial encounter
D - subsequent encounter
S - sequela

V19.Ø- **Pedal cycle driver injured in collision with other and unspecified motor vehicles in nontraffic accident**

V19.ØØx_ Unspecified
V19.Ø9x_ Other

V19.1- **Pedal cycle passenger injured in collision with other and unspecified motor vehicles in nontraffic accident**

V19.1Øx_ Unspecified
V19.19x_ Other

V19.2- **Unspecified pedal cyclist injured in collision with other and unspecified motor vehicles in nontraffic accident**

V19.2Øx_ Unspecified
Including: Collision NOS
V19.29x_ Other

V19.3xx_ Cyclist (driver) (passenger) in unspecified nontraffic accident
Including: Accident NOS, Injury NOS

V19.4- **Pedal cycle driver injured in collision with other and unspecified motor vehicles in traffic accident**

V19.4Øx_ Unspecified
V19.49x_ Other

V19.5- **Pedal cycle passenger injured in collision with other and unspecified motor vehicles in traffic accident**

V19.5Øx_ Unspecified
V19.59x_ Other

V19.6- **Unspecified pedal cyclist injured in collision with other and unspecified motor vehicles in traffic accident**

V19.6Øx_ Unspecified
Including: Collision NOS
V19.69x_ Other

V19.8- **Pedal cyclist (driver) (passenger) injured in other specified transport accidents**

V19.81x_ With military vehicle
V19.88x_ Other

V19.9xx_ Cyclist (driver) (passenger) in unspecified traffic accident
Including: Accident NOS

MOTORCYCLE RIDER INJURED IN TRANSPORT ACCIDENT (V2Ø-V29)

Includes:
electric bicycle
e-bike
e-bicycle
moped
motorcycle with sidecar
motorized bicycle
motor scooter
Excludes1:
three-wheeled motor vehicle (V3Ø-V39)
Indicator(s): POAEx

V2Ø- MOTORCYCLE RIDER INJURED IN COLLISION WITH PEDESTRIAN OR ANIMAL

Excludes1:
motorcycle rider collision with animal-drawn vehicle or animal being ridden (V26.-)

The appropriate 7th character is to be added to each code from category V2Ø
A - initial encounter
D - subsequent encounter
S - sequela

V2Ø.Ø- **Driver in nontraffic accident**

N **V2Ø.Ø1x_** **Electric (assisted) bicycle driver injured in collision with pedestrian or animal in nontraffic accident**

N **V2Ø.Ø9x_** **Other motorcycle driver injured in collision with pedestrian or animal in nontraffic accident**

V2Ø.1- **Passenger in nontraffic accident**

N **V2Ø.11x_** **Electric (assisted) bicycle passenger injured in collision with pedestrian or animal in nontraffic accident**

N **V2Ø.19x_** **Other motorcycle passenger injured in collision with pedestrian or animal in nontraffic accident**

V2Ø.2- **Unspecified rider in nontraffic accident**

N **V2Ø.21x_** **Unspecified electric (assisted) bicycle rider injured in collision with pedestrian or animal in nontraffic accident**

N **V2Ø.29x_** **Unspecified rider of other motorcycle injured in collision with pedestrian or animal in nontraffic accident**

V2Ø.3- **Person boarding or alighting a motorcycle**

N **V2Ø.31x_** **Person boarding or alighting an electric (assisted) bicycle injured in collision with pedestrian or animal**

N **V2Ø.39x_** **Person boarding or alighting other motorcycle injured in collision with pedestrian or animal**

V2Ø.4- **Driver in traffic accident**

N **V2Ø.41x_** **Electric (assisted) bicycle driver injured in collision with pedestrian or animal in traffic accident**

N **V2Ø.49x_** **Other motorcycle driver injured in collision with pedestrian or animal in traffic accident**

V2Ø.5- **Passenger in traffic accident**

N **V2Ø.51x_** **Electric (assisted) bicycle passenger injured in collision with pedestrian or animal in traffic accident**

N **V2Ø.59x_** **Other motorcycle passenger injured in collision with pedestrian or animal in traffic accident**

V2Ø.9- **Unspecified rider in traffic accident**

N **V2Ø.91x_** **Unspecified electric (assisted) bicycle rider injured in collision with pedestrian or animal in traffic accident**

N **V2Ø.99x_** **Unspecified rider of other motorcycle injured in collision with pedestrian or animal in traffic accident**

V21- MOTORCYCLE RIDER INJURED IN COLLISION WITH PEDAL CYCLE

The appropriate 7th character is to be added to each code from category V21
A - initial encounter
D - subsequent encounter
S - sequela

V21.Ø- **Driver in nontraffic accident**

N **V21.Ø1x_** **Electric (assisted) bicycle driver injured in collision with pedal cycle in nontraffic accident**

N **V21.Ø9x_** **Other motorcycle driver injured in collision with pedal cycle in nontraffic accident**

V21.1- **Passenger in nontraffic accident**

N **V21.11x_** **Electric (assisted) bicycle passenger injured in collision with pedal cycle in nontraffic accident**

N **V21.19x_** **Other motorcycle passenger injured in collision with pedal cycle in nontraffic accident**

V21.2- **Unspecified rider in nontraffic accident**

N **V21.21x_** **Unspecified electric (assisted) bicycle rider injured in collision with pedal cycle in nontraffic accident**

N **V21.29x_** **Unspecified rider of other motorcycle injured in collision with pedal cycle in nontraffic accident**

V21.3- **Person boarding or alighting a motorcycle**

N **V21.31x_** **Person boarding or alighting an electric (assisted) bicycle injured in collision with pedal cycle**

N **V21.39x_** **Person boarding or alighting other motorcycle injured in collision with pedal cycle**

V21.4- **Driver in traffic accident**

N **V21.41x_** **Electric (assisted) bicycle driver injured in collision with pedal cycle in traffic accident**

N **V21.49x_** **Other motorcycle driver injured in collision with pedal cycle in traffic accident**

V21.5- **Passenger in traffic accident**

N **V21.51x_** **Electric (assisted) bicycle passenger injured in collision with pedal cycle in traffic accident**

N **V21.59x_** **Other motorcycle passenger injured in collision with pedal cycle in traffic accident**

V21.9- **Unspecified rider in traffic accident**

N **V21.91x_** **Unspecified electric (assisted) bicycle rider injured in collision with pedal cycle in traffic accident**

N **V21.99x_** **Unspecified rider of other motorcycle injured in collision with pedal cycle in traffic accident**

V22- MOTORCYCLE RIDER INJURED IN COLLISION WITH TWO- OR THREE-WHEELED MOTOR VEHICLE

The appropriate 7th character is to be added to each code from category V22

A - initial encounter

D - subsequent encounter

S - sequela

V22.Ø- **Driver in nontraffic accident**

N **V22.Ø1x_** **Electric (assisted) bicycle driver injured in collision with two- or three-wheeled motor vehicle in nontraffic accident**

N **V22.Ø9x_** **Other motorcycle driver injured in collision with two- or three-wheeled motor vehicle in nontraffic accident**

V22.1- **Passenger in nontraffic accident**

N **V22.11x_** **Electric (assisted) bicycle passenger injured in collision with two- or three-wheeled motor vehicle in nontraffic accident**

N **V22.19x_** **Other motorcycle passenger injured in collision with two- or three-wheeled motor vehicle in nontraffic accident**

V22.2- **Unspecified rider in nontraffic accident**

N **V22.21x_** **Unspecified electric (assisted) bicycle rider injured in collision with two- or three-wheeled motor vehicle in nontraffic accident**

N **V22.29x_** **Unspecified rider of other motorcycle injured in collision with two- or three-wheeled motor vehicle in nontraffic accident**

V22.3- **Person boarding or alighting a motorcycle**

N **V22.31x_** **Person boarding or alighting an electric (assisted) bicycle injured in collision with two- or three-wheeled motor vehicle**

N **V22.39x_** **Person boarding or alighting other motorcycle injured in collision with two- or three-wheeled motor vehicle**

V22.4- **Driver in traffic accident**

N **V22.41x_** **Electric (assisted) bicycle driver injured in collision with two- or three-wheeled motor vehicle in traffic accident**

N **V22.49x_** **Other motorcycle driver injured in collision with two- or three-wheeled motor vehicle in traffic accident**

V22.5- **Passenger in traffic accident**

N **V22.51x_** **Electric (assisted) bicycle passenger injured in collision with two- or three-wheeled motor vehicle in traffic accident**

N **V22.59x_** **Other motorcycle passenger injured in collision with two- or three-wheeled motor vehicle in traffic accident**

V22.9- **Unspecified rider in traffic accident**

N **V22.91x_** **Unspecified electric (assisted) bicycle rider injured in collision with two- or three-wheeled motor vehicle in traffic accident**

N **V22.99x_** **Unspecified rider of other motorcycle injured in collision with two- or three-wheeled motor vehicle in traffic accident**

V23- MOTORCYCLE RIDER INJURED IN COLLISION WITH CAR, PICK-UP TRUCK OR VAN

The appropriate 7th character is to be added to each code from category V23

A - initial encounter

D - subsequent encounter

S - sequela

V23.Ø- **Driver in nontraffic accident**

N **V23.Ø1x_** **Electric (assisted) bicycle driver injured in collision with car, pick-up truck or van in nontraffic accident**

N **V23.Ø9x_** **Other motorcycle driver injured in collision with car, pick-up truck or van in nontraffic accident**

V23.1- **Passenger in nontraffic accident**

N **V23.11x_** **Electric (assisted) bicycle passenger injured in collision with car, pick-up truck or van in nontraffic accident**

N **V23.19x_** **Other motorcycle passenger injured in collision with car, pick-up truck or van in nontraffic accident**

V23.2- **Unspecified rider in nontraffic accident**

N **V23.21x_** **Unspecified electric (assisted) bicycle rider injured in collision with car, pick-up truck or van in nontraffic accident**

N **V23.29x_** **Unspecified rider of other motorcycle injured in collision with car, pick-up truck or van in nontraffic accident**

V23.3- **Person boarding or alighting a motorcycle**

N **V23.31x_** **Person boarding or alighting an electric (assisted) bicycle injured in collision with car, pick-up truck or van**

N **V23.39x_** **Person boarding or alighting other motorcycle injured in collision with car, pick-up truck or van**

V23.4- **Driver in traffic accident**

N **V23.41x_** **Electric (assisted) bicycle driver injured in collision with car, pick-up truck or van in traffic accident**

N **V23.49x_** **Other motorcycle driver injured in collision with car, pick-up truck or van in traffic accident**

V23.5- **Passenger in traffic accident**

N **V23.51x_** **Electric (assisted) bicycle passenger injured in collision with car, pick-up truck or van in traffic accident**

N **V23.59x_** **Other motorcycle passenger injured in collision with car, pick-up truck or van in traffic accident**

V23.9- **Unspecified rider in traffic accident**

N **V23.91x_** **Unspecified electric (assisted) bicycle rider injured in collision with car, pick-up truck or van in traffic accident**

N **V23.99x_** **Unspecified rider of other motorcycle injured in collision with car, pick-up truck or van in traffic accident**

V24- MOTORCYCLE RIDER INJURED IN COLLISION WITH HEAVY TRANSPORT VEHICLE OR BUS

Excludes1:

motorcycle rider injured in collision with military vehicle (V29.818)

The appropriate 7th character is to be added to each code from category V24

A - initial encounter

D - subsequent encounter

S - sequela

V24.Ø- **Driver in nontraffic accident**

N **V24.Ø1x_** **Electric (assisted) bicycle driver injured in collision with heavy transport vehicle or bus in nontraffic accident**

N **V24.Ø9x_** **Other motorcycle driver injured in collision with heavy transport vehicle or bus in nontraffic accident**

V24.1- **Passenger in nontraffic accident**

N **V24.11x_** **Electric (assisted) bicycle passenger injured in collision with heavy transport vehicle or bus in nontraffic accident**

N **V24.19x_** **Other motorcycle passenger injured in collision with heavy transport vehicle or bus in nontraffic accident**

V24.2- **Unspecified rider in nontraffic accident**

N **V24.21x_** **Unspecified electric (assisted) bicycle rider injured in collision with heavy transport vehicle or bus in nontraffic accident**

N **V24.29x_** **Unspecified rider of other motorcycle injured in collision with heavy transport vehicle or bus in nontraffic accident**

V24.3- **Person boarding or alighting a motorcycle**

N **V24.31x_** **Person boarding or alighting an electric (assisted) bicycle injured in collision with heavy transport vehicle or bus**

N **V24.39x_** **Person boarding or alighting other motorcycle injured in collision with heavy transport vehicle or bus**

V24.4- **Driver in traffic accident**

N **V24.41x_** **Electric (assisted) bicycle driver injured in collision with heavy transport vehicle or bus in traffic accident**

N **V24.49x_** **Other motorcycle driver injured in collision with heavy transport vehicle or bus in traffic accident**

V24.5- **Passenger in traffic accident**

N **V24.51x_** **Electric (assisted) bicycle passenger injured in collision with heavy transport vehicle or bus in traffic accident**

N **V24.59x_** **Other motorcycle passenger injured in collision with heavy transport vehicle or bus in traffic accident**

V24.9- **Unspecified rider in traffic accident**

N **V24.91x_** **Unspecified electric (assisted) bicycle rider injured in collision with heavy transport vehicle or bus in traffic accident**

N **V24.99x_** **Unspecified rider of other motorcycle injured in collision with heavy transport vehicle or bus in traffic accident**

V25- MOTORCYCLE RIDER INJURED IN COLLISION WITH RAILWAY TRAIN OR RAILWAY VEHICLE

The appropriate 7th character is to be added to each code from category V25

A - initial encounter

D - subsequent encounter

S - sequela

V25.Ø- **Driver in nontraffic accident**

N **V25.Ø1x_** **Electric (assisted) bicycle driver injured in collision with railway train or railway vehicle in nontraffic accident**

N **V25.Ø9x_** **Other motorcycle driver injured in collision with railway train or railway vehicle in nontraffic accident**

V25.1- **Passenger in nontraffic accident**

N **V25.11x_** **Electric (assisted) bicycle passenger injured in collision with railway train or railway vehicle in nontraffic accident**

N **V25.19x_** **Other motorcycle passenger injured in collision with railway train or railway vehicle in nontraffic accident**

V25.2- **Unspecified rider in nontraffic accident**

N **V25.21x_** **Unspecified electric (assisted) bicycle rider injured in collision with railway train or railway vehicle in nontraffic accident**

N **V25.29x_** **Unspecified rider of other motorcycle injured in collision with railway train or railway vehicle in nontraffic accident**

V25.3- **Person boarding or alighting a motorcycle**

N **V25.31x_** **Person boarding or alighting an electric (assisted) bicycle injured in collision with railway train or railway vehicle**

N **V25.39x_** **Person boarding or alighting other motorcycle injured in collision with railway train or railway vehicle**

V25.4- **Driver in traffic accident**

N **V25.41x_** **Electric (assisted) bicycle driver injured in collision with railway train or railway vehicle in traffic accident**

N **V25.49x_** **Other motorcycle driver injured in collision with railway train or railway vehicle in traffic accident**

V25.5- **Passenger in traffic accident**

N **V25.51x_** **Electric (assisted) bicycle passenger injured in collision with railway train or railway vehicle in traffic accident**

N **V25.59x_** **Other motorcycle passenger injured in collision with railway train or railway vehicle in traffic accident**

V25.9- **Unspecified rider in traffic accident**

N **V25.91x_** **Unspecified electric (assisted) bicycle rider injured in collision with railway train or railway vehicle in traffic accident**

N **V25.99x_** **Unspecified rider of other motorcycle injured in collision with railway train or railway vehicle in traffic accident**

V26- MOTORCYCLE RIDER INJURED IN COLLISION WITH OTHER NONMOTOR VEHICLE

Includes:

collision with animal-drawn vehicle, animal being ridden, streetcar

The appropriate 7th character is to be added to each code from category V26

A - initial encounter

D - subsequent encounter

S - sequela

V26.Ø- **Driver in nontraffic accident**

N **V26.Ø1x_** **Electric (assisted) bicycle driver injured in collision with other nonmotor vehicle in nontraffic accident**

N **V26.Ø9x_** **Other motorcycle driver injured in collision with other nonmotor vehicle in nontraffic accident**

V26.1- **Passenger in nontraffic accident**

N **V26.11x_** **Electric (assisted) bicycle passenger injured in collision with other nonmotor vehicle in nontraffic accident**

N **V26.19x_** **Other motorcycle passenger injured in collision with other nonmotor vehicle in nontraffic accident**

V26.2- **Unspecified rider in nontraffic accident**

N **V26.21x_** **Unspecified electric (assisted) bicycle rider injured in collision with other nonmotor vehicle in nontraffic accident**

N **V26.29x_** **Unspecified rider of other motorcycle injured in collision with other nonmotor vehicle in nontraffic accident**

V26.3- **Person boarding or alighting a motorcycle**

N **V26.31x_** **Person boarding or alighting an electric (assisted) bicycle injured in collision with other nonmotor vehicle**

N **V26.39x_** **Person boarding or alighting other motorcycle injured in collision with other nonmotor vehicle**

V26.4- **Driver in traffic accident**

N **V26.41x_** **Electric (assisted) bicycle driver injured in collision with other nonmotor vehicle in traffic accident**

N **V26.49x_** **Other motorcycle driver injured in collision with other nonmotor vehicle in traffic accident**

V26.5- **Passenger in traffic accident**

N **V26.51x_** **Electric (assisted) bicycle passenger injured in collision with other nonmotor vehicle in traffic accident**

N **V26.59x_** **Other motorcycle passenger injured in collision with other nonmotor vehicle in traffic accident**

V26.9- **Unspecified rider in traffic accident**

N **V26.91x_** **Unspecified electric (assisted) bicycle rider injured in collision with other nonmotor vehicle in traffic accident**

N **V26.99x_** **Unspecified rider of other motorcycle injured in collision with other nonmotor vehicle in traffic accident**

V27- MOTORCYCLE RIDER INJURED IN COLLISION WITH FIXED OR STATIONARY OBJECT

The appropriate 7th character is to be added to each code from category V27

A - initial encounter

D - subsequent encounter

S - sequela

V27.Ø- **Driver in nontraffic accident**

N **V27.Ø1x_** **Electric (assisted) bicycle driver injured in collision with fixed or stationary object in nontraffic accident**

N **V27.Ø9x_** **Other motorcycle driver injured in collision with fixed or stationary object in nontraffic accident**

V27.1- **Passenger in nontraffic accident**

N **V27.11x_** **Electric (assisted) bicycle passenger injured in collision with fixed or stationary object in nontraffic accident**

N **V27.19x_** **Other motorcycle passenger injured in collision with fixed or stationary object in nontraffic accident**

V27.2- **Unspecified rider in nontraffic accident**

N **V27.21x_** **Unspecified electric (assisted) bicycle rider injured in collision with fixed or stationary object in nontraffic accident**

N **V27.29x_** **Unspecified rider of other motorcycle injured in collision with fixed or stationary object in nontraffic accident**

V27.3- **Person boarding or alighting a motorcycle**

N **V27.31x_ Person boarding or alighting an electric (assisted) bicycle injured in collision with fixed or stationary object**

N **V27.39x_ Person boarding or alighting other motorcycle injured in collision with fixed or stationary object**

V27.4- **Driver in traffic accident**

N **V27.41x_ Electric (assisted) bicycle driver injured in collision with fixed or stationary object in traffic accident**

N **V27.49x_ Other motorcycle driver injured in collision with fixed or stationary object in traffic accident**

V27.5- **Passenger in traffic accident**

N **V27.51x_ Electric (assisted) bicycle passenger injured in collision with fixed or stationary object in traffic accident**

N **V27.59x_ Other motorcycle passenger injured in collision with fixed or stationary object in traffic accident**

V27.9- **Unspecified rider in traffic accident**

N **V27.91x_ Unspecified electric (assisted) bicycle rider injured in collision with fixed or stationary object in traffic accident**

N **V27.99x_ Unspecified rider of other motorcycle injured in collision with fixed or stationary object in traffic accident**

V28- MOTORCYCLE RIDER INJURED IN NONCOLLISION TRANSPORT ACCIDENT

Includes:
fall or thrown from motorcycle (without antecedent collision)
overturning motorcycle NOS
overturning motorcycle without collision

The appropriate 7th character is to be added to each code from category V28
A - initial encounter
D - subsequent encounter
S - sequela

V28.Ø- **Driver in nontraffic accident**

N **V28.Ø1x_ Electric (assisted) bicycle driver injured in noncollision transport accident in nontraffic accident**

N **V28.Ø9x_ Other motorcycle driver injured in noncollision transport accident in nontraffic accident**

V28.1- **Passenger in nontraffic accident**

N **V28.11x_ Electric (assisted) bicycle passenger injured in noncollision transport accident in nontraffic accident**

N **V28.19x_ Other motorcycle passenger injured in noncollision transport accident in nontraffic accident**

V28.2- **Unspecified rider in nontraffic accident**

N **V28.21x_ Unspecified electric (assisted) bicycle rider injured in noncollision transport accident in nontraffic accident**

N **V28.29x_ Unspecified rider of other motorcycle injured in noncollision transport accident in nontraffic accident**

V28.3- **Person boarding or alighting a motorcycle**

N **V28.31x_ Person boarding or alighting an electric (assisted) bicycle injured in noncollision transport accident**

N **V28.39x_ Person boarding or alighting other motorcycle injured in noncollision transport accident**

V28.4- **Driver in traffic accident**

N **V28.41x_ Electric (assisted) bicycle driver injured in noncollision transport accident in traffic accident**

N **V28.49x_ Other motorcycle driver injured in noncollision transport accident in traffic accident**

V28.5- **Passenger in traffic accident**

N **V28.51x_ Electric (assisted) bicycle passenger injured in noncollision transport accident in traffic accident**

N **V28.59x_ Other motorcycle passenger injured in noncollision transport accident in traffic accident**

V28.9- **Unspecified rider in traffic accident**

N **V28.91x_ Unspecified electric (assisted) bicycle rider injured in noncollision transport accident in traffic accident**

N **V28.99x_ Unspecified rider of other motorcycle injured in noncollision transport accident in traffic accident**

V29- MOTORCYCLE RIDER INJURED IN OTHER AND UNSPECIFIED TRANSPORT ACCIDENTS

The appropriate 7th character is to be added to each code from category V29
A - initial encounter
D - subsequent encounter
S - sequela

V29.Ø- **Motorcycle driver injured in collision with other and unspecified motor vehicles in nontraffic accident**

V29.ØØ- **Unspecified**

N **V29.ØØ1_ Electric (assisted) bicycle driver injured in collision with unspecified motor vehicles in nontraffic accident**

N **V29.ØØ8_ Other motorcycle driver injured in collision with unspecified motor vehicles in nontraffic accident**

V29.Ø9- **Other**

N **V29.Ø91_ Electric (assisted) bicycle driver injured in collision with other motor vehicles in nontraffic accident**

N **V29.Ø98_ Other motorcycle driver injured in collision with other motor vehicles in nontraffic accident**

Ch5

5. The Tabular List

V29.1- **Motorcycle passenger injured in collision with other and unspecified motor vehicles in nontraffic accident**

V29.1Ø- **Unspecified**

N **V29.1Ø1_** **Electric (assisted) bicycle passenger injured in collision with unspecified motor vehicles in nontraffic accident**

N **V29.1Ø8_** **Other motorcycle passenger injured in collision with unspecified motor vehicles in nontraffic accident**

V29.19- **Other**

N **V29.191_** **Electric (assisted) bicycle passenger injured in collision with other motor vehicles in nontraffic accident**

N **V29.198_** **Other motorcycle passenger injured in collision with other motor vehicles in nontraffic accident**

V29.2- **Unspecified motorcycle rider injured in collision with other and unspecified motor vehicles in nontraffic accident**

V29.2Ø- **Unspecified**

N **V29.2Ø1_** **Unspecified electric (assisted) bicycle rider injured in collision with unspecified motor vehicles in nontraffic accident**

N **V29.2Ø8_** **Unspecified rider of other motorcycle injured in collision with unspecified motor vehicles in nontraffic accident**

Including: Motorcycle collision NOS, nontraffic

V29.29- **Other**

N **V29.291_** **Unspecified electric (assisted) bicycle rider injured in collision with other motor vehicles in nontraffic accident**

N **V29.298_** **Unspecified rider of other motorcycle injured in collision with other motor vehicles in nontraffic accident**

V29.3- **Rider (driver) (passenger) in unspecified nontraffic accident**

N **V29.31x_** **Electric (assisted) bicycle (driver) (passenger) injured in unspecified nontraffic accident**

N **V29.39x_** **Other motorcycle (driver) (passenger) injured in unspecified nontraffic accident**

Including: accident NOS, nontraffic; rider injured in nontraffic accident NOS

V29.4- **Motorcycle driver injured in collision with other and unspecified motor vehicles in traffic accident**

V29.4Ø- **Unspecified**

N **V29.4Ø1_** **Electric (assisted) bicycle driver injured in collision with unspecified motor vehicles in traffic accident**

N **V29.4Ø8_** **Other motorcycle driver injured in collision with unspecified motor vehicles in traffic accident**

V29.49- **Other**

N **V29.491_** **Electric (assisted) bicycle driver injured in collision with other motor vehicles in traffic accident**

N **V29.498_** **Other motorcycle driver injured in collision with other motor vehicles in traffic accident**

V29.5- **Motorcycle passenger injured in collision with other and unspecified motor vehicles in traffic accident**

V29.5Ø- **Unspecified**

N **V29.5Ø1_** **Electric (assisted) bicycle passenger injured in collision with unspecified motor vehicles in traffic accident**

N **V29.5Ø8_** **Other motorcycle passenger injured in collision with unspecified motor vehicles in traffic accident**

V29.59- **Other**

N **V29.591_** **Electric (assisted) bicycle passenger injured in collision with other motor vehicles in traffic accident**

N **V29.598_** **Other motorcycle passenger injured in collision with other motor vehicles in traffic accident**

V29.6- **Unspecified motorcycle rider injured in collision with other and unspecified motor vehicles in traffic accident**

V29.6Ø- **Unspecified**

N **V29.6Ø1_** **Unspecified electric (assisted) bicycle rider injured in collision with unspecified motor vehicles in traffic accident**

N **V29.6Ø8_** **Unspecified rider of other motorcycle injured in collision with unspecified motor vehicles in traffic accident**

Including: Motorcycle collision NOS (traffic)

V29.69- **Other**

N **V29.691_** **Unspecified electric (assisted) bicycle rider injured in collision with other motor vehicles in traffic accident**

N **V29.698_** **Unspecified rider of other motorcycle injured in collision with other motor vehicles in traffic accident**

V29.8- **Motorcycle rider (driver) (passenger) injured in other specified transport accidents**

V29.81- **With military vehicle**

N **V29.811_** **Electric (assisted) bicycle rider (driver) (passenger) injured in transport accident with military vehicle**

N **V29.818_** **Rider (driver) (passenger) of other motorcycle injured in transport accident with military vehicle**

V29.88- **Other**

N **V29.881_** **Electric (assisted) bicycle rider (driver) (passenger) injured in other specified transport accidents**

N **V29.888_** **Rider (driver) (passenger) of other motorcycle injured in other specified transport accidents**

V29.9- **Rider (driver) (passenger) in unspecified traffic accident**

N **V29.91x_ Electric (assisted) bicycle rider (driver) (passenger) injured in unspecified traffic accident**

N **V29.99x_ Rider (driver) (passenger) of other motorcycle injured in unspecified traffic accident**
Including: Motorcycle accident NOS

OCCUPANT OF THREE-WHEELED MOTOR VEHICLE INJURED IN TRANSPORT ACCIDENT (V3Ø-V39)

Includes:
motorized tricycle
motorized rickshaw
three-wheeled motor car
Excludes1:
all-terrain vehicles (V86.-)
motorcycle with sidecar (V2Ø-V29)
vehicle designed primarily for off-road use (V86.-)
Indicator(s): POAEx

V3Ø- OCCUPANT OF THREE-WHEELED MOTOR VEHICLE INJURED IN COLLISION WITH PEDESTRIAN OR ANIMAL

Excludes1:
three-wheeled motor vehicle collision with animal-drawn vehicle or animal being ridden (V36.-)

The appropriate 7th character is to be added to each code from category V3Ø
A - initial encounter
D - subsequent encounter
S - sequela

V3Ø.Øxx_ Driver in nontraffic accident
V3Ø.1xx_ Passenger in nontraffic accident
V3Ø.2xx_ Person on outside of vehicle in nontraffic accident
V3Ø.3xx_ Unspecified occupant in nontraffic accident
V3Ø.4xx_ Person boarding or alighting vehicle
V3Ø.5xx_ Driver in traffic accident
V3Ø.6xx_ Passenger in traffic accident
V3Ø.7xx_ Person on outside of vehicle in traffic accident
V3Ø.9xx_ Unspecified occupant in traffic accident

V31- OCCUPANT OF THREE-WHEELED MOTOR VEHICLE INJURED IN COLLISION WITH PEDAL CYCLE

The appropriate 7th character is to be added to each code from category V31
A - initial encounter
D - subsequent encounter
S - sequela

V31.Øxx_ Driver in nontraffic accident
V31.1xx_ Passenger in nontraffic accident
V31.2xx_ Person on outside of vehicle in nontraffic accident
V31.3xx_ Unspecified occupant in nontraffic accident
V31.4xx_ Person boarding or alighting vehicle
V31.5xx_ Driver in traffic accident
V31.6xx_ Passenger in traffic accident
V31.7xx_ Person on outside of vehicle in traffic accident
V31.9xx_ Unspecified occupant in traffic accident

V32- OCCUPANT OF THREE-WHEELED MOTOR VEHICLE INJURED IN COLLISION WITH TWO- OR THREE-WHEELED MOTOR VEHICLE

The appropriate 7th character is to be added to each code from category V32
A - initial encounter
D - subsequent encounter
S - sequela

V32.Øxx_ Driver in nontraffic accident
V32.1xx_ Passenger in nontraffic accident
V32.2xx_ Person on outside of vehicle in nontraffic accident
V32.3xx_ Unspecified occupant in nontraffic accident
V32.4xx_ Person boarding or alighting vehicle
V32.5xx_ Driver in traffic accident
V32.6xx_ Passenger in traffic accident
V32.7xx_ Person on outside of vehicle in traffic accident
V32.9xx_ Unspecified occupant in traffic accident

V33- OCCUPANT OF THREE-WHEELED MOTOR VEHICLE INJURED IN COLLISION WITH CAR, PICK-UP TRUCK OR VAN

The appropriate 7th character is to be added to each code from category V33
A - initial encounter
D - subsequent encounter
S - sequela

V33.Øxx_ Driver in nontraffic accident
V33.1xx_ Passenger in nontraffic accident
V33.2xx_ Person on outside of vehicle in nontraffic accident
V33.3xx_ Unspecified occupant in nontraffic accident
V33.4xx_ Person boarding or alighting vehicle
V33.5xx_ Driver in traffic accident
V33.6xx_ Passenger in traffic accident
V33.7xx_ Person on outside of vehicle in traffic accident
V33.9xx_ Unspecified occupant in traffic accident

V34- OCCUPANT OF THREE-WHEELED MOTOR VEHICLE INJURED IN COLLISION WITH HEAVY TRANSPORT VEHICLE OR BUS

Excludes1:
occupant of three-wheeled motor vehicle injured in collision with military vehicle (V39.81)

The appropriate 7th character is to be added to each code from category V34
A - initial encounter
D - subsequent encounter
S - sequela

V34.Øxx_ Driver motor vehicle in nontraffic accident
V34.1xx_ Passenger in nontraffic accident
V34.2xx_ Person on outside of vehicle in nontraffic accident
V34.3xx_ Unspecified occupant in nontraffic accident
V34.4xx_ Person boarding or alighting vehicle
V34.5xx_ Driver in traffic accident
V34.6xx_ Passenger in traffic accident
V34.7xx_ Person on outside of vehicle in traffic accident
V34.9xx_ Unspecified occupant in traffic accident

V35- OCCUPANT OF THREE-WHEELED MOTOR VEHICLE INJURED IN COLLISION WITH RAILWAY TRAIN OR RAILWAY VEHICLE

The appropriate 7th character is to be added to each code from category V35
A - initial encounter
D - subsequent encounter
S - sequela

V35.Øxx_ Driver in nontraffic accident
V35.1xx_ Passenger in nontraffic accident
V35.2xx_ Person on outside of vehicle in nontraffic accident
V35.3xx_ Unspecified occupant in nontraffic accident
V35.4xx_ Person boarding or alighting vehicle
V35.5xx_ Driver in traffic accident
V35.6xx_ Passenger in traffic accident
V35.7xx_ Person on outside of vehicle in traffic accident
V35.9xx_ Unspecified occupant in traffic accident

V36- OCCUPANT OF THREE-WHEELED MOTOR VEHICLE INJURED IN COLLISION WITH OTHER NONMOTOR VEHICLE

Includes:
collision with animal-drawn vehicle, animal being ridden, streetcar

The appropriate 7th character is to be added to each code from category V36
A - initial encounter
D - subsequent encounter
S - sequela

V36.Øxx_ Driver in nontraffic accident
V36.1xx_ Passenger in nontraffic accident
V36.2xx_ Person on outside of vehicle in nontraffic accident
V36.3xx_ Unspecified occupant in nontraffic accident
V36.4xx_ Person boarding or alighting vehicle
V36.5xx_ Driver in traffic accident
V36.6xx_ Passenger in traffic accident
V36.7xx_ Person on outside of vehicle in traffic accident
V36.9xx_ Unspecified occupant in traffic accident

V37- OCCUPANT OF THREE-WHEELED MOTOR VEHICLE INJURED IN COLLISION WITH FIXED OR STATIONARY OBJECT

The appropriate 7th character is to be added to each code from category V37
A - initial encounter
D - subsequent encounter
S - sequela

V37.Øxx_ Driver in nontraffic accident
V37.1xx_ Passenger in nontraffic accident
V37.2xx_ Person on outside of vehicle in nontraffic accident
V37.3xx_ Unspecified occupant in nontraffic accident
V37.4xx_ Person boarding or alighting vehicle
V37.5xx_ Driver in traffic accident
V37.6xx_ Passenger in traffic accident
V37.7xx_ Person on outside of vehicle in traffic accident
V37.9xx_ Unspecified occupant in traffic accident

V38- OCCUPANT OF THREE-WHEELED MOTOR VEHICLE INJURED IN NONCOLLISION TRANSPORT ACCIDENT

Includes:
fall or thrown from three-wheeled motor vehicle
overturning of three-wheeled motor vehicle NOS
overturning of three-wheeled motor vehicle without collision

The appropriate 7th character is to be added to each code from category V38
A - initial encounter
D - subsequent encounter
S - sequela

V38.Øxx_ Driver in nontraffic accident
V38.1xx_ Passenger in nontraffic accident
V38.2xx_ Person on outside of vehicle in nontraffic accident
V38.3xx_ Unspecified occupant in nontraffic accident
V38.4xx_ Person boarding or alighting vehicle
V38.5xx_ Driver in traffic accident
V38.6xx_ Passenger in traffic accident
V38.7xx_ Person on outside of vehicle in traffic accident
V38.9xx_ Unspecified occupant in traffic accident

V39- OCCUPANT OF THREE-WHEELED MOTOR VEHICLE INJURED IN OTHER AND UNSPECIFIED TRANSPORT ACCIDENTS

The appropriate 7th character is to be added to each code from category V39
A - initial encounter
D - subsequent encounter
S - sequela

V39.Ø- **Driver of three-wheeled motor vehicle injured in collision with other and unspecified motor vehicles in nontraffic accident**
- **V39.ØØx_ Unspecified**
- **V39.Ø9x_ Other**

V39.1- **Passenger in three-wheeled motor vehicle injured in collision with other and unspecified motor vehicles in nontraffic accident**
- **V39.1Øx_ Unspecified**
- **V39.19x_ Other**

V39.2- **Unspecified occupant of three-wheeled motor vehicle injured in collision with other and unspecified motor vehicles in nontraffic accident**
- **V39.2Øx_ Unspecified**
  Including: Collision NOS
- **V39.29x_ Other**

V39.3xx_ Occupant (driver) (passenger) injured in unspecified nontraffic accident
Including: Accident NOS, Injury NOS

V39.4- **Driver of three-wheeled motor vehicle injured in collision with other and unspecified motor vehicles in traffic accident**
- **V39.4Øx_ Unspecified**
- **V39.49x_ Other**

V39.5- **Passenger in three-wheeled motor vehicle injured in collision with other and unspecified motor vehicles in traffic accident**
- **V39.5Øx_ Unspecified**
- **V39.59x_ Other**

V39.6- **Unspecified occupant of three-wheeled motor vehicle injured in collision with other and unspecified motor vehicles in traffic accident**

V39.6Øx_ Unspecified

Including: Collision NOS

V39.69x_ Other

V39.8- **Occupant (driver) (passenger) of three-wheeled motor vehicle injured in other specified transport accidents**

V39.81x_ With military vehicle

V39.89x_ Other

V39.9xx_ Unspecified

Including: Accident NOS

CAR OCCUPANT INJURED IN TRANSPORT ACCIDENT (V4Ø-V49)

Includes:
a four-wheeled motor vehicle designed primarily for carrying passengers
automobile (pulling a trailer or camper)
Excludes1:
bus (V5Ø-V59)
minibus (V5Ø-V59)
minivan (V5Ø-V59)
motorcoach (V7Ø-V79)
pick-up truck (V5Ø-V59)
sport utility vehicle (SUV) (V5Ø-V59)
Indicator(s): POAEx

V4Ø- CAR OCCUPANT INJURED IN COLLISION WITH PEDESTRIAN OR ANIMAL

Excludes1:
car collision with animal-drawn vehicle or animal being ridden (V46.-)

The appropriate 7th character is to be added to each code from category V4Ø
A - initial encounter
D - subsequent encounter
S - sequela

V4Ø.Øxx_ Driver in nontraffic accident
V4Ø.1xx_ Passenger in nontraffic accident
V4Ø.2xx_ Person on outside of car in nontraffic accident
V4Ø.3xx_ Unspecified occupant in nontraffic accident
V4Ø.4xx_ Person boarding or alighting a car
V4Ø.5xx_ Driver in traffic accident
V4Ø.6xx_ Passenger in traffic accident
V4Ø.7xx_ Person on outside of car in traffic accident
V4Ø.9xx_ Unspecified occupant in traffic accident

V41- CAR OCCUPANT INJURED IN COLLISION WITH PEDAL CYCLE

The appropriate 7th character is to be added to each code from category V41
A - initial encounter
D - subsequent encounter
S - sequela

V41.Øxx_ Driver in nontraffic accident
V41.1xx_ Passenger in nontraffic accident
V41.2xx_ Person on outside of car in nontraffic accident
V41.3xx_ Unspecified occupant in nontraffic accident
V41.4xx_ Person boarding or alighting a car
V41.5xx_ Driver in traffic accident
V41.6xx_ Passenger in traffic accident
V41.7xx_ Person on outside of car in traffic accident
V41.9xx_ Unspecified occupant in traffic accident

V42- CAR OCCUPANT INJURED IN COLLISION WITH TWO- OR THREE-WHEELED MOTOR VEHICLE

The appropriate 7th character is to be added to each code from category V42
A - initial encounter
D - subsequent encounter
S - sequela

V42.Øxx_ Driver in nontraffic accident
V42.1xx_ Passenger in nontraffic accident
V42.2xx_ Person on outside of car in nontraffic accident
V42.3xx_ Unspecified occupant in nontraffic accident
V42.4xx_ Person boarding or alighting a car
V42.5xx_ Driver in traffic accident
V42.6xx_ Passenger in traffic accident
V42.7xx_ Person on outside of car in traffic accident
V42.9xx_ Unspecified occupant in traffic accident

V43- CAR OCCUPANT INJURED IN COLLISION WITH CAR, PICK-UP TRUCK OR VAN

The appropriate 7th character is to be added to each code from category V43
A - initial encounter
D - subsequent encounter
S - sequela

V43.Ø- **Car driver injured in collision with car, pick-up truck or van in nontraffic accident**

V43.Ø1x_ Sport utility vehicle
V43.Ø2x_ Other type car
V43.Ø3x_ Pick-up truck
V43.Ø4x_ Van

V43.1- **Car passenger injured in collision with car, pick-up truck or van in nontraffic accident**

V43.11x_ Sport utility vehicle
V43.12x_ Other type car
V43.13x_ Pick-up truck
V43.14x_ Van

V43.2- **Person on outside of car injured in collision with car, pick-up truck or van in nontraffic accident**

V43.21x_ Sport utility vehicle
V43.22x_ Other type car
V43.23x_ Pick-up truck
V43.24x_ Van

V43.3- **Unspecified car occupant injured in collision with car, pick-up truck or van in nontraffic accident**

V43.31x_ Sport utility vehicle
V43.32x_ Other type car
V43.33x_ Pick-up truck
V43.34x_ Van

V43.4- **Person boarding or alighting a car injured in collision with car, pick-up truck or van**

V43.41x_ Sport utility vehicle
V43.42x_ Other type car
V43.43x_ Pick-up truck
V43.44x_ Van

V43.5- **Car driver injured in collision with car, pick-up truck or van in traffic accident**

V43.51x_ **Sport utility vehicle**

V43.52x_ **Other type car**

V43.53x_ **Pick-up truck**

V43.54x_ **Van**

V43.6- **Car passenger injured in collision with car, pick-up truck or van in traffic accident**

V43.61x_ **Sport utility vehicle**

V43.62x_ **Other type car**

V43.63x_ **Pick-up truck**

V43.64x_ **Van**

V43.7- **Person on outside of car injured in collision with car, pick-up truck or van in traffic accident**

V43.71x_ **Sport utility vehicle**

V43.72x_ **Other type car**

V43.73x_ **Pick-up truck**

V43.74x_ **Van**

V43.9- **Unspecified car occupant injured in collision with car, pick-up truck or van in traffic accident**

V43.91x_ **Sport utility vehicle**

V43.92x_ **Other type car**

V43.93x_ **Pick-up truck**

V43.94x_ **Van**

V44- CAR OCCUPANT INJURED IN COLLISION WITH HEAVY TRANSPORT VEHICLE OR BUS

Excludes1:

car occupant injured in collision with military vehicle (V49.81)

The appropriate 7th character is to be added to each code from category V44

A - initial encounter

D - subsequent encounter

S - sequela

V44.Øxx_ **Driver in nontraffic accident**

V44.1xx_ **Passenger or in nontraffic accident**

V44.2xx_ **Person on outside of car in nontraffic accident**

V44.3xx_ **Unspecified occupant in nontraffic accident**

V44.4xx_ **Person boarding or alighting a car**

V44.5xx_ **Driver in traffic accident**

V44.6xx_ **Passenger in traffic accident**

V44.7xx_ **Person on outside of car in traffic accident**

V44.9xx_ **Unspecified occupant in traffic accident**

V45- CAR OCCUPANT INJURED IN COLLISION WITH RAILWAY TRAIN OR RAILWAY VEHICLE

The appropriate 7th character is to be added to each code from category V45

A - initial encounter

D - subsequent encounter

S - sequela

V45.Øxx_ **Driver in nontraffic accident**

V45.1xx_ **Passenger in nontraffic accident**

V45.2xx_ **Person on outside of car in nontraffic accident**

V45.3xx_ **Unspecified occupant in nontraffic accident**

V45.4xx_ **Person boarding or alighting a car**

V45.5xx_ **Driver in traffic accident**

V45.6xx_ **Passenger in traffic accident**

V45.7xx_ **Person on outside of car in traffic accident**

V45.9xx_ **Unspecified occupant in traffic accident**

V46- CAR OCCUPANT INJURED IN COLLISION WITH OTHER NONMOTOR VEHICLE

Includes:

collision with animal-drawn vehicle, animal being ridden, streetcar

The appropriate 7th character is to be added to each code from category V46

A - initial encounter

D - subsequent encounter

S - sequela

V46.Øxx_ **Driver in nontraffic accident**

V46.1xx_ **Passenger in nontraffic accident**

V46.2xx_ **Person on outside of car in nontraffic accident**

V46.3xx_ **Unspecified occupant in nontraffic accident**

V46.4xx_ **Person boarding or alighting a car**

V46.5xx_ **Driver in traffic accident**

V46.6xx_ **Passenger in traffic accident**

V46.7xx_ **Person on outside of car in traffic accident**

V46.9xx_ **Unspecified occupant in traffic accident**

V47- CAR OCCUPANT INJURED IN COLLISION WITH FIXED OR STATIONARY OBJECT

The appropriate 7th character is to be added to each code from category V47

A - initial encounter

D - subsequent encounter

S - sequela

V47.Øxx_ **Driver in nontraffic accident**

V47.1xx_ **Passenger in nontraffic accident**

V47.2xx_ **Person on outside of car in nontraffic accident**

V47.3xx_ **Unspecified occupant in nontraffic accident**

V47.4xx_ **Person boarding or alighting a car**

V47.5xx_ **Driver in traffic accident**

V47.6xx_ **Passenger in traffic accident**

V47.7xx_ **Person on outside of car in traffic accident**

V47.9xx_ **Unspecified occupant in traffic accident**

V48- CAR OCCUPANT INJURED IN NONCOLLISION TRANSPORT ACCIDENT

Includes:

overturning car NOS

overturning car without collision

The appropriate 7th character is to be added to each code from category V48

A - initial encounter

D - subsequent encounter

S - sequela

V48.Øxx_ **Driver in nontraffic accident**

V48.1xx_ **Passenger in nontraffic accident**

V48.2xx_ **Person on outside of car in nontraffic accident**

V48.3xx_ **Unspecified occupant in nontraffic accident**

V48.4xx_ **Person boarding or alighting a car**

V48.5xx_ **Driver in traffic accident**

V48.6xx_ **Passenger in traffic accident**

V48.7xx_ **Person on outside of car in traffic accident**

V48.9xx_ **Unspecified occupant in traffic accident**

V49- CAR OCCUPANT INJURED IN OTHER AND UNSPECIFIED TRANSPORT ACCIDENTS

The appropriate 7th character is to be added to each code from category V49
A - initial encounter
D - subsequent encounter
S - sequela

V49.Ø- **Driver injured in collision with other and unspecified motor vehicles in nontraffic accident**

V49.ØØx_ Unspecified motor vehicles

V49.Ø9x_ Other motor vehicles

V49.1- **Passenger injured in collision with other and unspecified motor vehicles in nontraffic accident**

V49.1Øx_ Unspecified motor vehicles

V49.19x_ Other motor vehicles

V49.2- **Unspecified car occupant injured in collision with other and unspecified motor vehicles in nontraffic accident**

V49.2Øx_ Unspecified motor vehicles
Including: Collision NOS

V49.29x_ Other motor vehicles

V49.3xx_ Occupant (driver) (passenger) in unspecified nontraffic accident
Including: Accident NOS, Injury NOS

V49.4- **Driver injured in collision with other and unspecified motor vehicles in traffic accident**

V49.4Øx_ Unspecified motor vehicles

V49.49x_ Other motor vehicles

V49.5- **Passenger injured in collision with other and unspecified motor vehicles in traffic accident**

V49.5Øx_ Unspecified motor vehicles

V49.59x_ Other motor vehicles

V49.6- **Unspecified car occupant injured in collision with other and unspecified motor vehicles in traffic accident**

V49.6Øx_ Unspecified motor vehicles
Including: Collision NOS

V49.69x_ Other motor vehicles

V49.8- **Car occupant (driver) (passenger) injured in other specified transport accidents**

V49.81x_ With military vehicle

V49.88x_ Other

V49.9xx_ Occupant (driver) (passenger) in unspecified traffic accident
Including: Accident NOS

OCCUPANT OF PICK-UP TRUCK OR VAN INJURED IN TRANSPORT ACCIDENT (V5Ø-V59)

Includes:
a four or six wheel motor vehicle designed primarily for carrying passengers and property but weighing less than the local limit for classification as a heavy goods vehicle
minibus
minivan
sport utility vehicle (SUV)
truck
van
Excludes1:
heavy transport vehicle (V6Ø-V69)
Indicator(s): POAEx

V5Ø- OCCUPANT OF PICK-UP TRUCK OR VAN INJURED IN COLLISION WITH PEDESTRIAN OR ANIMAL

Excludes1:
pick-up truck or van collision with animal-drawn vehicle or animal being ridden (V56.-)

The appropriate 7th character is to be added to each code from category V5Ø
A - initial encounter
D - subsequent encounter
S - sequela

V5Ø.Øxx_ Driver in nontraffic accident
V5Ø.1xx_ Passenger in nontraffic accident
V5Ø.2xx_ Person on outside in nontraffic accident
V5Ø.3xx_ Unspecified occupant in nontraffic accident
V5Ø.4xx_ Person boarding or alighting
V5Ø.5xx_ Driver in traffic accident
V5Ø.6xx_ Passenger in traffic accident
V5Ø.7xx_ Person on outside in traffic accident
V5Ø.9xx_ Unspecified occupant in traffic accident

V51- OCCUPANT OF PICK-UP TRUCK OR VAN INJURED IN COLLISION WITH PEDAL CYCLE

The appropriate 7th character is to be added to each code from category V51
A - initial encounter
D - subsequent encounter
S - sequela

V51.Øxx_ Driver in nontraffic accident
V51.1xx_ Passenger in nontraffic accident
V51.2xx_ Person on outside in nontraffic accident
V51.3xx_ Unspecified occupant in nontraffic accident
V51.4xx_ Person boarding or alighting
V51.5xx_ Driver in traffic accident
V51.6xx_ Passenger in traffic accident
V51.7xx_ Person on outside in traffic accident
V51.9xx_ Unspecified occupant in traffic accident

V52- OCCUPANT OF PICK-UP TRUCK OR VAN INJURED IN COLLISION WITH TWO- OR THREE-WHEELED MOTOR VEHICLE

The appropriate 7th character is to be added to each code from category V52
A - initial encounter
D - subsequent encounter
S - sequela

V52.Øxx_ Driver in nontraffic accident
V52.1xx_ Passenger in nontraffic accident
V52.2xx_ Person on outside in nontraffic accident
V52.3xx_ Unspecified occupant in nontraffic accident
V52.4xx_ Person boarding or alighting
V52.5xx_ Driver in traffic accident
V52.6xx_ Passenger in traffic accident
V52.7xx_ Person on outside in traffic accident
V52.9xx_ Unspecified occupant in traffic accident

V53- OCCUPANT OF PICK-UP TRUCK OR VAN INJURED IN COLLISION WITH CAR, PICK-UP TRUCK OR VAN

The appropriate 7th character is to be added to each code from category V53
A - initial encounter
D - subsequent encounter
S - sequela

V53.Øxx_ Driver in nontraffic accident
V53.1xx_ Passenger in nontraffic accident
V53.2xx_ Person on outside in nontraffic accident
V53.3xx_ Unspecified occupant in nontraffic accident
V53.4xx_ Person boarding or alighting
V53.5xx_ Driver in traffic accident
V53.6xx_ Passenger in traffic accident
V53.7xx_ Person on outside in traffic accident
V53.9xx_ Unspecified occupant in traffic accident

V54- OCCUPANT OF PICK-UP TRUCK OR VAN INJURED IN COLLISION WITH HEAVY TRANSPORT VEHICLE OR BUS

Excludes1:
occupant of pick-up truck or van injured in collision with military vehicle (V59.81)

The appropriate 7th character is to be added to each code from category V54
A - initial encounter
D - subsequent encounter
S - sequela

V54.Øxx_ Driver in nontraffic accident
V54.1xx_ Passenger in nontraffic accident
V54.2xx_ Person on outside in nontraffic accident
V54.3xx_ Unspecified occupant in nontraffic accident
V54.4xx_ Person boarding or alighting
V54.5xx_ Driver in traffic accident
V54.6xx_ Passenger in traffic accident
V54.7xx_ Person on outside in traffic accident
V54.9xx_ Unspecified occupant in traffic accident

V55- OCCUPANT OF PICK-UP TRUCK OR VAN INJURED IN COLLISION WITH RAILWAY TRAIN OR RAILWAY VEHICLE

The appropriate 7th character is to be added to each code from category V55
A - initial encounter
D - subsequent encounter
S - sequela

V55.Øxx_ Driver in nontraffic accident
V55.1xx_ Passenger in nontraffic accident
V55.2xx_ Person on outside in nontraffic accident
V55.3xx_ Unspecified occupant in nontraffic accident
V55.4xx_ Person boarding or alighting
V55.5xx_ Driver in traffic accident
V55.6xx_ Passenger in traffic accident
V55.7xx_ Person on outside in traffic accident
V55.9xx_ Unspecified occupant in traffic accident

V56- OCCUPANT OF PICK-UP TRUCK OR VAN INJURED IN COLLISION WITH OTHER NONMOTOR VEHICLE

Includes:
collision with animal-drawn vehicle, animal being ridden, streetcar

The appropriate 7th character is to be added to each code from category V56
A - initial encounter
D - subsequent encounter
S - sequela

V56.Øxx_ Driver in nontraffic accident
V56.1xx_ Passenger in nontraffic accident
V56.2xx_ Person on outside in nontraffic accident
V56.3xx_ Unspecified occupant in nontraffic accident
V56.4xx_ Person boarding or alighting
V56.5xx_ Driver in traffic accident
V56.6xx_ Passenger in traffic accident
V56.7xx_ Person on outside in traffic accident
V56.9xx_ Unspecified occupant in traffic accident

V57- OCCUPANT OF PICK-UP TRUCK OR VAN INJURED IN COLLISION WITH FIXED OR STATIONARY OBJECT

The appropriate 7th character is to be added to each code from category V57
A - initial encounter
D - subsequent encounter
S - sequela

V57.Øxx_ Driver in nontraffic accident
V57.1xx_ Passenger in nontraffic accident
V57.2xx_ Person on outside in nontraffic accident
V57.3xx_ Unspecified occupant in nontraffic accident
V57.4xx_ Person boarding or alighting
V57.5xx_ Driver in traffic accident
V57.6xx_ Passenger in traffic accident
V57.7xx_ Person on outside in traffic accident
V57.9xx_ Unspecified occupant in traffic accident

V58- OCCUPANT OF PICK-UP TRUCK OR VAN INJURED IN NONCOLLISION TRANSPORT ACCIDENT

Includes:
overturning pick-up truck or van NOS
overturning pick-up truck or van without collision

The appropriate 7th character is to be added to each code from category V58
A - initial encounter
D - subsequent encounter
S - sequela

V58.Øxx_ Driver in nontraffic accident
V58.1xx_ Passenger in nontraffic accident
V58.2xx_ Person on outside in nontraffic accident
V58.3xx_ Unspecified occupant in nontraffic accident
V58.4xx_ Person boarding or alighting
V58.5xx_ Driver in traffic accident
V58.6xx_ Passenger in traffic accident
V58.7xx_ Person on outside in traffic accident
V58.9xx_ Unspecified occupant in traffic accident

V59- OCCUPANT OF PICK-UP TRUCK OR VAN INJURED IN OTHER AND UNSPECIFIED TRANSPORT ACCIDENTS

The appropriate 7th character is to be added to each code from category V59
A - initial encounter
D - subsequent encounter
S - sequela

V59.Ø- **Driver of pick-up truck or van injured in collision with other and unspecified motor vehicles in nontraffic accident**

V59.ØØx_ Unspecified motor vehicles

V59.Ø9x_ Other motor vehicles

V59.1- **Passenger in pick-up truck or van injured in collision with other and unspecified motor vehicles in nontraffic accident**

V59.1Øx_ Unspecified motor vehicles

V59.19x_ Other motor vehicles

V59.2- **Unspecified occupant of pick-up truck or van injured in collision with other and unspecified motor vehicles in nontraffic accident**

V59.2Øx_ Unspecified motor vehicles
Including: Collision NOS

V59.29x_ Other motor vehicles

V59.3xx_ Occupant (driver) (passenger) in unspecified nontraffic accident
Including: Accident NOS, Injury NOS

V59.4- **Driver of pick-up truck or van injured in collision with other and unspecified motor vehicles in traffic accident**

V59.4Øx_ Unspecified motor vehicles

V59.49x_ Other motor vehicles

V59.5- **Passenger in pick-up truck or van injured in collision with other and unspecified motor vehicles in traffic accident**

V59.5Øx_ Unspecified motor vehicles

V59.59x_ Other motor vehicles

V59.6- **Unspecified occupant of pick-up truck or van injured in collision with other and unspecified motor vehicles in traffic accident**

V59.6Øx_ Unspecified motor vehicles
Including: Collision NOS

V59.69x_ Other motor vehicles

V59.8- **Occupant (driver) (passenger) of pick-up truck or van injured in other specified transport accidents**

V59.81x_ With military vehicle

V59.88x_ Other

V59.9xx_ Occupant (driver) (passenger) in unspecified traffic accident
Including: Accident NOS

OCCUPANT OF HEAVY TRANSPORT VEHICLE INJURED IN TRANSPORT ACCIDENT (V6Ø-V69)

Includes:
18 wheeler
armored car
panel truck
Excludes1:
bus
motorcoach
Indicator(s): POAEx

V6Ø- OCCUPANT OF HEAVY TRANSPORT VEHICLE INJURED IN COLLISION WITH PEDESTRIAN OR ANIMAL

Excludes1:
heavy transport vehicle collision with animal-drawn vehicle or animal being ridden (V66.-)

The appropriate 7th character is to be added to each code from category V6Ø
A - initial encounter
D - subsequent encounter
S - sequela

V6Ø.Øxx_ Driver in nontraffic accident
V6Ø.1xx_ Passenger in nontraffic accident
V6Ø.2xx_ Person on outside in nontraffic accident
V6Ø.3xx_ Unspecified occupant in nontraffic accident
V6Ø.4xx_ Person boarding or alighting
V6Ø.5xx_ Driver in traffic accident
V6Ø.6xx_ Passenger in traffic accident
V6Ø.7xx_ Person on outside in traffic accident
V6Ø.9xx_ Unspecified occupant in traffic accident

V61- OCCUPANT OF HEAVY TRANSPORT VEHICLE INJURED IN COLLISION WITH PEDAL CYCLE

The appropriate 7th character is to be added to each code from category V61
A - initial encounter
D - subsequent encounter
S - sequela

V61.Øxx_ Driver in nontraffic accident
V61.1xx_ Passenger in nontraffic accident
V61.2xx_ Person on outside in nontraffic accident
V61.3xx_ Unspecified occupant in nontraffic accident
V61.4xx_ Person boarding or alighting
V61.5xx_ Driver in traffic accident
V61.6xx_ Passenger in traffic accident
V61.7xx_ Person on outside in traffic accident
V61.9xx_ Unspecified occupant in traffic accident

V62- OCCUPANT OF HEAVY TRANSPORT VEHICLE INJURED IN COLLISION WITH TWO- OR THREE-WHEELED MOTOR VEHICLE

The appropriate 7th character is to be added to each code from category V62
A - initial encounter
D - subsequent encounter
S - sequela

V62.Øxx_ Driver in nontraffic accident
V62.1xx_ Passenger in nontraffic accident
V62.2xx_ Person on outside in nontraffic accident
V62.3xx_ Unspecified occupant in nontraffic accident
V62.4xx_ Person boarding or alighting
V62.5xx_ Driver in traffic accident
V62.6xx_ Passenger in traffic accident
V62.7xx_ Person on outside in traffic accident
V62.9xx_ Unspecified occupant in traffic accident

V63- OCCUPANT OF HEAVY TRANSPORT VEHICLE INJURED IN COLLISION WITH CAR, PICK-UP TRUCK OR VAN

The appropriate 7th character is to be added to each code from category V63
A - initial encounter
D - subsequent encounter
S - sequela

V63.Øxx_ **Driver in nontraffic accident**
V63.1xx_ **Passenger in nontraffic accident**
V63.2xx_ **Person on outside in nontraffic accident**
V63.3xx_ **Unspecified occupant in nontraffic accident**
V63.4xx_ **Person boarding or alighting**
V63.5xx_ **Driver in traffic accident**
V63.6xx_ **Passenger in traffic accident**
V63.7xx_ **Person on outside in traffic accident**
V63.9xx_ **Unspecified occupant in traffic accident**

V64- OCCUPANT OF HEAVY TRANSPORT VEHICLE INJURED IN COLLISION WITH HEAVY TRANSPORT VEHICLE OR BUS

Excludes1:
occupant of heavy transport vehicle injured in collision with military vehicle (V69.81)

The appropriate 7th character is to be added to each code from category V64
A - initial encounter
D - subsequent encounter
S - sequela

V64.Øxx_ **Driver in nontraffic accident**
V64.1xx_ **Passenger in nontraffic accident**
V64.2xx_ **Person on outside in nontraffic accident**
V64.3xx_ **Unspecified occupant in nontraffic accident**
V64.4xx_ **Person boarding or alighting**
V64.5xx_ **Driver in traffic accident**
V64.6xx_ **Passenger in traffic accident**
V64.7xx_ **Person on outside in traffic accident**
V64.9xx_ **Unspecified occupant in traffic accident**

V65- OCCUPANT OF HEAVY TRANSPORT VEHICLE INJURED IN COLLISION WITH RAILWAY TRAIN OR RAILWAY VEHICLE

The appropriate 7th character is to be added to each code from category V65
A - initial encounter
D - subsequent encounter
S - sequela

V65.Øxx_ **Driver in nontraffic accident**
V65.1xx_ **Passenger in nontraffic accident**
V65.2xx_ **Person on outside in nontraffic accident**
V65.3xx_ **Unspecified occupant in nontraffic accident**
V65.4xx_ **Person boarding or alighting**
V65.5xx_ **Driver in traffic accident**
V65.6xx_ **Passenger in traffic accident**
V65.7xx_ **Person on outside in traffic accident**
V65.9xx_ **Unspecified occupant in traffic accident**

V66- OCCUPANT OF HEAVY TRANSPORT VEHICLE INJURED IN COLLISION WITH OTHER NONMOTOR VEHICLE

Includes:
collision with animal-drawn vehicle, animal being ridden, streetcar

The appropriate 7th character is to be added to each code from category V66
A - initial encounter
D - subsequent encounter
S - sequela

V66.Øxx_ **Driver in nontraffic accident**
V66.1xx_ **Passenger in nontraffic accident**
V66.2xx_ **Person on outside in nontraffic accident**
V66.3xx_ **Unspecified occupant in nontraffic accident**
V66.4xx_ **Person boarding or alighting**
V66.5xx_ **Driver in traffic accident**
V66.6xx_ **Passenger in traffic accident**
V66.7xx_ **Person on outside in traffic accident**
V66.9xx_ **Unspecified occupant in traffic accident**

V67- OCCUPANT OF HEAVY TRANSPORT VEHICLE INJURED IN COLLISION WITH FIXED OR STATIONARY OBJECT

The appropriate 7th character is to be added to each code from category V67
A - initial encounter
D - subsequent encounter
S - sequela

V67.Øxx_ **Driver in nontraffic accident**
V67.1xx_ **Passenger in nontraffic accident**
V67.2xx_ **Person on outside in nontraffic accident**
V67.3xx_ **Unspecified occupant in nontraffic accident**
V67.4xx_ **Person boarding or alighting**
V67.5xx_ **Driver in traffic accident**
V67.6xx_ **Passenger in traffic accident**
V67.7xx_ **Person on outside in traffic accident**
V67.9xx_ **Unspecified occupant in traffic accident**

V68- OCCUPANT OF HEAVY TRANSPORT VEHICLE INJURED IN NONCOLLISION TRANSPORT ACCIDENT

Includes:
overturning heavy transport vehicle NOS
overturning heavy transport vehicle without collision

The appropriate 7th character is to be added to each code from category V68
A - initial encounter
D - subsequent encounter
S - sequela

V68.Øxx_ **Driver in nontraffic accident**
V68.1xx_ **Passenger in nontraffic accident**
V68.2xx_ **Person on outside in nontraffic accident**
V68.3xx_ **Unspecified occupant in nontraffic accident**
V68.4xx_ **Person boarding or alighting**
V68.5xx_ **Driver in traffic accident**
V68.6xx_ **Passenger in traffic accident**
V68.7xx_ **Person on outside in traffic accident**
V68.9xx_ **Unspecified occupant in traffic accident**

V69- OCCUPANT OF HEAVY TRANSPORT VEHICLE INJURED IN OTHER AND UNSPECIFIED TRANSPORT ACCIDENTS

The appropriate 7th character is to be added to each code from category V69
A - initial encounter
D - subsequent encounter
S - sequela

V69.Ø- **Driver of heavy transport vehicle injured in collision with other and unspecified motor vehicles in nontraffic accident**

V69.ØØx_ Unspecified motor vehicles

V69.Ø9x_ Other motor vehicles

V69.1- **Passenger in heavy transport vehicle injured in collision with other and unspecified motor vehicles in nontraffic accident**

V69.1Øx_ Unspecified motor vehicles

V69.19x_ Other motor vehicles

V69.2- **Unspecified occupant of heavy transport vehicle injured in collision with other and unspecified motor vehicles in nontraffic accident**

V69.2Øx_ Unspecified motor vehicles
Including: Collision NOS

V69.29x_ Other motor vehicles

V69.3xx_ Occupant (driver) (passenger) in unspecified nontraffic accident
Including: Accident NOS, Injury NOS

V69.4- **Driver of heavy transport vehicle injured in collision with other and unspecified motor vehicles in traffic accident**

V69.4Øx_ Unspecified motor vehicles

V69.49x_ Other motor vehicles

V69.5- **Passenger in heavy transport vehicle injured in collision with other and unspecified motor vehicles in traffic accident**

V69.5Øx_ Unspecified motor vehicles

V69.59x_ Other motor vehicles

V69.6- **Unspecified occupant of heavy transport vehicle injured in collision with other and unspecified motor vehicles in traffic accident**

V69.6Øx_ Unspecified motor vehicles
Including: Collision NOS

V69.69x_ Other motor vehicles

V69.8- **Occupant (driver) (passenger) of heavy transport vehicle injured in other specified transport accidents**

V69.81x_ Military vehicle

V69.88x_ Other

V69.9xx_ Occupant (driver) (passenger) in unspecified traffic accident
Including: Accident NOS

BUS OCCUPANT INJURED IN TRANSPORT ACCIDENT (V7Ø-V79)

Includes:
motorcoach
Excludes1:
minibus (V5Ø-V59)
Indicator(s): POAEx

V7Ø- BUS OCCUPANT INJURED IN COLLISION WITH PEDESTRIAN OR ANIMAL

The appropriate 7th character is to be added to each code from category V7Ø
A - initial encounter
D - subsequent encounter
S - sequela

Excludes1:
bus collision with animal-drawn vehicle or animal being ridden (V76.-)

V7Ø.Øxx_ Driver in nontraffic accident
V7Ø.1xx_ Passenger in nontraffic accident
V7Ø.2xx_ Person on outside in nontraffic accident
V7Ø.3xx_ Unspecified occupant in nontraffic accident
V7Ø.4xx_ Person boarding or alighting
V7Ø.5xx_ Driver in traffic accident
V7Ø.6xx_ Passenger in traffic accident
V7Ø.7xx_ Person on outside in traffic accident
V7Ø.9xx_ Unspecified occupant in traffic accident

V71- BUS OCCUPANT INJURED IN COLLISION WITH PEDAL CYCLE

The appropriate 7th character is to be added to each code from category V71
A - initial encounter
D - subsequent encounter
S - sequela

V71.Øxx_ Driver in nontraffic accident
V71.1xx_ Passenger in nontraffic accident
V71.2xx_ Person on outside in nontraffic accident
V71.3xx_ Unspecified occupant in nontraffic accident
V71.4xx_ Person boarding or alighting
V71.5xx_ Driver in traffic accident
V71.6xx_ Passenger in traffic accident
V71.7xx_ Person on outside in traffic accident
V71.9xx_ Unspecified occupant in traffic accident

V72- BUS OCCUPANT INJURED IN COLLISION WITH TWO- OR THREE-WHEELED MOTOR VEHICLE

The appropriate 7th character is to be added to each code from category V72
A - initial encounter
D - subsequent encounter
S - sequela

V72.Øxx_ Driver in nontraffic accident
V72.1xx_ Passenger in nontraffic accident
V72.2xx_ Person on outside in nontraffic accident
V72.3xx_ Unspecified occupant in nontraffic accident
V72.4xx_ Person boarding or alighting
V72.5xx_ Driver in traffic accident
V72.6xx_ Passenger in traffic accident
V72.7xx_ Person on outside in traffic accident
V72.9xx_ Unspecified occupant in traffic accident

See Appendix A — Coding Reference Tables for lists of the ICD-10-CM Tabular indicators, HAC categories, and HCC codes.

V73- BUS OCCUPANT INJURED IN COLLISION WITH CAR, PICK-UP TRUCK OR VAN

The appropriate 7th character is to be added to each code from category V73
A - initial encounter
D - subsequent encounter
S - sequela

V73.Øxx_ Driver in nontraffic accident
V73.1xx_ Passenger in nontraffic accident
V73.2xx_ Person on outside in nontraffic accident
V73.3xx_ Unspecified occupant in nontraffic accident
V73.4xx_ Person boarding or alighting
V73.5xx_ Driver in traffic accident
V73.6xx_ Passenger in traffic accident
V73.7xx_ Person on outside in traffic accident
V73.9xx_ Unspecified occupant in traffic accident

V74- BUS OCCUPANT INJURED IN COLLISION WITH HEAVY TRANSPORT VEHICLE OR BUS

Excludes1:
bus occupant injured in collision with military vehicle (V79.81)

The appropriate 7th character is to be added to each code from category V74
A - initial encounter
D - subsequent encounter
S - sequela

V74.Øxx_ Driver in nontraffic accident
V74.1xx_ Passenger in nontraffic accident
V74.2xx_ Person on outside in nontraffic accident
V74.3xx_ Unspecified occupant in nontraffic accident
V74.4xx_ Person boarding or alighting
V74.5xx_ Driver in traffic accident
V74.6xx_ Passenger in traffic accident
V74.7xx_ Person on outside in traffic accident
V74.9xx_ Unspecified occupant in traffic accident

V75- BUS OCCUPANT INJURED IN COLLISION WITH RAILWAY TRAIN OR RAILWAY VEHICLE

The appropriate 7th character is to be added to each code from category V75
A - initial encounter
D - subsequent encounter
S - sequela

V75.Øxx_ Driver in nontraffic accident
V75.1xx_ Passenger in nontraffic accident
V75.2xx_ Person on outside in nontraffic accident
V75.3xx_ Unspecified occupant in nontraffic accident
V75.4xx_ Person boarding or alighting
V75.5xx_ Driver in traffic accident
V75.6xx_ Passenger in traffic accident
V75.7xx_ Person on outside in traffic accident
V75.9xx_ Unspecified occupant in traffic accident

V76- BUS OCCUPANT INJURED IN COLLISION WITH OTHER NONMOTOR VEHICLE

Includes:
collision with animal-drawn vehicle, animal being ridden, streetcar

The appropriate 7th character is to be added to each code from category V76
A - initial encounter
D - subsequent encounter
S - sequela

V76.Øxx_ Driver in nontraffic accident
V76.1xx_ Passenger in nontraffic accident
V76.2xx_ Person on outside in nontraffic accident
V76.3xx_ Unspecified occupant in nontraffic accident
V76.4xx_ Person boarding or alighting
V76.5xx_ Driver in traffic accident
V76.6xx_ Passenger in traffic accident
V76.7xx_ Person on outside in traffic accident
V76.9xx_ Unspecified occupant in traffic accident

V77- BUS OCCUPANT INJURED IN COLLISION WITH FIXED OR STATIONARY OBJECT

The appropriate 7th character is to be added to each code from category V77
A - initial encounter
D - subsequent encounter
S - sequela

V77.Øxx_ Driver in nontraffic accident
V77.1xx_ Passenger in nontraffic accident
V77.2xx_ Person on outside in nontraffic accident
V77.3xx_ Unspecified occupant in nontraffic accident
V77.4xx_ Person boarding or alighting
V77.5xx_ Driver in traffic accident
V77.6xx_ Passenger in traffic accident
V77.7xx_ Person on outside in traffic accident
V77.9xx_ Unspecified occupant in traffic accident

V78- BUS OCCUPANT INJURED IN NONCOLLISION TRANSPORT ACCIDENT

Includes:
overturning bus NOS
overturning bus without collision

The appropriate 7th character is to be added to each code from category V78
A - initial encounter
D - subsequent encounter
S - sequela

V78.Øxx_ Driver in nontraffic accident
V78.1xx_ Passenger in nontraffic accident
V78.2xx_ Person on outside in nontraffic accident
V78.3xx_ Unspecified occupant in nontraffic accident
V78.4xx_ Person boarding or alighting
V78.5xx_ Driver in traffic accident
V78.6xx_ Passenger in traffic accident
V78.7xx_ Person on outside in traffic accident
V78.9xx_ Unspecified occupant in traffic accident

V79- BUS OCCUPANT INJURED IN OTHER AND UNSPECIFIED TRANSPORT ACCIDENTS

The appropriate 7th character is to be added to each code from category V79
A - initial encounter
D - subsequent encounter
S - sequela

V79.Ø- **Driver of bus injured in collision with other and unspecified motor vehicles in nontraffic accident**

V79.ØØx_ Unspecified motor vehicles

V79.Ø9x_ Other motor vehicles

V79.1- **Passenger on bus injured in collision with other and unspecified motor vehicles in nontraffic accident**

V79.1Øx_ Unspecified motor vehicles

V79.19x_ Other motor vehicles

V79.2- **Unspecified bus occupant injured in collision with other and unspecified motor vehicles in nontraffic accident**

V79.2Øx_ Unspecified motor vehicles
Including: Collision NOS

V79.29x_ Other motor vehicles

V79.3xx_ Occupant (driver) (passenger) in unspecified nontraffic accident
Including: Accident NOS, Injury NOS

V79.4- **Driver of bus injured in collision with other and unspecified motor vehicles in traffic accident**

V79.4Øx_ Unspecified motor vehicles

V79.49x_ Other motor vehicles

V79.5- **Passenger on bus injured in collision with other and unspecified motor vehicles in traffic accident**

V79.5Øx_ Unspecified motor vehicles

V79.59x_ Other motor vehicles

V79.6- **Unspecified bus occupant injured in collision with other and unspecified motor vehicles in traffic accident**

V79.6Øx_ Unspecified motor vehicles
Including: Collision NOS

V79.69x_ Other motor vehicles

V79.8- **Bus occupant (driver) (passenger) injured in other specified transport accidents**

V79.81x_ Military vehicle

V79.88x_ Other

V79.9xx_ Occupant (driver) (passenger) in unspecified traffic accident
Including: Accident NOS

OTHER LAND TRANSPORT ACCIDENTS (V8Ø-V89)

Indicator(s): POAEx

V8Ø- ANIMAL-RIDER OR OCCUPANT OF ANIMAL-DRAWN VEHICLE INJURED IN TRANSPORT ACCIDENT

The appropriate 7th character is to be added to each code from category V8Ø
A - initial encounter
D - subsequent encounter
S - sequela

V8Ø.Ø- **Animal-rider or occupant of animal drawn vehicle injured by fall from or being thrown from animal or animal-drawn vehicle in noncollision accident**

V8Ø.Ø1- **Animal-rider injured by fall from or being thrown from animal in noncollision accident**

V8Ø.Ø1Ø_ Horse

V8Ø.Ø18_ Other

V8Ø.Ø2x_ Occupant of animal-drawn vehicle
Including: Overturning NOS, Overturning without collision

V8Ø.1- **Animal-rider or occupant of animal-drawn vehicle injured in collision with pedestrian or animal**

Excludes1:
animal-rider or animal-drawn vehicle collision with animal-drawn vehicle or animal being ridden (V8Ø.7)

V8Ø.11x_ Animal-rider

V8Ø.12x_ Occupant of animal-drawn vehicle

V8Ø.2- **Animal-rider or occupant of animal-drawn vehicle injured in collision with pedal cycle**

V8Ø.21x_ Animal-rider

V8Ø.22x_ Occupant of animal-drawn vehicle

V8Ø.3- **Animal-rider or occupant of animal-drawn vehicle injured in collision with two- or three-wheeled motor vehicle**

V8Ø.31x_ Animal-rider

V8Ø.32x_ Occupant of animal-drawn vehicle

V8Ø.4- **Animal-rider or occupant of animal-drawn vehicle injured in collision with car, pick-up truck, van, heavy transport vehicle or bus**

Excludes1:
animal-rider injured in collision with military vehicle (V8Ø.91Ø)
occupant of animal-drawn vehicle injured in collision with military vehicle (V8Ø.92Ø)

V8Ø.41x_ Animal-rider

V8Ø.42x_ Occupant of animal-drawn vehicle

V8Ø.5- **Animal-rider or occupant of animal-drawn vehicle injured in collision with other specified motor vehicle**

V8Ø.51x_ Animal-rider

V8Ø.52x_ Occupant of animal-drawn vehicle

V8Ø.6- **Animal-rider or occupant of animal-drawn vehicle injured in collision with railway train or railway vehicle**

V8Ø.61x_ Animal-rider

V8Ø.62x_ Occupant of animal-drawn vehicle

V8Ø.7- **Animal-rider or occupant of animal-drawn vehicle injured in collision with other nonmotor vehicles**

V8Ø.71- **Animal-rider or occupant of animal-drawn vehicle injured in collision with animal being ridden**

V8Ø.71Ø_ Animal-rider

V8Ø.711_ Occupant

V8Ø.72- **Animal-rider or occupant of animal-drawn vehicle injured in collision with other animal-drawn vehicle**

V8Ø.72Ø_ **Animal-rider**

V8Ø.721_ **Occupant**

V8Ø.73- **Animal-rider or occupant of animal-drawn vehicle injured in collision with streetcar**

V8Ø.73Ø_ **Animal-rider**

V8Ø.731_ **Occupant**

V8Ø.79- **Animal-rider or occupant of animal-drawn vehicle injured in collision with other nonmotor vehicles**

V8Ø.79Ø_ **Animal-rider**

V8Ø.791_ **Occupant**

V8Ø.8- **Animal-rider or occupant of animal-drawn vehicle injured in collision with fixed or stationary object**

V8Ø.81x_ **Animal-rider**

V8Ø.82x_ **Occupant**

V8Ø.9- **Animal-rider or occupant of animal-drawn vehicle injured in other and unspecified transport accidents**

V8Ø.91- **Animal-rider injured in other and unspecified transport accidents**

V8Ø.91Ø_ **Accident with military vehicle**

V8Ø.918_ **Other**

V8Ø.919_ **Unspecified**

Including: Accident NOS

V8Ø.92- **Occupant of animal-drawn vehicle injured in other and unspecified transport accidents**

V8Ø.92Ø_ **Accident with military**

V8Ø.928_ **Other**

V8Ø.929_ **Unspecified**

Including: Accident NOS

V81- OCCUPANT OF RAILWAY TRAIN OR RAILWAY VEHICLE INJURED IN TRANSPORT ACCIDENT

Includes:

derailment of railway train or railway vehicle

person on outside of train

Excludes1:

streetcar (V82.-)

The appropriate 7th character is to be added to each code from category V81

A - initial encounter

D - subsequent encounter

S - sequela

V81.Øxx_ **Collision with motor vehicle in nontraffic accident**

Excludes1:

Occupant of railway train or railway vehicle injured due to collision with military vehicle (V81.83)

V81.1xx_ **Collision with motor vehicle in traffic accident**

Excludes1:

Occupant of railway train or railway vehicle injured due to collision with military vehicle (V81.83)

V81.2xx_ **Collision with or hit by rolling stock**

V81.3xx_ **Collision with other object**

Including: Collision NOS

V81.4xx_ **Person injured while boarding or alighting**

V81.5xx_ **Fall in railway train or railway vehicle**

V81.6xx_ **Fall from railway train or railway vehicle**

V81.7xx_ **Derailment without antecedent collision**

V81.8- **Occupant of railway train or railway vehicle injured in other specified railway accidents**

V81.81x_ **Due to explosion or fire on train**

V81.82x_ **Due to object falling onto train**

Including: Falling earth, rocks, snow, trees

V81.83x_ **Due to collision with military vehicle**

V81.89x_ **Due to other specified railway accident**

V81.9xx_ **Unspecified railway accident**

Including: Accident NOS

V82- OCCUPANT OF POWERED STREETCAR INJURED IN TRANSPORT ACCIDENT

Includes:

interurban electric car

person on outside of streetcar

tram (car)

trolley (car)

Excludes1:

bus (V7Ø-V79)

motorcoach (V7Ø-V79)

nonpowered streetcar (V76.-)

train (V81.-)

The appropriate 7th character is to be added to each code from category V82

A - initial encounter

D - subsequent encounter

S - sequela

V82.Øxx_ **Collision with motor vehicle in nontraffic accident**

V82.1xx_ **Collision with motor vehicle in traffic accident**

V82.2xx_ **Collision with or hit by rolling stock**

V82.3xx_ **Collision with other object**

Excludes1:

collision with animal-drawn vehicle or animal being ridden (V82.8)

V82.4xx_ **Person injured while boarding or alighting**

V82.5xx_ **Fall in streetcar**

Excludes1:

fall in streetcar:

while boarding or alighting (V82.4)

with antecedent collision (V82.Ø-V82.3)

V82.6xx_ **Fall from streetcar**

Excludes1:

fall from streetcar:

while boarding or alighting (V82.4)

with antecedent collision (V82.Ø-V82.3)

V82.7xx_ **Derailment without antecedent collision**

Excludes1:

occupant of streetcar injured in derailment with antecedent collision (V82.Ø-V82.3)

V82.8xx_ **Other specified transport accidents**

Including: Collision with military vehicle, Collision with train or nonmotor vehicles

V82.9xx_ **Unspecified traffic accident**

Including: Accident NOS

V83- OCCUPANT OF SPECIAL VEHICLE MAINLY USED ON INDUSTRIAL PREMISES INJURED IN TRANSPORT ACCIDENT

Includes:
battery-powered airport passenger vehicle
battery-powered truck (baggage) (mail)
coal-car in mine
forklift (truck)
logging car
self-propelled industrial truck
station baggage truck (powered)
tram, truck, or tub (powered) in mine or quarry

Excludes1:
special construction vehicles (V85.-)
special industrial vehicle in stationary use or maintenance (W31.-)

The appropriate 7th character is to be added to each code from category V83
A - initial encounter
D - subsequent encounter
S - sequela

V83.Øxx_ Driver in traffic accident
V83.1xx_ Passenger in traffic accident
V83.2xx_ Person on outside in traffic accident
V83.3xx_ Unspecified occupant in traffic accident
V83.4xx_ Person injured while boarding or alighting
V83.5xx_ Driver in nontraffic accident
V83.6xx_ Passenger in nontraffic accident
V83.7xx_ Person on outside in nontraffic accident
V83.9xx_ Unspecified occupant in nontraffic accident
Including: Accident NOS

V84- OCCUPANT OF SPECIAL VEHICLE MAINLY USED IN AGRICULTURE INJURED IN TRANSPORT ACCIDENT

Includes:
self-propelled farm machinery
tractor (and trailer)

Excludes1:
animal-powered farm machinery accident (W3Ø.8-)
contact with combine harvester (W3Ø.Ø)
special agricultural vehicle in stationary use or maintenance (W3Ø.-)

The appropriate 7th character is to be added to each code from category V84
A - initial encounter
D - subsequent encounter
S - sequela

V84.Øxx_ Driver in traffic accident
V84.1xx_ Passenger in traffic accident
V84.2xx_ Person on outside in traffic accident
V84.3xx_ Unspecified occupant in traffic accident
V84.4xx_ Person injured while boarding or alighting
V84.5xx_ Driver in nontraffic accident
V84.6xx_ Passenger in nontraffic accident
V84.7xx_ Person on outside in nontraffic accident
V84.9xx_ Unspecified occupant in nontraffic accident
Including: Accident NOS

V85- OCCUPANT OF SPECIAL CONSTRUCTION VEHICLE INJURED IN TRANSPORT ACCIDENT

Includes:
bulldozer
digger
dump truck
earth-leveller
mechanical shovel
road-roller

Excludes1:
special industrial vehicle (V83.-)
special construction vehicle in stationary use or maintenance (W31.-)

The appropriate 7th character is to be added to each code from category V85
A - initial encounter
D - subsequent encounter
S - sequela

V85.Øxx_ Driver in traffic accident
V85.1xx_ Passenger in traffic accident
V85.2xx_ Person on outside in traffic accident
V85.3xx_ Unspecified occupant in traffic accident
V85.4xx_ Person injured while boarding or alighting
V85.5xx_ Driver in nontraffic accident
V85.6xx_ Passenger in nontraffic accident
V85.7xx_ Person on outside in nontraffic accident
V85.9xx_ Unspecified occupant in nontraffic accident
Including: Accident NOS

V86- OCCUPANT OF SPECIAL ALL-TERRAIN OR OTHER OFF-ROAD MOTOR VEHICLE, INJURED IN TRANSPORT ACCIDENT

Excludes1:
special all-terrain vehicle in stationary use or maintenance (W31.-)
sport-utility vehicle (V5Ø-V59)
three-wheeled motor vehicle designed for on-road use (V3Ø-V39)

The appropriate 7th character is to be added to each code from category V86
A - initial encounter
D - subsequent encounter
S - sequela

V86.Ø- **Driver of special all-terrain or other off-road motor vehicle injured in traffic accident**
V86.Ø1x_ Ambulance or fire engine
V86.Ø2x_ Snowmobile
V86.Ø3x_ Dune buggy
V86.Ø4x_ Military vehicle
V86.Ø5x_ 3- or 4- wheeled all-terrain vehicle (ATV)
V86.Ø6x_ Dirt bike or motor/cross bike
V86.Ø9x_ Other special all-terrain or other off-road motor vehicle
Including: Go cart, golf cart

V86.1- **Passenger of special all-terrain or other off-road motor vehicle injured in traffic accident**
V86.11x_ Ambulance or fire engine injured
V86.12x_ Snowmobile
V86.13x_ Dune buggy
V86.14x_ Military vehicle
V86.15x_ 3- or 4- wheeled all-terrain vehicle (ATV)
V86.16x_ Dirt bike or motor/cross bike
V86.19x_ Other special all-terrain or other off-road motor vehicle
Including: Go cart, golf cart

Ch5

5. The Tabular List

V86.2- **Person on outside of special all-terrain or other off-road motor vehicle injured in traffic accident**

- **V86.21x_** **Ambulance or fire engine**
- **V86.22x_** **Snowmobile**
- **V86.23x_** **Dune buggy**
- **V86.24x_** **Military vehicle injured in traffic accident**
- **V86.25x_** **Person on outside of 3- or 4- wheeled all-terrain vehicle (ATV) injured in traffic accident**
- **V86.26x_** **Person on outside of dirt bike or motor/cross bike injured in traffic accident**
- **V86.29x_** **Other special all-terrain or other off-road motor vehicle**
  Including: Go cart, golf cart

V86.3- **Unspecified occupant of special all-terrain or other off-road motor vehicle injured in traffic accident**

- **V86.31x_** **Ambulance or fire engine**
- **V86.32x_** **Snowmobile**
- **V86.33x_** **Dune buggy**
- **V86.34x_** **Military vehicle**
- **V86.35x_** **Unspecified occupant of 3- or 4- wheeled all-terrain vehicle (ATV) injured in traffic accident**
- **V86.36x_** **Unspecified occupant of dirt bike or motor/cross bike injured in traffic accident**
- **V86.39x_** **Other special all-terrain or other off-road motor vehicle**
  Including: Go cart, golf cart

V86.4- **Person injured while boarding or alighting from special all-terrain or other off-road motor vehicle**

- **V86.41x_** **Ambulance or fire engine**
- **V86.42x_** **Snowmobile**
- **V86.43x_** **Dune buggy**
- **V86.44x_** **Military vehicle**
- **V86.45x_** **Person injured while boarding or alighting from a 3- or 4- wheeled all-terrain vehicle (ATV)**
- **V86.46x_** **Person injured while boarding or alighting from a dirt bike or motor/cross bike**
- **V86.49x_** **Other special all-terrain or other off-road motor vehicle**
  Including: Go cart, golf cart

V86.5- **Driver of special all-terrain or other off-road motor vehicle injured in nontraffic accident**

- **V86.51x_** **Ambulance or fire engine**
- **V86.52x_** **Snowmobile**
- **V86.53x_** **Dune buggy**
- **V86.54x_** **Military vehicle**
- **V86.55x_** **Driver of 3- or 4- wheeled all-terrain vehicle (ATV) injured in nontraffic accident**
- **V86.56x_** **Driver of dirt bike or motor/cross bike injured in nontraffic accident**
- **V86.59x_** **Other special all-terrain or other off-road motor vehicle**
  Including: Go cart, golf cart

V86.6- **Passenger of special all-terrain or other off-road motor vehicle injured in nontraffic accident**

- **V86.61x_** **Ambulance or fire engine**
- **V86.62x_** **Snowmobile**
- **V86.63x_** **Dune buggy**
- **V86.64x_** **Military vehicle**
- **V86.65x_** **Passenger of 3- or 4- wheeled all-terrain vehicle (ATV) injured in nontraffic accident**
- **V86.66x_** **Passenger of dirt bike or motor/cross bike injured in nontraffic accident**
- **V86.69x_** **Other special all-terrain or other off-road motor vehicle**
  Including: Go cart, golf cart

V86.7- **Person on outside of special all-terrain or other off-road motor vehicle injured in nontraffic accident**

- **V86.71x_** **Ambulance or fire engine**
- **V86.72x_** **Snowmobile**
- **V86.73x_** **Dune buggy**
- **V86.74x_** **Military vehicle**
- **V86.75x_** **Person on outside of 3- or 4- wheeled all-terrain vehicle (ATV) injured in nontraffic accident**
- **V86.76x_** **Person on outside of dirt bike or motor/cross bike injured in nontraffic accident**
- **V86.79x_** **Other special all-terrain or other off-road motor vehicles**
  Including: Go cart, golf cart

V86.9- **Unspecified occupant of special all-terrain or other off-road motor vehicle injured in nontraffic accident**

- **V86.91x_** **Ambulance or fire engine**
- **V86.92x_** **Snowmobile**
- **V86.93x_** **Dune buggy**
- **V86.94x_** **Military vehicle**
- **V86.95x_** **Unspecified occupant of 3- or 4- wheeled all-terrain vehicle (ATV) injured in nontraffic accident**
- **V86.96x_** **Unspecified occupant of dirt bike or motor/cross bike injured in nontraffic accident**
- **V86.99x_** **Other special all-terrain or other off-road motor vehicle**
  Including: Off-road, Other motor-vehicle accident NOS; Unspecified occupant of go cart or golf cart injured

V87- TRAFFIC ACCIDENT OF SPECIFIED TYPE BUT VICTIM'S MODE OF TRANSPORT UNKNOWN

Excludes1:
collision involving:
pedal cycle (V1Ø-V19)
pedestrian (VØ1-VØ9)

The appropriate 7th character is to be added to each code from category V87
A - initial encounter
D - subsequent encounter
S - sequela

V87.Øxx_ **Collision between car and two- or three-wheeled powered vehicle (traffic)**
V87.1xx_ **Collision between other motor vehicle and two- or three-wheeled motor vehicle (traffic)**
V87.2xx_ **Collision between car and pick-up truck or van (traffic)**
V87.3xx_ **Collision between car and bus (traffic)**
V87.4xx_ **Collision between car and heavy transport vehicle (traffic)**
V87.5xx_ **Collision between heavy transport vehicle and bus (traffic)**
V87.6xx_ **Collision between railway train or railway vehicle and car (traffic)**
V87.7xx_ **Collision between other specified motor vehicles (traffic)**
V87.8xx_ **Other specified noncollision transport accidents involving motor vehicle (traffic)**
V87.9xx_ **Other specified (collision)(noncollision) transport accidents involving nonmotor vehicle (traffic)**

V88- NONTRAFFIC ACCIDENT OF SPECIFIED TYPE BUT VICTIM'S MODE OF TRANSPORT UNKNOWN

Excludes1:
collision involving:
pedal cycle (V1Ø-V19)
pedestrian (VØ1-VØ9)

The appropriate 7th character is to be added to each code from category V88
A - initial encounter
D - subsequent encounter
S - sequela

V88.Øxx_ **Collision between car and two- or three-wheeled motor vehicle, nontraffic**
V88.1xx_ **Collision between other motor vehicle and two- or three-wheeled motor vehicle, nontraffic**
V88.2xx_ **Collision between car and pick-up truck or van, nontraffic**
V88.3xx_ **Collision between car and bus, nontraffic**
V88.4xx_ **Collision between car and heavy transport vehicle, nontraffic**
V88.5xx_ **Collision between heavy transport vehicle and bus, nontraffic**
V88.6xx_ **Collision between railway train or railway vehicle and car, nontraffic**
V88.7xx_ **Collision between other specified motor vehicle, nontraffic**
V88.8xx_ **Other specified noncollision transport accidents involving motor vehicle, nontraffic**
V88.9xx_ **Other specified (collision)(noncollision) transport accidents involving nonmotor vehicle, nontraffic**

V89- MOTOR- OR NONMOTOR-VEHICLE ACCIDENT, TYPE OF VEHICLE UNSPECIFIED

The appropriate 7th character is to be added to each code from category V89
A - initial encounter
D - subsequent encounter
S - sequela

V89.Øxx_ **Person injured in unspecified motor-vehicle accident, nontraffic**
Including: Accident NOS
V89.1xx_ **Unspecified nonmotor-vehicle accident, nontraffic**
Including: Accident NOS
V89.2xx_ **Unspecified motor-vehicle accident, traffic**
Including: Motor-vehicle accident [MVA] NOS, Road (traffic) accident [RTA] NOS
V89.3xx_ **Unspecified nonmotor-vehicle accident, traffic**
Including: Accident NOS
V89.9xx_ **Unspecified vehicle accident**
Including: Collision NOS

WATER TRANSPORT ACCIDENTS (V9Ø-V94)

Indicator(s): POAEx

V9Ø- DROWNING AND SUBMERSION DUE TO ACCIDENT TO WATERCRAFT

Excludes1:
civilian water transport accident involving military watercraft (V94.81-)
fall into water not from watercraft (W16.-)
military watercraft accident in military or war operations (Y36.Ø-, Y37.Ø-)
water-transport-related drowning or submersion without accident to watercraft (V92.-)

The appropriate 7th character is to be added to each code from category V9Ø
A - initial encounter
D - subsequent encounter
S - sequela

V9Ø.Ø- **Drowning and submersion due to watercraft overturning**
V9Ø.ØØx_ **Merchant ship**
V9Ø.Ø1x_ **Passenger ship**
Including: Ferry-boat, Liner
V9Ø.Ø2x_ **Fishing boat**
V9Ø.Ø3x_ **Other powered watercraft**
Including: Hovercraft (on open water), Jet ski
V9Ø.Ø4x_ **Sailboat**
V9Ø.Ø5x_ **Canoe or kayak**
V9Ø.Ø6x_ **(nonpowered) inflatable craft**
V9Ø.Ø8x_ **Other unpowered watercraft**
Including: Windsurfer
V9Ø.Ø9x_ **Unspecified watercraft**
Including: Boat NOS, ship NOS, watercraft NOS

V9Ø.1- **Drowning and submersion due to watercraft sinking**
V9Ø.1Øx_ **Merchant ship**
V9Ø.11x_ **Passenger ship**
Including: Ferry-boat, Liner
V9Ø.12x_ **Fishing boat**
V9Ø.13x_ **Other powered watercraft**
Including: Hovercraft (on open water), Jet ski

V9Ø.14x_ Sailboat

V9Ø.15x_ Canoe or kayak

V9Ø.16x_ (nonpowered) inflatable craft

V9Ø.18x_ Other unpowered watercraft

V9Ø.19x_ Unspecified watercraft
Including: Boat NOS, ship NOS, watercraft NOS

V9Ø.2- **Drowning and submersion due to falling or jumping from burning watercraft**

V9Ø.2Øx_ Merchant ship

V9Ø.21x_ Passenger ship
Including: Ferry-boat, Liner

V9Ø.22x_ Fishing boat

V9Ø.23x_ Other powered watercraft
Including: Hovercraft (on open water), Jet ski

V9Ø.24x_ Sailboat

V9Ø.25x_ Canoe or kayak

V9Ø.26x_ (nonpowered) inflatable craft

V9Ø.27x_ Water-skis

V9Ø.28x_ Other unpowered watercraft
Including: Surf-board, Windsurfer

V9Ø.29x_ Unspecified watercraft
Including: Boat NOS, ship NOS, watercraft NOS

V9Ø.3- **Drowning and submersion due to falling or jumping from crushed watercraft**

V9Ø.3Øx_ Merchant ship

V9Ø.31x_ Passenger ship
Including: Ferry boat, Liner

V9Ø.32x_ Fishing boat

V9Ø.33x_ Other powered watercraft
Including: Hovercraft, Jet ski

V9Ø.34x_ Sailboat

V9Ø.35x_ Canoe or kayak

V9Ø.36x_ (nonpowered) inflatable craft

V9Ø.37x_ Water-skis

V9Ø.38x_ Other unpowered watercraft
Including: Surf-board, Windsurfer

V9Ø.39x_ Unspecified watercraft
Including: Boat NOS, Ship NOS, Watercraft NOS

V9Ø.8- **Drowning and submersion due to other accident to watercraft**

V9Ø.8Øx_ Merchant ship

V9Ø.81x_ Passenger ship
Including: Ferry-boat, Liner

V9Ø.82x_ Fishing boat

V9Ø.83x_ Other powered watercraft
Including: Hovercraft (on open water), Jet ski

V9Ø.84x_ Sailboat

V9Ø.85x_ Canoe or kayak

V9Ø.86x_ (nonpowered) inflatable craft

V9Ø.87x_ Water-skis

V9Ø.88x_ Other unpowered watercraft
Including: Surf-board, windsurfer

V9Ø.89x_ Unspecified watercraft
Including: Boat NOS, ship NOS, watercraft NOS

V91- OTHER INJURY DUE TO ACCIDENT TO WATERCRAFT

Includes:
any injury except drowning and submersion as a result of an accident to watercraft

Excludes1:
civilian water transport accident involving military watercraft (V94.81-)
military watercraft accident in military or war operations (Y36, Y37.-)

Excludes2:
drowning and submersion due to accident to watercraft (V9Ø.-)

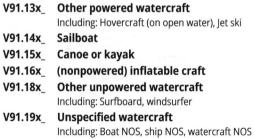

The appropriate 7th character is to be added to each code from category V91
A - initial encounter
D - subsequent encounter
S - sequela

V91.Ø- **Burn due to watercraft on fire**

Excludes1:
burn from localized fire or explosion on board ship without accident to watercraft (V93.-)

V91.ØØx_ Merchant ship

V91.Ø1x_ Passenger ship
Including: Ferry-boat, Liner

V91.Ø2x_ Fishing boat

V91.Ø3x_ Other powered watercraft
Including: Hovercraft (on open water), Jet ski

V91.Ø4x_ Sailboat

V91.Ø5x_ Canoe or kayak

V91.Ø6x_ (nonpowered) inflatable craft

V91.Ø7x_ Water-skis

V91.Ø8x_ Other unpowered watercraft

V91.Ø9x_ Unspecified watercraft
Including: Boat NOS, ship NOS, watercraft NOS

V91.1- **Crushed between watercraft and other watercraft or other object due to collision**
Including: Crushed by lifeboat after abandoning ship

Notes:
select the specified type of watercraft that the victim was on at the time of the collision

V91.1Øx_ Merchant ship

V91.11x_ Passenger ship
Including: Ferry-boat, Liner

V91.12x_ Fishing boat

V91.13x_ Other powered watercraft
Including: Hovercraft (on open water), Jet ski

V91.14x_ Sailboat

V91.15x_ Canoe or kayak

V91.16x_ (nonpowered) inflatable craft

V91.18x_ Other unpowered watercraft
Including: Surfboard, windsurfer

V91.19x_ Unspecified watercraft
Including: Boat NOS, ship NOS, watercraft NOS

V91.2- **Fall due to collision between watercraft and other watercraft or other object**
Including: Fall while remaining on watercraft after collision
Notes:
select the specified type of watercraft that the victim was on at the time of the collision
Excludes1:
crushed between watercraft and other watercraft and other object due to collision (V91.1-)
drowning and submersion due to falling from crushed watercraft (V9Ø.3-)

V91.2Øx_ Merchant ship
V91.21x_ Passenger ship
Including: Ferry-boat, Liner
V91.22x_ Fishing boat
V91.23x_ Other powered watercraft
Including: Hovercraft (on open water), Jet ski
V91.24x_ Sailboat
V91.25x_ Canoe or kayak
V91.26x_ (nonpowered) inflatable craft
V91.29x_ Unspecified watercraft
Including: Boat NOS, ship NOS, watercraft NOS

V91.3- **Hit or struck by falling object due to accident to watercraft**
Including: Hit or struck by falling object (part of damaged watercraft or other object) after falling or jumping from damaged watercraft
Excludes2:
drowning or submersion due to fall or jumping from damaged watercraft (V9Ø.2-, V9Ø.3-)

V91.3Øx_ Merchant ship
V91.31x_ Passenger ship
Including: Ferry-boat, Liner
V91.32x_ Fishing boat
V91.33x_ Other powered watercraft
Including: Hovercraft (on open water), Jet ski
V91.34x_ Sailboat
V91.35x_ Canoe or kayak
V91.36x_ (nonpowered) inflatable craft
V91.37x_ Water-skis
Including: Hit by water-skis after jumping off of water-skis
V91.38x_ Other unpowered watercraft
Including: Surf-board after falling off damaged surf-board, object after falling off damaged windsurfer
V91.39x_ Unspecified watercraft
Including: Boat NOS, ship NOS, watercraft NOS

V91.8- **Other injury due to other accident to watercraft**
V91.8Øx_ Merchant ship
V91.81x_ Passenger ship
Including: Ferry-boat, Liner
V91.82x_ Fishing boat
V91.83x_ Other powered watercraft
Including: Hovercraft (on open water), Jet ski
V91.84x_ Sailboat
V91.85x_ Canoe or kayak
V91.86x_ (nonpowered) inflatable craft
V91.87x_ Water-skis
V91.88x_ Other unpowered watercraft
Including: Surf-board, windsurfer
V91.89x_ Unspecified watercraft
Including: Boat NOS, ship NOS, watercraft NOS

V92- DROWNING AND SUBMERSION DUE TO ACCIDENT ON BOARD WATERCRAFT, WITHOUT ACCIDENT TO WATERCRAFT
Excludes1:
civilian water transport accident involving military watercraft (V94.81-)
drowning or submersion due to accident to watercraft (V9Ø-V91)
drowning or submersion of diver who voluntarily jumps from boat not involved in an accident (W16.711, W16.721)
fall into water without watercraft (W16.-)
military watercraft accident in military or war operations (Y36, Y37)

The appropriate 7th character is to be added to each code from category V92
A - initial encounter
D - subsequent encounter
S - sequela

V92.Ø- **Drowning and submersion due to fall off watercraft**
Including: Drowning and submersion due to fall from gangplank of watercraft, fall overboard watercraft
Excludes2:
hitting head on object or bottom of body of water due to fall from watercraft (V94.Ø-)

V92.ØØx_ Merchant ship
V92.Ø1x_ Passenger ship
Including: Ferry-boat, Liner
V92.Ø2x_ Fishing boat
V92.Ø3x_ Other powered watercraft
Including: Hovercraft (on open water), Jet ski
V92.Ø4x_ Sailboat
V92.Ø5x_ Canoe or kayak
V92.Ø6x_ (nonpowered) inflatable craft
V92.Ø7x_ Water-skis
Excludes1:
drowning and submersion due to falling off burning water-skis (V9Ø.27)
drowning and submersion due to falling off crushed water-skis (V9Ø.37)
hit by boat while water-skiing NOS (V94.X)
V92.Ø8x_ Other unpowered watercraft
Including: Surf-board, windsurfer
Excludes1:
drowning and submersion due to fall off burning unpowered watercraft (V9Ø.28)
drowning and submersion due to fall off crushed unpowered watercraft (V9Ø.38)
drowning and submersion due to fall off damaged unpowered watercraft (V9Ø.88)
drowning and submersion due to rider of nonpowered watercraft being hit by other watercraft (V94.-)
other injury due to rider of nonpowered watercraft being hit by other watercraft (V94.-)
V92.Ø9x_ Unspecified watercraft
Including: Boat NOS, ship, watercraft NOS

See Appendix A — Coding Reference Tables for lists of the ICD-10-CM Tabular indicators, HAC categories, and HCC codes.

V92.1- **Drowning and submersion due to being thrown overboard by motion of watercraft**

Excludes1:
drowning and submersion due to fall off surf-board (V92.Ø8)
drowning and submersion due to fall off water-skis (V92.Ø7)
drowning and submersion due to fall off windsurfer (V92.Ø8)

V92.1Øx_ Merchant ship

V92.11x_ Passenger ship
Including: Ferry-boat, Liner

V92.12x_ Fishing boat

V92.13x_ Other powered watercraft
Including: Hovercraft

V92.14x_ Sailboat

V92.15x_ Canoe or kayak

V92.16x_ (nonpowered) inflatable craft

V92.19x_ Unspecified watercraft
Including: Boat NOS, ship NOS, watercraft NOS

V92.2- **Drowning and submersion due to being washed overboard from watercraft**

Code First:
any associated cataclysm (X37.Ø-)

V92.2Øx_ Merchant ship

V92.21x_ Passenger ship
Including: Ferry-boat, Liner

V92.22x_ Fishing boat

V92.23x_ Other powered watercraft
Including: Hovercraft (on open water), Jet ski

V92.24x_ Sailboat

V92.25x_ Canoe or kayak

V92.26x_ (nonpowered) inflatable craft

V92.27x_ Water-skis
Excludes1:
drowning and submersion due to fall off water-skis (V92.Ø7)

V92.28x_ Other unpowered watercraft
Including: Surf-board, windsurfer

V92.29x_ Unspecified watercraft
Including: Boat NOS, ship NOS, watercraft NOS

V93- OTHER INJURY DUE TO ACCIDENT ON BOARD WATERCRAFT, WITHOUT ACCIDENT TO WATERCRAFT

Excludes1:
civilian water transport accident involving military watercraft (V94.81-)
other injury due to accident to watercraft (V91.-)
military watercraft accident in military or war operations (Y36, Y37.-)

Excludes2:
drowning and submersion due to accident on board watercraft, without accident to watercraft (V92.-)

The appropriate 7th character is to be added to each code from category V93
A - initial encounter
D - subsequent encounter
S - sequela

V93.Ø- **Burn due to localized fire on board watercraft**

Excludes1:
burn due to watercraft on fire (V91.Ø-)

V93.ØØx_ Merchant vessel

V93.Ø1x_ Passenger vessel
Including: Ferry-boat, Liner

V93.Ø2x_ Fishing boat

V93.Ø3x_ Other powered watercraft
Including: Hovercraft, Jet ski

V93.Ø4x_ Sailboat

V93.Ø9x_ Unspecified watercraft
Including: Boat NOS, ship NOS, watercraft NOS

V93.1- **Other burn on board watercraft**
Including: Burn due to source other than fire

Excludes1:
burn due to watercraft on fire (V91.Ø-)

V93.1Øx_ Merchant vessel

V93.11x_ Passenger vessel
Including: Ferry-boat, Liner

V93.12x_ Fishing boat

V93.13x_ Other powered watercraft
Including: Hovercraft, Jet ski

V93.14x_ Sailboat

V93.19x_ Unspecified watercraft
Including: Boat NOS, ship NOS, watercraft NOS

V93.2- **Heat exposure on board watercraft**

Excludes1:
exposure to man-made heat not aboard watercraft (W92)
exposure to natural heat while on board watercraft (X3Ø)
exposure to sunlight while on board watercraft (X32)

Excludes2:
burn due to fire on board watercraft (V93.Ø-)

V93.2Øx_ Merchant ship

V93.21x_ Passenger ship
Including: Ferry-boat, Liner

V93.22x_ Fishing boat

V93.23x_ Other powered watercraft
Including: Hovercraft

V93.24x_ Sailboat

V93.29x_ Unspecified watercraft
Including: Boat NOS, ship NOS, watercraft NOS

V93.3- **Fall on board watercraft**

Excludes1:
fall due to collision of watercraft (V91.2-)

V93.3Øx_ Merchant ship

V93.31x_ Passenger ship
Including: Ferry-boat, Liner

V93.32x_ Fishing boat

V93.33x_ Other powered watercraft
Including: Hovercraft (on open water), Jet ski

V93.34x_ Sailboat

V93.35x_ Canoe or kayak

V93.36x_ (nonpowered) inflatable craft

V93.38x_ Other unpowered watercraft

V93.39x_ Unspecified watercraft
Including: Boat NOS, ship NOS, watercraft NOS

V93.4- **Struck by falling object on board watercraft**
Including: Hit by falling object
Excludes1:
struck by falling object due to accident to watercraft (V91.3)

V93.40x_ Merchant ship

V93.41x_ Passenger ship
Including: Ferry-boat, Liner

V93.42x_ Fishing boat

V93.43x_ Other powered watercraft
Including: Hovercraft

V93.44x_ Sailboat

V93.48x_ Other unpowered watercraft

V93.49x_ Unspecified watercraft

V93.5- **Explosion on board watercraft**
Including: Boiler explosion on steamship
Excludes2:
fire on board watercraft (V93.0-)

V93.50x_ Merchant ship

V93.51x_ Passenger ship
Including: Ferry-boat, Liner

V93.52x_ Fishing boat

V93.53x_ Other powered watercraft
Including: Hovercraft, Jet ski

V93.54x_ Sailboat

V93.59x_ Unspecified watercraft
Including: Boat NOS, ship NOS, watercraft NOS

V93.6- **Machinery accident on board watercraft**
Excludes1:
machinery explosion on board watercraft (V93.4-)
machinery fire on board watercraft (V93.0-)

V93.60x_ Merchant ship

V93.61x_ Passenger ship
Including: Ferry-boat, Liner

V93.62x_ Fishing boat

V93.63x_ Other powered watercraft
Including: Hovercraft

V93.64x_ Sailboat

V93.69x_ Unspecified watercraft
Including: Boat NOS, ship NOS, watercraft NOS

V93.8- **Other injury due to other accident on board watercraft**
Including: Accidental poisoning by gases or fumes

V93.80x_ Merchant ship

V93.81x_ Passenger ship
Including: Ferry-boat, Liner

V93.82x_ Fishing boat

V93.83x_ Other powered watercraft
Including: Hovercraft, Jet ski

V93.84x_ Sailboat

V93.85x_ Canoe or kayak

V93.86x_ (nonpowered) inflatable craft

V93.87x_ Water-skis
Including: Hit or struck by object

V93.88x_ Other unpowered watercraft
Including: Hit or struck by object while surfing, while on board windsurfer

V93.89x_ Unspecified watercraft
Including: Boat NOS, ship NOS, watercraft NOS

V94- OTHER AND UNSPECIFIED WATER TRANSPORT ACCIDENTS
Excludes1:
military watercraft accidents in military or war operations (Y36, Y37)

The appropriate 7th character is to be added to each code from category V94
A - initial encounter
D - subsequent encounter
S - sequela

V94.0xx_ Hitting object or bottom of body of water due to fall from watercraft
Excludes2:
drowning and submersion due to fall from watercraft (V92.0-)

V94.1- **Bather struck by watercraft**
Including: Swimmer hit by watercraft

V94.11x_ Powered

V94.12x_ Nonpowered

V94.2- **Rider of nonpowered watercraft struck by other watercraft**

V94.21x_ Nonpowered
Including: Canoer, Surfer, Windsurfer

V94.22x_ Powered
Including: Canoer, Surfer, Windsurfer

V94.3- **Injury to rider of (inflatable) watercraft being pulled behind other watercraft**

V94.31x_ Recreational watercraft
Including: Rider of inner-tube pulled behind motor boat

V94.32x_ Non-recreational watercraft
Including: Occupant of dingy, occupant of life-raft

V94.4xx_ Injury to barefoot water-skier
Including: Person being pulled behind boat or ship

V94.8- **Other water transport accident**

V94.81- **Water transport accident involving military watercraft**

V94.810_ Civilian watercraft involved in water transport accident with military watercraft
Including: Passenger on civilian watercraft injured

V94.811_ Civilian in water injured by military watercraft

V94.818_ Other

V94.89x_ Other

V94.9xx_ Unspecified
Including: Accident NOS

Ch5

5. The Tabular List

AIR AND SPACE TRANSPORT ACCIDENTS (V95-V97)

Excludes1:
military aircraft accidents in military or war operations (Y36, Y37)
Indicator(s): POAEx

V95- ACCIDENT TO POWERED AIRCRAFT CAUSING INJURY TO OCCUPANT

The appropriate 7th character is to be added to each code from category V95
A - initial encounter
D - subsequent encounter
S - sequela

V95.Ø- **Helicopter accident injuring occupant**
- **V95.ØØx_ Unspecified accident**
- **V95.Ø1x_ Crash**
- **V95.Ø2x_ Forced landing**
- **V95.Ø3x_ Collision**
  Including: Collision with any object, fixed, movable or moving
- **V95.Ø4x_ Fire**
- **V95.Ø5x_ Explosion**
- **V95.Ø9x_ Other accident**

V95.1- **Ultralight, microlight or powered-glider accident injuring occupant**
- **V95.1Øx_ Unspecified accident**
- **V95.11x_ Crash**
- **V95.12x_ Forced landing**
- **V95.13x_ Collision**
  Including: Collision with any object, fixed, movable or moving
- **V95.14x_ Fire**
- **V95.15x_ Explosion**
- **V95.19x_ Other accident**

V95.2- **Other private fixed-wing aircraft accident injuring occupant**
- **V95.2Øx_ Unspecified accident**
- **V95.21x_ Crash**
- **V95.22x_ Forced landing**
- **V95.23x_ Collision**
  Including: Collision with any object, fixed, movable or moving
- **V95.24x_ Fire**
- **V95.25x_ Explosion**
- **V95.29x_ Other accident**

V95.3- **Commercial fixed-wing aircraft accident injuring occupant**
- **V95.3Øx_ Unspecified accident**
- **V95.31x_ Crash**
- **V95.32x_ Forced landing**
- **V95.33x_ Collision**
  Including: Collision with any object, fixed, movable or moving
- **V95.34x_ Fire**
- **V95.35x_ Explosion**
- **V95.39x_ Other accident**

V95.4- **Spacecraft accident injuring occupant**
- **V95.4Øx_ Unspecified accident**
- **V95.41x_ Crash**
- **V95.42x_ Forced landing**
- **V95.43x_ Collision**
  Including: Collision with any object, fixed, moveable or moving
- **V95.44x_ Fire**
- **V95.45x_ Explosion**
- **V95.49x_ Other accident**

V95.8xx_ Other powered aircraft accidents

V95.9xx_ Unspecified aircraft accident
Including: Accident NOS, Air transport accident NOS

V96- ACCIDENT TO NONPOWERED AIRCRAFT CAUSING INJURY TO OCCUPANT

The appropriate 7th character is to be added to each code from category V96
A - initial encounter
D - subsequent encounter
S - sequela

V96.Ø- **Balloon accident injuring occupant**
- **V96.ØØx_ Unspecified accident**
- **V96.Ø1x_ Crash**
- **V96.Ø2x_ Forced landing**
- **V96.Ø3x_ Collision**
  Including: Collision with any object, fixed, moveable or moving
- **V96.Ø4x_ Fire**
- **V96.Ø5x_ Explosion**
- **V96.Ø9x_ Other accident**

V96.1- **Hang-glider accident injuring occupant**
- **V96.1Øx_ Unspecified accident**
- **V96.11x_ Crash**
- **V96.12x_ Forced landing**
- **V96.13x_ Collision**
  Including: Collision with any object, fixed, moveable or moving
- **V96.14x_ Fire**
- **V96.15x_ Explosion**
- **V96.19x_ Other accident**

V96.2- **Glider (nonpowered) accident injuring occupant**
- **V96.2Øx_ Unspecified accident**
- **V96.21x_ Crash**
- **V96.22x_ Forced landing**
- **V96.23x_ Collision**
  Including: Collision with any object, fixed, moveable or moving
- **V96.24x_ Fire**
- **V96.25x_ Explosion**
- **V96.29x_ Other accident**

V96.8xx_ Other nonpowered-aircraft accidents
Including: Kite carrying a person

V96.9xx_ Unspecified nonpowered-aircraft accident
Including: Accident NOS

V97- OTHER SPECIFIED AIR TRANSPORT ACCIDENTS

The appropriate 7th character is to be added to each code from category V97
A - initial encounter
D - subsequent encounter
S - sequela

V97.Øxx_ Occupant of aircraft injured in other specified air transport accidents
Including: Fall in, on or from aircraft in air transport accident
Excludes1:
accident while boarding or alighting aircraft (V97.1)

V97.1xx_ Person injured while boarding or alighting from aircraft

V97.2- **Parachutist accident**

V97.21x_ Entangled in object
Including: Landing in tree

V97.22x_ Injured on landing

V97.29x_ Other accident

V97.3- **Person on ground injured in air transport accident**

V97.31x_ Hit by object falling from aircraft
Including: Crashing aircraft, Injured by aircraft hitting house, Injured by aircraft hitting car

V97.32x_ Injured by rotating propeller

V97.33x_ Sucked into jet engine

V97.39x_ Other injury

V97.8- **Other air transport accidents, not elsewhere classified**
Excludes1:
aircraft accident NOS (V95.9)
exposure to changes in air pressure during ascent or descent (W94.-)

V97.81- **Air transport accident involving military aircraft**

V97.81Ø_ Civilian aircraft involved in air transport accident with military aircraft
Including: Passenger in civilian aircraft injured

V97.811_ Civilian injured by military aircraft

V97.818_ Other

V97.89x_ Other
Including: Injury from machinery on aircraft

OTHER AND UNSPECIFIED TRANSPORT ACCIDENTS (V98-V99)

Excludes1:
vehicle accident, type of vehicle unspecified (V89.-)
Indicator(s): POAEx

V98- OTHER SPECIFIED TRANSPORT ACCIDENTS

The appropriate 7th character is to be added to each code from category V98
A - initial encounter
D - subsequent encounter
S - sequela

V98.Øxx_ Cable-car, not on rails
Including: Caught or dragged by, Fall or jump from, Object thrown from or in cable-car, not on rails

V98.1xx_ Involving land-yacht

V98.2xx_ Involving ice yacht

V98.3xx_ Involving ski lift
Including: Chair-lift, ski-lift with gondola

V98.8xx_ Other accidents

V99.xxx_ Unspecified transport accident

The appropriate 7th character is to be added to code V99
A - initial encounter
D - subsequent encounter
S - sequela

OTHER EXTERNAL CAUSES OF ACCIDENTAL INJURY (WØØ-X58)

SLIPPING, TRIPPING, STUMBLING AND FALLS (WØØ-W19)

Excludes1:
assault involving a fall (YØ1-YØ2)
fall from animal (V8Ø.-)
fall (in) (from) machinery (in operation) (W28-W31)
fall (in) (from) transport vehicle (VØ1-V99)
intentional self-harm involving a fall (X8Ø-X81)
Excludes2:
at risk for fall (history of fall) Z91.81
fall (in) (from) burning building (XØØ.-)
fall into fire (XØØ-XØ4, XØ8)

The appropriate 7th character is to be added to each code from this category
A - initial encounter
D - subsequent encounter
S - sequela

WØØ- FALL DUE TO ICE AND SNOW

Includes:
pedestrian on foot falling (slipping) on ice and snow
Excludes1:
fall on (from) ice and snow involving pedestrian conveyance (VØØ.-)
fall from stairs and steps not due to ice and snow (W1Ø.-)

WØØ.Øxx_ Fall on same level

WØØ.1xx_ Fall from stairs and steps

WØØ.2xx_ Other fall from one level to another

WØØ.9xx_ Unspecified fall

WØ1- FALL ON SAME LEVEL FROM SLIPPING, TRIPPING AND STUMBLING

Includes:
fall on moving sidewalk
Excludes1:
fall due to bumping (striking) against object (W18.Ø-)
fall in shower or bathtub (W18.2-)
fall on same level NOS (W18.3Ø)
fall on same level from slipping, tripping and stumbling due to ice or snow (WØØ.Ø)
fall off or from toilet (W18.1-)
slipping, tripping and stumbling NOS (W18.4Ø)
slipping, tripping and stumbling without falling (W18.4-)

WØ1.Øxx_ Without subsequent striking against object
Including: Falling over animal

WØ1.1- **Subsequent striking against object**

WØ1.1Øx_ Unspecified object

WØ1.11- **Sharp object**

WØ1.11Ø_ Glass

WØ1.111_ Power tool or machine

WØ1.118_ Other sharp object

WØ1.119_ Unspecified

WØ1.19- **Other object**

WØ1.19Ø_ Furniture

WØ1.198_ Other object

WØ3.xxx_ Other fall on same level due to collision with another person
Including: Non-transport collision
Excludes1:
collision with another person without fall (W51)
crushed or pushed by a crowd or human stampede (W52)
fall involving pedestrian conveyance (VØØ-VØ9)
fall due to ice or snow (WØØ)
fall on same level NOS (W18.3Ø)

WØ4.xxx_ Fall while being carried or supported by other persons
Including: Accidentally dropped while being carried

WØ5- FALL FROM NON-MOVING WHEELCHAIR, NONMOTORIZED SCOOTER AND MOTORIZED MOBILITY SCOOTER
Excludes1:
fall from moving wheelchair (powered) (VØØ.811)
fall from moving motorized mobility scooter (VØØ.831)
fall from nonmotorized scooter (VØØ.141)

WØ5.Øxx_ Non-moving wheelchair
WØ5.1xx_ Non-moving nonmotorized scooter
WØ5.2xx_ Non-moving motorized mobility scooter
WØ6.xxx_ Fall from bed
WØ7.xxx_ Fall from chair
WØ8.xxx_ Fall from other furniture

WØ9- FALL ON AND FROM PLAYGROUND EQUIPMENT
Excludes1:
fall involving recreational machinery (W31)
Indicator(s): *POAEx (7th D/S)*

WØ9.Øxx_ Playground slide
WØ9.1xx_ Playground swing
WØ9.2xx_ Jungle gym
WØ9.8xx_ Other playground equipment

W1Ø- FALL ON AND FROM STAIRS AND STEPS
Excludes1:
Fall from stairs and steps due to ice and snow (WØØ.1)

W1Ø.Øxx_ Escalator
W1Ø.1xx_ Sidewalk curb
W1Ø.2xx_ Incline
Including: Ramp
W1Ø.8xx_ Other stairs and steps
W1Ø.9xx_ Unspecified stairs and steps
W11.xxx_ Fall on and from ladder
W12.xxx_ Fall on and from scaffolding

W13- FALL FROM, OUT OF OR THROUGH BUILDING OR STRUCTURE

W13.Øxx_ Balcony
Including: Railing
W13.1xx_ Bridge
W13.2xx_ Roof
W13.3xx_ Through floor
W13.4xx_ Window
Excludes2:
fall with subsequent striking against sharp glass (WØ1.11Ø-)
W13.8xx_ Other building or structure
Including: Viaduct, wall, flag-pole
W13.9xx_ Building, not otherwise specified
Excludes1:
collapse of a building or structure (W2Ø.-)
fall or jump from burning building or structure (XØØ.-)
W14.xxx_ Fall from tree
W15.xxx_ Fall from cliff

W16- FALL, JUMP OR DIVING INTO WATER
Excludes1:
accidental non-watercraft drowning and submersion not involving fall (W65-W74)
effects of air pressure from diving (W94.-)
fall into water from watercraft (V9Ø-V94)
hitting an object or against bottom when falling from watercraft (V94.Ø)
Excludes2:
striking or hitting diving board (W21.4)

W16.Ø- **Fall into swimming pool**
Including: Fall NOS
Excludes1:
fall into empty swimming pool (W17.3)
Indicator(s): *POAEx (7th D/S)*
W16.Ø1- **Striking water surface**
W16.Ø12_ Causing other injury
W16.Ø2- **Striking bottom**
W16.Ø22_ Causing other injury
W16.Ø3- **Striking wall**
W16.Ø32_ Causing other injury

W16.1- **Fall into natural body of water**
Including: Lake, open sea, river, stream
Indicator(s): *POAEx (7th D/S)*
W16.11- **Striking water surface**
W16.112_ Causing other injury
W16.12- **Striking bottom**
W16.122_ Causing other injury
W16.13- **Striking side**
W16.132_ Causing other injury

W16.2- **Fall in (into) filled bathtub or bucket of water**
Indicator(s): *POAEx (7th D/S)*
W16.21- **Filled bathtub**
Excludes1:
fall into empty bathtub (W18.2)
W16.212_ Causing other injury
W16.22- **Bucket of water**
W16.222_ Causing other injury

W16.3- **Fall into other water**
Including: Fountain, reservoir
W16.31- **Striking water surface**
Indicator(s): *POAEx (7th D/S)*
W16.312_ Causing other injury
W16.32- **Striking bottom**
W16.322_ Causing other injury
W16.33- **Striking wall**
Indicator(s): *POAEx (7th D/S)*
W16.332_ Causing other injury

W16.4- **Fall into unspecified water**
Indicator(s): *POAEx (7th D/S)*
W16.42x_ Causing other injury

W16.5- **Jumping or diving into swimming pool**
Indicator(s): *POAEx (7th D/S)*
W16.51- **Striking water surface**
W16.512_ Causing other injury
W16.52- **Striking bottom**
W16.522_ Causing other injury
W16.53- **Striking wall**
W16.532_ Causing other injury

W16.6- **Jumping or diving into natural body of water**
Including: Lake, open sea, river, stream
Indicator(s): POAEx (7th D/S)
W16.61- **Striking water surface**
W16.612_ Causing other injury
W16.62- **Striking bottom**
W16.622_ Causing other injury
W16.7- **Jumping or diving from boat**
Excludes1:
Fall from boat into water -see watercraft accident (V9Ø-V94)
Indicator(s): POAEx
W16.71- **Striking water surface**
W16.712_ Causing other injury
W16.72- **Striking bottom**
W16.722_ Causing other injury
W16.8- **Jumping or diving into other water**
Including: Fountain, reservoir
Indicator(s): POAEx
W16.81- **Striking water surface**
W16.812_ Causing other injury
W16.82- **Striking bottom**
W16.822_ Causing other injury
W16.83- **Striking wall**
W16.832_ Causing other injury
W16.9- **Jumping or diving into unspecified water**
Indicator(s): POAEx
W16.92x_ Causing other injury

W17- OTHER FALL FROM ONE LEVEL TO ANOTHER
W17.Øxx_ Into well
W17.1xx_ Into storm drain or manhole
W17.2xx_ Into hole
Including: Pit
W17.3xx_ Into empty swimming pool
Excludes1:
fall into filled swimming pool (W16.Ø-)
W17.4xx_ From dock
W17.8- **Other fall from one level to another**
W17.81x_ Down embankment (hill)
W17.82x_ From (out of) grocery cart
Including: Grocery cart tipping over
W17.89x_ Other fall
Including: Cherry picker, lifting device, mobile elevated work platform [MEWP], sky lift

W18- OTHER SLIPPING, TRIPPING AND STUMBLING AND FALLS
W18.Ø- **Fall due to bumping against object**
Including: Striking against object with subsequent fall
Excludes1:
fall on same level due to slipping, tripping, or stumbling with subsequent striking against object (WØ1.1-)
W18.ØØx_ Striking against unspecified object with subsequent fall
W18.Ø1x_ Striking against sports equipment with subsequent fall
W18.Ø2x_ Striking against glass with subsequent fall
W18.Ø9x_ Striking against other object with subsequent fall
W18.1- **Fall from or off toilet**
Indicator(s): POAEx (7th D/S)
W18.11x_ Without subsequent striking against object
Including: Fall NOS
W18.12x_ With subsequent striking against object
W18.2xx_ Fall in (into) shower or empty bathtub
Excludes1:
fall in full bathtub causing drowning or submersion (W16.21-)
W18.3- **Other and unspecified fall on same level**
Indicator(s): POAEx (7th D/S)
W18.3Øx_ Unspecified
W18.31x_ Due to stepping on an object
Including: Stepping on an animal
Excludes1:
slipping, tripping and stumbling without fall due to stepping on animal (W18.41)
W18.39x_ Other fall
W18.4- **Slipping, tripping and stumbling without falling**
Excludes1:
collision with another person without fall (W51)
Indicator(s): POAEx (7th D/S)
W18.4Øx_ Unspecified
W18.41x_ Due to stepping on object
Including: Stepping on an animal
Excludes1:
slipping, tripping and stumbling with fall due to stepping on animal (W18.31)
W18.42x_ Due to stepping into hole or opening
W18.43x_ Due to stepping from one level to another
W18.49x_ Other
W19.xxx_ Unspecified fall
Including: Accidental fall NOS

EXPOSURE TO INANIMATE MECHANICAL FORCES (W2Ø-W49)

Excludes1:
assault (X92-YØ9)
contact or collision with animals or persons (W5Ø-W64)
exposure to inanimate mechanical forces involving military or war operations (Y36.-, Y37.-)
intentional self-harm (X71-X83)
The appropriate 7th character is to be added to each code from this category
A - initial encounter
D - subsequent encounter
S - sequela

W2Ø- STRUCK BY THROWN, PROJECTED OR FALLING OBJECT
Code First:
any associated:
cataclysm (X34-X39)
lightning strike (T75.ØØ)
Excludes1:
falling object in machinery accident (W24, W28-W31)
falling object in transport accident (VØ1-V99)
object set in motion by explosion (W35-W4Ø)
object set in motion by firearm (W32-W34)
struck by thrown sports equipment (W21.-)

W2Ø.Øxx_ Falling object in cave-in

Excludes2:

asphyxiation due to cave-in (T71.21)

W2Ø.1xx_ Due to collapse of building

Excludes1:

struck by object due to collapse of burning building (XØØ.2, XØ2.2)

W2Ø.8xx_ Other cause of strike

Excludes1:

struck by thrown sports equipment (W21.-)

W21- STRIKING AGAINST OR STRUCK BY SPORTS EQUIPMENT

Excludes1:

assault with sports equipment (YØ8.Ø-)

striking against or struck by sports equipment with subsequent fall (W18.Ø1)

Indicator(s): POAEx

W21.Ø- **Struck by hit or thrown ball**

W21.ØØx_ Unspecified type

W21.Ø1x_ Football

W21.Ø2x_ Soccer ball

W21.Ø3x_ Baseball

W21.Ø4x_ Golf ball

W21.Ø5x_ Basketball

W21.Ø6x_ Volleyball

W21.Ø7x_ Softball

W21.Ø9x_ Other hit or thrown ball

W21.1- **Struck by bat, racquet or club**

W21.11x_ Baseball bat

W21.12x_ Tennis racquet

W21.13x_ Golf club

W21.19x_ Other

W21.2- **Struck by hockey stick or puck**

W21.21- **Hockey stick**

W21.21Ø_ Ice

W21.211_ Field

W21.22- **Hockey puck**

W21.22Ø_ Ice

W21.221_ Field

W21.3- **Struck by sports foot wear**

W21.31x_ Shoe cleats

Including: Stepped on by shoe cleats

W21.32x_ Skate blades

Including: Skated over by skate blades

W21.39x_ Other

W21.4xx_ Diving board

Use additional code for subsequent falling into water, if applicable (W16.-)

W21.8- **Other sports equipment**

W21.81x_ Football helmet

W21.89x_ Other sports equipment

W21.9xx_ Unspecified

W22- STRIKING AGAINST OR STRUCK BY OTHER OBJECTS

Excludes1:

striking against or struck by object with subsequent fall (W18.Ø9)

W22.Ø- **Stationary object**

Excludes1:

striking against stationary sports equipment (W21.8)

W22.Ø1x_ Walked into wall

W22.Ø2x_ Walked into lamppost

W22.Ø3x_ Walked into furniture

W22.Ø4- **Wall of swimming pool**

W22.Ø42_ Causing other injury

W22.Ø9x_ Other stationary object

W22.1- **Automobile airbag**

Indicator(s): POAEx

W22.1Øx_ Unspecified

W22.11x_ Driver side

W22.12x_ Front passenger side

W22.19x_ Other airbag

W22.8xx_ Other objects

Including: Object NOS

Excludes1:

struck by thrown, projected or falling object (W2Ø.-)

W23- CAUGHT, CRUSHED, JAMMED OR PINCHED IN OR BETWEEN OBJECTS

Excludes1:

injury caused by cutting or piercing instruments (W25-W27)

injury caused by firearms malfunction (W32.1, W33.1-, W34.1-)

injury caused by lifting and transmission devices (W24.-)

injury caused by machinery (W28-W31)

injury caused by nonpowered hand tools (W27.-)

injury caused by transport vehicle being used as a means of transportation (VØ1-V99)

injury caused by struck by thrown, projected or falling object (W2Ø.-)

W23.Øxx_ Moving objects

W23.1xx_ Stationary objects

N **W23.2xx_ Caught, crushed, jammed or pinched between a moving and stationary object**

W24- CONTACT WITH LIFTING AND TRANSMISSION DEVICES, NOT ELSEWHERE CLASSIFIED

Excludes1:

transport accidents (VØ1-V99)

W24.Øxx_ Lifting devices

Including: Chain hoist, drive belt, pulley (block)

W24.1xx_ Transmission devices

Including: Belt or cable

EXPOSURE TO ANIMATE MECHANICAL FORCES (W5Ø-W64)

Excludes1:

Toxic effect of contact with venomous animals and plants (T63.-)

The appropriate 7th character is to be added to each code from this category

A - initial encounter

D - subsequent encounter

S - sequela

W5Ø- ACCIDENTAL HIT, STRIKE, KICK, TWIST, BITE OR SCRATCH BY ANOTHER PERSON

Includes:
hit, strike, kick, twist, bite, or scratch by another person NOS

Excludes1:
assault by bodily force (YØ4)
struck by objects (W2Ø-W22)

W5Ø.Øxx_ **Hit or strike**
Including: Hit or strike NOS

W5Ø.1xx_ **Kick**
Including: Kick NOS

W5Ø.2xx_ **Twist**
Including: Twist NOS

W5Ø.3xx_ **Bite**
Including: Human bite, Bite NOS

W5Ø.4xx_ **Scratch**
Including: Scratch NOS

W51.xxx_ **Accidental striking against or bumped into by another person**
Excludes1:
assault by striking against or bumping into by another person (YØ4.2)
fall due to collision with another person (WØ3)

W52.xxx_ **Crushed, pushed or stepped on by crowd or human stampede**
Including: With or without fall

X5Ø OVEREXERTION AND STRENUOUS OR REPETITIVE MOVEMENTS (X5Ø) (X5Ø-X5Ø)

Indicator(s): *POAEx*

X5Ø- OVEREXERTION AND STRENUOUS OR REPETITIVE MOVEMENTS

The appropriate 7th character is to be added to each code from category X5Ø
A - initial encounter
D - subsequent encounter
S - sequela
The appropriate 7th character is to be added to each code from category X5Ø
A - initial encounter
D - subsequent encounter
S - sequela

X5Ø.Øxx_ **Overexertion from strenuous movement or load**
Including: Lifting heavy objects, Lifting weights

X5Ø.1xx_ **Overexertion from prolonged static or awkward postures**
Including: Prolonged or static bending, kneeling, reaching, sitting, standing, twisting

X5Ø.9xx_ **Other and unspecified overexertion or strenuous movements or postures**
Including: Contact pressure, Contact stress

EVENT OF UNDETERMINED INTENT (Y21-Y33)

Undetermined intent is only for use when there is specific documentation in the record that the intent of the injury cannot be determined. If no such documentation is present, code to accidental (unintentional)

The appropriate 7th character is to be added to each code from this category
A - initial encounter
D - subsequent encounter
S - sequela

Y3Ø.xxx_ **Falling, jumping or pushed from a high place, undetermined intent**
Including: Falling from one level to another

Y31.xxx_ **Falling, lying or running before or into moving object, undetermined intent**

Y32.xxx_ **Crashing of motor vehicle, undetermined intent**

Y33.xxx_ **Other specified events, undetermined intent**

SUPPLEMENTARY FACTORS RELATED TO CAUSES OF MORBIDITY CLASSIFIED ELSEWHERE (Y9Ø-Y99)

Notes:
These categories may be used to provide supplementary information concerning causes of morbidity. They are not to be used for single-condition coding.

Y92- PLACE OF OCCURRENCE OF THE EXTERNAL CAUSE

The following category is for use, when relevant, to identify the place of occurrence of the external cause. Use in conjunction with an activity code.

Place of occurrence should be recorded only at the initial encounter for treatment.

See Guidelines: 1;C.2Ø.b | 1;C.2Ø.j

Y92.Ø- **Non-institutional (private) residence**
Excludes1:
abandoned or derelict house (Y92.89)
home under construction but not yet occupied (Y92.6-)
institutional place of residence (Y92.1-)
Indicator(s): *POAEx*

Y92.ØØ- **Unspecified**

Y92.ØØØ **Kitchen**
Y92.ØØ1 **Dining room**
Y92.ØØ2 **Bathroom**
Y92.ØØ3 **Bedroom**
Y92.ØØ7 **Garden or yard**
Y92.ØØ8 **Other place**
Y92.ØØ9 **Unspecified place**
Including: Home (NOS)

Y92.Ø1- **Single-family**
Including: Farmhouse
Excludes1:
barn (Y92.71)
chicken coop or hen house (Y92.72)
farm field (Y92.73)
orchard (Y92.74)
single family mobile home or trailer (Y92.Ø2-)
slaughter house (Y92.86)

Y92.Ø1Ø **Kitchen**
Y92.Ø11 **Dining room**
Y92.Ø12 **Bathroom**
Y92.Ø13 **Bedroom**
Y92.Ø14 **Private driveway**
Y92.Ø15 **Private garage**

Y92.Ø16 **Swimming-pool or garden**
Y92.Ø17 **Garden or yard**
Y92.Ø18 **Other place**
Y92.Ø19 **Unspecified place**

Y92.Ø2- **Mobile home**
Y92.Ø2Ø **Kitchen**
Y92.Ø21 **Dining room**
Y92.Ø22 **Bathroom**
Y92.Ø23 **Bedroom**
Y92.Ø24 **Driveway**
Y92.Ø25 **Garage**
Y92.Ø26 **Swimming-pool**
Y92.Ø27 **Garden or yard**
Y92.Ø28 **Other place**
Y92.Ø29 **Unspecified place**

Y92.Ø3- **Apartment**
Including: Condominium, Co-op
Y92.Ø3Ø **Kitchen**
Y92.Ø31 **Bathroom**
Y92.Ø32 **Bedroom**
Y92.Ø38 **Other place**
Y92.Ø39 **Unspecified place**

Y92.Ø4- **Boarding-house**
Y92.Ø4Ø **Kitchen**
Y92.Ø41 **Bathroom**
Y92.Ø42 **Bedroom**
Y92.Ø43 **Driveway**
Y92.Ø44 **Garage**
Y92.Ø45 **Swimming-pool**
Y92.Ø46 **Garden or yard**
Y92.Ø48 **Other place**
Y92.Ø49 **Unspecified place**

Y92.Ø9- **Other**
Y92.Ø9Ø **Kitchen**
Y92.Ø91 **Bathroom**
Y92.Ø92 **Bedroom**
Y92.Ø93 **Driveway**
Y92.Ø94 **Garage**
Y92.Ø95 **Swimming-pool**
Y92.Ø96 **Garden or yard**
Y92.Ø98 **Other place**
Y92.Ø99 **Unspecified place**

Y92.1- **Institutional (nonprivate) residence**
<u>*Indicator(s):*</u> *POAEx*

Y92.1Ø **Unspecified residential institution**

Y92.11- **Children's home and orphanage**
Y92.11Ø **Kitchen**
Y92.111 **Bathroom**
Y92.112 **Bedroom**
Y92.113 **Driveway**
Y92.114 **Garage**
Y92.115 **Swimming-pool**
Y92.116 **Garden or yard**
Y92.118 **Other place**
Y92.119 **Unspecified place**

Y92.12- **Nursing home**
Including: Home for the sick, Hospice
Y92.12Ø **Kitchen**
Y92.121 **Bathroom**
Y92.122 **Bedroom**
Y92.123 **Driveway**
Y92.124 **Garage**
Y92.125 **Swimming-pool**
Y92.126 **Garden or yard**
Y92.128 **Other place**
Y92.129 **Unspecified place**

Y92.13- **Military base**
<u>*Excludes1:*</u>
military training grounds (Y92.83)
Y92.13Ø **Kitchen**
Y92.131 **Mess hall**
Y92.133 **Barracks**
Y92.135 **Garage**
Y92.136 **Swimming-pool**
Y92.137 **Garden or yard**
Y92.138 **Other place**
Y92.139 **Unspecified place**

Y92.14- **Prison**
Y92.14Ø **Kitchen**
Y92.141 **Dining room**
Y92.142 **Bathroom**
Y92.143 **Cell**
Y92.146 **Swimming-pool**
Y92.147 **Courtyard**
Y92.148 **Other place**
Y92.149 **Unspecified place**

Y92.15- **Reform school as the place**
Y92.15Ø **Kitchen**
Y92.151 **Dining room**
Y92.152 **Bathroom**
Y92.153 **Bedroom**
Y92.154 **Driveway**
Y92.155 **Garage**
Y92.156 **Swimming-pool**
Y92.157 **Garden or yard**
Y92.158 **Other place**
Y92.159 **Unspecified place**

Y92.16- **School dormitory**
<u>*Excludes1:*</u>
reform school as the place of occurrence of the external cause (Y92.15-)
school buildings and grounds as the place of occurrence of the external cause (Y92.2-)
school sports and athletic areas as the place of occurrence of the external cause (Y92.3-)
Y92.16Ø **Kitchen**
Y92.161 **Dining room**
Y92.162 **Bathroom**
Y92.163 **Bedroom**
Y92.168 **Other place**
Y92.169 **Unspecified place**

Y92.19- **Other specified residential institution**

Y92.190 Kitchen

Y92.191 Dining room

Y92.192 Bathroom

Y92.193 Bedroom

Y92.194 Driveway

Y92.195 Garage

Y92.196 Pool

Y92.197 Garden or yard

Y92.198 Other place

Y92.199 Unspecified place

Y92.2- **School, other institution and public administrative area**

Including: Building and adjacent grounds used by the general public or by a particular group of the public

Excludes1:

building under construction as the place of occurrence of the external cause (Y92.6)

residential institution as the place of occurrence of the external cause (Y92.1)

school dormitory as the place of occurrence of the external cause (Y92.16-)

sports and athletics area of schools as the place of occurrence of the external cause (Y92.3-)

Y92.21- **School (private) (public) (state)**

Indicator(s): *POAEx*

Y92.210 Daycare center

Y92.211 Elementary school

Including: Kindergarten

Y92.212 Middle school

Y92.213 High school

Y92.214 College

Including: University

Y92.215 Trade school

Y92.218 Other school

Y92.219 Unspecified school

Y92.22 Religious institution

Including: Church, Mosque, Synagogue

Indicator(s): *POAEx*

Y92.23- **Hospital**

Excludes1:

ambulatory (outpatient) health services establishments (Y92.53-)

home for the sick as the place of occurrence of the external cause (Y92.12-)

hospice as the place of occurrence of the external cause (Y92.12-)

nursing home as the place of occurrence of the external cause (Y92.12-)

Y92.230 Patient room

Y92.231 Patient bathroom

Y92.232 Corridor

Y92.233 Cafeteria

Y92.234 Operating room

Y92.238 Other place

Y92.239 Unspecified place

Y92.24- **Public administrative building**

Indicator(s): *POAEx*

Y92.240 Courthouse

Y92.241 Library

Y92.242 Post office

Y92.243 City hall

Y92.248 Other public administrative building

Y92.25- **Cultural building**

Indicator(s): *POAEx*

Y92.250 Art Gallery

Y92.251 Museum

Y92.252 Music hall

Y92.253 Opera house

Y92.254 Theater (live)

Y92.258 Other cultural public building

Y92.26 Movie house or cinema

Indicator(s): *POAEx*

Y92.29 Other specified public building

Including: Assembly hall, Clubhouse

Indicator(s): *POAEx*

Y92.3- **Sports and athletics area**

Indicator(s): *POAEx*

Y92.31- **Athletic court**

Excludes1:

tennis court in private home or garden (Y92.09)

Y92.310 Basketball court

Y92.311 Squash court

Y92.312 Tennis court

Y92.318 Other athletic court

Y92.32- **Athletic field**

Y92.320 Baseball field

Y92.321 Football field

Y92.322 Soccer field

Y92.328 Other athletic field

Including: Cricket, Hockey

Y92.33- **Skating rink**

Y92.330 Ice skating rink (indoor) (outdoor)

Y92.331 Roller skating rink

Y92.34 Swimming pool (public)

Excludes1:

swimming pool in private home or garden (Y92.016)

Y92.39 Other area

Including: Golf-course, Gymnasium, Riding-school, Stadium

Y92.4- **Street , highway and other paved roadways**

Excludes1:

private driveway of residence (Y92.014, Y92.024, Y92.043, Y92.093, Y92.113, Y92.123, Y92.154, Y92.194)

Indicator(s): *POAEx*

Y92.41- **Street and highway**

Y92.410 Unspecified street and highway

Including: Road NOS

Y92.411 Interstate highway

Including: Freeway, Motorway

Y92.412 Parkway

Y92.413 State road

Y92.414 Local residential or business street

Y92.415 Exit ramp or entrance ramp of street or highway

Y92.48- **Other paved roadways**

Y92.48Ø Sidewalk

Y92.481 Parking lot

Y92.482 Bike path

Y92.488 Other paved roadways

Y92.5- **Trade and service area**

Excludes1:

garage in private home (Y92.Ø15)

schools and other public administration buildings (Y92.2-)

Y92.51- **Private commercial establishments**

Indicator(s): POAEx

Y92.51Ø Bank

Y92.511 Restaurant or café

Y92.512 Supermarket, store or market

Y92.513 Shop (commercial)

Y92.52- **Service areas**

Indicator(s): POAEx

Y92.52Ø Airport

Y92.521 Bus station

Y92.522 Railway station

Y92.523 Highway rest stop

Y92.524 Gas station

Including: Petroleum station, Service station

Y92.53- **Ambulatory health services establishments**

Y92.53Ø Ambulatory surgery center

Including: Outpatient and same day surgery centers (including that connected with a hospital)

Y92.531 Health care provider office

Including: Physician office

Indicator(s): POAEx

Y92.532 Urgent care center

Indicator(s): POAEx

Y92.538 Other establishments

Y92.59 Other trade areas

Including: Office building, Casino, Garage (commercial), Hotel, Radio or television station, Shopping mall, Warehouse

Indicator(s): POAEx

Y92.6- **Industrial and construction area**

Indicator(s): POAEx

Y92.61 Building [any] under construction

Y92.62 Dock or shipyard

Including: Dockyard, Dry dock

Y92.63 Factory

Including: Factory building, Factory premises, Industrial yard

Y92.64 Mine or pit

Y92.65 Oil rig

Including: Pit (coal) (gravel) (sand)

Y92.69 Other area

Including: Gasworks, Power-station (coal) (nuclear) (oil), Tunnel under construction, Workshop

Y92.7- **Farm**

Including: Ranch

Excludes1:

farmhouse and home premises of farm (Y92.Ø1-)

Indicator(s): POAEx

Y92.71 Barn

Y92.72 Chicken coop

Including: Hen house

Y92.73 Farm field

Y92.74 Orchard

Y92.79 Other farm location

Y92.8- **Other places**

Indicator(s): POAEx

Y92.81- **Transport vehicle**

Excludes1:

transport accidents (VØØ-V99)

Y92.81Ø Car

Y92.811 Bus

Y92.812 Truck

Y92.813 Airplane

Y92.814 Boat

Y92.815 Train

Y92.816 Subway car

Y92.818 Other transport vehicle

Y92.82- **Wilderness area**

Y92.82Ø Desert

Y92.821 Forest

Y92.828 Other wilderness area

Including: Swamp, Mountain, Marsh, Prairie

Y92.83- **Recreation area**

Y92.83Ø Public park

Y92.831 Amusement park

Y92.832 Beach

Including: Seashore

Y92.833 Campsite

Y92.834 Zoological garden (Zoo)

Y92.838 Other recreation area

Y92.84 Military training ground

Y92.85 Railroad track

Y92.86 Slaughter house

Y92.89 Other specified places

Including: Derelict house

Y92.9 Unspecified place or not applicable

See Guidelines: 1;C.2Ø.b-c

Indicator(s): POAEx

Y93- ACTIVITY CODES

Notes:

Category Y93 is provided for use to indicate the activity of the person seeking healthcare for an injury or health condition, such as a heart attack while shoveling snow, which resulted from, or was contributed to, by the activity. These codes are appropriate for use for both acute injuries, such as those from chapter 19, and conditions that are due to the long-term, cumulative effects of an activity, such as those from chapter 13. They are also appropriate for use with external cause codes for cause and intent if identifying the activity provides additional information on the event. These codes should be used in conjunction with codes for external cause status (Y99) and place of occurrence (Y92).

This section contains the following broad activity categories:

Y93.Ø Activities involving walking and running
Y93.1 Activities involving water and water craft
Y93.2 Activities involving ice and snow
Y93.3 Activities involving climbing, rappelling, and jumping off
Y93.4 Activities involving dancing and other rhythmic movement
Y93.5 Activities involving other sports and athletics played individually
Y93.6 Activities involving other sports and athletics played as a team or group
Y93.7 Activities involving other specified sports and athletics
Y93.A Activities involving other cardiorespiratory exercise
Y93.B Activities involving other muscle strengthening exercises
Y93.C Activities involving computer technology and electronic devices
Y93.D Activities involving arts and handcrafts
Y93.E Activities involving personal hygiene and interior property and clothing maintenance
Y93.F Activities involving caregiving
Y93.G Activities involving food preparation, cooking and grilling
Y93.H Activities involving exterior property and land maintenance, building and construction
Y93.I Activities involving roller coasters and other types of external motion
Y93.J Activities involving playing musical instrument
Y93.K Activities involving animal care
Y93.8 Activities, other specified
Y93.9 Activity, unspecified

See Guidelines: 1;C.2Ø.b | 1;C.2Ø.c

Y93.Ø- **Involving walking and running**
Excludes1:
activity, walking an animal (Y93.K1)
activity, walking or running on a treadmill (Y93.A1)

Y93.Ø1 Walking, marching and hiking
Including: On level or elevated terrain
Excludes1:
activity, mountain climbing (Y93.31)

Y93.Ø2 Running

Y93.1- **Involving water and water craft**
Excludes1:
activities involving ice (Y93.2-)

Y93.11 Swimming

Y93.12 Springboard and platform diving
Indicator(s): POAEx

Y93.13 Water polo
Indicator(s): POAEx

Y93.14 Water aerobics and water exercise
Indicator(s): POAEx

Y93.15 Underwater diving and snorkeling
Including: SCUBA diving
Indicator(s): POAEx

Y93.16 Rowing, canoeing, kayaking, rafting and tubing
Including: In calm and turbulent water
Indicator(s): POAEx

Y93.17 Water skiing and wake boarding
Indicator(s): POAEx

Y93.18 Surfing, windsurfing and boogie boarding
Including: Water sliding
Indicator(s): POAEx

Y93.19 Other
Including: Activity involving water NOS, parasailing, water survival training and testing
Indicator(s): POAEx

Y93.2- **Involving ice and snow**
Excludes1:
activity, shoveling ice and snow (Y93.H1)
Indicator(s): POAEx

Y93.21 Ice skating
Including: Figure skating (singles) (pairs), Ice dancing
Excludes1:
activity, ice hockey (Y93.22)

Y93.22 Ice hockey

Y93.23 Snow (alpine) (downhill) skiing, snowboarding, sledding, tobogganing and snow tubing
Excludes1:
activity, cross country skiing (Y93.24)

Y93.24 Cross country skiing
Including: Nordic skiing

Y93.29 Other
Including: Activity NOS

Y93.3- **Involving climbing, rappelling and jumping off**
Excludes1:
activity, hiking on level or elevated terrain (Y93.Ø1)
activity, jumping rope (Y93.56)
activity, trampoline jumping (Y93.44)
Indicator(s): POAEx

Y93.31 Mountain climbing, rock climbing and wall climbing

Y93.32 Rappelling

Y93.33 BASE jumping
Including: Building, Antenna, Span, Earth jumping

Y93.34 Bungee jumping

Y93.35 Hang gliding

Y93.39 Other

Y93.4- **Involving dancing and other rhythmic movement**
Excludes1:
activity, martial arts (Y93.75)
Indicator(s): POAEx

Y93.41 Dancing

Y93.42 Yoga

Y93.43 Gymnastics
Including: Rhythmic gymnastics
Excludes1:
activity, trampolining (Y93.44)

Y93.44 Trampolining

Y93.45 Cheerleading

Y93.49 Other

Y93.5- **Involving other sports and athletics played individually**
Excludes1:
activity, dancing (Y93.41)
activity, gymnastic (Y93.43)
activity, trampolining (Y93.44)
activity, yoga (Y93.42)
Indicator(s): POAEx

Y93.51 Roller skating (inline) and skateboarding
Y93.52 Horseback riding
Y93.53 Golf
Y93.54 Bowling
Y93.55 Bike riding
Y93.56 Jumping rope
Y93.57 Non-running track and field events
Excludes1:
activity, running (any form) (Y93.Ø2)
Y93.59 Other
Excludes1:
activities involving climbing, rappelling, and jumping (Y93.3-)
activities involving ice and snow (Y93.2-)
activities involving walking and running (Y93.Ø-)
activities involving water and watercraft (Y93.1-)

Y93.6- **Involving other sports and athletics played as a team or group**
Excludes1:
activity, ice hockey (Y93.22)
activity, water polo (Y93.13)
Indicator(s): POAEx

Y93.61 American tackle football
Including: Football NOS
Y93.62 American flag or touch football
Y93.63 Rugby
Y93.64 Baseball
Including: Softball
Y93.65 Lacrosse and field hockey
Y93.66 Soccer
Y93.67 Basketball
Y93.68 Volleyball (beach) (court)
Y93.69 Other
Including: Cricket
Y93.6A Physical games generally associated with school recess, summer camp and children
Including: Capture the flag, dodge ball, four square, kickball

Y93.7- **Involving other specified sports and athletics**
Indicator(s): POAEx

Y93.71 Boxing
Y93.72 Wrestling
Y93.73 Racquet and hand sports
Including: Handball, racquetball, squash, tennis
Y93.74 Frisbee
Including: Ultimate frisbee
Y93.75 Martial arts
Including: Combatives
Y93.79 Other
Excludes1:
sports and athletics activities specified in categories Y93.Ø-Y93.6

Y93.8- **Activities, other specified**
Indicator(s): POAEx

Y93.81 Refereeing a sports activity
Y93.82 Spectator at an event
Y93.83 Rough housing and horseplay
Y93.84 Sleeping
Y93.85 Choking game
Including: Blackout, fainting, pass out game
Y93.89 Other

Y93.9 Activity, unspecified
See Guidelines: *1;C.2Ø.c*
Indicator(s): POAEx

Y93.A- **Involving other cardiorespiratory exercise**
Including: Activities involving physical training
Indicator(s): POAEx

Y93.A1 Exercise machines primarily for cardiorespiratory conditioning
Including: Elliptical and stepper machines, stationary bike, treadmill
Y93.A2 Calisthenics
Including: Jumping jacks, warm up and cool down
Y93.A3 Aerobic and step
Y93.A4 Circuit training
Y93.A5 Obstacle course
Including: Challenge course, confidence course
Y93.A6 Grass drills
Including: Guerilla drills
Y93.A9 Other
Excludes1:
activities involving cardiorespiratory exercise specified in categories Y93.Ø-Y93.7

Y93.B- **Involving other muscle strengthening exercises**
Indicator(s): POAEx

Y93.B1 Exercise machines primarily for muscle strengthening
Y93.B2 Push-ups, pull-ups, sit-ups
Y93.B3 Free weights
Including: Barbells, dumbbells
Y93.B4 Pilates
Y93.B9 Other
Excludes1:
activities involving muscle strengthening specified in categories Y93.Ø-Y93.A

Y93.C- **Involving computer technology and electronic devices**
Excludes1:
activity, electronic musical keyboard or instruments (Y93.J-)
Indicator(s): POAEx

Y93.C1 Computer keyboarding
Including: Electronic game playing using keyboard or other stationary device
Y93.C2 Hand held interactive electronic device
Including: Cellular telephone and communication device, electronic game playing using interactive device
Excludes1:
activity, electronic game playing using keyboard or other stationary device (Y93.C1)
Y93.C9 Other

Y93.D- **Involving arts and handcrafts**
<u>Excludes1:</u>
activities involving playing musical instrument (Y93.J-)
<u>Indicator(s):</u> *POAEx*
Y93.D1 Knitting and crocheting
Y93.D2 Sewing
Y93.D3 Furniture building and finishing
Including: Furniture repair
Y93.D9 Other

Y93.E- **Involving personal hygiene and interior property and clothing maintenance**
<u>Excludes1:</u>
activities involving cooking and grilling (Y93.G-)
activities involving exterior property and land maintenance, building and construction (Y93.H-)
activities involving caregiving (Y93.F-)
activity, dishwashing (Y93.G1)
activity, food preparation (Y93.G1)
activity, gardening (Y93.H2)
<u>Indicator(s):</u> *POAEx*
Y93.E1 Personal bathing and showering
Y93.E2 Laundry
Y93.E3 Vacuuming
Y93.E4 Ironing
Y93.E5 Floor mopping and cleaning
Y93.E6 Residential relocation
Including: Packing and unpacking
Y93.E8 Other personal hygiene
Y93.E9 Other interior property and clothing maintenance

Y93.F- **Involving caregiving**
Including: Activity involving the provider of caregiving
<u>Indicator(s):</u> *POAEx*
Y93.F1 Bathing
Y93.F2 Lifting
Y93.F9 Other

Y93.G- **Involving food preparation, cooking and grilling**
<u>Indicator(s):</u> *POAEx*
Y93.G1 Food preparation and clean up
Including: Dishwashing
Y93.G2 Grilling and smoking food
Y93.G3 Cooking and baking
Including: Use of stove, oven and microwave oven
Y93.G9 Other

Y93.H- **Involving exterior property and land maintenance, building and construction**
<u>Indicator(s):</u> *POAEx*
Y93.H1 Digging, shoveling and raking
Including: Dirt digging, raking leaves, snow shoveling
Y93.H2 Gardening and landscaping
Including: Pruning, trimming shrubs, weeding
Y93.H3 Building and construction
Y93.H9 Other

Y93.I- **Involving roller coasters and other types of external motion**
<u>Indicator(s):</u> *POAEx*
Y93.I1 Roller coaster riding
Y93.I9 Other

Y93.J- **Involving playing musical instrument**
Including: Electric musical instrument
<u>Indicator(s):</u> *POAEx*
Y93.J1 Piano
Including: Musical keyboard (electronic)
Y93.J2 Drum and other percussion
Y93.J3 String
Y93.J4 Winds and brass

Y93.K- **Involving animal care**
<u>Excludes1:</u>
activity, horseback riding (Y93.52)
<u>Indicator(s):</u> *POAEx*
Y93.K1 Walking animal
Y93.K2 Milking
Y93.K3 Grooming and shearing
Y93.K9 Other

Y99- EXTERNAL CAUSE STATUS
<u>Notes:</u>
A single code from category Y99 should be used in conjunction with the external cause code(s) assigned to a record to indicate the status of the person at the time the event occurred.
<u>See Guidelines:</u> *1;C.20.k*
<u>Indicator(s):</u> *POAEx*

Y99.0 Civilian activity done for income or pay
Including: Financial or other compensation
<u>Excludes1:</u>
military activity (Y99.1)
volunteer activity (Y99.2)

Y99.1 Military activity
<u>Excludes1:</u>
activity of off duty military personnel (Y99.8)

Y99.2 Volunteer activity
<u>Excludes1:</u>
activity of child or other family member assisting in compensated work of other family member (Y99.8)

Y99.8 Other external cause status
Including: Activity NEC, Activity of child or other family member assisting in compensated work of other family member, Hobby not done for income, Leisure activity, Off-duty activity of military personnel, Recreation or sport not for income or while a student, Student activity
<u>Excludes1:</u>
civilian activity done for income or compensation (Y99.0)
military activity (Y99.1)

Y99.9 Unspecified external cause status

21. Factors influencing health status and contact with health services (ZØØ-Z99)

Notes:

Z codes represent reasons for encounters. A corresponding procedure code must accompany a Z code if a procedure is performed. Categories ZØØ-Z99 are provided for occasions when circumstances other than a disease, injury or external cause classifiable to categories AØØ-Y89 are recorded as 'diagnoses' or 'problems'. This can arise in two main ways:

(a) When a person who may or may not be sick encounters the health services for some specific purpose, such as to receive limited care or service for a current condition, to donate an organ or tissue, to receive prophylactic vaccination (immunization), or to discuss a problem which is in itself not a disease or injury.

(b) When some circumstance or problem is present which influences the person's health status but is not in itself a current illness or injury.

See Guidelines: *1;C.2Ø.a.1 | 1;C.21.a-b | 4;E*

PERSONS ENCOUNTERING HEALTH SERVICES FOR EXAMINATIONS (ZØØ-Z13)

Notes:

Nonspecific abnormal findings disclosed at the time of these examinations are classified to categories R7Ø-R94.

Excludes1:

examinations related to pregnancy and reproduction (Z3Ø-Z36, Z39.-)

ZØØ- ENCOUNTER FOR GENERAL EXAMINATION WITHOUT COMPLAINT, SUSPECTED OR REPORTED DIAGNOSIS

Excludes1:

encounter for examination for administrative purposes (ZØ2.-)

Excludes2:

encounter for pre-procedural examinations (ZØ1.81-)

special screening examinations (Z11-Z13)

See Guidelines: *1;C.21.c.13 | 1;C.21.c.16*

Indicator(s): *POAEx*

ZØØ.Ø- **Adult medical examination**

Including: Encounter for adult periodic examination (annual) (physical) and any associated laboratory and radiologic examinations

Excludes1:

encounter for examination of sign or symptom- code to sign or symptom

general health check-up of infant or child (ZØØ.12.-)

See Guidelines: *4;P*

Indicator(s): *NoPDx/M | Z-PDx*

ZØØ.ØØ Without abnormal findings

Including: Health check-up NOS

Indicator(s): *Adult*

ZØØ.Ø1 With abnormal findings

Use additional *code to identify abnormal findings*

Indicator(s): *Adult*

ZØØ.1- **Newborn, infant and child health examinations**

See Guidelines: *1;C.21.c.12*

Indicator(s): *NoPDx/M | Z-PDx*

ZØØ.11- **Newborn**

Including: Health check for child under 29 days old

Use additional *code to identify any abnormal findings*

Excludes1:

health check for child over 28 days old (ZØØ.12-)

ZØØ.11Ø Under 8 days old

Including: Health check

Indicator(s): *Newborn*

ZØØ.111 8 to 28 days old

Including: Health check, Newborn weight check

Indicator(s): *Newborn*

ZØØ.12- **Routine child health examination**

Including: Health check (routine) for child over 28 days old, Immunizations appropriate for age, Routine developmental screening of infant or child, Routine vision and hearing testing

Excludes1:

health check for child under 29 days old (ZØØ.11-)

health supervision of foundling or other healthy infant or child (Z76.1-Z76.2)

newborn health examination (ZØØ.11-)

See Guidelines: *4;P*

ZØØ.121 With abnormal findings

Use additional *code to identify abnormal findings*

Indicator(s): *Pediatric*

ZØØ.129 Without abnormal findings

Including: Encounter NOS

Indicator(s): *Pediatric*

ZØØ.8 Other general examination

Including: Health examination in population surveys

Indicator(s): *NoPDx/M | Z-PDx*

ZØ2- ENCOUNTER FOR ADMINISTRATIVE EXAMINATION

See Guidelines: *1;C.21.c.13 | 1;C.21.c.16*

Indicator(s): *Z-PDx | POAEx*

ZØ2.Ø Admission to educational institution

Including: Preschool (education), re-admission to school following illness or medical treatment

Indicator(s): *NoPDx/M*

ZØ2.1 Pre-employment

ZØ2.2 Admission to residential institution

Excludes1:

examination for admission to prison (ZØ2.89)

Indicator(s): *NoPDx/M*

ZØ2.3 Recruitment to armed forces

ZØ2.4 Driving license

Indicator(s): *NoPDx/M*

ZØ2.5 Participation in sport

Excludes1:

blood-alcohol and blood-drug test (ZØ2.83)

Indicator(s): *NoPDx/M*

ZØ2.6 Insurance purposes

Indicator(s): *NoPDx/M*

ZØ2.7- **Issue of medical certificate**

Excludes1:

encounter for general medical examination (ZØØ-ZØ1, ZØ2.Ø-ZØ2.6, ZØ2.8-ZØ2.9)

Indicator(s): *NoPDx/M*

ZØ2.71 Disability determination

Including: Issue of medical certificate of incapacity or invalidity

ZØ2.79 Other

Z02.8- **Other administrative examinations**

Z02.83 **Blood-alcohol and blood-drug test**

Use additional code for findings of alcohol or drugs in blood (R78.-)

Z02.89 **Other**

Including: Examination for admission to prison, admission to summer camp, immigration examination, naturalization examination, premarital examination

Excludes1:

health supervision of foundling or other healthy infant or child (Z76.1-Z76.2)

Indicator(s): NoPDx/M

Z02.9 **Unspecified administrative examinations**

See Guidelines: 1;C.21.c.15

Indicator(s): NoPDx/M

Z04- ENCOUNTER FOR EXAMINATION AND OBSERVATION FOR OTHER REASONS

Includes:

encounter for examination for medicolegal reasons

This category is to be used when a person without a diagnosis is suspected of having an abnormal condition, without signs or symptoms, which requires study, but after examination and observation, is ruled-out. This category is also for use for administrative and legal observation status.

See Guidelines: 1;C.21.c.6 | 1;C.21.c.16

Indicator(s): Z-PDx

Z04.1 **Following transport accident**

Excludes1:

encounter for examination and observation following work accident (Z04.2)

Z04.2 **Following work accident**

Z04.3 **Following other accident**

Z04.9 **Unspecified reason**

Including: Encounter for observation NOS

See Guidelines: 1;C.21.c.6 | 1;C.21.c.15

Indicator(s): NoPDx/M

Z13- ENCOUNTER FOR SCREENING FOR OTHER DISEASES AND DISORDERS

Including: Screening is the testing for disease or disease precursors in asymptomatic individuals so that early detection and treatment can be provided for those who test positive for the disease.

Excludes1:

encounter for diagnostic examination-code to sign or symptom

See Guidelines: 1;C.21.c.5

Indicator(s): NoPDx/M | POAEx

Z13.0 **Diseases of the blood and blood-forming organs and certain disorders involving the immune mechanism**

Z13.1 **Diabetes mellitus**

Z13.2- **Nutritional, metabolic and other endocrine disorders**

Z13.21 **Nutritional disorder**

Z13.22- **Metabolic disorder**

Z13.220 **Lipoid disorders**

Including: Cholesterol level, hypercholesterolemia, hyperlipidemia

Z13.228 **Other metabolic disorders**

Z13.29 **Other suspected endocrine disorder**

Excludes2:

encounter for screening for diabetes mellitus (Z13.1)

Z13.8- **Other specified diseases and disorders**

Excludes2:

screening for malignant neoplasms (Z12.-)

Z13.82- **Musculoskeletal disorder**

Z13.820 **Osteoporosis**

Z13.828 **Other musculoskeletal disorder**

Z13.85- **Nervous system disorders**

Z13.850 **Traumatic brain injury**

Z13.858 **Other nervous system disorders**

Z13.88 **Disorder due to exposure to contaminants**

Excludes1:

those exposed to contaminants without suspected disorders (Z57.-, Z77.-)

Z13.89 **Other disorder**

Including: Genitourinary disorders

Z13.9 **Encounter for screening, unspecified**

See Guidelines: 1;C.21.c.15

PERSONS ENCOUNTERING HEALTH SERVICES IN CIRCUMSTANCES RELATED TO REPRODUCTION (Z30-Z39)

Z33- PREGNANT STATE

See Guidelines: 1;C.21.c.11

Z33.1 **Incidental**

Including: Pregnant state NOS, Pregnancy NOS

Excludes1:

complications of pregnancy (O00-O9A)

pregnant state, gestational carrier (Z33.3)

See Guidelines: 1;C.15.a.1 | 1;C.21.c.3

Indicator(s): Female | NoPDx/M | HHS07: 212

Z34- ENCOUNTER FOR SUPERVISION OF NORMAL PREGNANCY

Excludes1:

any complication of pregnancy (O00-O9A)

encounter for pregnancy test (Z32.0-)

encounter for supervision of high risk pregnancy (O09.-)

See Guidelines: 1;C.15.b.1 | 1;C.21.c.11 | 1;C.21.c.16

Indicator(s): NoPDx/M | Z-PDx | POAEx | HHS07: 212

Z34.0- **First pregnancy**

Z34.00 **Unspecified trimester**

Indicator(s): Female

Z34.01 **First trimester**

Indicator(s): Female

Z34.02 **Second trimester**

Indicator(s): Female

Z34.03 **Third trimester**

Indicator(s): Female

Z34.8- **Other normal pregnancy**

Z34.80 **Unspecified trimester**

Indicator(s): Female

Z34.81 **First trimester**

Indicator(s): Female

Z34.82 **Second trimester**

Indicator(s): Female

Z34.83 **Third trimester**

Indicator(s): Female

Z34.9- **Unspecified**

Z34.90 **Unspecified trimester**
Indicator(s): Female

Z34.91 **First trimester**
Indicator(s): Female

Z34.92 **Second trimester**
Indicator(s): Female

Z34.93 **Third trimester**
Indicator(s): Female

Z3A- WEEKS OF GESTATION

Notes:
Codes from category Z3A are for use, only on the maternal record, to indicate the weeks of gestation of the pregnancy, if known.
Code First:
obstetric condition or encounter for delivery (O09-O60, O80-O82)
See Guidelines: 1;C.21.c.11
Indicator(s): NoPDx/M | POAEx | HHS07: 212

Z3A.0- **Weeks of gestation of pregnancy, unspecified or less than 10 weeks**

Z3A.00 **Not specified**
Indicator(s): Female

Z3A.01 **Less than 8 weeks**
Indicator(s): Female

Z3A.08 **8 weeks**
Indicator(s): Female

Z3A.09 **9 weeks**
Indicator(s): Female

Z3A.1- **Weeks of gestation of pregnancy, weeks 10-19**

Z3A.10 **10 weeks**
Indicator(s): Female

Z3A.11 **11 weeks**
Indicator(s): Female

Z3A.12 **12 weeks**
Indicator(s): Female

Z3A.13 **13 weeks**
Indicator(s): Female

Z3A.14 **14 weeks**
Indicator(s): Female

Z3A.15 **15 weeks**
Indicator(s): Female

Z3A.16 **16 weeks**
Indicator(s): Female

Z3A.17 **17 weeks**
Indicator(s): Female

Z3A.18 **18 weeks**
Indicator(s): Female

Z3A.19 **19 weeks**
Indicator(s): Female

Z3A.2- **Weeks of gestation of pregnancy, weeks 20-29**

Z3A.20 **20 weeks**
Indicator(s): Female

Z3A.21 **21 weeks**
Indicator(s): Female

Z3A.22 **22 weeks**
Indicator(s): Female

Z3A.23 **23 weeks**
Indicator(s): Female

Z3A.24 **24 weeks**
Indicator(s): Female

Z3A.25 **25 weeks**
Indicator(s): Female

Z3A.26 **26 weeks**
Indicator(s): Female

Z3A.27 **27 weeks**
Indicator(s): Female

Z3A.28 **28 weeks**
Indicator(s): Female

Z3A.29 **29 weeks**
Indicator(s): Female

Z3A.3- **Weeks of gestation of pregnancy, weeks 30-39**

Z3A.30 **30 weeks**
Indicator(s): Female

Z3A.31 **31 weeks**
Indicator(s): Female

Z3A.32 **32 weeks**
Indicator(s): Female

Z3A.33 **33 weeks**
Indicator(s): Female

Z3A.34 **34 weeks**
Indicator(s): Female

Z3A.35 **35 weeks**
Indicator(s): Female

Z3A.36 **36 weeks**
Indicator(s): Female

Z3A.37 **37 weeks**
Indicator(s): Female

Z3A.38 **38 weeks**
Indicator(s): Female

Z3A.39 **39 weeks**
Indicator(s): Female

Z3A.4- **Weeks of gestation of pregnancy, weeks 40 or greater**

Z3A.40 **40 weeks**
Indicator(s): Female

Z3A.41 **41 weeks**
Indicator(s): Female

Z3A.42 **42 weeks**
Indicator(s): Female

Z3A.49 **Greater than 42 weeks**
Indicator(s): Female

ENCOUNTERS FOR OTHER SPECIFIC HEALTH CARE (Z40-Z53)

Including: Categories Z40-Z53 are intended for use to indicate a reason for care. They may be used for patients who have already been treated for a disease or injury, but who are receiving aftercare or prophylactic care, or care to consolidate the treatment, or to deal with a residual state
Excludes2:
follow-up examination for medical surveillance after treatment (Z08-Z09)

Z41- ENCOUNTER FOR PROCEDURES FOR PURPOSES OTHER THAN REMEDYING HEALTH STATE

See Guidelines: 1;C.21.c.14
Indicator(s): POAEx

Z41.8 **Other procedures**

Z41.9 **Unspecified**
See Guidelines: 1;C.21.c.15
Indicator(s): NoPDx/M

Ch5

5. The Tabular List

Z47- ORTHOPEDIC AFTERCARE

Excludes1:
aftercare for healing fracture-code to fracture with 7th character D
See Guidelines: 1;C.21.c.7
Indicator(s): POAEx

Z47.8- **Other orthopedic aftercare**

Z47.81 **Following surgical amputation**
Use additional code to identify the limb amputated (Z89.-)

Z47.82 **Following scoliosis surgery**

Z47.89 **Other orthopedic aftercare**

Z53- PERSONS ENCOUNTERING HEALTH SERVICES FOR SPECIFIC PROCEDURES AND TREATMENT, NOT CARRIED OUT

See Guidelines: 1;C.21.c.14
Indicator(s): NoPDx/M

Z53.Ø- **Because of contraindication**

Z53.Ø1 **Due to patient smoking**

Z53.Ø9 **Because of other contraindication**

Z53.1 **Because of patient's decision for reasons of belief and group pressure**

Z53.2- **Because of patient's decision for other and unspecified reasons**

Z53.2Ø **Unspecified reasons**

Z53.21 **Due to patient leaving prior to being seen by health care provider**

Z53.29 **Other reasons**

Z53.8 **Other reasons**

Z53.9 **Unspecified reason**

PERSONS WITH POTENTIAL HEALTH HAZARDS RELATED TO SOCIOECONOMIC AND PSYCHOSOCIAL CIRCUMSTANCES (Z55-Z65)

Indicator(s): NoPDx/M

Z55- PROBLEMS RELATED TO EDUCATION AND LITERACY

Excludes1:
disorders of psychological development (F8Ø-F89)
See Guidelines: 1;C.21.c.14
Indicator(s): POAEx

Z55.Ø **Illiteracy and low-level literacy**

Z55.1 **Schooling unavailable and unattainable**

Z55.2 **Failed school examinations**

Z55.3 **Underachievement in school**

Z55.4 **Educational maladjustment and discord with teachers and classmates**

Z55.8 **Other problems**
Including: Problems related to inadequate teaching

Z55.9 **Unspecified**
Including: Academic problems NOS
Indicator(s): DSM-5

Z56- PROBLEMS RELATED TO EMPLOYMENT AND UNEMPLOYMENT

Excludes2:
occupational exposure to risk factors (Z57.-)
problems related to housing and economic circumstances (Z59.-)
See Guidelines: 1;C.21.c.14
Indicator(s): POAEx

Z56.Ø **Unemployment, unspecified**

Z56.1 **Change of job**
Indicator(s): Adult

Z56.2 **Threat of job loss**

Z56.3 **Stressful work schedule**

Z56.4 **Discord with boss and workmates**

Z56.5 **Uncongenial work environment**
Including: Difficult conditions at work

Z56.6 **Other physical and mental strain related to work**

Z56.8- **Other problems related to employment**

Z56.81 **Sexual harassment on the job**

Z56.82 **Military deployment status**
Including: Individual (civilian or military) currently deployed in theater or in support of military war, peacekeeping and humanitarian operations
Indicator(s): DSM-5

Z56.89 **Other problems**

Z56.9 **Unspecified problems related to employment**
Including: Occupational problems NOS
Indicator(s): DSM-5

Z57- OCCUPATIONAL EXPOSURE TO RISK FACTORS

See Guidelines: 1;C.21.c.14
Indicator(s): POAEx

Z57.Ø **Noise**

Z57.1 **Radiation**

Z57.2 **Dust**

Z57.3- **Other air contaminants**

Z57.31 **Environmental tobacco smoke**
Excludes2:
exposure to environmental tobacco smoke (Z77.22)

Z57.39 **Other contaminants**

Z57.4 **Toxic agents in agriculture**
Including: Solids, liquids, gases or vapors

Z57.5 **Toxic agents in other industries**
Including: Solids, liquids, gases or vapors

Z57.6 **Extreme temperature**

Z57.7 **Vibration**

Z57.8 **Other risk factors**

Z57.9 **Unspecified risk factor**

Z59- PROBLEMS RELATED TO HOUSING AND ECONOMIC CIRCUMSTANCES

Excludes2:
problems related to upbringing (Z62.-)
See Guidelines: 1;C.21.c.14
Indicator(s): POAEx

Z59.1 **Inadequate housing**
Including: Lack of heating, Restriction of space, Technical defects in home preventing adequate care, Unsatisfactory surroundings
Excludes1:
problems related to the natural and physical environment (Z77.1-)
Indicator(s): DSM-5

Z59.2 **Discord with neighbors, lodgers and landlord**
Indicator(s): DSM-5

Z59.3 **Problems related to living in residential institution**
Including: Boarding-school resident
Excludes1:
institutional upbringing (Z62.2)
Indicator(s): DSM-5

Z59.5 **Extreme poverty**
Indicator(s): DSM-5

Z59.6 **Low income**
Indicator(s): DSM-5

Z59.7 **Insufficient social insurance and welfare support**
Indicator(s): DSM-5

Z59.8- **Other problems**
Including: Foreclosure on loan, Isolated dwelling, Problems with creditors
Indicator(s): POAEx | POAEx

N **Z59.86** **Financial insecurity**
Including: Bankruptcy, Burdensome debt, Economic strain, strain, Money problems, Running out of money, Unable to make ends meet
Excludes2:
extreme poverty (Z59.5)
low income (Z59.6)
material hardship, not elsewhere classified (Z59.87)

Z59.9 **Unspecified**
Indicator(s): DSM-5

Z60- PROBLEMS RELATED TO SOCIAL ENVIRONMENT

See Guidelines: 1;C.21.c.14

Z60.0 **Adjustment to life-cycle transitions**
Including: Empty nest syndrome, Phase of life problem, Problem with adjustment to retirement [pension]
Indicator(s): DSM-5

Z60.2 **Living alone**
Indicator(s): DSM-5

Z60.3 **Acculturation difficulty**
Including: Problem with migration, Problem with social transplantation
Indicator(s): DSM-5

Z60.4 **Exclusion and rejection**
Including: on the basis of personal characteristics, such as unusual physical appearance, illness or behavior
Excludes1:
target of adverse discrimination such as for racial or religious reasons (Z60.5)
Indicator(s): DSM-5

Z60.5 **Target of (perceived) adverse discrimination and persecution**
Excludes1:
social exclusion and rejection (Z60.4)
Indicator(s): DSM-5

Z60.8 **Other problems**

Z60.9 **Unspecified**
Indicator(s): DSM-5

Z62- PROBLEMS RELATED TO UPBRINGING

Includes:
current and past negative life events in childhood
current and past problems of a child related to upbringing
Excludes2:
maltreatment syndrome (T74.-)
problems related to housing and economic circumstances (Z59.-)
See Guidelines: 1;C.21.c.14

Z62.0 **Inadequate parental supervision and control**

Z62.1 **Parental overprotection**

Z62.2- **Away from parents**
Excludes1:
problems with boarding school (Z59.3)

Z62.21 **Child in welfare custody**
Including: In care of non-parental family member, foster care
Excludes2:
problem for parent due to child in welfare custody (Z63.5)
Indicator(s): Pediatric

Z62.22 **Institutional upbringing**
Including: Child living in orphanage or group home

Z62.29 **Other upbringing away from parents**
Indicator(s): DSM-5

Z62.3 **Hostility towards and scapegoating of child**
Indicator(s): Pediatric

Z62.6 **Inappropriate (excessive) parental pressure**

Z62.8- **Other specified problems**

Z62.81- **Personal history of abuse in childhood**

Z62.810 **Physical and sexual**
Excludes1:
current child physical abuse (T74.12, T76.12)
current child sexual abuse (T74.22, T76.22)
Indicator(s): DSM-5

Z62.811 **Psychological**
Excludes1:
current child psychological abuse (T74.32, T76.32)
Indicator(s): DSM-5

Z62.812 **Neglect**
Excludes1:
current child neglect (T74.02, T76.02)
Indicator(s): DSM-5

Z62.819 **Unspecified abuse**
Excludes1:
current child abuse NOS (T74.92, T76.92)

Z62.82- **Parent-child conflict**

Z62.820 **Biological child**
Including: Parent-child problem NOS
Indicator(s): DSM-5

Z62.821 **Adopted child**

Z62.822 **Foster child**

Z62.89- **Other specified problems**

Z62.89Ø **Parent-child estrangement NEC**

Z62.891 **Sibling rivalry**
Indicator(s): DSM-5

Z62.898 **Other problems**
Indicator(s): DSM-5

Z62.9 **Problem related to upbringing, unspecified**

Z63- OTHER PROBLEMS RELATED TO PRIMARY SUPPORT GROUP, INCLUDING FAMILY CIRCUMSTANCES

Excludes2:
maltreatment syndrome (T74.-, T76)
parent-child problems (Z62.-)
problems related to negative life events in childhood (Z62.-)
problems related to upbringing (Z62.-)
See Guidelines: 1;C.21.c.14
Indicator(s): POAEx

Z63.Ø **Problems in relationship with spouse or partner**
Including: Relationship distress with spouse or intimate partner
Excludes1:
counseling for spousal or partner abuse problems (Z69.1)
counseling related to sexual attitude, behavior, and orientation (Z7Ø.-)
Indicator(s): DSM-5

Z63.1 **Problems in relationship with in-laws**

Z63.3- **Absence of family member**
Excludes1:
absence of family member due to disappearance and death (Z63.4)
absence of family member due to separation and divorce (Z63.5)

Z63.31 **Due to military deployment**
Including: Individual or family affected by other family member being on deployment
Excludes1:
family disruption due to return of family member from military deployment (Z63.71)

Z63.32 **Other absence**

Z63.4 **Disappearance and death of family member**
Including: Assumed death, Bereavement
Indicator(s): DSM-5

Z63.5 **Disruption of family by separation and divorce**
Including: Marital estrangement
Indicator(s): DSM-5

Z63.6 **Dependent relative needing care at home**

Z63.7- **Other stressful life events affecting family and household**

Z63.71 **Stress on family due to return of family member from military deployment**
Including: Individual or family affected by family member having returned from military deployment (current or past conflict)

Z63.72 **Alcoholism and drug addiction in family**

Z63.79 **Other stressful life events**
Including: Anxiety (normal) about sick person in family, Health problems within family, Ill or disturbed family member, Isolated family

Z63.8 **Other problems**
Including: Family discord NOS, Family estrangement NOS, High expressed emotional level within family, Inadequate family support NOS, Inadequate or distorted communication within family
Indicator(s): DSM-5

Z63.9 **Unspecified**
Including: Relationship disorder NOS

Z64- PROBLEMS RELATED TO CERTAIN PSYCHOSOCIAL CIRCUMSTANCES
See Guidelines: 1;C.21.c.14
Indicator(s): POAEx | DSM-5

Z64.Ø **Unwanted pregnancy**
Indicator(s): Female

Z64.1 **Multiparity**
Indicator(s): Female

Z64.4 **Discord with counselors**
Including: Probation officer, social worker

Z65- PROBLEMS RELATED TO OTHER PSYCHOSOCIAL CIRCUMSTANCES
See Guidelines: 1;C.21.c.14
Indicator(s): POAEx | DSM-5

Z65.Ø **Conviction in civil and criminal proceedings without imprisonment**

Z65.1 **Imprisonment and other incarceration**

Z65.2 **Release from prison**

Z65.3 **Legal circumstances**
Including: Arrest, Child custody or support proceedings, Litigation, Prosecution

Z65.4 **Victim of crime and terrorism**
Including: Torture

Z65.5 **Exposure to disaster, war and other hostilities**
Excludes1:
target of perceived discrimination or persecution (Z6Ø.5)

Z65.8 **Other problems**
Including: Religious or spiritual problem

Z65.9 **Unspecified**

Z68 BODY MASS INDEX [BMI] (Z68) (Z68-Z68)

Z68- BODY MASS INDEX [BMI]
Including: Kilograms per meters squared
Notes:
BMI adult codes are for use for persons 2Ø years of age or older
BMI pediatric codes are for use for persons 2-19 years of age.
These percentiles are based on the growth charts published by the Centers for Disease Control and Prevention (CDC)
See Guidelines: 1;C.21.c.3
Indicator(s): NoPDx/M | POAEx

Z68.1 **19.9 or less, adult**
Indicator(s): Adult | CC

Z68.2- **2Ø-29, adult**

Z68.2Ø **2Ø.Ø-2Ø.9**
Indicator(s): Adult

Z68.21 **21.Ø-21.9**
Indicator(s): Adult

Z68.22 **22.Ø-22.9**
Indicator(s): Adult

Z68.23 **23.Ø-23.9**
Indicator(s): Adult

Z68.24 **24.Ø-24.9**
Indicator(s): Adult

Z68.25 **25.Ø-25.9**
Indicator(s): Adult

Z68.26 **26.Ø-26.9**
Indicator(s): Adult

Z68.27 **27.Ø-27.9**
Indicator(s): Adult

Z68.28 **28.0-28.9**
Indicator(s): Adult

Z68.29 **29.0-29.9**
Indicator(s): Adult

Z68.3- **30-39, adult**

Z68.30 **30.0-30.9**
Indicator(s): Adult

Z68.31 **31.0-31.9**
Indicator(s): Adult

Z68.32 **32.0-32.9**
Indicator(s): Adult

Z68.33 **33.0-33.9**
Indicator(s): Adult

Z68.34 **34.0-34.9**
Indicator(s): Adult

Z68.35 **35.0-35.9**
Indicator(s): Adult

Z68.36 **36.0-36.9**
Indicator(s): Adult

Z68.37 **37.0-37.9**
Indicator(s): Adult

Z68.38 **38.0-38.9**
Indicator(s): Adult

Z68.39 **39.0-39.9**
Indicator(s): Adult

Z68.4- **40 or greater, adult**
Indicator(s): CC | CMS22: 22 | CMS24: 22 | Rx05: 43 | ESRD21: 22

Z68.41 **40.0-44.9**
Indicator(s): Adult

Z68.42 **45.0-49.9**
Indicator(s): Adult

Z68.43 **50.0-59.9**
Indicator(s): Adult

Z68.44 **60.0-69.9**
Indicator(s): Adult

Z68.45 **70 or greater**
Indicator(s): Adult

Z68.5- **Pediatric**

Z68.51 **Less than 5th percentile for age**

Z68.52 **5th percentile to less than 85th percentile for age**

Z68.53 **85th percentile to less than 95th percentile for age**

Z68.54 **Greater than or equal to 95th percentile for age**

PERSONS ENCOUNTERING HEALTH SERVICES IN OTHER CIRCUMSTANCES (Z69-Z76)

Z71- PERSONS ENCOUNTERING HEALTH SERVICES FOR OTHER COUNSELING AND MEDICAL ADVICE, NOT ELSEWHERE CLASSIFIED

Excludes2:
contraceptive or procreation counseling (Z30-Z31)
sex counseling (Z70.-)
See Guidelines: 1;C.21.c.10
Indicator(s): POAEx

Z71.0 **Person encountering health services to consult on behalf of another person**
Including: Seeking advice or treatment for non-attending third party
Excludes2:
anxiety (normal) about sick person in family (Z63.7)
expectant (adoptive) parent(s) pre-birth pediatrician visit (Z76.81)
Indicator(s): NoPDx/M

Z71.1 **Person with feared health complaint in whom no diagnosis is made**
Including: Person encountering health services with feared condition which was not demonstrated, in which problem was normal state, 'Worried well'
Excludes1:
medical observation for suspected diseases and conditions proven not to exist (Z03.-)
Indicator(s): NoPDx/M

Z71.2 **Person consulting for explanation of examination or test findings**
Indicator(s): NoPDx/M

Z71.3 **Dietary counseling and surveillance**
Use additional code for any associated underlying medical condition
Use additional code to identify body mass index (BMI), if known (Z68.-)
Indicator(s): NoPDx/M

Z71.4- **Alcohol abuse counseling and surveillance**
Use additional code for alcohol abuse or dependence (F10.-)
Indicator(s): NoPDx/M

Z71.41 **Alcoholic**

Z71.42 **Family member of alcoholic**
Including: Significant other, partner, or friend

Z71.5- **Drug abuse counseling and surveillance**
Use additional code for drug abuse or dependence (F11-F16, F18-F19)
Indicator(s): NoPDx/M

Z71.51 **Drug abuser**

Z71.52 **Family member of drug abuser**
Including: Significant other, partner, or friend

Z71.6 **Tobacco abuse counseling**
Use additional code for nicotine dependence (F17.-)
Indicator(s): NoPDx/M

Z71.7 **Human immunodeficiency virus [HIV] counseling**
See Guidelines: 1;C.1.a.2.h
Indicator(s): NoPDx/M

Z71.8- **Other specified counseling**
Excludes2:
counseling for contraception (Z30.0-)

Z71.81 **Spiritual or religious counseling**
Indicator(s): NoPDx/M

Z71.82 **Exercise counseling**
Indicator(s): NoPDx/M

Z71.89 **Other**
Indicator(s): NoPDx/M

Z72- PROBLEMS RELATED TO LIFESTYLE

Excludes2:
problems related to life-management difficulty (Z73.-)
problems related to socioeconomic and psychosocial circumstances (Z55-Z65)
See Guidelines: 1;C.21.c.14

Z72.Ø **Tobacco use**
Including: Tobacco use NOS
Excludes1:
history of tobacco dependence (Z87.891)
nicotine dependence (F17.2-)
tobacco dependence (F17.2-)
tobacco use during pregnancy (O99.33-)
See Guidelines: 1;C.15.l.2
Indicator(s): NoPDx/M | POAEx | DSM-5

Z72.3 **Lack of physical exercise**
Indicator(s): NoPDx/M | POAEx

Z72.4 **Inappropriate diet and eating habits**
Excludes1:
behavioral eating disorders of infancy or childhood (F98.2.-F98.3)
eating disorders (F5Ø.-)
lack of adequate food (Z59.48)
malnutrition and other nutritional deficiencies (E4Ø-E64)
Indicator(s): NoPDx/M | POAEx

Z72.5- **High risk sexual behavior**
Including: Promiscuity
Excludes1:
paraphilias (F65)
Indicator(s): NoPDx/M | POAEx

Z72.51 **Heterosexual**

Z72.52 **Homosexual**

Z72.53 **Bisexual**

Z72.6 **Gambling and betting**
Excludes1:
compulsive or pathological gambling (F63.Ø)
Indicator(s): NoPDx/M | POAEx

Z72.8- **Other problems**

Z72.81- **Antisocial behavior**
Excludes1:
conduct disorders (F91.-)
Indicator(s): POAEx | DSM-5

Z72.81Ø **Child and adolescent**
Including: Without manifest psychiatric disorder, Delinquency NOS, Group delinquency, Offenses in the context of gang membership, Stealing in company with others, Truancy from school
Indicator(s): Pediatric

Z72.811 **Adult**
Including: Without manifest psychiatric disorder
Indicator(s): Adult

Z72.82- **Sleep**

Z72.82Ø **Sleep deprivation**
Including: Lack of adequate sleep
Excludes1:
insomnia (G47.Ø-)
Indicator(s): POAEx

Z72.821 **Inadequate sleep hygiene**
Including: Bad sleep habits, Irregular sleep habits, Unhealthy sleep wake schedule
Excludes1:
insomnia (F51.Ø-, G47.Ø-)
Indicator(s): NoPDx/M | POAEx

Z72.89 **Other problems related to lifestyle**
Including: Self-damaging behavior
Indicator(s): NoPDx/M | POAEx

Z72.9 **Problem related to lifestyle, unspecified**
Indicator(s): NoPDx/M | POAEx | DSM-5

Z73- PROBLEMS RELATED TO LIFE MANAGEMENT DIFFICULTY

Excludes2:
problems related to socioeconomic and psychosocial circumstances (Z55-Z65)
See Guidelines: 1;C.21.c.14
Indicator(s): NoPDx/M | POAEx

Z73.Ø **Burn-out**

Z73.1 **Type A behavior pattern**

Z73.2 **Lack of relaxation and leisure**

Z73.3 **Stress, NEC**
Including: Physical and mental strain NOS
Excludes1:
stress related to employment or unemployment (Z56.-)

Z73.4 **Inadequate social skills, NEC**

Z73.5 **Social role conflict, NEC**

Z73.6 **Limitation of activities due to disability**
Excludes1:
care-provider dependency (Z74.-)

Z74- PROBLEMS RELATED TO CARE PROVIDER DEPENDENCY

Excludes2:
dependence on enabling machines or devices NEC (Z99.-)
See Guidelines: 1;C.21.c.14
Indicator(s): NoPDx/M

Z74.Ø- **Reduced mobility**

Z74.Ø1 **Bed confinement status**
Including: Bedridden
See Guidelines: 1;C.21.c.3
Indicator(s): POAEx

Z74.Ø9 **Other reduced mobility**
Including: Chairridden, Reduced mobility NOS
Excludes2:
wheelchair dependence (Z99.3)

Z74.1 **Need for assistance with personal care**

Z74.2 **Need for assistance at home and no other household member able to render care**

Z74.3 **Need for continuous supervision**

Z74.8 **Other problems**

Z74.9 **Unspecified**

Z76- PERSONS ENCOUNTERING HEALTH SERVICES IN OTHER CIRCUMSTANCES

Indicator(s): POAEx

Z76.5 **Malingerer [conscious simulation]**
Including: Person feigning illness (with obvious motivation)
Excludes1:
factitious disorder (F68.1-, F68.A)
peregrinating patient (F68.1-)
See Guidelines: 1;C.21.c.14
Indicator(s): DSM-5

Z76.8- **Other specified circumstances**
Indicator(s): NoPDx/M

Z76.89 **Other circumstances**
Including: Persons encountering health services NOS

PERSONS WITH POTENTIAL HEALTH HAZARDS RELATED TO FAMILY AND PERSONAL HISTORY AND CERTAIN CONDITIONS INFLUENCING HEALTH STATUS (Z77-Z99)

Code Also
any follow-up examination (Z08-Z09)

Z79- LONG TERM (CURRENT) DRUG THERAPY

Includes:
long term (current) drug use for prophylactic purposes
Code Also
any therapeutic drug level monitoring (Z51.81)
Excludes2:
drug abuse and dependence (F11-F19)
drug use complicating pregnancy, childbirth, and the puerperium (O99.32-)
See Guidelines: 1;C.4.a.3 | 1;C.4.a.6.a | 1;C.21.c.3
Indicator(s): POAEx

R **Z79.4** **Insulin**
Excludes2:
long-term (current) use of injectable non-insulin antidiabetic drugs (Z79.85)
long term (current) use of oral antidiabetic drugs (Z79.84)
long term (current) use of oral hypoglycemic drugs (Z79.84)
See Guidelines: 1;C.4.a.2 | 1;C.15.g-i | 1;C.15.h-i
Indicator(s): CMS22: 19 | CMS24: 19 | Rx05: 31 | ESRD21: 19 | HHS05: 21 | HHS07: 21

Z79.8- **Other long term (current) drug therapy**

Z79.82 **Aspirin**

R **Z79.84** **Oral hypoglycemic drugs**
Including: antidiabetic drugs
Excludes2:
long-term (current) use of injectable non-insulin antidiabetic drugs (Z79.85)
long term (current) use of insulin (Z79.4)
See Guidelines: 1;C.15.g-i
Indicator(s): NoPDx/M

Z79.89- **Other**

Z79.890 **Hormone replacement**
Indicator(s): NoPDx/M

Z79.899 **Other drug therapy**

Z80- FAMILY HISTORY OF PRIMARY MALIGNANT NEOPLASM

See Guidelines: 1;C.21.c.4 | 3;A | 4;J
Indicator(s): NoPDx/M | POAEx

Z80.0 **Digestive organs**
Including: Conditions classifiable to C15-C26

Z80.1 **Trachea, bronchus and lung**
Including: Conditions classifiable to C33-C34

Z80.2 **Other respiratory and intrathoracic organs**
Including: Conditions classifiable to C30-C32, C37-C39

Z80.3 **Breast**
Including: Conditions classifiable to C50.-

Z80.4- **Genital organs**
Including: Conditions classifiable to C51-C63

Z80.41 **Ovary**

Z80.42 **Prostate**

Z80.43 **Testis**

Z80.49 **Other genital organs**

Z80.5- **Urinary tract**
Including: Conditions classifiable to C64-C68

Z80.51 **Kidney**

Z80.52 **Bladder**

Z80.59 **Other urinary tract organ**

Z80.6 **Leukemia**
Including: Conditions classifiable to C91-C95

Z80.7 **Other lymphoid, hematopoietic and related tissues**
Including: Conditions classifiable to C81-C90, C96.-

Z80.8 **Other organs or systems**
Including: Conditions classifiable to C00-C14, C40-C49, C69-C79

Z80.9 **Unspecified**
Including: Conditions classifiable to C80.1

Z81- FAMILY HISTORY OF MENTAL AND BEHAVIORAL DISORDERS

See Guidelines: 1;C.21.c.4 | 3;A | 4;J
Indicator(s): NoPDx/M | POAEx

Z81.0 **Intellectual disabilities**
Including: Conditions classifiable to F70-F79

Z81.1 **Alcohol abuse and dependence**
Including: Conditions classifiable to F10.-

Z81.2 **Tobacco abuse and dependence**
Including: Conditions classifiable to F17.-

Z81.3 **Other psychoactive substance abuse and dependence**
Including: Conditions classifiable to F11-F16, F18-F19

Z81.4 **Other substance abuse and dependence**
Including: Conditions classifiable to F55

Z81.8 **Other mental and behavioral disorders**
Including: Conditions classifiable elsewhere in F01-F99

Z82- FAMILY HISTORY OF CERTAIN DISABILITIES AND CHRONIC DISEASES (LEADING TO DISABLEMENT)

See Guidelines: 1;C.21.c.4 | 3;A | 4;J
Indicator(s): NoPDx/M | POAEx

Z82.0 **Epilepsy and other diseases of the nervous system**
Including: Conditions classifiable to G00-G99

Z82.1 **Blindness and visual loss**
Including: Conditions classifiable to H54.-

Z82.2 **Deafness and hearing loss**
Including: Conditions classifiable to H90-H91

Z82.3 **Stroke**
Including: Conditions classifiable to I60-I64

Z82.4- **Ischemic heart disease and other diseases of the circulatory system**
Including: Conditions classifiable to I00-I5A, I65-I99

Z82.41 **Sudden cardiac death**

Z82.49 **Ischemic heart disease and other diseases of the circulatory system**

Z82.5 **Asthma and other chronic lower respiratory diseases**
Including: Conditions classifiable to J40-J47
Excludes2:
family history of other diseases of the respiratory system (Z83.6)

Ch5

5. The Tabular List

Z82.6- **Arthritis and other diseases of the musculoskeletal system and connective tissue**
Including: Conditions classifiable to MØØ-M99

Z82.61 **Arthritis**

Z82.62 **Osteoporosis**

Z82.69 **Other diseases of the musculoskeletal system and connective tissue**

Z82.7- **Congenital malformations, deformations and chromosomal abnormalities**
Including: Conditions classifiable to QØØ-Q99

Z82.71 **Polycystic kidney**

Z82.79 **Other**

Z82.8 **Other, NEC**

Z83- FAMILY HISTORY OF OTHER SPECIFIC DISORDERS

<u>Excludes2:</u>
contact with and (suspected) exposure to communicable disease in the family (Z2Ø.-)
<u>See Guidelines:</u> *1;C.21.c.4 | 3;A | 4;J*
<u>Indicator(s):</u> *NoPDx/M | POAEx*

Z83.Ø **Human immunodeficiency virus [HIV] disease**
Including: Conditions classifiable to B2Ø

Z83.1 **Infectious and parasitic diseases**
Including: Conditions classifiable to AØØ-B19, B25-B94, B99

Z83.2 **Diseases of the blood and blood-forming organs and certain disorders involving the immune mechanism**
Including: Conditions classifiable to D5Ø-D89

Z83.3 **Diabetes mellitus**
Including: Conditions classifiable to EØ8-E13

Z83.4- **Other endocrine, nutritional and metabolic diseases**
Including: Conditions classifiable to EØØ-EØ7, E15-E88

Z83.41 **Multiple endocrine neoplasia [MEN] syndrome**

Z83.49 **Other diseases**

Z83.5- **Eye and ear disorders**

Z83.51- **Eye disorders**
Including: Conditions classifiable to HØØ-H53, H55-H59
<u>Excludes2:</u>
family history of blindness and visual loss (Z82.1)

Z83.511 **Glaucoma**

Z83.518 **Other eye disorder**

Z83.52 **Ear disorders**
Including: Conditions classifiable to H6Ø-H83, H92-H95
<u>Excludes2:</u>
family history of deafness and hearing loss (Z82.2)

Z83.6 **Other diseases of the respiratory system**
Including: Conditions classifiable to JØØ-J39, J6Ø-J99
<u>Excludes2:</u>
family history of asthma and other chronic lower respiratory diseases (Z82.5)

Z83.7- **Diseases of the digestive system**
Including: Conditions classifiable to KØØ-K93

Z83.71 **Colonic polyps**
<u>Excludes2:</u>
family history of malignant neoplasm of digestive organs (Z8Ø.Ø)

Z83.79 **Other diseases**

Z84- FAMILY HISTORY OF OTHER CONDITIONS

<u>See Guidelines:</u> *1;C.21.c.4 | 3;A | 4;J*
<u>Indicator(s):</u> *NoPDx/M | POAEx*

Z84.Ø **Diseases of the the skin and subcutaneous tissue**
Including: Conditions classifiable to LØØ-L99

Z84.1 **Disorders of the kidney and ureter**
Including: Conditions classifiable to NØØ-N29

Z84.2 **Diseases of the genitourinary system**
Including: Conditions classifiable to N3Ø-N99

Z84.3 **Consanguinity**

Z85- PERSONAL HISTORY OF MALIGNANT NEOPLASM

<u>Code First:</u>
any follow-up examination after treatment of malignant neoplasm (ZØ8)
<u>Use additional</u> *code to identify:*
alcohol use and dependence (F1Ø.-)
exposure to environmental tobacco smoke (Z77.22)
history of tobacco dependence (Z87.891)
occupational exposure to environmental tobacco smoke (Z57.31)
tobacco dependence (F17.-)
tobacco use (Z72.Ø)
<u>Excludes2:</u>
personal history of benign neoplasm (Z86.Ø1-)
personal history of carcinoma-in-situ (Z86.ØØ-)
<u>See Guidelines:</u> *1;C.2.d | 1;C.2.m | 1;C.21.c.4 | 3;A | 4;J*
<u>Indicator(s):</u> *NoPDx/M | POAEx*

Z85.Ø- **Personal history of malignant neoplasm of digestive organs**

Z85.ØØ **Unspecified digestive organ**

Z85.Ø1 **Esophagus**
Including: Conditions classifiable to C15

Z85.Ø2- **Stomach**

Z85.Ø2Ø **Carcinoid tumor**
Including: Conditions classifiable to C7A.Ø92

Z85.Ø28 **Other malignant neoplasm**
Including: Conditions classifiable to C16

Z85.Ø3- **Large intestine**

Z85.Ø3Ø **Carcinoid tumor**
Including: Conditions classifiable to C7A.Ø22-C7A.Ø25, C7A.Ø29

Z85.Ø38 **Other malignant neoplasm**
Including: Conditions classifiable to C18

Z85.Ø4- **Rectum, rectosigmoid junction, and anus**

Z85.Ø4Ø **Carcinoid tumor of rectum**
Including: Conditions classifiable to C7A.Ø26

Z85.Ø48 **Other malignant neoplasm**
Including: Conditions classifiable to C19-C21

Z85.Ø5 **Liver**
Including: Conditions classifiable to C22

Z85.Ø6- **Small intestine**

Z85.Ø6Ø **Carcinoid tumor**
Including: Conditions classifiable to C7A.Ø1-

Z85.Ø68 **Other malignant neoplasm**
Including: Conditions classifiable to C17

Z85.Ø7 **Pancreas**
Including: Conditions classifiable to C25

Z85.Ø9 **Other malignant neoplasm**

Z85.1- **Personal history of malignant neoplasm of trachea, bronchus and lung**

Z85.11- **Bronchus and lung**

Z85.11Ø **Carcinoid tumor**
Including: Conditions classifiable to C7A.Ø9Ø

Z85.118 **Other malignant neoplasm**
Including: Conditions classifiable to C34

Z85.12 **Trachea**
Including: Conditions classifiable to C33

Z85.2- **Personal history of malignant neoplasm of other respiratory and intrathoracic organs**

Z85.2Ø **Unspecified respiratory organ**

Z85.21 **Larynx**
Including: Conditions classifiable to C32

Z85.22 **Nasal cavities, middle ear, and accessory sinuses**
Including: Conditions classifiable to C3Ø-C31

Z85.23- **Thymus**

Z85.23Ø **Carcinoid tumor**
Including: Conditions classifiable to C7A.Ø91

Z85.238 **Other malignant neoplasm**
Including: Conditions classifiable to C37

Z85.29 **Other organs**

Z85.3 **Personal history of malignant neoplasm of breast**
Including: Conditions classifiable to C5Ø.-

Z85.4- **Personal history of malignant neoplasm of genital organs**
Including: Conditions classifiable to C51-C63

Z85.4Ø **Unspecified female genital organ**
Indicator(s): Female

Z85.41 **Cervix uteri**
Indicator(s): Female

Z85.42 **Other parts of uterus**
Indicator(s): Female

Z85.43 **Ovary**
Indicator(s): Female

Z85.44 **Other female genital organs**
Indicator(s): Female

Z85.45 **Unspecified male genital organ**
Indicator(s): Male

Z85.46 **Prostate**
Indicator(s): Male

Z85.47 **Testis**
Indicator(s): Male

Z85.48 **Epididymis**
Indicator(s): Male

Z85.49 **Other male genital organs**
Indicator(s): Male

Z85.5- **Personal history of malignant neoplasm of urinary tract**
Including: Conditions classifiable to C64-C68

Z85.5Ø **Unspecified urinary tract organ**

Z85.51 **Bladder**

Z85.52- **Kidney**
Excludes1:
personal history of malignant neoplasm of renal pelvis (Z85.53)

Z85.52Ø **Carcinoid tumor**
Including: Conditions classifiable to C7A.Ø93

Z85.528 **Other malignant neoplasm**
Including: Conditions classifiable to C64

Z85.53 **Renal pelvis**

Z85.54 **Ureter**

Z85.59 **Other urinary tract organ**

Z85.6 **Personal history of leukemia**
Including: Conditions classifiable to C91-C95
Excludes1:
leukemia in remission C91.Ø-C95.9 with 5th character 1
See Guidelines: 1;C.2.n

Z85.7- **Personal history of other malignant neoplasms of lymphoid, hematopoietic and related tissues**

Z85.71 **Hodgkin lymphoma**
Including: Conditions classifiable to C81

Z85.72 **Non-Hodgkin lymphomas**
Including: Conditions classifiable to C82-C85

Z85.79 **Other malignant neoplasm**
Including: Conditions classifiable to C88-C9Ø, C96
Excludes1:
multiple myeloma in remission (C9Ø.Ø1)
plasma cell leukemia in remission (C9Ø.11)
plasmacytoma in remission (C9Ø.21)
See Guidelines: 1;C.2.n

Z85.8- **Personal history of malignant neoplasms of other organs and systems**
Including: Conditions classifiable to CØØ-C14, C4Ø-C49, C69-C75, C7A.Ø98, C76-C79

Z85.81- **Personal history of malignant neoplasm of lip, oral cavity, and pharynx**
Including: Conditions classifiable to CØØ-C14

Z85.81Ø **Tongue**

Z85.818 **Other sites**

Z85.819 **Unspecified site**

Z85.82- **Personal history of malignant neoplasm of skin**

Z85.82Ø **Melanoma**
Including: Conditions classifiable to C43

Z85.821 **Merkel cell carcinoma**
Including: Conditions classifiable to C4A

Z85.828 **Other malignant neoplasm**
Including: Conditions classifiable to C44

Z85.83- **Personal history of malignant neoplasm of bone and soft tissue**
Including: Conditions classifiable to C4Ø-C41; C45-C49

Z85.83Ø **Bone**

Z85.831 **Soft tissue**
Excludes2:
personal history of malignant neoplasm of skin (Z85.82-)

Z85.84- **Personal history of malignant neoplasm of eye and nervous tissue**
Including: Conditions classifiable to C69-C72

Z85.84Ø Eye

Z85.841 Brain

Z85.848 Other parts of nervous tissue

Z85.85- **Personal history of malignant neoplasm of endocrine glands**
Including: Conditions classifiable to C73-C75

Z85.85Ø Thyroid

Z85.858 Other endocrine glands

Z85.89 Other organs and systems
Including: Conditions classifiable to C7A.Ø98, C76, C77-C79

Z85.9 Personal history of malignant neoplasm, unspecified
Including: Conditions classifiable to C7A.ØØ, C8Ø.1

Z86- PERSONAL HISTORY OF CERTAIN OTHER DISEASES
Code First:
any follow-up examination after treatment (ZØ9)
See Guidelines: *1;C.21.c.4 | 3;A | 4;J*
Indicator(s): *POAEx*

Z86.Ø- **Personal history of in-situ and benign neoplasms and neoplasms of uncertain behavior**
Excludes2:
personal history of malignant neoplasms (Z85.-)
Indicator(s): *NoPDx/M*

Z86.ØØ- **In-situ neoplasm**
Including: Conditions classifiable to DØØ-DØ9

Z86.ØØØ Breast
Including: Conditions classifiable to DØ5

Z86.ØØ1 Cervix uteri
Including: Conditions classifiable to DØ6, cervical intraepithelial neoplasia III [CIN III]
Indicator(s): *Female*

Z86.ØØ8 Other site
Including: Conditions classifiable to DØ9

Z86.Ø1- **Benign neoplasm**

Z86.Ø1Ø Colonic polyps

Z86.Ø11 Brain

Z86.Ø12 Carcinoid tumor

Z86.Ø18 Other benign neoplasm

Z86.Ø3 Neoplasm of uncertain behavior

Z86.1- **Personal history of infectious and parasitic diseases**
Including: Conditions classifiable to AØØ-B89, B99
Excludes1:
personal history of infectious diseases specific to a body system
sequelae of infectious and parasitic diseases (B9Ø-B94)

Z86.11 Tuberculosis
Indicator(s): *NoPDx/M*

Z86.12 Poliomyelitis
Indicator(s): *NoPDx/M*

Z86.13 Malaria
Indicator(s): *NoPDx/M*

Z86.14 Methicillin resistant Staphylococcus aureus infection
Including: MRSA infection
See Guidelines: *1;C.1.e*
Indicator(s): *NoPDx/M*

Z86.19 Other diseases
Indicator(s): *NoPDx/M*

Z86.2 Personal history of diseases of the blood and blood-forming organs and certain disorders involving the immune mechanism
Including: Conditions classifiable to D5Ø-D89
Indicator(s): *NoPDx/M*

Z86.3- **Personal history of endocrine, nutritional and metabolic diseases**
Including: Conditions classifiable to EØØ-E88
Indicator(s): *NoPDx/M*

Z86.31 Diabetic foot ulcer
Excludes2:
current diabetic foot ulcer (EØ8.621, EØ9.621, E1Ø.621, E11.621, E13.621)

Z86.32 Gestational diabetes
Including: Conditions classifiable to O24.4-
Excludes1:
gestational diabetes mellitus in current pregnancy (O24.4-)
Indicator(s): *Female*

Z86.39 Other disease

Z86.5- **Personal history of mental and behavioral disorders**
Including: Conditions classifiable to F4Ø-F59
Indicator(s): *NoPDx/M*

Z86.51 Combat and operational stress reaction
Indicator(s): *Adult*

Z86.59 Other disorders
See Guidelines: *1;C.21.c.15*

Z86.6- **Personal history of diseases of the nervous system and sense organs**
Including: Conditions classifiable to GØØ-G99, HØØ-H95
Indicator(s): *NoPDx/M*

Z86.61 Infections of the central nervous system
Including: Encephalitis, meningitis

Z86.69 Other diseases

Z86.7- **Personal history of diseases of the circulatory system**
Including: Conditions classifiable to IØØ-I99
Excludes2:
old myocardial infarction (I25.2)
personal history of anaphylactic shock (Z87.892)
postmyocardial infarction syndrome (I24.1)
Indicator(s): *NoPDx/M*

Z86.71- **Venous thrombosis and embolism**

Z86.711 Pulmonary embolism

Z86.718 Other venous thrombosis and embolism

Z86.72 Thrombophlebitis

Z86.73 Transient ischemic attack (TIA), and cerebral infarction without residual deficits
Including: Prolonged reversible ischemic neurological deficit (PRIND), stroke NOS
Excludes1:
personal history of traumatic brain injury (Z87.82Ø)
sequelae of cerebrovascular disease (I69.-)
See Guidelines: *1;C.d.3 | 1;C.9.d.3*

Z86.74 Sudden cardiac arrest
Including: Cardiac death successfully resuscitated

Z86.79 Other diseases

Z87- PERSONAL HISTORY OF OTHER DISEASES AND CONDITIONS

Code First:
any follow-up examination after treatment (ZØ9)
See Guidelines: 1;C.21.c.4 | 3;A | 4;J
Indicator(s): POAEx

Z87.Ø- **Personal history of diseases of the respiratory system**
Including: Conditions classifiable to JØØ-J99
Indicator(s): NoPDx/M

Z87.Ø1 **Pneumonia (recurrent)**

Z87.Ø9 **Other diseases**

Z87.1- **Personal history of diseases of the digestive system**
Including: Conditions classifiable to KØØ-K93
Indicator(s): NoPDx/M

Z87.11 **Peptic ulcer disease**

Z87.19 **Other diseases**

Z87.2 **Personal history of diseases of the skin and subcutaneous tissue**
Including: Conditions classifiable to LØØ-L99
Excludes2:
personal history of diabetic foot ulcer (Z86.31)
Indicator(s): NoPDx/M

Z87.3- **Personal history of diseases of the musculoskeletal system and connective tissue**
Including: Conditions classifiable to MØØ-M99
Excludes2:
personal history of (healed) traumatic fracture (Z87.81)
Indicator(s): NoPDx/M

Z87.31- **(healed) nontraumatic fracture**

Z87.31Ø **Osteoporosis fracture**
Including: Fragility, collapsed vertebra due to osteoporosis
See Guidelines: 1;C.13.d | 1;C.13.d.1

Z87.311 **Other pathological fracture**
Including: Collapsed vertebra NOS
Excludes2:
personal history of osteoporosis fracture (Z87.31Ø)

Z87.312 **Stress fracture**
Including: Fatigue fracture

Z87.39 **Other diseases**

Z87.4- **Personal history of diseases of genitourinary system**
Including: Conditions classifiable to NØØ-N99
Indicator(s): NoPDx/M

Z87.41- **Dysplasia of the female genital tract**
Excludes1:
personal history of intraepithelial neoplasia III of female genital tract (Z86.ØØ1, Z86.ØØ8)
personal history of malignant neoplasm of female genital tract (Z85.4Ø-Z85.44)

Z87.41Ø **Cervical dysplasia**
Indicator(s): Female

Z87.411 **Vaginal dysplasia**
Indicator(s): Female

Z87.412 **Vulvar dysplasia**
Indicator(s): Female

Z87.42 **Other diseases of the female genital tract**
Indicator(s): Female

Z87.43- **Male genital organs**

Z87.43Ø **Prostatic dysplasia**
Excludes1:
personal history of malignant neoplasm of prostate (Z85.46)
Indicator(s): Male

Z87.438 **Other diseases**
Indicator(s): Male

Z87.44- **Urinary system**
Excludes1:
personal history of malignant neoplasm of cervix uteri (Z85.41)

Z87.44Ø **Urinary (tract) infections**

Z87.441 **Nephrotic syndrome**

Z87.442 **Urinary calculi**
Including: Kidney stones

Z87.448 **Other diseases**

Z87.5- **Personal history of complications of pregnancy, childbirth and the puerperium**
Including: Conditions classifiable to OØØ-O9A
Excludes2:
recurrent pregnancy loss (N96)
Indicator(s): NoPDx/M

Z87.51 **Pre-term labor**
Excludes1:
current pregnancy with history of pre-term labor (OØ9.21-)
Indicator(s): Female

Z87.59 **Other complications**
Including: Trophoblastic disease
Indicator(s): Female

Z87.7- **Personal history of (corrected) congenital malformations**
Including: Conditions classifiable to QØØ-Q89 that have been repaired or corrected
Excludes1:
congenital malformations that have been partially corrected or repair but which still require medical treatment - code to condition
Excludes2:
other postprocedural states (Z98.-)
personal history of medical treatment (Z92.-)
presence of cardiac and vascular implants and grafts (Z95.-)
presence of other devices (Z97.-)
presence of other functional implants (Z96.-)
transplanted organ and tissue status (Z94.-)
Indicator(s): NoPDx/M

Z87.71- **Genitourinary system**
Indicator(s): NoPDx/M

Z87.71Ø **Hypospadias**
Indicator(s): Male

Z87.718 **Other specified malformations**

Z87.72- **Nervous system and sense organs**
Indicator(s): NoPDx/M

Z87.72Ø **Eye**

Z87.721 **Ear**

Z87.728 **Other specified malformations**

Z87.73- **Digestive system**
Indicator(s): NoPDx/M

Z87.73Ø **Cleft lip and palate**

Z87.738 **Other specified**

Z87.74 **Heart and circulatory system**

Z87.75 **Respiratory system**

Z87.79- **Other (corrected) congenital malformations**
Indicator(s): NoPDx/M

Z87.790 **Face and neck**

Z87.798 **Other malformations**

Z87.8- **Personal history of other specified conditions**
Excludes2:
personal history of self harm (Z91.5-)

Z87.81 **(healed) traumatic fracture**
Excludes2:
personal history of (healed) nontraumatic fracture (Z87.31-)
Indicator(s): NoPDx/M

Z87.82- **Other (healed) physical injury and trauma**
Including: Conditions classifiable to SØØ-T88, except traumatic fractures
Indicator(s): NoPDx/M

Z87.82Ø **Traumatic brain injury**
Excludes1:
personal history of transient ischemic attack (TIA), and cerebral infarction without residual deficits (Z86.73)

Z87.821 **Retained foreign body fully removed**

Z87.828 **Other injury and trauma**

Z87.89- **Other specified conditions**

Z87.89Ø **Sex reassignment**

Z87.891 **Nicotine dependence**
Excludes1:
current nicotine dependence (F17.2-)
Indicator(s): NoPDx/M

Z87.892 **Anaphylaxis**
Code Also
allergy status such as:
allergy status to drugs, medicaments and biological substances (Z88.-)
allergy status, other than to drugs and biological substances (Z91.Ø-)
Indicator(s): NoPDx/M

Z87.898 **Other conditions**
Indicator(s): NoPDx/M

Z89- ACQUIRED ABSENCE OF LIMB
Includes:
amputation status
postprocedural loss of limb
post-traumatic loss of limb
Excludes1:
acquired deformities of limbs (M2Ø-M21)
congenital absence of limbs (Q71-Q73)
See Guidelines: 1;C.21.c.3
Indicator(s): NoPDx/M | POAEx

Z89.Ø- **Thumb and other finger(s)**

Z89.Ø1- **Thumb**

Z89.Ø11 **Right thumb**

Z89.Ø12 **Left thumb**

Z89.Ø19 **Unspecified thumb**

Z89.Ø2- **Other finger(s)**
Excludes2:
acquired absence of thumb (Z89.Ø1-)

Z89.Ø21 **Right finger(s)**

Z89.Ø22 **Left finger(s)**

Z89.Ø29 **Unspecified finger(s)**

Z89.1- **Hand and wrist**
Indicator(s): HHSØ7: 254

Z89.11- **Hand**

Z89.111 **Right hand**

Z89.112 **Left hand**

Z89.119 **Unspecified hand**

Z89.12- **Wrist**
Including: Disarticulation

Z89.121 **Right wrist**

Z89.122 **Left wrist**

Z89.129 **Unspecified wrist**

Z89.2- **Upper limb above wrist**

Z89.2Ø- **Upper limb, unspecified level**
Indicator(s): HHSØ7: 254

Z89.2Ø1 **Right limb**

Z89.2Ø2 **Left limb**

Z89.2Ø9 **Unspecified limb**
Including: Arm NOS

Z89.21- **Upper limb below elbow**
Indicator(s): HHSØ7: 254

Z89.211 **Right limb**

Z89.212 **Left limb**

Z89.219 **Unspecified limb**

Z89.22- **Upper limb above elbow**
Including: Disarticulation
Indicator(s): HHSØ7: 254

Z89.221 **Right limb**

Z89.222 **Left limb**

Z89.229 **Unspecified limb**

Z89.23- **Shoulder**
Including: Acquired absence of shoulder joint following explantation of shoulder joint prosthesis, with or without presence of antibiotic-impregnated cement spacer

Z89.231 **Right shoulder**

Z89.232 **Left shoulder**

Z89.239 **Unspecified shoulder**

Z89.4- **Toe(s), foot, and ankle**
Indicator(s): CMS22: 189 | CMS24: 189 | ESRD21: 189 | HHSØ5: 254

Z89.41- **Great toe**

Z89.411 **Right toe**

Z89.412 **Left toe**

Z89.419 **Unspecified toe**

Z89.42- **Other toe(s)**
Excludes2:
acquired absence of great toe (Z89.41-)

Z89.421 **Right toe(s)**

Z89.422 **Left toe(s)**

Z89.429 **Unspecified side toe(s)**

Z89.43- **Foot**

Z89.431 **Right foot**

Z89.432 **Left foot**

Z89.439 **Unspecified foot**

Z89.44- **Ankle**

Including: Disarticulation

Z89.441 **Right ankle**

Z89.442 **Left ankle**

Z89.449 **Unspecified ankle**

Z89.5- **Leg below knee**

Z89.51- **Leg below knee**

Indicator(s): CMS22: 189 | CMS24: 189 | ESRD21: 189 | HHSØ5: 254 | HHSØ7: 254

Z89.511 **Right leg**

Z89.512 **Left leg**

Z89.519 **Unspecified leg**

Z89.52- **Knee**

Including: Acquired absence of knee joint following explantation of knee joint prosthesis, with or without presence of antibiotic-impregnated cement spacer

Z89.521 **Right knee**

Z89.522 **Left knee**

Z89.529 **Unspecified knee**

Z89.6- **Leg above knee**

Z89.61- **Leg above knee**

Including: Acquired absence NOS, Disarticulation at knee

Indicator(s): CMS22: 189 | CMS24: 189 | ESRD21: 189 | HHSØ5: 254 | HHSØ7: 254

Z89.611 **Right leg**

Z89.612 **Left leg**

Z89.619 **Unspecified leg**

Z89.62- **Hip**

Including: Acquired absence of hip joint following explantation of hip joint prosthesis (with or without presence of antibiotic-impregnated cement spacer), Disarticulation at hip

Z89.621 **Right hip joint**

Z89.622 **Left hip joint**

Z89.629 **Unspecified hip joint**

Z89.9 **Acquired absence of limb, unspecified**

Indicator(s): HHSØ7: 254

Z9Ø- ACQUIRED ABSENCE OF ORGANS, NOT ELSEWHERE CLASSIFIED

Includes:

postprocedural or post-traumatic loss of body part NEC

Excludes1:

congenital absence - see Alphabetical Index

Excludes2:

postprocedural absence of endocrine glands (E89.-)

See Guidelines: 1;C.21.c.3

Indicator(s): POAEx

Z9Ø.Ø- **Head and neck**

Indicator(s): NoPDx/M

Z9Ø.Ø1 **Eye**

Z9Ø.Ø2 **Larynx**

Z9Ø.Ø9 **Other part**

Including: Nose

Excludes2:

teeth (KØ8.1)

Z9Ø.1- **Breast and nipple**

Z9Ø.1Ø **Unspecified breast and nipple**

Z9Ø.11 **Right breast and nipple**

Z9Ø.12 **Left breast and nipple**

Z9Ø.13 **Bilateral breasts and nipples**

Z9Ø.2 **Lung [part of]**

Indicator(s): NoPDx/M

Z9Ø.3 **Stomach [part of]**

Indicator(s): NoPDx/M

Z9Ø.4- **Other specified parts of digestive tract**

Indicator(s): NoPDx/M

Z9Ø.41- **Pancreas**

Code Also

exocrine pancreatic insufficiency (K86.81)

Use additional code to identify any associated:

diabetes mellitus, postpancreatectomy (E13.-)

insulin use (Z79.4)

See Guidelines: 1;C.4.a.6.b | 1;C.4.a.6.b.i

Z9Ø.41Ø **Total absence**

Including: Acquired absence NOS

Z9Ø.411 **Partial absence**

Z9Ø.49 **Other parts of digestive tract**

Z9Ø.5 **Kidney**

Indicator(s): NoPDx/M

Z9Ø.6 **Other parts of urinary tract**

Including: Bladder

Indicator(s): NoPDx/M

Z9Ø.7- **Genital organ(s)**

Excludes1:

personal history of sex reassignment (Z87.89Ø)

Excludes2:

female genital mutilation status (N9Ø.81-)

Indicator(s): NoPDx/M

Z9Ø.71- **Cervix and uterus**

Z9Ø.71Ø **Both cervix and uterus**

Including: Uterus NOS, Status post total hysterectomy

Indicator(s): Female

Z9Ø.711 **Uterus with remaining cervical stump**

Including: Status post partial hysterectomy

Indicator(s): Female

Z9Ø.712 **Cervix with remaining uterus**

Indicator(s): Female

Z9Ø.72- **Ovaries**

Z9Ø.721 **Unilateral**

Indicator(s): Female

Z9Ø.722 **Bilateral**

Indicator(s): Female

Z9Ø.79 **Other genital organ(s)**

Z9Ø.8- **Other organs**

Indicator(s): NoPDx/M

Z9Ø.81 **Spleen**

Z9Ø.89 **Other organs**

Z91- PERSONAL RISK FACTORS, NOT ELSEWHERE CLASSIFIED

Excludes2:
contact with and (suspected) exposures hazardous to health (Z77.-)
exposure to pollution and other problems related to physical environment (Z77.1-)
female genital mutilation status (N9Ø.81-)
occupational exposure to risk factors (Z57.-)
personal history of physical injury and trauma (Z87.81, Z87.82-)

Z91.1- **Patient's noncompliance with medical treatment and regimen**
Including: Excludes 2: caregiver noncompliance with patient's medical treatment and regimen (Z91.A-)
See Guidelines: 1;C.21.c.14
Indicator(s): NoPDx/M | POAEx

Z91.11- **Dietary regimen**
Code Also
if applicable, food insecurity (Z59.4-)
Indicator(s): POAEx

N **Z91.11Ø Due to financial hardship**

N **Z91.118 For other reason**
Including: Inability to comply with dietary regimen

N **Z91.119 Due to unspecified reason**

Z91.12- **Intentional underdosing of medication regimen**
Code First:
underdosing of medication (T36-T5Ø) with fifth or sixth character 6
Excludes1:
adverse effect of prescribed drug taken as directed- code to adverse effect
poisoning (overdose) -code to poisoning
See Guidelines: 1;C.19.e.5.c
Indicator(s): POAEx

Z91.12Ø Due to financial hardship

Z91.128 For other reason

Z91.13- **Unintentional underdosing of medication regimen**
Code First:
underdosing of medication (T36-T5Ø) with fifth or sixth character 6
Excludes1:
adverse effect of prescribed drug taken as directed- code to adverse effect
poisoning (overdose) -code to poisoning
See Guidelines: 1;C.19.e.5.c
Indicator(s): POAEx

Z91.13Ø Due to age-related debility

Z91.138 For other reason

Z91.14 Other noncompliance with medication regimen
Including: Underdosing of medication NOS
See Guidelines: 1;C.19.e.5.c

Z91.15 Noncompliance with renal dialysis
Indicator(s): CMS22: 134 | CMS24: 134 | RxØ5: 261 | ESRD21: 134

Z91.19- **Patient's noncompliance with other medical treatment and regimen**
Including: Nonadherence to medical treatment
Indicator(s): POAEx | DSM-5

N **Z91.19Ø Due to financial hardship**

N **Z91.198 For other reason**

N **Z91.199 Due to unspecified reason**

Z91.8- **Other specified**
Indicator(s): POAEx

Z91.81 History of falling
Including: At risk for falling
See Guidelines: 1;C.18.d | 1;C.21.c.4
Indicator(s): NoPDx/M

Z91.82 History of military deployment
Including: Individual (civilian or military) with past history of military war, peacekeeping and humanitarian deployment (current or past conflict); Returned from deployment
See Guidelines: 1;C.21.c.4
Indicator(s): Adult | NoPDx/M | DSM-5

R **Z91.83 Wandering in diseases classified elsewhere**
Code First:
underlying disorder such as:
Alzheimer's disease (G3Ø.-)
autism or pervasive developmental disorder (F84.-)
intellectual disabilities (F7Ø-F79)
unspecified dementia with behavioral disturbance (FØ3.9-, FØ3.A-, FØ3.B-, FØ3.C-)
See Guidelines: 1;C.21.c.14
Indicator(s): Manifestation | DSM-5

Z91.89 Other
See Guidelines: 1;C.21.c.14
Indicator(s): NoPDx/M | DSM-5

Z91.A- **Unintentional noncompliance**
Indicator(s): NoPDx/M | POAEx

Z91.A1- **Dietary regimen**
Including: inability to comply
Code Also
if applicable, food insecurity (Z59.4-)

N **Z91.A1Ø Due to financial hardship**

N **Z91.A18 For other reason**

Z91.A2- **Intentional underdosing of medication regimen**
Code First:
underdosing of medication (T36-T5Ø) with fifth or sixth character 6

N **Z91.A2Ø Due to financial hardship**

N **Z91.A28 For other reason**

N **Z91.A3 Unintentional underdosing**
Code First:
underdosing of medication (T36-T5Ø) with fifth or sixth character 6

N **Z91.A4 Other noncompliance**
Including: Caregiver's underdosing of patient's medication NOS

N **Z91.A9 Other medical treatment and regimen**
Including: nonadherence to patient's medical treatment

Z92- PERSONAL HISTORY OF MEDICAL TREATMENT

Excludes2:
postprocedural states (Z98.-)
See Guidelines: 1;C.21.c.4
Indicator(s): NoPDx/M | POAEx

Z92.8- **Other medical treatment**
Indicator(s): NoPDx/M | POAEx

Z92.89 Other medical treatment

Z96- PRESENCE OF OTHER FUNCTIONAL IMPLANTS

Excludes2:
complications of internal prosthetic devices, implants and grafts (T82-T85)
fitting and adjustment of prosthetic and other devices (Z44-Z46)
See Guidelines: 1;C.21.c.3
Indicator(s): NoPDx/M

Z96.6- **Orthopedic joint implants**

Z96.6Ø **Unspecified**

Z96.61- **Artificial shoulder joint**

Z96.611 **Right shoulder**

Z96.612 **Left shoulder**

Z96.619 **Unspecified shoulder**

Z96.62- **Artificial elbow joint**

Z96.621 **Right elbow**

Z96.622 **Left elbow**

Z96.629 **Unspecified elbow**

Z96.63- **Artificial wrist joint**

Z96.631 **Right wrist**

Z96.632 **Left wrist**

Z96.639 **Unspecified wrist**

Z96.64- **Artificial hip joint**
Including: Hip-joint replacement (partial) (total)

Z96.641 **Right hip**

Z96.642 **Left hip**

Z96.643 **Bilateral**

Z96.649 **Unspecified hip**

Z96.65- **Artificial knee joint**

Z96.651 **Right knee**

Z96.652 **Left knee**

Z96.653 **Bilateral**

Z96.659 **Unspecified knee**

Z96.66- **Artificial ankle joint**

Z96.661 **Right ankle**

Z96.662 **Left ankle**

Z96.669 **Unspecified ankle**

Z96.69- **Other orthopedic joint implants**

Z96.691 **Finger-joint replacement of right hand**

Z96.692 **Finger-joint replacement of left hand**

Z96.693 **Finger-joint replacement, bilateral**

Z96.698 **Other implants**

Z96.7 **Bone and tendon implants**
Including: Skull plate

Z96.8- **Other specified functional implants**

Z96.81 **Artificial skin**

Z96.82 **Neurostimulator**
Including: Brain, gastric, peripheral nerve, sacral nerve, spinal cord, vagus nerve neurostimulators
Indicator(s): POAEx

Z96.89 **Other implants**

Z96.9 **Presence of functional implant, unspecified**

Z97- PRESENCE OF OTHER DEVICES

Excludes1:
complications of internal prosthetic devices, implants and grafts (T82-T85)
Excludes2:
fitting and adjustment of prosthetic and other devices (Z44-Z46)
presence of cerebrospinal fluid drainage device (Z98.2)
See Guidelines: 1;C.21.c.3
Indicator(s): NoPDx/M | POAEx

Z97.Ø **Artificial eye**

Z97.1- **Artificial limb (complete) (partial)**
Indicator(s): HHSØ7: 254

Z97.1Ø **Unspecified**

Z97.11 **Right arm**

Z97.12 **Left arm**

Z97.13 **Right leg**

Z97.14 **Left leg**

Z97.15 **Arms, bilateral**

Z97.16 **Legs, bilateral**

Z99- DEPENDENCE ON ENABLING MACHINES AND DEVICES, NOT ELSEWHERE CLASSIFIED

See Guidelines: 1;C.21.c.3
Indicator(s): POAEx

Z99.Ø **Aspirator**
Indicator(s): NoPDx/M

Z99.1- **Respirator**
Including: Dependence on ventilator
Indicator(s): CC | CMS22: 82 | CMS24: 82 | ESRD21: 82 | HHSØ5: 125 | HHSØ7: 125

Z99.11 **Respirator [ventilator] status**

Z99.12 **Encounter for respirator [ventilator] dependence during power failure**
Excludes1:
mechanical complication of respirator [ventilator] (J95.85Ø)
See Guidelines: 1;C.21.c.16
Indicator(s): Z-PDx

Z99.2 **Renal dialysis**
Including: Hemodialysis status, Peritoneal dialysis status, Presence of arteriovenous shunt for dialysis, Renal dialysis status NOS
Excludes1:
encounter for fitting and adjustment of dialysis catheter (Z49.Ø-)
Excludes2:
noncompliance with renal dialysis (Z91.15)
Indicator(s): NoPDx/M | CMS22: 134 | CMS24: 134 | RxØ5: 261 | ESRD21: 134

Z99.3 **Wheelchair**
Including: Wheelchair confinement status
Code First:
cause of dependence, such as:
muscular dystrophy (G71.Ø-)
obesity (E66.-)
Indicator(s): NoPDx/M

Z99.8- **Other enabling machines and devices**
Indicator(s): NoPDx/M

Z99.81 **Supplemental oxygen**
Including: Long-term dependence

Z99.89 **Other**
Including: Dependence NOS

22. Codes for special purposes (UØØ-U85)

PROVISIONAL ASSIGNMENT OF NEW DISEASES OF UNCERTAIN ETIOLOGY OR EMERGENCY USE (UØØ-U49)

UØ7- EMERGENCY USE OF UØ7

UØ7.1 **COVID-19**

<u>Use additional</u> *code to identify pneumonia or other manifestations, such as:*

pneumonia due to COVID-19 (J12.82)

<u>Excludes2:</u>

coronavirus as the cause of diseases classified elsewhere (B97.2-)

coronavirus infection, unspecified (B34.2)

pneumonia due to SARS-associated coronavirus (J12.81)

<u>Indicator(s):</u> MCC

UØ9- POST COVID-19 CONDITION

UØ9.9 **Post COVID-19 condition, unspecified**

Including: Post-acute sequela of COVID-19

<u>Code First:</u>

the specific condition related to COVID-19 if known, such as:

chronic respiratory failure (J96.1-)

loss of smell (R43.8)

loss of taste (R43.8)

multisystem inflammatory syndrome (M35.81)

pulmonary embolism (I26.-)

pulmonary fibrosis (J84.1Ø)

<u>Notes:</u>

This code enables establishment of a link with COVID-19.

This code is not to be used in cases that are still presenting with active COVID-19. However, an exception is made in cases of re-infection with COVID-19, occurring with a condition related to prior COVID-19.

See Appendix A — Coding Reference Tables for lists of the ICD-10-CM Tabular indicators, HAC categories, and HCC codes.

Notes:

Notes:

Notes

Appendix A. Coding Reference Tables

Disclaimer: The indicators were current at the time of publication. Changes may occur after printing. Find-ACode.com subscribers have access to the most current information including any changes or updates to the indicators included in this book.

Figure A.1

ICD-10-CM Tabular Indicators

Abbreviation	Title	Source	Description
Adult	Adult	CMS	Age range 15-24 years inclusive
CC	Complication or Comorbidity	MS-DRG v40.0	Presence of a complication or condition that increases the severity of a patient's condition, affects DRG assignment, and increases the resources needed to care for the patient appropriately.
DSM-5	DSM-5	APA	Codes mentioned in the American Psychiatric Association's DSM-5 publication. This indicator is useful for those working in the field of behavioral health or in an integrated care practice. At the time of publication, it seemed likely that the APA would add the new codes in categories F01- and F02- to the DSM-5 so they have been flagged as such. Watch for further notification of any differences.
Female	Female only	CMS	Female-related diagnoses only
HAC: #	Hospital Acquired Condition	MS-DRG v40.0	A condition that arises during a hospital stay that affects the patient negatively and may affect DRG assignation.
CMS22: # **CMS24: #**	CMS Hierarchical Condition Categories; v22, v24	CMS	Payment model for Medicare Advantage plans used to identify and calculate enrollee health status; versions 22 and 24
ESRD21: # **ESRD24: #**	CMS-ESRD Hierarchical Condition Categories: v21, v24	CMS	Payment model for Medicare ESRD plans used to identify and calculate enrollee health status; versions 21 and 24
HHS04: # **HHS05: #**	HHS Hierarchical Condition Categories; v04, v05	HHS	Payment model for Affordable Care Act plans used to identify and calculate enrollee health status; versions 04 and 05
Male	Male only	CMS	Male-related diagnoses only
Manifestation	Manifestation	CMS	Describes the manifestation of an underlying disease, not the disease itself. Code first the underlying disease followed by the manifestation code.
Maternity	Maternity	CMS	Age-range 12-55 years only
MCC	Major Complication or Comorbidity	MS-DRG v40.0	Presence of a major complication or condition that increases the severity of the patient's condition, affects DRG assignment, and significantly increases the resources needed to care for the patient appropriately.
Newborn	Newborn	CMS	Only reported for newborns 0-28 days old
NoPDx/M	Unacceptable principal diagnosis (for Medicare)	CMS	There are selected codes that describe a circumstance which influences an individual's health status, but not a current illness or injury, or codes that are not specific manifestation but they may be due to an underlying cause. These codes are considered unacceptable as a principal diagnosis. The following unacceptable principal diagnosis code is considered "acceptable" when a secondary diagnosis is also coded on the record. Example: **Z51.89** "Encounter for other specified aftercare"
PDx/CC	Primary diagnosis is its own CC	MS-DRG v40.0	Diagnosis is a combination code in ICD-10-CM, which also represents the CC. In ICD-9-CM, it was represented by two or more codes, one of which was the CC.
PDx/MCC	Primary diagnosis is its own MCC	MS-DRG v40.0	Diagnosis is a combination code in ICD-10-CM, which also represents the MCC. In ICD-9-CM, it was represented by two or more codes, one of which was the MCC.
Pediatric	Pediatric	CMS	Age range 0-17 inclusive
POAEx	Present on Admission Exempt	CDC/CMS	Diagnosis codes that cannot be listed as Present on Admission. They are exempt from POA use.
QAdmit	Questionable Admission	CMS	Some diagnoses are not usually sufficient justification for admission to an acute care hospital. For example, if a patient is given code **R03.0** for elevated blood pressure reading, without diagnosis of hypertension, then the patient would have a questionable admission, since an elevated blood pressure reading is not normally sufficient justification for admission to a hospital.
Rx05: # **Rx08: #**	Prescription Drug Hierarchical Condition Categories: v05, v08	MS-DRG v40.0	A risk adjustment payment model utilized by prescription drug plans for Medicare Part D beneficiaries; versions 05 and 08
Z-PDx	Only as Principal/ First-Listed Diagnosis	ICD-10-CM Guidelines	Codes located in Chapter 21 that begin with the letter "Z" and can only be reported as first-listed or principal diagnosis.

Figure A.2

HCC Codes and Descriptions (CMS-HCC v22)

1	HIV/AIDs	82	Respirator Dependence/Tracheostomy Status
2	Septicemia, Sepsis, Systemic Inflammatory Response Syndrome/Shock	83	Respiratory Arrest
6	Opportunistic Infections	84	Cardio-Respiratory Failure and Shock
8	Metastatic Cancer and Acute Leukemia	85	Congestive Heart Failure
9	Lung and Other Severe Cancers	86	Acute Myocardial Infarction
10	Lymphoma and Other Cancers	87	Unstable Angina and Other Acute Ischemic Heart Disease
11	Colorectal, Bladder, and Other Cancers	88	Angina Pectoris
12	Breast, Prostate, and Other Cancers and Tumors	96	Specified Heart Arrhythmias
17	Diabetes with Acute Complications	99	Cerebral Hemorrhage
18	Diabetes with Chronic Complications	100	Ischemic or Unspecified Stroke
19	Diabetes without Complication	103	Hemiplegia/Hemiparesis
21	Protein-Calorie Malnutrition	104	Monoplegia, Other Paralytic Syndromes
22	Morbid Obesity	106	Atherosclerosis of the Extremities with Ulceration or Gangrene
23	Other Significant Endocrine and Metabolic Disorders	107	Vascular Disease with Complications
27	End-Stage Liver Disease	108	Vascular Disease
28	Cirrhosis of Liver	110	Cystic Fibrosis
29	Chronic Hepatitis	111	Chronic Obstructive Pulmonary Disease
33	Intestinal Obstruction/Perforation	112	Fibrosis of Lung and Other Chronic Lung Disorders
34	Chronic Pancreatitis	114	Aspiration and Specified Bacterial Pneumonias
35	Inflammatory Bowel Disease	115	Pneumococcal Pneumonia, Empyema, Lung Abscess
39	Bone/Joint/Muscle Infections/Necrosis	122	Proliferative Diabetic Retinopathy and Vitreous Hemorrhage
40	Rheumatoid Arthritis and Inflammatory Connective Tissue Disease	124	Exudative Macular Degeneration
46	Severe Hematological Disorders	134	Dialysis Status
47	Disorders of Immunity	135	Acute Renal Failure
48	Coagulation Defects and Other Specified Hematological Disorders	136	Chronic Kidney Disease, Stage 5
54	Drug/Alcohol Psychosis	137	Chronic Kidney Disease, Severe (Stage 4)
55	Drug/Alcohol Dependence	157	Pressure Ulcer of Skin with Necrosis Through to Muscle, Tendon, or Bone
57	Schizophrenia	158	Pressure Ulcer of Skin with Full Thickness Skin Loss
58	Major Depressive, Bipolar, and Paranoid Disorders	161	Chronic Ulcer of Skin, Except Pressure
70	Quadriplegia	162	Severe Skin Burn or Condition
71	Paraplegia	166	Severe Head Injury
72	Spinal Cord Disorders/Injuries	167	Major Head Injury
73	Amyotrophic Lateral Sclerosis and Other Motor Neuron Disease	169	Vertebral Fractures without Spinal Cord Injury
74	Cerebral Palsy	170	Hip Fracture/Dislocation
75	Myasthenia Gravis/Myoneural Disorders, Inflammatory and Toxic Neuropathy	173	Traumatic Amputations and Complications
76	Muscular Dystrophy	176	Complications of Specified Implanted Device or Graft
77	Multiple Sclerosis	186	Major Organ Transplant or Replacement Status
78	Parkinson's and Huntington's Diseases	188	Artificial Openings for Feeding or Elimination
79	Seizure Disorders and Convulsions	189	Amputation Status, Lower Limb/Amputation Complications
80	Coma, Brain Compression/Anoxic Damage		

Notes

HCC Codes and Descriptions (CMS-HCC v24)

1	HIV/AIDS	79	Seizure Disorders and Convulsions
2	Septicemia, Sepsis, Systemic Inflammatory Response Syndrome/Shock	80	Coma, Brain Compression/Anoxic Damage
6	Opportunistic Infections	82	Respirator Dependence/Tracheostomy Status
8	Metastatic Cancer and Acute Leukemia	83	Respiratory Arrest
9	Lung and Other Severe Cancers	84	Cardio-Respiratory Failure and Shock
10	Lymphoma and Other Cancers	85	Congestive Heart Failure
11	Colorectal, Bladder, and Other Cancers	86	Acute Myocardial Infarction
12	Breast, Prostate, and Other Cancers and Tumors	87	Unstable Angina and Other Acute Ischemic Heart Disease
17	Diabetes with Acute Complications	88	Angina Pectoris
18	Diabetes with Chronic Complications	96	Specified Heart Arrhythmias
19	Diabetes without Complication	99	Intracranial Hemorrhage
21	Protein-Calorie Malnutrition	100	Ischemic or Unspecified Stroke
22	Morbid Obesity	103	Hemiplegia/Hemiparesis
23	Other Significant Endocrine and Metabolic Disorders	104	Monoplegia, Other Paralytic Syndromes
27	End-Stage Liver Disease	106	Atherosclerosis of the Extremities with Ulceration or Gangrene
28	Cirrhosis of Liver	107	Vascular Disease with Complications
29	Chronic Hepatitis	108	Vascular Disease
33	Intestinal Obstruction/Perforation	110	Cystic Fibrosis
34	Chronic Pancreatitis	111	Chronic Obstructive Pulmonary Disease
35	Inflammatory Bowel Disease	112	Fibrosis of Lung and Other Chronic Lung Disorders
39	Bone/Joint/Muscle Infections/Necrosis	114	Aspiration and Specified Bacterial Pneumonias
40	Rheumatoid Arthritis and Inflammatory Connective Tissue Disease	115	Pneumococcal Pneumonia, Empyema, Lung Abscess
46	Severe Hematological Disorders	122	Proliferative Diabetic Retinopathy and Vitreous Hemorrhage
47	Disorders of Immunity	124	Exudative Macular Degeneration
48	Coagulation Defects and Other Specified Hematological Disorders	134	Dialysis Status
51	Dementia With Complications	135	Acute Renal Failure
52	Dementia Without Complication	136	Chronic Kidney Disease, Stage 5
54	Substance Use with Psychotic Complications	137	Chronic Kidney Disease, Severe (Stage 4)
55	Substance Use Disorder, Moderate/Severe, or Substance Use with Complications	138	Chronic Kidney Disease, Moderate (Stage 3)
56	Substance Use Disorder, Mild, Except Alcohol and Cannabis	157	Pressure Ulcer of Skin with Necrosis Through to Muscle, Tendon, or Bone
57	Schizophrenia	158	Pressure Ulcer of Skin with Full Thickness Skin Loss
58	Reactive and Unspecified Psychosis	159	Pressure Ulcer of Skin with Partial Thickness Skin Loss
59	Major Depressive, Bipolar, and Paranoid Disorders	161	Chronic Ulcer of Skin, Except Pressure
60	Personality Disorders	162	Severe Skin Burn or Condition
70	Quadriplegia	166	Severe Head Injury
71	Paraplegia	167	Major Head Injury
72	Spinal Cord Disorders/Injuries	169	Vertebral Fractures without Spinal Cord Injury
73	Amyotrophic Lateral Sclerosis and Other Motor Neuron Disease	170	Hip Fracture/Dislocation
74	Cerebral Palsy	173	Traumatic Amputations and Complications
75	Myasthenia Gravis/Myoneural Disorders and Guillain-Barre Syndrome/Inflammatory and Toxic Neuropathy	176	Complications of Specified Implanted Device or Graft
76	Muscular Dystrophy	186	Major Organ Transplant or Replacement Status
77	Multiple Sclerosis	188	Artificial Openings for Feeding or Elimination
78	Parkinson's and Huntington's Diseases	189	Amputation Status, Lower Limb/Amputation Complications

HCC Codes and Descriptions (HHS-HCC v07)

1	HIV/AIDS	61	Osteogenesis Imperfecta and Other Osteodystrophies
2	Septicemia, Sepsis, Systemic Inflammatory Response Syndrome/Shock	62	Congenital/Developmental Skeletal and Connective Tissue Disorders
3	Central Nervous System Infections, Except Viral Meningitis	63	Cleft Lip/Cleft Palate
4	Viral or Unspecified Meningitis	64	Major Congenital Anomalies of Diaphragm, Abdominal Wall, and Esophagus, Age < 2
6	Opportunistic Infections	66	Hemophilia
8	Metastatic Cancer	67	Myelodysplastic Syndromes and Myelofibrosis
9	Lung, Brain, and Other Severe Cancers, Including Pediatric Acute Lymphoid Leukemia	68	Aplastic Anemia
10	Non-Hodgkin Lymphomas and Other Cancers and Tumors	69	Acquired Hemolytic Anemia, Including Hemolytic Disease of Newborn
11	Colorectal, Breast (Age < 50), Kidney, and Other Cancers	70	Sickle Cell Anemia (Hb-SS)
12	Breast (Age 50+) and Prostate Cancer, Benign/Uncertain Brain Tumors, and Other Cancers and Tumors	71	Beta Thalassemia Major
13	Thyroid Cancer, Melanoma, Neurofibromatosis, and Other Cancers and Tumors	73	Combined and Other Severe Immunodeficiencies
18	Pancreas Transplant Status	74	Disorders of the Immune Mechanism
19	Diabetes with Acute Complications	75	Coagulation Defects and Other Specified Hematological Disorders
20	Diabetes with Chronic Complications	81	Drug Use with Psychotic Complications
21	Diabetes without Complication	82	Drug Use Disorder, Moderate/Severe, or Drug Use with Non-Psychotic Complications
22	Type 1 Diabetes Mellitus, add-on to Diabetes HCCs 19-21	83	Alcohol Use with Psychotic Complications
23	Protein-Calorie Malnutrition	84	Alcohol Use Disorder, Moderate/Severe, or Alcohol Use with Specified Non-Psychotic Complications
26	Mucopolysaccharidosis	87.1	Schizophrenia
27	Lipidoses and Glycogenosis	87.2	Delusional and Other Specified Psychotic Disorders, Unspecified Psychosis
28	Congenital Metabolic Disorders, Not Elsewhere Classified	88	Major Depressive Disorder, Severe, and Bipolar Disorders
29	Amyloidosis, Porphyria, and Other Metabolic Disorders	90	Personality Disorders
30	Adrenal, Pituitary, and Other Significant Endocrine Disorders	94	Anorexia/Bulimia Nervosa
34	Liver Transplant Status/Complications	96	Prader-Willi, Patau, Edwards, and Autosomal Deletion Syndromes
35.1	Acute Liver Failure/Disease, Including Neonatal Hepatitis	97	Down Syndrome, Fragile X, Other Chromosomal Anomalies, and Congenital Malformation Syndromes
35.2	Chronic Liver Failure/End-Stage Liver Disorders	102	Autistic Disorder
36	Cirrhosis of Liver	103	Pervasive Developmental Disorders, Except Autistic Disorder
37.1	Chronic Viral Hepatitis C	106	Traumatic Complete Lesion Cervical Spinal Cord
37.2	Chronic Hepatitis, Except Chronic Viral Hepatitis C	107	Quadriplegia
41	Intestine Transplant Status/Complications	108	Traumatic Complete Lesion Dorsal Spinal Cord
42	Peritonitis/Gastrointestinal Perforation/Necrotizing Enterocolitis	109	Paraplegia
45	Intestinal Obstruction	110	Spinal Cord Disorders/Injuries
46	Chronic Pancreatitis	111	Amyotrophic Lateral Sclerosis and Other Anterior Horn Cell Disease
47	Acute Pancreatitis	112	Quadriplegic Cerebral Palsy
48	Inflammatory Bowel Disease	113	Cerebral Palsy, Except Quadriplegic
54	Necrotizing Fasciitis	114	Spina Bifida and Other Brain/Spinal/Nervous System Congenital Anomalies
55	Bone/Joint/Muscle Infections/Necrosis	115	Myasthenia Gravis/Myoneural Disorders and Guillain-Barre Syndrome/Inflammatory and Toxic Neuropathy
56	Rheumatoid Arthritis and Specified Autoimmune Disorders	117	Muscular Dystrophy

HCC Codes and Descriptions (HHS-HCC v07)

57	Systemic Lupus Erythematosus and Other Autoimmune Disorders	118	Multiple Sclerosis
119	Parkinson's, Huntington's, and Spinocerebellar Disease, and Other Neurodegenerative Disorders	188	Chronic Kidney Disease, Severe (Stage 4)
120	Seizure Disorders and Convulsions	203	Ectopic and Molar Pregnancy
121	Hydrocephalus	204	Miscarriage with Complications
122	Coma, Brain Compression/Anoxic Damage	205	Miscarriage with No or Minor Complications
123	Narcolepsy and Cataplexy	207	Pregnancy with Delivery with Major Complications
125	Respirator Dependence/Tracheostomy Status	208	Pregnancy with Delivery with Complications
126	Respiratory Arrest	209	Pregnancy with Delivery with No or Minor Complications
127	Cardio-Respiratory Failure and Shock, Including Respiratory Distress Syndromes	210	(Ongoing) Pregnancy without Delivery with Major Complications
128	Heart Assistive Device/Artificial Heart	211	(Ongoing) Pregnancy without Delivery with Complications
129	Heart Transplant Status/Complications	212	(Ongoing) Pregnancy without Delivery with No or Minor Complications
130	Heart Failure	217	Chronic Ulcer of Skin, Except Pressure
131	Acute Myocardial Infarction	218	Extensive Third Degree Burns
132	Unstable Angina and Other Acute Ischemic Heart Disease	219	Major Skin Burn or Condition
135	Heart Infection/Inflammation, Except Rheumatic	223	Severe Head Injury
137	Hypoplastic Left Heart Syndrome and Other Severe Congenital Heart Disorders	226	Hip and Pelvic Fractures
138	Major Congenital Heart/Circulatory Disorders	228	Vertebral Fractures without Spinal Cord Injury
139	Atrial and Ventricular Septal Defects, Patent Ductus Arteriosus, and Other Congenital Heart/Circulatory Disorders	234	Traumatic Amputations and Amputation Complications
142	Specified Heart Arrhythmias	242	Extremely Immature Newborns, Birthweight < 500 Grams
145	Intracranial Hemorrhage	243	Extremely Immature Newborns, Including Birthweight 500-749 Grams
146	Ischemic or Unspecified Stroke	244	Extremely Immature Newborns, Including Birthweight 750-999 Grams
149	Cerebral Aneurysm and Arteriovenous Malformation	245	Premature Newborns, Including Birthweight 1000-1499 Grams
150	Hemiplegia/Hemiparesis	246	Premature Newborns, Including Birthweight 1500-1999 Grams
151	Monoplegia, Other Paralytic Syndromes	247	Premature Newborns, Including Birthweight 2000-2499 Grams
153	Atherosclerosis of the Extremities with Ulceration or Gangrene	248	Other Premature, Low Birthweight, Malnourished, or Multiple Birth Newborns
154	Vascular Disease with Complications	249	Term or Post-Term Singleton Newborn, Normal or High Birthweight
156	Pulmonary Embolism and Deep Vein Thrombosis	251	Stem Cell, Including Bone Marrow, Transplant Status/Complications
158	Lung Transplant Status/Complications	253	Artificial Openings for Feeding or Elimination
159	Cystic Fibrosis	254	Amputation Status, Upper Limb or Lower Limb
160	Chronic Obstructive Pulmonary Disease, Including Bronchiectasis		
161.1	Severe Asthma		
161.2	Asthma, Except Severe		
162	Fibrosis of Lung and Other Lung Disorders		
163	Aspiration and Specified Bacterial Pneumonias and Other Severe Lung Infections		
174	Exudative Macular Degeneration		
183	Kidney Transplant Status/Complications		
184	End Stage Renal Disease		
187	Chronic Kidney Disease, Stage 5		

HCC Codes and Descriptions (ESRD-HCC v21)

1	HIV/AIDS	86	Acute Myocardial Infarction
2	Septicemia, Sepsis, Systemic Inflammatory Response Syndrome/Shock	87	Unstable Angina and Other Acute Ischemic Heart Disease
6	Opportunistic Infections	88	Angina Pectoris
8	Metastatic Cancer and Acute Leukemia	96	Specified Heart Arrhythmias
9	Lung, Brain, and Other Severe Cancers	99	Cerebral Hemorrhage
10	Lymphoma and Other Cancers	100	Ischemic or Unspecified Stroke
11	Colorectal, Bladder, and Other Cancers	103	Hemiplegia/Hemiparesis
12	Breast, Prostate, and Other Cancers and Tumors	104	Monoplegia, Other Paralytic Syndromes
17	Diabetes with Acute Complications	106	Atherosclerosis of the Extremities with Ulceration or Gangrene
18	Diabetes with Chronic Complications	107	Vascular Disease with Complications
19	Diabetes without Complication	108	Vascular Disease
21	Protein-Calorie Malnutrition	110	Cystic Fibrosis
22	Morbid Obesity	111	Chronic Obstructive Pulmonary Disease
23	Other Significant Endocrine and Metabolic Disorders	112	Fibrosis of Lung and Other Chronic Lung Disorders
27	End-Stage Liver Disease	114	Aspiration and Specified Bacterial Pneumonias
28	Cirrhosis of Liver	115	Pneumococcal Pneumonia, Empyema, Lung Abscess
29	Chronic Hepatitis	122	Proliferative Diabetic Retinopathy and Vitreous Hemorrhage
33	Intestinal Obstruction/Perforation	124	Exudative Macular Degeneration
34	Chronic Pancreatitis	134	Dialysis Status
35	Inflammatory Bowel Disease	135	Acute Renal Failure
39	Bone/Joint/Muscle Infections/Necrosis	136	Chronic Kidney Disease, Stage 5
40	Rheumatoid Arthritis and Inflammatory Connective Tissue Disease	137	Chronic Kidney Disease, Severe (Stage 4)
46	Severe Hematological Disorders	138	Chronic Kidney Disease, Moderate (Stage 3)
47	Disorders of Immunity	139	Chronic Kidney Disease, Mild or Unspecified (Stages 1-2 or Unspecified)
48	Coagulation Defects and Other Specified Hematological Disorders	140	Unspecified Renal Failure
51	Dementia With Complications	141	Nephritis
52	Dementia Without Complication	157	Pressure Ulcer of Skin with Necrosis Through to Muscle, Tendon, or Bone
54	Drug/Alcohol Psychosis	158	Pressure Ulcer of Skin with Full Thickness Skin Loss
55	Drug/Alcohol Dependence	159	Pressure Ulcer of Skin with Partial Thickness Skin Loss
57	Schizophrenia	160	Pressure Pre-Ulcer Skin Changes or Unspecified Stage
58	Major Depressive, Bipolar, and Paranoid Disorders	161	Chronic Ulcer of Skin, Except Pressure
70	Quadriplegia	162	Severe Skin Burn or Condition
71	Paraplegia	166	Severe Head Injury
72	Spinal Cord Disorders/Injuries	167	Vertebral Fractures without Spinal Cord Injury
73	Amyotrophic Lateral Sclerosis and Other Motor Neuron Disease	169	Pathological Fractures, Except of Vertebrae, Hip, or Humerus
74	Cerebral Palsy	170	Hip Fracture/Dislocation
75	Polyneuropathy	173	Traumatic Amputations and Complications
76	Muscular Dystrophy	176	Complications of Specified Implanted Device or Graft
77	Multiple Sclerosis	186	Major Organ Transplant or Replacement Status
78	Parkinson's and Huntington's Diseases	188	Artificial Openings for Feeding or Elimination
79	Seizure Disorders and Convulsions	189	Amputation Status, Lower Limb/Amputation Complications
80	Coma, Brain Compression/Anoxic Damage		
82	Respirator Dependence/Tracheostomy Status		
83	Respiratory Arrest		
84	Cardio-Respiratory Failure and Shock		
85	Congestive Heart Failure		

Notes

HCC Codes and Descriptions (ESRD-HCC v24)

1	HIV/AIDS	80	Coma, Brain Compression/Anoxic Damage
2	Septicemia, Sepsis, Systemic Inflammatory Response Syndrome/Shock	82	Respirator Dependence/Tracheostomy Status
6	Opportunistic Infections	83	Respiratory Arrest
8	Metastatic Cancer and Acute Leukemia	84	Cardio-Respiratory Failure and Shock
9	Lung and Other Severe Cancers	85	Congestive Heart Failure
10	Lymphoma and Other Cancers	86	Acute Myocardial Infarction
11	Colorectal, Bladder, and Other Cancers	87	Unstable Angina and Other Acute Ischemic Heart Disease
12	Breast, Prostate, and Other Cancers and Tumors	88	Angina Pectoris
17	Diabetes with Acute Complications	96	Specified Heart Arrhythmias
18	Diabetes with Chronic Complications	99	Intracranial Hemorrhage
19	Diabetes without Complication	100	Ischemic or Unspecified Stroke
21	Protein-Calorie Malnutrition	103	Hemiplegia/Hemiparesis
22	Morbid Obesity	104	Monoplegia, Other Paralytic Syndromes
23	Other Significant Endocrine and Metabolic Disorders	106	Atherosclerosis of the Extremities with Ulceration or Gangrene
27	End-Stage Liver Disease	107	Vascular Disease with Complications
28	Cirrhosis of Liver	108	Vascular Disease
29	Chronic Hepatitis	110	Cystic Fibrosis
33	Intestinal Obstruction/Perforation	111	Chronic Obstructive Pulmonary Disease
34	Chronic Pancreatitis	112	Fibrosis of Lung and Other Chronic Lung Disorders
35	Inflammatory Bowel Disease	114	Aspiration and Specified Bacterial Pneumonias
39	Bone/Joint/Muscle Infections/Necrosis	115	Pneumococcal Pneumonia, Empyema, Lung Abscess
40	Rheumatoid Arthritis and Inflammatory Connective Tissue Disease	122	Proliferative Diabetic Retinopathy and Vitreous Hemorrhage
46	Severe Hematological Disorders	124	Exudative Macular Degeneration
47	Disorders of Immunity	134	Dialysis Status
48	Coagulation Defects and Other Specified Hematological Disorders	135	Acute Renal Failure
51	Dementia With Complications	136	Chronic Kidney Disease, Stage 5
52	Dementia Without Complication	137	Chronic Kidney Disease, Severe (Stage 4)
54	Substance Use with Psychotic Complications	138	Chronic Kidney Disease, Moderate (Stage 3)
55	Substance Use Disorder, Moderate/Severe, or Substance Use with Complications	157	Pressure Ulcer of Skin with Necrosis Through to Muscle, Tendon, or Bone
56	Substance Use Disorder, Mild, Except Alcohol and Cannabis	158	Pressure Ulcer of Skin with Full Thickness Skin Loss
57	Schizophrenia	159	Pressure Ulcer of Skin with Partial Thickness Skin Loss
58	Reactive and Unspecified Psychosis	161	Chronic Ulcer of Skin, Except Pressure
59	Major Depressive, Bipolar, and Paranoid Disorders	162	Severe Skin Burn or Condition
60	Personality Disorders	166	Severe Head Injury
70	Quadriplegia	167	Major Head Injury
71	Paraplegia	169	Vertebral Fractures without Spinal Cord Injury
72	Spinal Cord Disorders/Injuries	170	Hip Fracture/Dislocation
73	Amyotrophic Lateral Sclerosis and Other Motor Neuron Disease	173	Traumatic Amputations and Complications
74	Cerebral Palsy	176	Complications of Specified Implanted Device or Graft
75	Myasthenia Gravis/Myoneural Disorders and Guillain-Barre Syndrome/Inflammatory and Toxic Neuropathy	186	Major Organ Transplant or Replacement Status
76	Muscular Dystrophy	188	Artificial Openings for Feeding or Elimination
77	Multiple Sclerosis	189	Amputation Status, Lower Limb/Amputation Complications
78	Parkinson's and Huntington's Diseases		
79	Seizure Disorders and Convulsions		

HCC Codes and Descriptions (Rx-HCC v05)

1	HIV/AIDS	148	Mild or Unspecified Intellectual Disability/ Developmental Disorder
5	Opportunistic Infections	156	Myasthenia Gravis, Amyotrophic Lateral Sclerosis and Other Motor Neuron Disease
15	Chronic Myeloid Leukemia	157	Spinal Cord Disorders
16	Multiple Myeloma and Other Neoplastic Disorders	159	Inflammatory and Toxic Neuropathy
17	Secondary Cancers of Bone, Lung, Brain, and Other Specified Sites; Liver Cancer	160	Multiple Sclerosis
18	Lung, Kidney, and Other Cancers	161	Parkinson's and Huntington's Diseases
19	Breast and Other Cancers and Tumors	163	Intractable Epilepsy
30	Diabetes with Complications	164	Epilepsy and Other Seizure Disorders, Except Intractable Epilepsy
31	Diabetes without Complication	165	Convulsions
40	Specified Hereditary Metabolic/Immune Disorders	166	Migraine Headaches
41	Pituitary, Adrenal Gland, and Other Endocrine and Metabolic Disorders	168	Trigeminal and Postherpetic Neuralgia
42	Thyroid Disorders	185	Primary Pulmonary Hypertension
43	Morbid Obesity	186	Congestive Heart Failure
45	Disorders of Lipoid Metabolism	187	Hypertension
54	Chronic Viral Hepatitis C	188	Coronary Artery Disease
55	Chronic Viral Hepatitis, Except Hepatitis C	193	Atrial Arrhythmias
65	Chronic Pancreatitis	206	Cerebrovascular Disease, Except Hemorrhage or Aneurysm
66	Pancreatic Disorders and Intestinal Malabsorption, Except Pancreatitis	207	Spastic Hemiplegia
67	Inflammatory Bowel Disease	215	Venous Thromboembolism
68	Esophageal Reflux and Other Disorders of Esophagus	216	Peripheral Vascular Disease
80	Aseptic Necrosis of Bone	225	Cystic Fibrosis
82	Psoriatic Arthropathy and Systemic Sclerosis	226	Chronic Obstructive Pulmonary Disease and Asthma
83	Rheumatoid Arthritis and Other Inflammatory Polyarthropathy	227	Pulmonary Fibrosis and Other Chronic Lung Disorders
84	Systemic Lupus Erythematosus, Other Connective Tissue Disorders, and Inflammatory Spondylopathies	241	Diabetic Retinopathy
87	Osteoporosis, Vertebral and Pathological Fractures	243	Open-Angle Glaucoma
95	Sickle Cell Anemia	260	Kidney Transplant Status
96	Myelodysplastic Syndromes and Myelofibrosis	261	Dialysis Status
97	Immune Disorders	262	Chronic Kidney Disease Stage 5
98	Aplastic Anemia and Other Significant Blood Disorders	263	Chronic Kidney Disease Stage 4
111	Alzheimer's Disease	311	Chronic Ulcer of Skin, Except Pressure
112	Dementia, Except Alzheimer's Disease	314	Pemphigus
130	Schizophrenia	316	Psoriasis, Except with Arthropathy
131	Bipolar Disorders	355	Narcolepsy and Cataplexy
132	Major Depression	395	Lung Transplant Status
133	Specified Anxiety, Personality, and Behavior Disorders	396	Major Organ Transplant Status, Except Lung, Kidney, and Pancreas
134	Depression	397	Pancreas Transplant Status
135	Anxiety Disorders	395	Lung Transplant Status
145	Autism	396	Major Organ Transplant Status, Except Lung, Kidney, and Pancreas
146	Profound or Severe Intellectual Disability/ Developmental Disorder	397	Pancreas Transplant Status
147	Moderate Intellectual Disability/Developmental Disorder		

HCC Codes and Descriptions (Rx-HCC v08)

1	HIV/AIDS	146	Profound or Severe Intellectual Disability/Developmental Disorder
5	Opportunistic Infections	147	Moderate Intellectual Disability/Developmental Disorder
15	Chronic Myeloid Leukemia	148	Mild or Unspecified Intellectual Disability/Developmental Disorder
16	Multiple Myeloma and Other Hematologic Cancers	153	Myasthenia Gravis and Other Myoneural Disorders
17	Secondary Cancer of Bone and Kidney	154	Amyotrophic Lateral Sclerosis and Other Motor Neuron Disease
18	Secondary Cancer of Lung, Liver, Brain, and Other Sites	155	Spinal Cord Disorders
19	Leukemias and Other Hematologic Cancers	157	Chronic Inflammatory Demyelinating Polyneuritis
20	Lung, Kidney, and Other Cancers; Secondary Cancer of Lymph Nodes and Other Sites	158	Inflammatory and Toxic Neuropathy
21	Lymphomas and Other Hematologic Cancers	159	Multiple Sclerosis
22	Prostate, Breast, Bladder, and Other Cancers and Tumors	160	Huntington Disease
30	Diabetes with Complications	161	Parkinson Disease
31	Diabetes without Complication	163	Intractable Epilepsy
40	Alpha-1-Antitrypsin Deficiency	164	Epilepsy and Other Seizure Disorders, Except Intractable Epilepsy
41	Lysosomal Storage Disorders	166	Migraine Headaches
42	Acromegaly and Other Endocrine and Metabolic Disorders	168	Trigeminal and Postherpetic Neuralgia
43	Pituitary, Adrenal Gland, and Other Endocrine and Metabolic Disorders	183	Pulmonary Arterial Hypertension
44	Thyroid Disorders	184	Pulmonary Hypertension, Except Arterial, and Other Pulmonary Heart Disease
47	Disorders of Lipoid Metabolism	186	Heart Failure
54	Chronic Viral Hepatitis C	187	Hypertension
55	Acute or Unspecified Viral Hepatitis C	188	Coronary Artery Disease
56	Chronic Viral Hepatitis B and Other Specified Chronic Viral Hepatitis	191	Ventricular Septal Defect and Major Congenital Heart Disorders
59	Primary Biliary Cirrhosis	193	Atrial Arrhythmias
65	Chronic Pancreatitis	207	Spastic Hemiplegia
66	Pancreatic Disorders and Intestinal Malabsorption, Except Pancreatitis	215	Venous Thromboembolism
67	Inflammatory Bowel Disease	225	Cystic Fibrosis
80	Aseptic Necrosis of Bone	226	Idiopathic Pulmonary Fibrosis and Systemic Sclerosis with Lung Involvement
81	Psoriatic Arthropathy	227	Pulmonary Fibrosis, Except Idiopathic
82	Systemic Sclerosis	228	Severe Persistent Asthma
83	Rheumatoid Arthritis and Other Inflammatory Polyarthropathy	229	Chronic Obstructive Pulmonary Disease, Bronchiectasis, and Other Asthma
84	Systemic Lupus Erythematosus and Other Systemic Connective Tissue Disorders	243	Glaucoma, Open-Angle or Moderate/Severe Stage
87	Osteoporosis, Vertebral and Pathological Fractures	244	Other Non-Acute Glaucoma
95	Sickle Cell Anemia	260	Kidney Transplant Status
96	Acquired Hemolytic, Aplastic, and Sideroblastic Anemias	261	Dialysis Status, Including End Stage Renal Disease
98	Hereditary Angioedema and Other Defects in the Complement System	262	Chronic Kidney Disease Stage 5
99	Immune Disorders	263	Chronic Kidney Disease Stage 4
100	Immune Thrombocytopenic Purpura	311	Chronic Ulcer of Skin, Except Pressure
111	Alzheimer's Disease	314	Pemphigus, Pemphigoid, and Other Bullous Skin Disorders
112	Dementia, Except Alzheimer's Disease	316	Psoriasis, Except with Arthropathy
130	Schizophrenia and Other Psychosis	317	Discoid Lupus Erythematosus
131	Bipolar Disorders	355	Narcolepsy and Cataplexy
132	Depression	395	Stem Cell, Including Bone Marrow, Transplant Status/Complications
133	Anxiety and Other Psychiatric Disorders	396	Heart, Lung, Liver, Intestine, or Pancreas Transplant Status

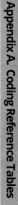

Figure A.3

Hospital-acquired Condition (HAC)	
01	Foreign Object Retained After Surgery
02	Air Embolism
03	Blood Incompatibility
04	Stage III and IV Pressure Ulcers
05	Falls and Trauma
06	Catheter-Associated Urinary Tract Infection (UTI)
07	Vascular Catheter-Associated Infection
08	Surgical Site Infection, Mediastinitis following Coronary Artery Bypass Graft (CABG)
09	Manifestations of Poor Glycemic Control
10	Deep Vein Thrombosis (DVT) / Pulmonary Embolism (PE) with Total Knee or Hip Replacement
11	Surgical Site Infection Following Bariatric Surgery
12	Surgical Site Infection Following Certain Orthopedic Procedures of Spine, Shoulder and Elbow
13	Surgical Site Infection (SSI) Following Cardiac Implantable Electronic Device (CIED)
14	Iatrogenic Pneumothorax with Venous Catheterization

Notes:

Notes:

Notes

Appendix B. ICD-10-CM Abridged Official Guidelines

Introduction

One of the first steps to learning a new language is to become familiar with the rules of grammar. Official coding guidelines include conventions and directions that are like the rules of grammar for ICD-10-CM. Once they are understood, the user can become "fluent" in the new language. Knowing the codes (vocabulary) is not enough, because without the knowledge of grammar structure (guidelines), errors in code selection could happen. Guidelines aid providers and coders to ensure accurate coding. Therefore, it is imperative that providers and support staff know and understand them. Chapter 1 – Diagnosis Coding Essentials contains a discussion of many of these guidelines, along with examples.

Providers are usually not interested in coding guidelines, however; these are the rules that payers play by, and can ultimately use to deny payment. The complete guidelines contain information about circumstances and codes that may not be needed for your specialty. In an attempt to make this section slightly more appealing, many guidelines were not included. The text of Chapter 1 – Diagnosis Coding Essentials reviews the important guidelines from Section *I*, *A* and *B*, but not *C*. Section *I.C* is, by far, the longest portion of the guidelines. They cover rules specific to each chapter.

> **Alert:** This introduction is created by ChiroCode. The remainder of this chapter is excerpted directly from the Official ICD-10-CM Guidelines.

Table of Contents

Table of Contents (continued)

Table of Contents (continued)

ICD-10-CM Official Guidelines for Coding and Reporting FY 2023 (October 1, 2022 - September 30, 2023)

Narrative changes appear in **bold** text

Items underlined have been moved within the guidelines since the FY 2021 version

Italics are used to indicate revisions to heading changes

The Centers for Medicare and Medicaid Services (CMS) and the National Center for Health Statistics (NCHS), two departments within the U.S. Federal Government's Department of Health and Human Services (DHHS) provide the following guidelines for coding and reporting using the International Classification of Diseases, 10th Revision, Clinical Modification (ICD-10-CM). These guidelines should be used as a companion document to the official version of the ICD-10- CM as published on the NCHS website. The ICD-10-CM is a morbidity classification published by the United States for classifying diagnoses and reason for visits in all health care settings. The ICD-10-CM is based on the ICD-10, the statistical classification of disease published by the World Health Organization (WHO).

These guidelines have been approved by the four organizations that make up the Cooperating Parties for the ICD-10-CM: the American Hospital Association (AHA), the American Health Information Management Association (AHIMA), CMS, and NCHS.

These guidelines are a set of rules that have been developed to accompany and complement the official conventions and instructions provided within the ICD-10-CM itself. The instructions and conventions of the classification take precedence over guidelines. These guidelines are based on the coding and sequencing instructions in the Tabular List and Alphabetic Index of ICD-10-CM, but provide additional instruction. Adherence to these guidelines when assigning ICD-10-CM diagnosis codes is required under the Health Insurance Portability and Accountability Act (HIPAA). The diagnosis codes (Tabular List and Alphabetic Index) have been adopted under HIPAA for all healthcare settings. A joint effort between the healthcare provider and the coder is essential to achieve complete and accurate documentation, code assignment, and reporting of diagnoses and procedures. These guidelines have been developed to assist both the healthcare provider and the coder in identifying those diagnoses that are to be reported. The importance of consistent, complete documentation in the medical record cannot be overemphasized. Without such documentation accurate coding cannot be achieved. The entire record should be reviewed to determine the specific reason for the encounter and the conditions treated.

The term encounter is used for all settings, including hospital admissions. In the context of these guidelines, the term provider is used throughout the guidelines to mean physician or any qualified health care practitioner who is legally accountable for establishing the patient's diagnosis. Only this set of guidelines, approved by the Cooperating Parties, is official.

The guidelines are organized into sections. Section I includes the structure and conventions of the classification and general guidelines that apply to the entire classification, and chapter-specific guidelines that correspond to the chapters as they are arranged in the classification. Section II includes guidelines for selection of principal diagnosis for non-outpatient settings. Section III includes guidelines for reporting additional diagnoses in non-outpatient settings. Section IV is for outpatient coding and reporting. It is necessary to review all sections of the guidelines to fully understand all of the rules and instructions needed to code properly.

Section I. Conventions, general coding guidelines and chapter specific guidelines

The conventions, general guidelines and chapter-specific guidelines are applicable to all health care settings unless otherwise indicated. The conventions and instructions of the classification take precedence over guidelines.

A. Conventions for the ICD-10-CM

The conventions for the ICD-10-CM are the general rules for use of the classification independent of the guidelines. These conventions are incorporated within the Alphabetic Index and Tabular List of the ICD-10-CM as instructional notes.

1. The Alphabetic Index and Tabular List

The ICD-10-CM is divided into the Alphabetic Index, an alphabetical list of terms and their corresponding code, and the Tabular List, a structured list of codes divided into chapters based on body system or condition. The Alphabetic Index consists of the following parts: the Index of Diseases and Injury, the Index of External Causes of Injury, the Table of Neoplasms and the Table of Drugs and Chemicals.

See Section I.C2. General guidelines
See Section I.C.19. Adverse effects, poisoning, underdosing and toxic effects

2. Format and Structure:

The ICD-10-CM Tabular List contains categories, subcategories and codes. Characters for categories, subcategories and codes may be either a letter or a number. All categories are 3 characters. A three-character category that has no further subdivision is equivalent to a code. Subcategories are either 4 or 5 characters. Codes may be 3, 4, 5, 6 or 7 characters. That is, each level of subdivision after a category is a subcategory. The final level of subdivision is a code. Codes that have applicable 7th characters are still referred to as codes, not subcategories. A code that has an applicable 7th character is considered invalid without the 7th character.

The ICD-10-CM uses an indented format for ease in reference.

3. Use of codes for reporting purposes

For reporting purposes only codes are permissible, not categories or subcategories, and any applicable 7th character is required.

4. Placeholder character

The ICD-10-CM utilizes a placeholder character "X". The "X" is used as a placeholder at certain codes to allow for future expansion. An example of this is at the poisoning, adverse effect and underdosing codes, categories T36-T50.

Where a placeholder exists, the X must be used in order for the code to be considered a valid code.

5. 7th Characters

Certain ICD-10-CM categories have applicable 7th characters. The applicable 7th character is required for all codes within the category, or as the notes in the Tabular List instruct. The 7th character must always be the 7th character in the data field. If a code that requires a 7th character is not 6 characters, a placeholder X must be used to fill in the empty characters.

6. Abbreviations

a. Alphabetic Index abbreviations

NEC — "Not elsewhere classifiable"

This abbreviation in the Alphabetic Index represents "other specified." When a specific code is not available for a condition, the Alphabetic Index directs the coder to the "other specified" code in the Tabular List.

NOS — "Not otherwise specified"

This abbreviation is the equivalent of unspecified.

b. Tabular List abbreviations

NEC — "Not elsewhere classifiable"

This abbreviation in the Tabular List represents "other specified." When a specific code is not available for a condition, the Tabular List includes an NEC entry under a code to identify the code as the "other specified" code.

NOS — "Not otherwise specified"

This abbreviation is the equivalent of unspecified.

7. Punctuation

[ ] — Brackets are used in the Tabular List to enclose synonyms, alternative wording or explanatory phrases. Brackets are used in the Alphabetic Index to identify manifestation codes.

( ) — Parentheses are used in both the Alphabetic Index and Tabular List to enclose supplementary words that may be present or absent in the statement of a disease or procedure without affecting the code number to which it is assigned. The terms within the parentheses are referred to as nonessential modifiers. The nonessential modifiers in the Alphabetic Index to Diseases apply to subterms following a main term except when a nonessential modifier and a subentry are mutually exclusive, the subentry takes precedence. For example, in the ICD-10-CM Alphabetic Index under the main term Enteritis, "acute" is a nonessential modifier and "chronic" is a subentry. In this case, the nonessential modifier "acute" does not apply to the subentry "chronic".

: — Colons are used in the Tabular List after an incomplete term which needs one or more of the modifiers following the colon to make it assignable to a given category.

8. Use of "and".

See Section I.A.14. Use of the term "And"

9. Other and Unspecified codes

a. "Other" codes

Codes titled "other" or "other specified" are for use when the information in the medical record provides detail for which a specific code does not exist. Alphabetic Index entries with NEC in the line designate "other" codes in the Tabular List. These Alphabetic Index entries represent specific disease entities for which no specific code exists so the term is included within an "other" code.

b. "Unspecified" codes

Codes titled "unspecified" are for use when the information in the medical record is insufficient to assign a more specific code. For those categories for which an unspecified code is not provided, the "other specified" code may represent both other and unspecified.

See Section I.B.18 Use of Signs/Symptom/Unspecified Codes

10. Includes Notes

This note appears immediately under a three character code title to further define, or give examples of, the content of the category.

11. Inclusion terms

List of terms is included under some codes. These terms are the conditions for which that code is to be used. The terms may be synonyms of the code title, or, in the case of "other specified" codes, the terms are a list of the various conditions assigned to that code. The inclusion terms are not necessarily exhaustive. Additional terms found only in the Alphabetic Index may also be assigned to a code.

12. Excludes Notes

The ICD-10-CM has two types of excludes notes. Each type of note has a different definition for use but they are all similar in that they indicate that codes excluded from each other are independent of each other.

a. Excludes1

A type 1 Excludes note is a pure excludes note. It means "NOT CODED HERE!" An Excludes1 note indicates that the code excluded should never be used at the same time as the code above the Excludes1 note. An Excludes1 is used when two conditions cannot occur together, such as a congenital form versus an acquired form of the same condition.

An exception to the Excludes1 definition is the circumstance when the two conditions are unrelated to each other. If it is not clear whether the two conditions involving an Excludes1 note are related or not, query the provider. For example, code F45.8, Other somatoform disorders, has an Excludes1 note for "sleep related teeth grinding (G47.63)," because "teeth grinding" is an inclusion term under F45.8. Only one of these two codes should be assigned for teeth grinding. However psychogenic dysmenorrhea is also an inclusion term under F45.8, and a patient could have both this condition and sleep related teeth grinding. In this case, the two conditions are clearly unrelated to each other, and so it would be appropriate to report F45.8 and G47.63 together.

b. Excludes2

A type 2 Excludes note represents "Not included here." An excludes2 note indicates that the condition excluded is not part of the condition represented by the code, but a patient may have both conditions at the same time. When an Excludes2 note appears under a code, it is acceptable to use both the code and the excluded code together, when appropriate.

13. Etiology/manifestation convention ("code first", "use additional code" and "in diseases classified elsewhere" notes)

Certain conditions have both an underlying etiology and multiple body system manifestations due to the underlying etiology. For such conditions, the ICD-10-CM has a coding convention that requires the underlying condition be sequenced first, if applicable, followed by the manifestation. Wherever such a combination exists, there is a "use additional code" note at the etiology code, and a "code first" note at the manifestation code. These instructional notes indicate the proper sequencing order of the codes, etiology followed by manifestation.

In most cases the manifestation codes will have in the code title, "in diseases classified elsewhere." Codes with this title are a component of the etiology/ manifestation convention. The code title indicates that it is a manifestation code. "In diseases classified elsewhere" codes are never permitted to be used as first-listed or principal diagnosis codes. They must be used in conjunction with an underlying condition code and they must be listed following the underlying condition. See category F02, Dementia in other diseases classified elsewhere, for an example of this convention.

There are manifestation codes that do not have "in diseases classified elsewhere" in the title. For such codes, there is a "use additional code" note at the etiology code and a "code first" note at the manifestation code, and the rules for sequencing apply.

In addition to the notes in the Tabular List, these conditions also have a specific Alphabetic Index entry structure. In the Alphabetic Index both conditions are listed together with the etiology code first followed by the manifestation codes in brackets. The code in brackets is always to be sequenced second.

An example of the etiology/manifestation convention is dementia in Parkinson's disease. In the Alphabetic Index, code G20 is listed first, followed by code F02.80 or F02.81 in brackets. Code G20 represents the underlying etiology, Parkinson's disease, and must be sequenced first, whereas codes F02.80 and F02.81 represent the manifestation of dementia in diseases classified elsewhere, with or without behavioral disturbance.

"Code first" and "Use additional code" notes are also used as sequencing rules in the classification for certain codes that are not part of an etiology/manifestation combination.

See Section I.B.7. Multiple coding for a single condition.

14. "And"

The word "and" should be interpreted to mean either "and" or "or" when it appears in a title.

For example, cases of "tuberculosis of bones", "tuberculosis of joints" and "tuberculosis of bones and joints" are classified to subcategory A18.0, Tuberculosis of bones and joints.

15. "With"

The word "with" or "in" should be interpreted to mean "associated with" or "due to" when it appears in a code title, the Alphabetic Index (either under a main term or subterm), or an instructional note in the Tabular List. The classification presumes a causal relationship between the two conditions linked by these terms in the Alphabetic Index or Tabular List. These conditions should be coded as related even in the absence of provider documentation explicitly linking them, unless the documentation clearly states the conditions are unrelated or when another guideline exists that specifically requires a documented linkage between two conditions (e.g., sepsis guideline for "acute organ dysfunction that is not clearly associated with the sepsis").

For conditions not specifically linked by these relational terms in the classification or when a guideline requires that a linkage between two conditions be explicitly documented, provider documentation must link the conditions in order to code them as related.

The word "with" in the Alphabetic Index is sequenced immediately following the main term **or subterm**, not in alphabetical order.

16. "See" and "See Also"

The "see" instruction following a main term in the Alphabetic Index indicates that another term should be referenced. It is necessary to go to the main term referenced with the "see" note to locate the correct code.

A "see also" instruction following a main term in the Alphabetic Index instructs that there is another main term that may also be referenced that may provide additional Alphabetic Index entries that may be useful. It is not necessary to follow the "see also" note when the original main term provides the necessary code.

17. "Code also" note

A "code also" note instructs that two codes may be required to fully describe a condition, but this note does not provide sequencing direction. The sequencing depends on the circumstances of the encounter.

18. Default codes

A code listed next to a main term in the ICD-10-CM Alphabetic Index is referred to as a default code. The default code represents that condition that is most commonly associated with the main term, or is the unspecified code for the condition. If a condition is documented in a medical record (for example, appendicitis) without any additional information, such as acute or chronic, the default code should be assigned.

19. Code assignment and Clinical Criteria

The assignment of a diagnosis code is based on the provider's diagnostic statement that the condition exists. The provider's statement that the patient has a particular condition is sufficient. **If there is conflicting medical record documentation, query the provider.** Code assignment is not based on clinical criteria used by the provider to establish the diagnosis.

B. General Coding Guidelines

1. Locating a code in the ICD-10-CM

To select a code in the classification that corresponds to a diagnosis or reason for visit documented in a medical record, first locate the term in the Alphabetic Index, and then verify the code in the Tabular List. Read and be guided by instructional notations that appear in both the Alphabetic Index and the Tabular List.

It is essential to use both the Alphabetic Index and Tabular List when locating and assigning a code. The Alphabetic Index does not always provide the full code. Selection of the full code, including laterality and any applicable 7th character can only be done in the Tabular List. A dash (-) at the end of an Alphabetic Index entry indicates that additional characters are required. Even if a dash is not included at the Alphabetic Index entry, it is necessary to refer to the Tabular List to verify that no 7th character is required.

2. Level of Detail in Coding

Diagnosis codes are to be used and reported at their highest number of characters available **and to the highest level of specificity documented in the medical record.**

ICD-10-CM diagnosis codes are composed of codes with 3, 4, 5, 6 or 7 characters. Codes with three characters are included in ICD-10-CM as the heading of a category of codes that may be further subdivided by the use of fourth and/or fifth characters and/or sixth characters, which provide greater detail.

A three-character code is to be used only if it is not further subdivided. A code is invalid if it has not been coded to the full number of characters required for that code, including the 7th character, ifapplicable.

3. Code or codes from A00.0 through T88.9, Z00-Z99.8, *U00-U85*

The appropriate code or codes from A00.0 through T88.9, Z00-Z99.8, **and U00-U85** must be used to identify diagnoses, symptoms, conditions, problems, complaints or other reason(s) for the encounter/ visit.

4. Signs and symptoms

Codes that describe symptoms and signs, as opposed to diagnoses, are acceptable for reporting purposes when a related definitive diagnosis has not been established (confirmed) by the provider. Chapter 18 of ICD-10-CM, Symptoms, Signs, and Abnormal Clinical and Laboratory Findings, Not Elsewhere Classified (codes R00.0 - R99) contains many, but not all, codes for symptoms.

See Section I.B.18 Use of Signs/Symptom/Unspecified Codes

5. Conditions that are an integral part of a disease process

Signs and symptoms that are associated routinely with a disease process should not be assigned as additional codes, unless otherwise instructed by the classification.

6. Conditions that are not an integral part of a disease process

Additional signs and symptoms that may not be associated routinely with a disease process should be coded when present.

7. Multiple coding for a single condition

In addition to the etiology/manifestation convention that requires two codes to fully describe a single condition that affects multiple body systems, there are other single conditions that also require more than one code. "Use additional code" notes are found in the Tabular List at codes that are not part of an etiology/manifestation pair where a secondary code is useful to fully describe a condition. The sequencing rule is the same as the etiology/manifestation pair, "use additional code" indicates that a secondary code should be added, if known.

For example, for bacterial infections that are not included in chapter 1, a secondary code from category B95, Streptococcus, Staphylococcus, and Enterococcus, as the cause of diseases classified elsewhere, or B96, Other bacterial agents as the cause of diseases classified elsewhere, may be required to identify the bacterial organism causing the infection. A "use additional code" note will normally be found at the infectious disease code, indicating a need for the organism code to be added as a secondary code.

"Code first" notes are also under certain codes that are not specifically manifestation codes but may be due to an underlying cause. When there is a "code first" note and an underlying condition is present, the underlying condition should be sequenced first, if known.

"Code, if applicable, any causal condition first" notes indicate that this code may be assigned as a principal diagnosis when the causal condition is unknown or not applicable. If a causal condition is known, then the code for that condition should be sequenced as the principal or first-listed diagnosis.

Multiple codes may be needed for sequela, complication codes and obstetric codes to more fully describe a condition. See the specific guidelines for these conditions for further instruction.

8. Acute and Chronic Conditions

If the same condition is described as both acute (subacute) and chronic, and separate subentries exist in the Alphabetic Index at the same indentation level, code both and sequence the acute (subacute) code first.

9. Combination Code

A combination code is a single code used to classify:

Two diagnoses, or

A diagnosis with an associated secondary process (manifestation)

A diagnosis with an associated complication

Combination codes are identified by referring to subterm entries in the Alphabetic Index and by reading the inclusion and exclusion notes in the Tabular List.

Assign only the combination code when that code fully identifies the diagnostic conditions involved or when the Alphabetic Index so directs. Multiple coding should not be used when the classification provides a combination code that clearly identifies all of the elements documented in the diagnosis. When the combination code lacks necessary specificity in describing the manifestation or complication, an additional code should be used as a secondary code.

10. Sequela (Late Effects)

A sequela is the residual effect (condition produced) after the acute phase of an illness or injury has terminated. There is no time limit on when a sequela code can be used. The residual may be apparent early, such as in cerebral infarction, or it may occur months or years later, such as that due to a previous injury. Examples of sequela include: scar formation resulting from a burn, deviated septum due to a nasal fracture, and infertility due to tubal occlusion from old tuberculosis. Coding of sequela generally requires two codes sequenced in the following order: the condition or nature of the sequela is sequenced first. The sequela code is sequenced second.

An exception to the above guidelines are those instances where the code for the sequela is followed by a manifestation code identified in the Tabular List and title, or the sequela code has been expanded (at the fourth, fifth or sixth character levels) to include the manifestation(s). The code for the acute phase of an illness or injury that led to the sequela is never used with a code for the late effect.

See Section I.C.9. Sequelae of cerebrovascular disease
See Section I.C.15. Sequelae of complication of pregnancy, childbirth and the puerperium
See Section I.C.19. Application of 7th characters for Chapter 19

11. Impending or Threatened Condition

Code any condition described at the time of discharge as "impending" or "threatened" as follows:

If it did occur, code as confirmed diagnosis.

If it did not occur, reference the Alphabetic Index to determine if the condition has a subentry term for "impending" or "threatened" and also reference main term entries for "Impending" and for "Threatened."

If the subterms are listed, assign the given code.

If the subterms are not listed, code the existing underlying condition(s) and not the condition described as impending or threatened.

12. Reporting Same Diagnosis Code More than Once

Each unique ICD-10-CM diagnosis code may be reported only once for an encounter. This applies to bilateral conditions when there are no distinct codes identifying laterality or two different conditions classified to the same ICD-10-CM diagnosis code.

13. Laterality

Some ICD-10-CM codes indicate laterality, specifying whether the condition occurs on the left, right or is bilateral. If no bilateral code is provided and the condition is bilateral, assign separate codes for both the left and right side. If the side is not identified in the medical record, assign the code for the unspecified side.

When a patient has a bilateral condition and each side is treated during separate encounters, assign the "bilateral" code (as the condition still exists on both sides), including for the encounter to treat the first side. For the second encounter for treatment after one side has previously been treated and the condition no longer exists on that side, assign the appropriate unilateral code for the side where the condition still exists (e.g., cataract surgery performed on each eye in separate encounters). The bilateral code would not be assigned for the subsequent encounter, as the patient no longer has the condition in the previously-treated site. If the treatment on the first side did not completely resolve the condition, then the bilateral code would still be appropriate.

When laterality is not documented by the patient's provider, code assignment for the affected side may be based on medical record documentation from other clinicians. If there is conflicting medical record documentation regarding the affected side, the patient's attending provider should be queried for clarification. Codes for "unspecified" side should rarely be used, such as when the documentation in the record is insufficient to determine the affected side and it is not possible to obtain clarification.

14. Documentation by Clinicians Other than the Patient's Provider

Code assignment is based on the documentation by the patient's provider (i.e., physician or other qualified healthcare practitioner legally accountable for establishing the patient's diagnosis). There are a few exceptions when code assignment may be based on medical record documentation from clinicians who are not the patient's provider (i.e., physician or other qualified healthcare practitioner legally accountable for establishing the patient's diagnosis). In this context, "clinicians" other than the patient's provider refer to healthcare professionals permitted, based on regulatory or accreditation requirements or internal hospital policies, to document in a patient's official medical record.

These exceptions include codes for:

- Body Mass Index (BMI)
- Depth of non-pressure chronic ulcers
- Pressure ulcer stage
- Coma scale
- NIH stroke scale (NIHSS)
- Social determinants of health (SDOH)
- Laterality
- Blood alcohol level
- **Underimmunization status**

This information is typically, or may be, documented by other clinicians involved in the care of the patient (e.g., a dietitian often documents the BMI, a nurse often documents the pressure ulcer stages, and an emergency medical technician often documents the coma scale). However, the associated diagnosis (such as overweight, obesity, acute stroke, pressure ulcer, or a condition classifiable to category F10, Alcohol related disorders) must be documented by the patient's provider. If there is conflicting medical record documentation, either from the same clinician or different clinicians, the patient's attending provider should be queried for clarification.

The BMI, coma scale, NIHSS, blood alcohol level codes and codes for social determinants of health **and underimmunization status** should only be reported as secondary diagnoses.

See Section I.C.21.c.17 for additional information regarding coding social determinants of health.

15. Syndromes

Follow the Alphabetic Index guidance when coding syndromes. In the absence of Alphabetic Index guidance, assign codes for the documented manifestations of the syndrome. Additional codes for manifestations that are not an integral part of the disease process may also be assigned when the condition does not have a unique code.

16. Documentation of Complications of Care

Code assignment is based on the provider's documentation of the relationship between the condition and the care or procedure, unless otherwise instructed by the classification. The guideline extends to any complications of care, regardless of the chapter the code is located in. It is important to note that not all conditions that occur during or following medical care or surgery are classified as complications. There must be a cause-and-effect relationship between the care provided and the condition, and **the documentation must support that the condition is clinically significant. It is not necessary for the provider to explicitly document the term "complication." For example, if the condition alters the course of the surgery as documented in the operative report, then it would be appropriate to report a complication code.**

Query the provider for clarification **if the documentation is not clear as to the relationship between the condition and the care or procedure.**

17. Borderline Diagnosis

If the provider documents a "borderline" diagnosis at the time of discharge, the diagnosis is coded as confirmed, unless the classification provides a specific entry (e.g., borderline diabetes). If a borderline condition has a specific index entry in ICD-10-CM, it should be coded as such. Since borderline conditions are not uncertain diagnoses, no distinction is made between the care setting (inpatient versus outpatient). Whenever the documentation is unclear regarding a borderline condition, coders are encouraged to query for clarification.

18. Use of Sign/Symptom/Unspecified Codes

Sign/symptom and "unspecified" codes have acceptable, even necessary, uses. While specific diagnosis codes should be reported when they are supported by the available medical record documentation and clinical knowledge of the patient's health condition, there are instances when signs/symptoms or unspecified codes are the best choices for accurately reflecting the healthcare encounter. Each healthcare encounter should be coded to the level of certainty known for that encounter.

As stated in the introductory section of these official coding guidelines, a joint effort between the healthcare provider and the coder is essential to achieve complete and accurate documentation, code assignment, and reporting of diagnoses and procedures. The importance of consistent, complete documentation in the medical record cannot be overemphasized. Without such documentation accurate coding cannot be achieved. The entire record should be reviewed to determine the specific reason for the encounter and the conditions treated.

If a definitive diagnosis has not been established by the end of the encounter, it is appropriate to report codes for sign(s) and/or symptom(s) in lieu of a definitive diagnosis. When sufficient clinical information isn't known or available about a particular health condition to assign a more specific code, it is acceptable to report the appropriate "unspecified" code (e.g., a diagnosis of pneumonia has been determined, but not the specific type). Unspecified codes should be reported when they are the codes that most accurately reflect what is known about the patient's condition at the time of that particular encounter. It would be inappropriate to select a specific code that is not supported by the medical record documentation or conduct medically unnecessary diagnostic testing in order to determine a more specific code.

19. Coding for Healthcare Encounters in Hurricane Aftermath

a. Use of External Cause of Morbidity Codes

An external cause of morbidity code should be assigned to identify the cause of the injury(ies) incurred as a result of the hurricane. The use of external cause of morbidity codes is supplemental to the application of ICD-10-CM codes. External cause of morbidity codes are never to be recorded as a principal diagnosis (first-listed in non-inpatient settings). The appropriate injury code should be sequenced before any external cause codes. The external cause of morbidity codes capture how the injury or health condition happened (cause), the intent (unintentional or accidental; or intentional, such as suicide or assault), the place where the event occurred, the activity of the patient at the time of the event, and the person's status (e.g., civilian, military). They should not be assigned for encounters to treat hurricane victims' medical conditions when no injury, adverse effect or poisoning is involved. External cause of morbidity codes should be assigned for each encounter for care and treatment of the injury. External cause of morbidity codes may be assigned in all health care settings. For the purpose of capturing complete and accurate ICD-10-CM data in the aftermath of the hurricane, a healthcare setting should be considered as any location where medical care is provided by licensed healthcare professionals.

b. Sequencing of External Causes of Morbidity Codes

Codes for cataclysmic events, such as a hurricane, take priority over all other external cause codes except child and adult abuse and terrorism and should be sequenced before other external cause of injury codes. Assign as many external cause of morbidity codes as necessary to fully explain each cause. For example, if an injury occurs as a result of a building collapse during the hurricane, external cause codes for both the hurricane and the building collapse should be assigned, with the external causes code for hurricane being sequenced as the first external cause code. For injuries incurred as a direct result of the hurricane, assign the appropriate code(s) for the injuries, followed by the code X37.0-, Hurricane (with the appropriate 7th character), and any other applicable external cause of injury codes. Code X37.0- also should be assigned when an injury is incurred as a result of flooding caused by a levee breaking related to the hurricane. Code X38.-, Flood (with the appropriate 7th character), should be assigned when an injury is from flooding resulting directly from the storm. Code X36.0.-, Collapse of dam or man-made structure, should not be assigned when the cause of the collapse is due to the hurricane. Use of code X36.0- is limited to collapses of man-made structures due to earth surface movements, not due to storm surges directly from a hurricane.

c. Other External Causes of Morbidity Code Issues

For injuries that are not a direct result of the hurricane, such as an evacuee that has incurred an injury as a result of a motor vehicle accident, assign the appropriate external cause of morbidity code(s) to describe the cause of the injury, but do not assign code X37.0-, Hurricane. If it is not clear whether the injury was a direct result of the hurricane, assume the injury is due to the hurricane and assign code X37.0-, Hurricane, as well as any other applicable external cause of morbidity codes. In addition to code X37.0-, Hurricane, other possible applicable external cause of morbidity codes include:

W54.0-, Bitten by dog

X30-, Exposure to excessive natural heat

X31-, Exposure to excessive natural cold

X38-, Flood

d. Use of Z codes

Z codes (other reasons for healthcare encounters) may be assigned as appropriate to further explain the reasons for presenting for healthcare services, including transfers between healthcare facilities **or provide additional information relevant to a patient encounter.** The ICD-10-CM Official Guidelines for Coding and Reporting identify which codes maybe assigned as principal or first-listed diagnosis only, secondary diagnosis only, or principal/first-listed or secondary (depending on the circumstances). Possible applicable Z codes include:

Z59.0, Homelessness

Z59.1, Inadequate housing

Z59.5, Extreme poverty

Z75.1, Person awaiting admission to adequate facility elsewhere

Z75.3, Unavailability and inaccessibility of health-care facilities

Z75.4, Unavailability and inaccessibility of other helping agencies

Z76.2, Encounter for health supervision and care of other healthy infant and child

Z99.12, Encounter for respirator [ventilator] dependence during power failure

The external cause of morbidity codes and the Z codes listed above are not an all-inclusive list. Other codes may be applicable to the encounter based upon the documentation. Assign as many codes as necessary to fully explain each healthcare encounter. Since patient history information may be very limited, use any available documentation to assign the appropriate external cause of morbidity and Z codes.

C. Chapter-Specific Coding Guidelines

In addition to general coding guidelines, there are guidelines for specific diagnoses and/or conditions in the classification. Unless otherwise indicated, these guidelines apply to all health care settings. Please refer to Section II for guidelines on the selection of principal diagnosis.

1. Chapter 1: Certain Infectious and Parasitic Diseases (A00-B99), U07.1, U09.9

Refer to the complete guidelines on FindACode.com

2. Chapter 2: Neoplasms (C00-D49)

Refer to the complete guidelines on FindACode.com

3. Chapter 3: Disease of the blood and blood-forming organs and certain disorders involving the immune mechanism (D50-D89)

Reserved for future guideline expansion

4. Chapter 4: Endocrine, Nutritional, and Metabolic Diseases (E00-E89)

Refer to the complete guidelines on FindACode.com

5. Chapter 5: Mental, Behavioral and Neurodevelopmental disorders (F01 – F99)

Refer to the complete guidelines on FindACode.com

6. Chapter 6: Diseases of the Nervous System (G00-G99)

a. Dominant/nondominant side

Codes from category G81, Hemiplegia and hemiparesis, and subcategories G83.1, Monoplegia of lower limb, G83.2, Monoplegia of upper limb, and G83.3, Monoplegia, unspecified, identify whether the dominant or nondominant side is affected. Should the affected side be documented, but not specified as dominant or nondominant, and the classification system does not indicate a default, code selection is as follows:

- For ambidextrous patients, the default should be dominant.
- If the left side is affected, the default is non-dominant.
- If the right side is affected, the default is dominant.

b. Pain - Category G89

1) General coding information

Codes in category G89, Pain, not elsewhere classified, may be used in conjunction with codes from other categories and chapters to provide more detail about acute or chronic pain and neoplasm-related pain, unless otherwise indicated below.

If the pain is not specified as acute or chronic, post-thoracotomy, postprocedural, or neoplasm-related, do not assign codes from category G89.

A code from category G89 should not be assigned if the underlying (definitive) diagnosis is known, unless the reason for the encounter is pain control/ management and not management of the underlying condition.

When an admission or encounter is for a procedure aimed at treating the underlying condition (e.g., spinal fusion, kyphoplasty), a code for the underlying condition (e.g., vertebral fracture, spinal stenosis) should be assigned as the principal diagnosis. No code from category G89 should be assigned.

(a) Category G89 Codes as Principal or First-Listed Diagnosis

Category G89 codes are acceptable as principal diagnosis or the first-listed code:

- When pain control or pain management is the reason for the admission/ encounter (e.g., a patient with displaced intervertebral disc, nerve impingement and severe back pain presents for injection of steroid into the spinal canal). The underlying cause of the pain should be reported as an additional diagnosis, if known.
- When a patient is admitted for the insertion of a neurostimulator for pain control, assign the appropriate pain code as the principal or first-listed diagnosis. When an admission or encounter is for a procedure aimed at treating the underlying condition and a neurostimulator is inserted for pain control during the same admission/encounter, a code for the underlying condition should be assigned as the principal diagnosis and the appropriate pain code should be assigned as a secondary diagnosis.

(b) Use of Category G89 Codes in Conjunction with Site Specific Pain Codes

(i) Assigning Category G89 and Site-Specific Pain Codes

Codes from category G89 may be used in conjunction with codes that identify the site of pain (including codes from chapter 18) if the category G89 code provides additional information. For example, if the code describes the site of the pain, but does not fully describe whether the pain is acute or chronic, then both codes should be assigned.

(ii) Sequencing of Category G89 Codes with Site- Specific Pain Codes

The sequencing of category G89 codes with site- specific pain codes (including chapter 18 codes), is dependent on the circumstances of the encounter/admission as follows:

- If the encounter is for pain control or pain management, assign the code from category G89 followed by the code identifying the specific site of pain (e.g., encounter for pain management for acute neck pain from trauma is assigned code G89.11, Acute pain due to trauma, followed by code M54.2, Cervicalgia, to identify the site of pain).
- If the encounter is for any other reason except pain control or pain management, and a related definitive diagnosis has not been established (confirmed) by the provider, assign the code for the specific site of pain first, followed by the appropriate code from category G89.

2) **Pain due to devices, implants and grafts**

See Section I.C.19. Pain due to medical devices

3) **Postoperative Pain**

The provider's documentation should be used to guide the coding of postoperative pain, as well as *Section III. Reporting Additional Diagnoses* and *Section IV. Diagnostic Coding and Reporting in the Outpatient Setting.*

The default for post-thoracotomy and other postoperative pain not specified as acute or chronic is the code for the acute form.

Routine or expected postoperative pain immediately after surgery should not be coded.

(a) **Postoperative pain not associated with specific postoperative complication**

Postoperative pain not associated with a specific postoperative complication is assigned to the appropriate postoperative pain code in category G89.

(b) **Postoperative pain associated with specific postoperative complication**

Postoperative pain associated with a specific postoperative complication (such as painful wire sutures) is assigned to the appropriate code(s) found in Chapter 19, Injury, poisoning, and certain other consequences of external causes. If appropriate, use additional code(s) from category G89 to identify acute or chronic pain (G89.18 or G89.28).

4) **Chronic pain**

Chronic pain is classified to subcategory G89.2. There is no time frame defining when pain becomes chronic pain. The provider's documentation should be used to guide use of these codes.

5) **Neoplasm Related Pain**

Code G89.3 is assigned to pain documented as being related, associated or due to cancer, primary or secondary malignancy, or tumor. This code is assigned regardless of whether the pain is acute or chronic.

This code may be assigned as the principal or first-listed code when the stated reason for the admission/encounter is documented as pain control/pain management. The underlying neoplasm should be reported as an additional diagnosis.

When the reason for the admission/encounter is management of the neoplasm and the pain associated with the neoplasm is also documented, code G89.3 may be assigned as an additional diagnosis. It is not necessary to assign an additional code for the site of the pain.

See Section I.C.2 for instructions on the sequencing of neoplasms for all other stated reasons for the admission/encounter (except for pain control/pain management).

6) **Chronic pain syndrome**

Central pain syndrome (G89.0) and chronic pain syndrome (G89.4) are different than the term "chronic pain," and therefore codes should only be used when the provider has specifically documented this condition.

See Section I.C.5. Pain disorders related to psychological factors

7. Chapter 7: Diseases of the Eye and Adnexa (H00-H59)

Refer to the complete guidelines on FindACode.com

8. Chapter 8: Diseases of the Ear and Mastoid Process (H60-H95)

Reserved for future guideline expansion

9. Chapter 9: Diseases of the Circulatory System (I00-I99)

Refer to the complete guidelines on FindACode.com

10. Chapter 10: Diseases of the Respiratory System (J00-J99), U07.0

Refer to the complete guidelines on FindACode.com

11. Chapter 11: Diseases of the Digestive System (K00-K95)

Reserved for future guideline expansion

12. Chapter 12: Diseases of the Skin and Subcutaneous Tissue (L00-L99)

Refer to the complete guidelines on FindACode.com

13. Chapter 13: Diseases of the Musculoskeletal System and Connective Tissue (M00-M99)

a. Site and laterality

Most of the codes within Chapter 13 have site and laterality designations. The site represents the bone, joint or the muscle involved. For some conditions where more than one bone, joint or muscle is usually involved, such as osteoarthritis, there is a "multiple sites" code available. For categories where no multiple site code is provided and more than one bone, joint or muscle is involved, multiple codes should be used to indicate the different sites involved.

1) Bone versus joint

For certain conditions, the bone may be affected at the upper or lower end, (e.g., avascular necrosis of bone, M87, Osteoporosis, M80, M81). Though the portion of the bone affected may be at the joint, the site designation will be the bone, not the joint.

b. Acute traumatic versus chronic or recurrent musculoskeletal conditions

Many musculoskeletal conditions are a result of previous injury or trauma to a site, or are recurrent conditions. Bone, joint or muscle conditions that are the result of a healed injury are usually found in chapter 13. Recurrent bone, joint or muscle conditions are also usually found in chapter 13. Any current, acute injury should be coded to the appropriate injury code from chapter 19. Chronic or recurrent conditions should generally be coded with a code from chapter 13. If it is difficult to determine from the documentation in the record which code is best to describe a condition, query the provider.

c. Coding of Pathologic Fractures

7th character A is for use as long as the patient is receiving active treatment for the fracture. While the patient may be seen by a new or different provider over the course of treatment for a pathological fracture, assignment of the 7th character is based on whether the patient is undergoing active treatment and not whether the provider is seeing the patient for the first time.

7th character D is to be used for encounters after the patient has completed active treatment for the fracture and is receiving routine care for the fracture during the healing or recovery phase. The other 7th characters, listed under each subcategory in the Tabular List, are to be used for subsequent encounters for treatment of problems associated with the healing, such as malunions, nonunions, and sequelae.

Care for complications of surgical treatment for fracture repairs during the healing or recovery phase should be coded with the appropriate complication codes.

See Section I.C.19. Coding of traumatic fractures.

d. Osteoporosis

Osteoporosis is a systemic condition, meaning that all bones of the musculoskeletal system are affected. Therefore, site is not a component of the codes under category M81, Osteoporosis without current pathological fracture. The site codes under category M80, Osteoporosis with current pathological fracture, identify the site of the fracture, not the osteoporosis.

1) Osteoporosis without pathological fracture

Category M81, Osteoporosis without current pathological fracture, is for use for patients with osteoporosis who do not currently have a pathologic fracture due to the osteoporosis, even if they have had a fracture in the past. For patients with a history of osteoporosis fractures, status code Z87.310, Personal history of (healed) osteoporosis fracture, should follow the code from M81.

2) Osteoporosis with current pathological fracture

Category M80, Osteoporosis with current pathological fracture, is for patients who have a current pathologic fracture at the time of an encounter. The codes under M80 identify the site of the fracture. A code from category M80, not a traumatic fracture code, should be used for any patient with known osteoporosis who suffers a fracture, even if the patient had a minor fall or trauma, if that fall or trauma would not usually break a normal, healthy bone.

e. Multisystem Inflammatory Syndrome

See Section I.C.1.g.1.l for Multisystem Inflammatory Syndrome

14. Chapter 14: Diseases of Genitourinary System (N00-N99)

Refer to the complete guidelines on FindACode.com

15. Chapter 15: Pregnancy, Childbirth, and the Puerperium (O00-O9A)

Refer to the complete guidelines on FindACode.com

16. Chapter 16: Certain Conditions Originating in the Perinatal Period (P00-P96)

Refer to the complete guidelines on FindACode.com

17. Chapter 17: Congenital malformations, deformations, and chromosomal abnormalities (Q00-Q99)

Assign an appropriate code(s) from categories Q00-Q99, Congenital malformations, deformations, and chromosomal abnormalities when a malformation/deformation or chromosomal abnormality is documented. A malformation/deformation/or chromosomal abnormality may be the principal/first-listed diagnosis on a record or a secondary diagnosis.

When a malformation/deformation or chromosomal abnormality does not have a unique code assignment, assign additional code(s) for any manifestations that may be present.

When the code assignment specifically identifies the malformation/deformation or chromosomal abnormality, manifestations that are an inherent component of the anomaly should not be coded separately. Additional codes should be assigned for manifestations that are not an inherent component.

Codes from Chapter 17 may be used throughout the life of the patient. If a congenital malformation or deformity has been corrected, a personal history code should be used to identify the history of the malformation or deformity. Although present at birth, **a** malformation/deformation/or chromosomal abnormality may not be identified until later in life. Whenever the condition is diagnosed by the **provider**, it is appropriate to assign a code from codes Q00-Q99.For the birth admission, the appropriate code from category Z38, Liveborn infants, according to place of birth and type of delivery, should be sequenced as the principal diagnosis, followed by any congenital anomaly codes, Q00-Q99.

18. Chapter 18: Symptoms, signs, and abnormal clinical and laboratory findings, not elsewhere classified (R00-R99)

Chapter 18 includes symptoms, signs, abnormal results of clinical or other investigative procedures, and ill-defined conditions regarding which no diagnosis classifiable elsewhere is recorded. Signs and symptoms that point to a specific diagnosis have been assigned to a category in other chapters of the classification.

a. Use of symptom codes

Codes that describe symptoms and signs are acceptable for reporting purposes when a related definitive diagnosis has not been established (confirmed) by the provider.

b. Use of a symptom code with a definitive diagnosis code

Codes for signs and symptoms may be reported in addition to a related definitive diagnosis when the sign or symptom is not routinely associated with that diagnosis, such as the various signs and symptoms associated with complex syndromes. The definitive diagnosis code should be sequenced before the symptom code.

Signs or symptoms that are associated routinely with a disease process should not be assigned as additional codes, unless otherwise instructed by the classification.

c. Combination codes that include symptoms

ICD-10-CM contains a number of combination codes that identify both the definitive diagnosis and common symptoms of that diagnosis. When using one of these combination codes, an additional code should not be assigned for the symptom.

d. Repeated falls

Code R29.6, Repeated falls, is for use for encounters when a patient has recently fallen and the reason for the fall is being investigated.

Code Z91.81, History of falling, is for use when a patient has fallen in the past and is at risk for future falls. When appropriate, both codes R29.6 and Z91.81 may be assigned together.

e. Coma

Code R40.20, Unspecified coma, may be assigned in conjunction with codes for any medical condition.

Do not report codes for unspecified coma, individual or total Glasgow coma scale scores for a patient with a medically induced coma or a sedated patient.

1) The Coma Scale

The coma scale codes **(R40.1- to R40.24-)** can be used in conjunction with traumatic brain injury codes, acute cerebrovascular disease or sequelae of cerebrovascular disease codes. These codes are primarily for use by trauma registries, but they may be used in any setting where this information is collected. The coma scale may also be used to assess the status of the central nervous system for other non-trauma conditions, such as monitoring patients in the intensive care unit regardless of medical condition. The coma scale codes should be sequenced after the diagnosis code(s).

These codes, one from each subcategory, are needed to complete the scale. The 7th character indicates when the scale was recorded. The 7th character should match for all three codes.

At a minimum, report the initial score documented on presentation at your facility. This may be a score from the emergency medicine technician (EMT) or in the emergency department. If desired, a facility may choose to capture multiple coma scale scores.

Assign code R40.24, Glasgow coma scale, total score, when only the total score is documented in the medical record and not the individual score(s).

If multiple coma scores are captured within the first 24 hours after hospital admission, assign only the code for the score at the time of admission. ICD-10-CM does not classify coma scores that are reported after admission but less than 24 hours later.

See Section I.B.14 for coma scale documentation by clinicians other than patient's provider

f. Functional quadriplegia

GUIDELINE HAS BEEN DELETED EFFECTIVE OCTOBER 1, 2017

g. SIRS due to Non-Infectious Process

The systemic inflammatory response syndrome (SIRS) can develop as a result of certain non-infectious disease processes, such as trauma, malignant neoplasm, or pancreatitis. When SIRS is documented with a noninfectious condition, and no subsequent infection is documented, the code for the underlying condition, such as an injury, should be assigned, followed by code R65.10, Systemic inflammatory response syndrome (SIRS) of non-infectious origin without acute organ dysfunction, or code R65.11, Systemic inflammatory response syndrome (SIRS) of non-infectious origin with acute organ dysfunction. If an associated acute organ dysfunction is documented, the appropriate code(s) for the specific type of organ dysfunction(s) should be assigned in addition to code R65.11. If acute organ dysfunction is documented, but it cannot be determined if the acute organ dysfunction is associated with SIRS or due to another condition (e.g., directly due to the trauma), the provider should be queried.

h. Death NOS

Code R99, Ill-defined and unknown cause of mortality, is only for use in the very limited circumstance when a patient who has already died is brought into an emergency department or other healthcare facility and is pronounced dead upon arrival. It does not represent the discharge disposition of death.

i. NIHSS Stroke Scale

The NIH stroke scale (NIHSS) codes (R29.7- -) can be used in conjunction with acute stroke codes (I63) to identify the patient's neurological status and the severity of the stroke. The stroke scale codes should be sequenced after the acute stroke diagnosis code(s).

At a minimum, report the initial score documented. If desired, a facility may choose to capture multiple stroke scale scores.

See Section I.B.14 for NIHSS stroke scale documentation by clinicians other than patient's provider

19. Chapter 19: Injury, poisoning, and certain other consequences of external causes (S00-T88)

a. Application of 7th Characters in Chapter 19

Most categories in chapter 19 have a 7th character requirement for each applicable code. Most categories in this chapter have three 7th character values (with the exception of fractures): A, initial encounter, D, subsequent encounter and S, sequela. Categories for traumatic fractures have additional 7th character values. While the patient may be seen by a new or different provider over the course of treatment for an injury, assignment of the 7th character is based on whether the patient is undergoing active treatment and not whether the provider is seeing the patient for the first time.

For complication codes, active treatment refers to treatment for the condition described by the code, even though it may be related to an earlier precipitating problem. For example, code T84.50XA, Infection and inflammatory reaction due to unspecified internal joint prosthesis, initial encounter, is used when active treatment is provided for the infection, even though the condition relates to the prosthetic device, implant or graft that was placed at a previous encounter.

7th character "A", initial encounter is used for each encounter where the patient is receiving active treatment for the condition.

7th character "D" subsequent encounter is used for encounters after the patient has completed active treatment of the condition and is receiving routine care for the condition during the healing or recovery phase.

The aftercare Z codes should not be used for aftercare for conditions such as injuries or poisonings, where 7th characters are provided to identify subsequent care. For example, for aftercare of an injury, assign the acute injury code with the 7th character "D" (subsequent encounter).

7th character "S", sequela, is for use for complications or conditions that arise as a direct result of a condition, such as scar formation after a burn. The scars are sequelae of the burn. When using 7th character "S", it is necessary to use both the injury code that precipitated the sequela and the code for the sequela itself. The "S" is added only to the injury code, not the sequela code. The 7th character "S" identifies the injury responsible for the sequela. The specific type of sequela (e.g. scar) is sequenced first, followed by the injury code.

See Section I.B.10 Sequelae, (Late Effects)

b. Coding of Injuries

When coding injuries, assign separate codes for each injury unless a combination code is provided, in which case the combination code is assigned. Codes from category T07, Unspecified multiple injuries should not be assigned in the inpatient setting unless information for a more specific code is not available. Traumatic injury codes (S00-T14.9) are not to be used for normal, healing surgical wounds or to identify complications of surgical wounds.

The code for the most serious injury, as determined by the provider and the focus of treatment, is sequenced first.

1) Superficial injuries

Superficial injuries such as abrasions or contusions are not coded when associated with more severe injuries of the same site.

2) Primary injury with damage to nerves/blood vessels

When a primary injury results in minor damage to peripheral nerves or blood vessels, the primary injury is sequenced first with additional code(s) for injuries to nerves and spinal cord (such as category S04), and/or injury to blood vessels (such as category S15). When the primary injury is to the blood vessels or nerves, that injury should be sequenced first.

3) Iatrogenic injuries

Injury codes from Chapter 19 should not be assigned for injuries that occur during, or as a result of, a medical intervention. Assign the appropriate complication code(s).

c. Coding of Traumatic Fractures

The principles of multiple coding of injuries should be followed in coding fractures. Fractures of specified sites are coded individually by site in accordance with both the provisions within categories S02, S12, S22, S32, S42, S49, S52, S59, S62, S72, S79, S82, S89, S92 and the level of detail furnished by medical record content.

A fracture not indicated as open or closed should be coded to closed. A fracture not indicated whether displaced or not displaced should be coded to displaced.

More specific guidelines are as follows:

1) **Initial vs. Subsequent Encounter for Fractures**

Traumatic fractures are coded using the appropriate 7th character for initial encounter (A, B, C) for each encounter where the patient is receiving active treatment for the fracture. The appropriate 7th character for initial encounter should also be assigned for a patient who delayed seeking treatment for the fracture or nonunion.

Fractures are coded using the appropriate 7th character for subsequent care for encounters after the patient has completed active treatment of the fracture and is receiving routine care for the fracture during the healing or recovery phase.

Care for complications of surgical treatment for fracture repairs during the healing or recovery phase should be coded with the appropriate complication codes.

Care of complications of fractures, such as malunion and nonunion, should be reported with the appropriate 7th character for subsequent care with nonunion (K, M, N,) or subsequent care with malunion (P, Q, R).

Malunion/nonunion: The appropriate 7th character for initial encounter should also be assigned for a patient who delayed seeking treatment for the fracture or nonunion.

The open fracture designations in the assignment of the 7th character for fractures of the forearm, femur and lower leg, including ankle are based on the Gustilo open fracture classification. When the Gustilo classification type is not specified for an open fracture, the 7th character for open fracture type I or II should be assigned (B, E, H, M, Q).

A code from category M80, not a traumatic fracture code, should be used for any patient with known osteoporosis who suffers a fracture, even if the patient had a minor fall or trauma, if that fall or trauma would not usually break a normal, healthy bone.

See Section I.C.13. Osteoporosis.

The aftercare Z codes should not be used for aftercare for traumatic fractures. For aftercare of a traumatic fracture, assign the acute fracture code with the appropriate 7th character.

2) **Multiple fractures sequencing**

Multiple fractures are sequenced in accordance with the severity of the fracture.

3) **Physeal fractures**

For physeal fractures, assign only the code identifying the type of physeal fracture. Do not assign a separate code to identify the specific bone that is fractured.

d. Coding of Burns and Corrosions

Refer to the complete guidelines on FindACode.com

e. Adverse Effects, Poisoning, Underdosing and Toxic Effects

Refer to the complete guidelines on FindACode.com

f. Adult and child abuse, neglect and other maltreatment

Refer to the complete guidelines on FindACode.com

g. Complications of care

1) General guidelines for complications of care

(a) Documentation of complications of care

See Section I.B.16. for information on documentation of complications of care.

2) Pain due to medical devices

Pain associated with devices, implants or grafts left in a surgical site (for example painful hip prosthesis) is assigned to the appropriate code(s) found in Chapter 19, Injury, poisoning, and certain other consequences of external causes. Specific codes for pain due to medical devices are found in the T code section of the ICD-10-CM. Use additional code(s) from category G89 to identify acute or chronic pain due to presence of the device, implant or graft (G89.18 or G89.28).

3) Transplant complications

(a) Transplant complications other than kidney

Codes under category T86, Complications of transplanted organs and tissues, are for use for both complications and rejection of transplanted organs. A transplant complication code is only assigned if the complication affects the function of the transplanted organ. Two codes are required to fully describe a transplant complication: the appropriate code from category T86 and a secondary code that identifies the complication.

Pre-existing conditions or conditions that develop after the transplant are not coded as complications unless they affect the function of the transplanted organs.

See I.C.21. for transplant organ removal status
See I.C.2. for malignant neoplasm associated with transplanted organ.

(b) Kidney transplant complications

Patients who have undergone kidney transplant may still have some form of chronic kidney disease (CKD) because the kidney transplant may not fully restore kidney function. Code T86.1- should be assigned for documented complications of a kidney transplant, such as transplant failure or rejection or other transplant complication. Code T86.1- should not be assigned for post kidney transplant patients who have chronic kidney (CKD) unless a transplant complication such as transplant failure or rejection is documented. If the documentation is unclear as to whether the patient has a complication of the transplant, query the provider.

Conditions that affect the function of the transplanted kidney, other than CKD, should be assigned a code from subcategory T86.1, Complications of transplanted organ, Kidney, and a secondary code that identifies the complication.

For patients with CKD following a kidney transplant, but who do not have a complication such as failure or rejection, *see section I.C.14. Chronic kidney disease and kidney transplant status.*

4) Complication codes that include the external cause

As with certain other T codes, some of the complications of care codes have the external cause included in the code. The code includes the nature of the complication as well as the type of procedure that caused the complication. No external cause code indicating the type of procedure is necessary for these codes.

5) **Complications of care codes within the body system chapters**

Intraoperative and postprocedural complication codes are found within the body system chapters with codes specific to the organs and structures of that body system. These codes should be sequenced first, followed by a code(s) for the specific complication, if applicable.

Complication codes from the body system chapters should be assigned for intraoperative and postprocedural complications (e.g., the appropriate complication code from chapter 9 would be assigned for a vascular intraoperative or postprocedural complication) unless the complication is specifically indexed to a T code in chapter 19.

20. Chapter 20: External Causes of Morbidity (V00-Y99)

The external causes of morbidity codes should never be sequenced as the first-listed or principal diagnosis.

External cause codes are intended to provide data for injury research and evaluation of injury prevention strategies. These codes capture how the injury or health condition happened (cause), the intent (unintentional or accidental; or intentional, such as suicide or assault), the place where the event occurred the activity of the patient at the time of the event, and the person's status (e.g., civilian, military).

There is no national requirement for mandatory ICD-10-CM external cause code reporting. Unless a provider is subject to a state-based external cause code reporting mandate or these codes are required by a particular payer, reporting of ICD-10-CM codes in Chapter 20, External Causes of Morbidity, is not required. In the absence of a mandatory reporting requirement, providers are encouraged to voluntarily report external cause codes, as they provide valuable data for injury research and evaluation of injury prevention strategies.

a. General External Cause Coding Guidelines

1) **Used with any code in the range of A00.0-T88.9, Z00-Z99**

An external cause code may be used with any code in the range of A00.0-T88.9, Z00-Z99, classification that represents a health condition due to an external cause. Though they are most applicable to injuries, they are also valid for use with such things as infections or diseases due to an external source, and other health conditions, such as a heart attack that occurs during strenuous physical activity.

2) **External cause code used for length of treatment**

Assign the external cause code, with the appropriate 7th character (initial encounter, subsequent encounter or sequela) for each encounter for which the injury or condition is being treated.

Most categories in chapter 20 have a 7th character requirement for each applicable code. Most categories in this chapter have three 7th character values: A, initial encounter, D, subsequent encounter and S, sequela. While the patient may be seen by a new or different provider over the course of treatment for an injury or condition, assignment of the 7th character for external cause should match the 7th character of the code assigned for the associated injury or condition for the encounter.

3) **Use the full range of external cause codes**

Use the full range of external cause codes to completely describe the cause, the intent, the place of occurrence, and if applicable, the activity of the patient at the time of the event, and the patient's status, for all injuries, and other health conditions due to an external cause.

4) **Assign as many external cause codes as necessary**

Assign as many external cause codes as necessary to fully explain each cause. If only one external code can be recorded, assign the code most related to the principal diagnosis.

5) **The selection of the appropriate external cause code**

The selection of the appropriate external cause code is guided by the Alphabetic Index of External Causes and by Inclusion and Exclusion notes in the Tabular List.

6) **External cause code can never be a principal diagnosis**

An external cause code can never be a principal (first-listed) diagnosis.

7) **Combination external cause codes**

Certain of the external cause codes are combination codes that identify sequential events that result in an injury, such as a fall which results in striking against an object. The injury may be due to either event or both. The combination external cause code used should correspond to the sequence of events regardless of which caused the most serious injury.

8) **No external cause code needed in certain circumstances**

No external cause code from Chapter 20 is needed if the external cause and intent are included in a code from another chapter (e.g. T36.0X1- Poisoning by penicillins, accidental (unintentional)).

b. Place of Occurrence Guideline

Codes from category Y92, Place of occurrence of the external cause, are secondary codes for use after other external cause codes to identify the location of the patient at the time of injury or other condition.

Generally, a place of occurrence code is assigned only once, at the initial encounter for treatment. However, in the rare instance that a new injury occurs during hospitalization, an additional place of occurrence code may be assigned. No 7th characters are used for Y92.

Do not use place of occurrence code Y92.9 if the place is not stated or is not applicable.

c. Activity Code

Assign a code from category Y93, Activity code, to describe the activity of the patient at the time the injury or other health condition occurred.

An activity code is used only once, at the initial encounter for treatment. Only one code from Y93 should be recorded on a medical record.

The activity codes are not applicable to poisonings, adverse effects, misadventures or sequela.

Do not assign Y93.9, Unspecified activity, if the activity is not stated.

A code from category Y93 is appropriate for use with external cause and intent codes if identifying the activity provides additional information about the event.

d. Place of Occurrence, Activity, and Status Codes Used with other External Cause Code

When applicable, place of occurrence, activity, and external cause status codes are sequenced after the main external cause code(s). Regardless of the number of external cause codes assigned, generally there should be only one place of occurrence code, one activity code, and one external cause status code assigned to an encounter. However, in the rare instance that a new injury occurs during hospitalization, an additional place of occurrence code may be assigned.

e. If the Reporting Format Limits the Number of External Cause Codes

If the reporting format limits the number of external cause codes that can be used in reporting clinical data, report the code for the cause/intent most related to the principal diagnosis. If the format permits capture of additional external cause codes, the cause/intent, including medical misadventures, of the additional events should be reported rather than the codes for place, activity, or external status.

f. Multiple External Cause Coding Guidelines

More than one external cause code is required to fully describe the external cause of an illness or injury. The assignment of external cause codes should be sequenced in the following priority:

If two or more events cause separate injuries, an external cause code should be assigned for each cause. The first-listed external cause code will be selected in the following order:

External codes for child and adult abuse take priority over all other external cause codes.

See Section I.C.19., Child and Adult abuse guidelines.

External cause codes for terrorism events take priority over all other external cause codes except child and adult abuse.

External cause codes for cataclysmic events take priority over all other external cause codes except child and adult abuse and terrorism.

External cause codes for transport accidents take priority over all other external cause codes except cataclysmic events, child and adult abuse and terrorism.

Activity and external cause status codes are assigned following all causal (intent) external cause codes.

The first-listed external cause code should correspond to the cause of the most serious diagnosis due to an assault, accident, or self-harm, following the order of hierarchy listed above.

g. Child and Adult Abuse Guideline

Adult and child abuse, neglect and maltreatment are classified as assault. Any of the assault codes may be used to indicate the external cause of any injury resulting from the confirmed abuse.

For confirmed cases of abuse, neglect and maltreatment, when the perpetrator is known, a code from Y07, Perpetrator of maltreatment and neglect, should accompany any other assault codes.

See Section I.C.19. Adult and child abuse, neglect and other maltreatment

h. Unknown or Undetermined Intent Guideline

If the intent (accident, self-harm, assault) of the cause of an injury or other condition is unknown or unspecified, code the intent as accidental intent. All transport accident categories assume accidental intent.

1) Use of undetermined intent

External cause codes for events of undetermined intent are only for use if the documentation in the record specifies that the intent cannot be determined.

i. Sequelae (Late Effects) of External Cause Guidelines

1) Sequelae external cause codes

Sequela are reported using the external cause code with the 7th character "S" for sequela. These codes should be used with any report of a late effect or sequela resulting from a previous injury.

See Section I.B.10 Sequela (Late Effects)

2) Sequela external cause code with a related current injury

A sequela external cause code should never be used with a related current nature of injury code.

3) Use of sequela external cause codes for subsequent visits

Use a late effect external cause code for subsequent visits when a late effect of the initial injury is being treated. Do not use a late effect external cause code for subsequent visits for follow-up care (e.g., to assess healing, to receive rehabilitative therapy) of the injury when no late effect of the injury has been documented.

j. Terrorism Guidelines

Refer to the complete guidelines on FindACode.com

k. External cause status

A code from category Y99, External cause status, should be assigned whenever any other external cause code is assigned for an encounter, including an Activity code, except for the events noted below. Assign a code from category Y99, External cause status, to indicate the work status of the person at the time the event occurred. The status code indicates whether the event occurred during military activity, whether a non-military person was at work, whether an individual including a student or volunteer was involved in a non-work activity at the time of the causal event.

A code from Y99, External cause status, should be assigned, when applicable, with other external cause codes, such as transport accidents and falls. The external cause status codes are not applicable to poisonings, adverse effects, misadventures or late effects.

Do not assign a code from category Y99 if no other external cause codes (cause, activity) are applicable for the encounter.

An external cause status code is used only once, at the initial encounter for treatment. Only one code from Y99 should be recorded on a medical record.

Do not assign code Y99.9, Unspecified external cause status, if the status is not stated.

21. Chapter 21: Factors influencing health status and contact with health services (Z00-Z99)

Note: The chapter specific guidelines provide additional information about the use of Z codes for specified encounters.

a. Use of Z codes in any healthcare setting

Z codes are for use in any healthcare setting. Z codes may be used as either a first-listed (principal diagnosis code in the inpatient setting) or secondary code, depending on the circumstances of the encounter.

Certain Z codes may only be used as first-listed or principal diagnosis.

b. Z Codes indicate a reason for an encounter *or Provide Additional Information about a Patient Encounter*

Z codes are not procedure codes. A corresponding procedure code must accompany a Z code to describe any procedure performed.

c. Categories of Z Codes

1) Contact/Exposure

Category Z20 indicates contact with, and suspected exposure to, communicable diseases. These codes are for patients who do not show any sign or symptom of a disease but are suspected to have been exposed to it by close personal contact with an infected individual or are in an area where a disease is epidemic.

Category Z77, Other contact with and (suspected) exposures hazardous to health, indicates contact with and suspected exposures hazardous to health.

Contact/exposure codes may be used as a first-listed code to explain an encounter for testing, or, more commonly, as a secondary code to identify a potential risk.

2) Inoculations and vaccinations

Code Z23 is for encounters for inoculations and vaccinations. It indicates that a patient is being seen to receive a prophylactic inoculation against a disease. Procedure codes are required to identify the actual administration of the injection and the type(s) of immunizations given. Code Z23 may be used as a secondary code if the inoculation is given as a routine part of preventive health care, such as a well-baby visit.

3) Status

Status codes indicate that a patient is either a carrier of a disease or has the sequelae or residual of a past disease or condition. This includes such things as the presence of prosthetic or mechanical devices resulting from past treatment. A status code is informative, because the status may affect the course of treatment and its outcome. A status code is distinct from a history code. The history code indicates that the patient no longer has the condition.

A status code should not be used with a diagnosis code from one of the body system chapters, if the diagnosis code includes the information provided by the status code. For example, code Z94.1, Heart transplant status, should not be used with a code from subcategory T86.2, Complications of heart transplant. The status code does not provide additional information. The complication code indicates that the patient is a heart transplant patient.

For encounters for weaning from a mechanical ventilator, assign a code from subcategory J96.1, Chronic respiratory failure, followed by code Z99.11, Dependence on respirator [ventilator] status.

The status Z codes/categories are:

Z14 Genetic carrier

Genetic carrier status indicates that a person carries a gene, associated with a particular disease, which may be passed to offspring who may develop that disease. The person does not have the disease and is not at risk of developing the disease.

Z15 Genetic susceptibility to disease

Genetic susceptibility indicates that a person has a gene that increases the risk of that person developing the disease.

Codes from category Z15 should not be used as principal or first-listed codes. If the patient has the condition to which he/she is susceptible, and that condition is the reason for the encounter, the code for the current condition should be sequenced first. If the patient is being seen for follow-up after completed treatment for this condition, and the condition no longer exists, a follow-up code should be sequenced first, followed by the appropriate personal history and genetic susceptibility codes. If the purpose of the encounter is genetic counseling associated with procreative management, code Z31.5, Encounter for genetic counseling, should be assigned as the first-listed code, followed by a code from category Z15. Additional codes should be assigned for any applicable family or personal history.

Z16 Resistance to antimicrobial drugs

This code indicates that a patient has a condition that is resistant to antimicrobial drug treatment. Sequence the infection code first.

Z17 Estrogen receptor status

Z18 Retained foreign body fragments

Z19 Hormone sensitivity malignancy status

Z21 Asymptomatic HIV infection status

This code indicates that a patient has tested positive for HIV but has manifested no signs or symptoms of the disease.

Z22	Carrier of infectious disease Carrier status indicates that a person harbors the specific organisms of a disease without manifest symptoms and is capable of transmitting the infection.
Z28.3	Underimmunization status ***See Section I.B.14. for underimmunization documentation by clinicians other than the patient's provider.***
Z33.1	Pregnant state, incidental This code is a secondary code only for use when the pregnancy is in no way complicating the reason for visit. Otherwise, a code from the obstetric chapter is required.
Z66	Do not resuscitate This code may be used when it is documented by the provider that a patient is on do not resuscitate status at any time during the stay.
Z67	Blood type
Z68	Body mass index (BMI) BMI codes should only be assigned when there is an associated, reportable diagnosis (such as obesity). Do not assign BMI codes during pregnancy. *See Section I.B.14 for BMI documentation by clinician's other than the patient's provider.*
Z74.01	Bed confinement status
Z76.82	Awaiting organ transplant status
Z78	Other specified health status Code Z78.1, Physical restraint status, may be used when it is documented by the provider that a patient has been put in restraints during the current encounter. Please note that this code should not be reported when it is documented by the provider that a patient is temporarily restrained during a procedure.
Z79	Long-term (current) drug therapy Codes from this category indicate a patient's continuous use of a prescribed drug (including such things as aspirin therapy) for the long-term treatment of a condition or for prophylactic use. It is not for use for patients who have addictions to drugs. This subcategory is not for use of medications for detoxification or maintenance programs to prevent withdrawal symptoms in patients with drug dependence (e.g., methadone maintenance for opiate dependence). Assign the appropriate code for the drug dependence instead. Assign a code from Z79 if the patient is receiving a medication for an extended period as a prophylactic measure (such as for the prevention of deep vein thrombosis) or as treatment of a chronic condition (such as arthritis) or a disease requiring a lengthy course of treatment (such as cancer). Do not assign a code from category Z79 for medication being administered for a brief period of time to treat an acute illness or injury (such as a course of antibiotics to treat acute bronchitis).
Z88	Allergy status to drugs, medicaments and biological substances Except: Z88.9, Allergy status to unspecified drugs, medicaments and biological substances status

Z89	Acquired absence of limb
Z90	Acquired absence of organs, not elsewhere classified
Z91.0-	Allergy status, other than to drugs and biological substances
Z92.82	Status post administration of tPA (rtPA) in a different facility within the last 24 hours prior to admission to a current facility

Assign code Z92.82, Status post administration of tPA (rtPA) in a different facility within the last 24 hours prior to admission to current facility, as a secondary diagnosis when a patient is received by transfer into a facility and documentation indicates they were administered tissue plasminogen activator (tPA) within the last 24 hours prior to admission to the current facility.

This guideline applies even if the patient is still receiving the tPA at the time they are received into the current facility.

The appropriate code for the condition for which the tPA was administered (such as cerebrovascular disease or myocardial infarction) should be assigned first.

Code Z92.82 is only applicable to the receiving facility record and not to the transferring facility record.

Z93	Artificial opening status
Z94	Transplanted organ and tissue status
Z95	Presence of cardiac and vascular implants and grafts
Z96	Presence of other functional implants
Z97	Presence of other devices
Z98	Other postprocedural states

Assign code Z98.85, Transplanted organ removal status, to indicate that a transplanted organ has been previously removed. This code should not be assigned for the encounter in which the transplanted organ is removed. The complication necessitating removal of the transplant organ should be assigned for that encounter.

See section I.C19. for information on the coding of organ transplant complications.

Z99	Dependence on enabling machines and devices, not elsewhere classified

Note: Categories Z89-Z90 and Z93-Z99 are for use only if there are no complications or malfunctions of the organ or tissue replaced, the amputation site or the equipment on which the patient is dependent.

4) History (of)

There are two types of history Z codes, personal and family. Personal history codes explain a patient's past medical condition that no longer exists and is not receiving any treatment, but that has the potential for recurrence, and therefore may require continued monitoring.

Family history codes are for use when a patient has a family member(s) who has had a particular disease that causes the patient to be at higher risk of also contracting the disease.

Personal history codes may be used in conjunction with follow-up codes and family history codes may be used in conjunction with screening codes to explain the need for a test or procedure. History codes are also acceptable on any medical record regardless of the reason for visit. A history of an illness, even if no longer present, is important information that may alter the type of treatment ordered.

The reason for the encounter (for example, screening or counseling) should be sequenced first and the appropriate personal and/or family history code(s) should be assigned as additional diagnos(es).

The history Z code categories are:

Z80	Family history of primary malignant neoplasm
Z81	Family history of mental and behavioral disorders
Z82	Family history of certain disabilities and chronic diseases (leading to disablement)
Z83	Family history of other specific disorders
Z84	Family history of other conditions
Z85	Personal history of malignant neoplasm
Z86	Personal history of certain other diseases
Z87	Personal history of other diseases and conditions
Z91.4-	Personal history of psychological trauma, not elsewhere classified
Z91.5-	Personal history of self-harm
Z91.81	History of falling
Z91.82	Personal history of military deployment
Z92	Personal history of medical treatment Except: Z92.0, Personal history of contraception Except: Z92.82, Status post administration of tPA (rtPA) in a different facility within the last 24 hours prior to admission to a current facility

5) **Screening**

Refer to the complete guidelines on FindACode.com

6) **Observation**

Refer to the complete guidelines on FindACode.com

7) **Aftercare**

Aftercare visit codes cover situations when the initial treatment of a disease has been performed and the patient requires continued care during the healing or recovery phase, or for the long-term consequences of the disease. The aftercare Z code should not be used if treatment is directed at a current, acute disease. The diagnosis code is to be used in these cases. Exceptions to this rule are codes Z51.0, Encounter for antineoplastic radiation therapy, and codes from subcategory Z51.1, Encounter for antineoplastic chemotherapy and immunotherapy. These codes are to be first-listed, followed by the diagnosis code when a patient's encounter is solely to receive radiation therapy, chemotherapy, or immunotherapy for the treatment of a neoplasm. If the reason for the encounter is more than one type of antineoplastic therapy, code Z51.0

and a code from subcategory Z51.1 may be assigned together, in which case one of these codes would be reported as a secondary diagnosis.

The aftercare Z codes should also not be used for aftercare for injuries. For aftercare of an injury, assign the acute injury code with the appropriate 7th character (for subsequent encounter).

The aftercare codes are generally first-listed to explain the specific reason for the encounter. An aftercare code may be used as an additional code when some type of aftercare is provided in addition to the reason for admission and no diagnosis code is applicable. An example of this would be the closure of a colostomy during an encounter for treatment of another condition.

Aftercare codes should be used in conjunction with other aftercare codes or diagnosis codes to provide better detail on the specifics of an aftercare encounter visit, unless otherwise directed by the classification. The sequencing of multiple aftercare codes depends on the circumstances of the encounter.

Certain aftercare Z code categories need a secondary diagnosis code to describe the resolving condition or sequelae. For others, the condition is included in the code title.

Additional Z code aftercare category terms include fitting and adjustment, and attention to artificial openings.

Status Z codes may be used with aftercare Z codes to indicate the nature of the aftercare. For example, code Z95.1, Presence of aortocoronary bypass graft, may be used with code Z48.812, Encounter for surgical aftercare following surgery on the circulatory system, to indicate the surgery for which the aftercare is being performed. A status code should not be used when the aftercare code indicates the type of status, such as using Z43.0, Encounter for attention to tracheostomy, with Z93.0, Tracheostomy status.

The aftercare Z category/codes:

Z42	Encounter for plastic and reconstructive surgery following medical procedure or healed injury
Z43	Encounter for attention to artificial openings
Z44	Encounter for fitting and adjustment of external prosthetic device
Z45	Encounter for adjustment and management of implanted device
Z46	Encounter for fitting and adjustment of other devices
Z47	Orthopedic aftercare
Z48	Encounter for other postprocedural aftercare Z49 Encounter for care involving renal dialysis
Z49	Encounter for care involving renal dialysis
Z51	Encounter for other aftercare and medical care

8) **Follow-up**

Refer to the complete guidelines on FindACode.com

9) **Donor**

Refer to the complete guidelines on FindACode.com

10) **Counseling**

Refer to the complete guidelines on FindACode.com

11) Encounters for Obstetrical and Reproductive Services

Refer to the complete guidelines on FindACode.com

12) Newborns and Infants

Refer to the complete guidelines on FindACode.com

13) Routine and administrative examinations

The Z codes allow for the description of encounters for routine examinations, such as, a general check-up, or, examinations for administrative purposes, such as, a pre-employment physical. The codes are not to be used if the examination is for diagnosis of a suspected condition or for treatment purposes. In such cases the diagnosis code is used. During a routine exam, should a diagnosis or condition be discovered, it should be coded as an additional code. Pre-existing and chronic conditions and history codes may also be included as additional codes as long as the examination is for administrative purposes and not focused on any particular condition.

Some of the codes for routine health examinations distinguish between "with" and "without" abnormal findings. Code assignment depends on the information that is known at the time the encounter is being coded. For example, if no abnormal findings were found during the examination, but the encounter is being coded before test results are back, it is acceptable to assign the code for "without abnormal findings." When assigning a code for "with abnormal findings," additional code(s) should be assigned to identify the specific abnormal finding(s).

Pre-operative examination and pre-procedural laboratory examination Z codes are for use only in those situations when a patient is being cleared for a procedure or surgery and no treatment is given.

The Z codes/categories for routine and administrative examinations:

Z00	Encounter for general examination without complaint, suspected or reported diagnosis
Z01	Encounter for other special examination without complaint, suspected or reported diagnosis
Z02	Encounter for administrative examination Except: Z02.9, Encounter for administrative examinations, unspecified
Z32.0-	Encounter for pregnancy test

14) Miscellaneous Z codes

The miscellaneous Z codes capture a number of other health care encounters that do not fall into one of the other categories. **Some** of these codes identify the reason for the encounter; others are for use as additional codes that provide useful information on circumstances that may affect a patient's care and treatment.

Prophylactic Organ Removal

For encounters specifically for prophylactic removal of an organ (such as prophylactic removal of breasts due to a genetic susceptibility to cancer or a family history of cancer), the principal or first-listed code should be a code from category Z40, Encounter for prophylactic surgery, followed by the appropriate codes to identify the associated risk factor (such as genetic susceptibility or family history).

If the patient has a malignancy of one site and is having prophylactic removal at another site to prevent either a new primary malignancy or metastatic disease, a code for the malignancy should also be assigned in addition to a code from subcategory Z40.0, Encounter for prophylactic surgery for risk factors related to malignant neoplasms. A Z40.0 code should not be assigned if the patient is having organ removal for treatment of a malignancy, such as the removal of the testes for the treatment of prostate cancer.

Miscellaneous Z codes/categories:

Z28	Immunization not carried out Except: Z28.3, Underimmunization status
Z29	Encounter for other prophylactic measures
Z40	Encounter for prophylactic surgery
Z41	Encounter for procedures for purposes other than remedying health state Except: Z41.9, Encounter for procedure for purposes other than remedying health state, unspecified
Z53	Persons encountering health services for specific procedures and treatment, not carried out
Z72	Problems related to lifestyle **Note:** These codes should be assigned only when the documentation specifies that the patient has an associated problem
Z73	Problems related to life management difficulty **Note: These codes should be assigned only when the documentation specifies that the patient has an associated problem.**
Z74	Problems related to care provider dependency Except: Z74.01, Bed confinement status
Z75	Problems related to medical facilities and other health care
Z76.0	Encounter for issue of repeat prescription
Z76.3	Healthy person accompanying sick person
Z76.4	Other boarder to healthcare facility
Z76.5	Malingerer [conscious simulation]
Z91.1-	Patient's noncompliance with medical treatment and regimen
Z91.83	Wandering in diseases classified elsewhere
Z91.84-	Oral health risk factors
Z91.89	Other specified personal risk factors, not elsewhere classified

See Section I.B.14 for Z55-Z65 Persons with potential health hazards related to socioeconomic and psychosocial circumstances, documentation by clinicians other than the patient's provider

15) Nonspecific Z codes

Certain Z codes are so non-specific, or potentially redundant with other codes in the classification, that there can be little justification for their use in the inpatient setting. Their use in the outpatient setting should be limited to those instances when there is no further documentation to permit more precise coding. Otherwise, any sign or symptom or any other reason for visit that is captured in another code should be used.

Nonspecific Z codes/categories:

Z02.9	Encounter for administrative examinations, unspecified
Z04.9	Encounter for examination and observation for unspecified reason
Z13.9	Encounter for screening, unspecified

Z41.9	Encounter for procedure for purposes other than remedying health state, unspecified
Z52.9	Donor of unspecified organ or tissue
Z86.59	Personal history of other mental and behavioral disorders
Z88.9	Allergy status to unspecified drugs, medicaments and biological substances status
Z92.0	Personal history of contraception

16) Z Codes That May Only be Principal/First-Listed Diagnosis

The following Z codes/categories may only be reported as the principal/first-listed diagnosis, except when there are multiple encounters on the same day and the medical records for the encounters are combined:

Z00	Encounter for general examination without complaint, suspected or reported diagnosis Except: Z00.6
Z01	Encounter for other special examination without complaint, suspected or reported diagnosis
Z02	Encounter for administrative examination
Z04	Encounter for examination and observation for other reasons
Z33.2	Encounter for elective termination of pregnancy
Z31.81	Encounter for male factor infertility in female patient
Z31.83	Encounter for assisted reproductive fertility procedure cycle
Z31.84	Encounter for fertility preservation procedure
Z34	Encounter for supervision of normal pregnancy
Z39	Encounter for maternal postpartum care and examination
Z38	Liveborn infants according to place of birth and type of delivery
Z40	Encounter for prophylactic surgery
Z42	Encounter for plastic and reconstructive surgery following medical procedure or healed injury
Z51.0	Encounter for antineoplastic radiation therapy
Z51.1-	Encounter for antineoplastic chemotherapy and immunotherapy
Z52	Donors of organs and tissues Except: Z52.9, Donor of unspecified organ or tissue
Z76.1	Encounter for health supervision and care of foundling
Z76.2	Encounter for health supervision and care of other healthy infant and child
Z99.12	Encounter for respirator [ventilator] dependence during power failure

17) Social Determinants of Health

Codes describing **problems or risk factors related to** social determinants of health **(SDOH) should be assigned when this information is documented. Assign as many SDOH codes as are necessary to describe all of the problems or risk factors. These codes should be assigned only when the documentation specifies that the patient has an associated problem or risk factor. For example, not every individual living alone would be assigned code Z60.2, Problems related to living alone.**

For social determinants of health, such as information found in categories Z55-Z65, Persons with potential health hazards related to socioeconomic and psychosocial circumstances, code assignment may be based on medical record documentation from clinicians involved in the care of the patient who are not the patient's provider since this information represents social information, rather than medical diagnoses For example, coding professionals may utilize documentation of social information from social workers, community health workers, case managers, or nurses, if their documentation is included in the official medical record.

Patient self-reported documentation may be used to assign codes for social determinants of health, as long as the patient self-reported information is signed-off by and incorporated into the medical record by either a clinician or provider.

Social determinants of health codes are located primarily in these Z code categories:

Z55	Problems related to education and literacy
Z56	Problems related to employment and unemployment
Z57	Occupational exposure to risk factors
Z58	Problems related to physical environment
Z59	Problems related to housing and economic circumstances
Z60	Problems related to social environment
Z62	Problems related to upbringing
Z63	Other problems related to primary support group,including family circumstances
Z64	Problems related to certain psychosocial circumstances
Z65	Problems related to other psychosocial circumstances

See Section I.B.14. Documentation by Clinicians Other than the Patient's Provider.

22. Chapter 22: Codes for Special Purposes (U00-U85)

Refer to the complete guidelines on FindACode.com

Section II. Selection of Principal Diagnosis

The circumstances of inpatient admission always govern the selection of principal diagnosis. The principal diagnosis is defined in the Uniform Hospital Discharge Data Set (UHDDS) as "that condition established after study to be chiefly responsible for occasioning the admission of the patient to the hospital for care."

The UHDDS definitions are used by hospitals to report inpatient data elements in a standardized manner. These data elements and their definitions can be found in the July 31, 1985, Federal Register (Vol. 50, No, 147), pp. 31038-40.

Since that time the application of the UHDDS definitions has been expanded to include all non-outpatient settings (acute care, short term, long term care and psychiatric hospitals; home health agencies; rehab facilities; nursing homes, etc). The UHDDS definitions also apply to hospice services (all levels of care).

In determining principal diagnosis, coding conventions in the ICD-10-CM, the Tabular List and Alphabetic Index take precedence over these official coding guidelines.

(See Section I.A., Conventions for the ICD-10-CM)

The importance of consistent, complete documentation in the medical record cannot be overemphasized. Without such documentation the application of all coding guidelines is a difficult, if not impossible, task.

A. Codes for symptoms, signs, and ill-defined conditions

Codes for symptoms, signs, and ill-defined conditions from Chapter 18 are not to be used as principal diagnosis when a related definitive diagnosis has been established.

B. Two or more interrelated conditions, each potentially meeting the definition for principal diagnosis.

When there are two or more interrelated conditions (such as diseases in the same ICD-10-CM chapter or manifestations characteristically associated with a certain disease) potentially meeting the definition of principal diagnosis, either condition may be sequenced first, unless the circumstances of the admission, the therapy provided, the Tabular List, or the Alphabetic Index indicate otherwise.

C. Two or more diagnoses that equally meet the definition for principal diagnosis

In the unusual instance when two or more diagnoses equally meet the criteria for principal diagnosis as determined by the circumstances of admission, diagnostic workup and/or therapy provided, and the Alphabetic Index, Tabular List, or another coding guidelines does not provide sequencing direction, any one of the diagnoses may be sequenced first.

D. Two or more comparative or contrasting conditions

In those rare instances when two or more contrasting or comparative diagnoses are documented as "either/or" (or similar terminology), they are coded as if the diagnoses were confirmed and the diagnoses are sequenced according to the circumstances of the admission. If no further determination can be made as to which diagnosis should be principal, either diagnosis may be sequenced first.

E. A symptom(s) followed by contrasting/comparative diagnoses

GUIDELINE HAS BEEN DELETED EFFECTIVE OCTOBER 1, 2014

F. Original treatment plan not carried out

Sequence as the principal diagnosis the condition, which after study occasioned the admission to the hospital, even though treatment may not have been carried out due to unforeseen circumstances.

G. Complications of surgery and other medical care

When the admission is for treatment of a complication resulting from surgery or other medical care, the complication code is sequenced as the principal diagnosis. If the complication is classified to the T80-T88 series and the code lacks the necessary specificity in describing the complication, an additional code for the specific complication should be assigned.

H. Uncertain Diagnosis

If the diagnosis documented at the time of discharge is qualified as "probable", "suspected", "likely", "questionable", "possible", or "still to be ruled out", "compatible with," "consistent with," or other similar terms indicating uncertainty, code the condition as if it existed or was established. The bases for these guidelines are the diagnostic workup, arrangements for further workup or observation, and initial therapeutic approach that correspond most closely with the established diagnosis.

Note: This guideline is applicable only to inpatient admissions to short-term, acute, long-term care and psychiatric hospitals.

I. Admission from Observation Unit

1. Admission Following Medical Observation

When a patient is admitted to an observation unit for a medical condition, which either worsens or does not improve, and is subsequently admitted as an inpatient of the same hospital for this same medical condition, the principal diagnosis would be the medical condition which led to the hospital admission.

2. Admission Following Post-Operative Observation

When a patient is admitted to an observation unit to monitor a condition (or complication) that develops following outpatient surgery, and then is subsequently admitted as an inpatient of the same hospital, hospitals should apply the Uniform Hospital Discharge Data Set (UHDDS) definition of principal diagnosis as "that condition established after study to be chiefly responsible for occasioning the admission of the patient to the hospital for care."

J. Admission from Outpatient Surgery

When a patient receives surgery in the hospital's outpatient surgery department and is subsequently admitted for continuing inpatient care at the same hospital, the following guidelines should be followed in selecting the principal diagnosis for the inpatient admission:

- If the reason for the inpatient admission is a complication, assign the complication as the principal diagnosis.
- If no complication, or other condition, is documented as the reason for the inpatient admission, assign the reason for the outpatient surgery as the principal diagnosis.
- If the reason for the inpatient admission is another condition unrelated to the surgery, assign the unrelated condition as the principal diagnosis.

K. Admissions/Encounters for Rehabilitation

When the purpose for the admission/encounter is rehabilitation, sequence first the code for the condition for which the service is being performed. For example, for an admission/encounter for rehabilitation for right-sided dominant hemiplegia following a cerebrovascular infarction, report code I69.351, Hemiplegia and hemiparesis following cerebral infarction affecting right dominant side, as the first-listed or principal diagnosis.

If the condition for which the rehabilitation service is being provided is no longer present, report the appropriate aftercare code as the first-listed or principal diagnosis, unless the rehabilitation service is being provided following an injury. For rehabilitation services following active treatment of an injury, assign the injury code with the appropriate seventh character for subsequent encounter as the first-listed or principal diagnosis. For example, if a patient with severe degenerative osteoarthritis of the hip, underwent hip replacement and the current encounter/admission is for rehabilitation, report code Z47.1, Aftercare following joint replacement surgery, as the first-listed or principal diagnosis. If the patient requires rehabilitation post hip replacement for right intertrochanteric femur fracture, report code S72.141D, Displaced intertrochanteric fracture of right femur, subsequent encounter for closed fracture with routine healing, as the first-listed or principal diagnosis.

See Section I.C.21.c.7, Factors influencing health states and contact with health services, Aftercare.
See Section I.C.19.a for additional information about the use of 7th characters for injury codes.

Section III. Reporting Additional Diagnoses

GENERAL RULES FOR OTHER (ADDITIONAL) DIAGNOSES

For reporting purposes the definition for "other diagnoses" is interpreted as additional conditions that affect patient care in terms of requiring:

clinical evaluation; or

therapeutic treatment; or

diagnostic procedures; or

extended length of hospital stay; or

increased nursing care and/or monitoring.

The UHDDS item #11-b defines Other Diagnoses as "all conditions that coexist at the time of admission, that develop subsequently, or that affect the treatment received and/or the length of stay. Diagnoses that relate to an earlier episode which have no bearing on the current hospital stay are to be excluded." UHDDS definitions apply to inpatients in acute care, short-term, long term care and psychiatric hospital setting. The UHDDS definitions are used by acute care short-term hospitals to report inpatient data elements in a standardized manner. These data elements and their definitions can be found in the July 31, 1985, Federal Register (Vol. 50, No, 147), pp. 31038-40.

Since that time the application of the UHDDS definitions has been expanded to include all non-outpatient settings (acute care, short term, long term care and psychiatric hospitals; home health agencies; rehab facilities; nursing homes, etc). The UHDDS definitions also apply to hospice services (all levels of care).

The following guidelines are to be applied in designating "other diagnoses" when neither the Alphabetic Index nor the Tabular List in ICD-10-CM provide direction. The listing of the diagnoses in the patient record is the responsibility of the attending provider.

A. Previous conditions

If the provider has included a diagnosis in the final diagnostic statement, such as the discharge summary or the face sheet, it should ordinarily be coded. Some providers include in the diagnostic statement resolved conditions or diagnoses and status-post procedures from previous admission that have no bearing on the current stay. Such conditions are not to be reported and are coded only if required by hospital policy.

However, history codes (categories Z80-Z87) may be used as secondary codes if the historical condition or family history has an impact on current care or influences treatment.

B. Abnormal findings

Abnormal findings (laboratory, x-ray, pathologic, and other diagnostic results) are not coded and reported unless the provider indicates their clinical significance. If the findings are outside the normal range and the attending provider has ordered other tests to evaluate the condition or prescribed treatment, it is appropriate to ask the provider whether the abnormal finding should be added.

Please note: This differs from the coding practices in the outpatient setting for coding encounters for diagnostic tests that have been interpreted by a provider.

C. Uncertain Diagnosis

If the diagnosis documented at the time of discharge is qualified as "probable", "suspected", "likely", "questionable", "possible", or "still to be ruled out", "compatible with," "consistent with," or other similar terms indicating uncertainty, code the condition as if it existed or was established. The bases for these guidelines are the diagnostic workup, arrangements for further workup or observation, and initial therapeutic approach that correspond most closely with the established diagnosis.

Note: This guideline is applicable only to inpatient admissions to short-term, acute, long-term care and psychiatric hospitals.

Section IV. Diagnostic Coding and Reporting Guidelines for Outpatient Services

These coding guidelines for outpatient diagnoses have been approved for use by hospitals/ providers in coding and reporting hospital-based outpatient services and provider-based office visits. Guidelines in Section I, Conventions, general coding guidelines and chapter-specific guidelines, should also be applied for outpatient services and office visits.

Information about the use of certain abbreviations, punctuation, symbols, and other conventions used in the ICD-10-CM Tabular List (code numbers and titles), can be found in Section IA of these guidelines, under "Conventions Used in the Tabular List." Section I.B. contains general guidelines that apply to the entire classification. Section I.C. contains chapter-specific guidelines that correspond to the chapters as they are arranged in the classification. Information about the correct sequence to use in finding a code is also described in Section I.

The terms encounter and visit are often used interchangeably in describing outpatient service contacts and, therefore, appear together in these guidelines without distinguishing one from the other.

Though the conventions and general guidelines apply to all settings, coding guidelines for outpatient and provider reporting of diagnoses will vary in a number of instances from those for inpatient diagnoses, recognizing that:

> The Uniform Hospital Discharge Data Set (UHDDS) definition of principal diagnosis does not apply to hospital-based outpatient services and provider-based office visits.
>
> Coding guidelines for inconclusive diagnoses (probable, suspected, rule out, etc.) were developed for inpatient reporting and do not apply to outpatients.

A. Selection of first-listed condition

In the outpatient setting, the term first-listed diagnosis is used in lieu of principal diagnosis.

In determining the first-listed diagnosis the coding conventions of ICD-10-CM, as well as the general and disease specific guidelines take precedence over the outpatient guidelines.

Diagnoses often are not established at the time of the initial encounter/visit. It may take two or more visits before the diagnosis is confirmed.

The most critical rule involves beginning the search for the correct code assignment through the Alphabetic Index. Never begin searching initially in the Tabular List as this will lead to coding errors.

1. Outpatient Surgery

When a patient presents for outpatient surgery (same day surgery), code the reason for the surgery as the first-listed diagnosis (reason for the encounter), even if the surgery is not performed due to a contraindication.

2. Observation Stay

When a patient is admitted for observation for a medical condition, assign a code for the medical condition as the first-listed diagnosis.

When a patient presents for outpatient surgery and develops complications requiring admission to observation, code the reason for the surgery as the first reported diagnosis (reason for the encounter), followed by codes for the complications as secondary diagnoses.

B. Codes from A00.0 through T88.9, Z00-Z99, *U00-U85*

The appropriate code(s) from A00.0 through T88.9, Z00-Z99, **and U00-U85** must be used to identify diagnoses, symptoms, conditions, problems, complaints, or other reason(s) for the encounter/visit.

C. Accurate reporting of ICD-10-CM diagnosis codes

For accurate reporting of ICD-10-CM diagnosis codes, the documentation should describe the patient's condition, using terminology which includes specific diagnoses as well as symptoms, problems, or reasons for the encounter. There are ICD-10-CM codes to describe all of these.

D. Codes that describe symptoms and signs

Codes that describe symptoms and signs, as opposed to diagnoses, are acceptable for reporting purposes when a diagnosis has not been established (confirmed) by the provider. Chapter 18 of ICD-10-CM, Symptoms, Signs, and Abnormal Clinical and Laboratory Findings Not Elsewhere Classified (codes R00-R99) contain many, but not all codes for symptoms.

E. Encounters for circumstances other than a disease or injury

ICD-10-CM provides codes to deal with encounters for circumstances other than a disease or injury. The Factors Influencing Health Status and Contact with Health Services codes (Z00-Z99) are provided to deal with occasions when circumstances other than a disease or injury are recorded as diagnosis or problems.

See Section I.C.21. Factors influencing health status and contact with health services.

F. Level of Detail in Coding

1. ICD-10-CM codes with 3, 4, 5, 6 or 7 characters

ICD-10-CM is composed of codes with 3, 4, 5, 6 or 7 characters. Codes with three characters are included in ICD-10-CM as the heading of a category of codes that may be further subdivided by the use of fourth, fifth, sixth or seventh characters to provide greater specificity.

2. Use of full number of characters required for a code

A three-character code is to be used only if it is not further subdivided. A code is invalid if it has not been coded to the full number of characters required for that code, including the 7th character, if applicable.

3. Highest level of specificity

Code to the highest level of specificity when supported by the medical record documentation.

G. ICD-10-CM code for the diagnosis, condition, problem, or other reason for encounter/visit

List first the ICD-10-CM code for the diagnosis, condition, problem, or other reason for encounter/visit shown in the medical record to be chiefly responsible for the services provided. List additional codes that describe any coexisting conditions. In some cases, the first-listed diagnosis may be a symptom when a diagnosis has not been established (confirmed) by the provider.

H. Uncertain diagnosis

Do not code diagnoses documented as "probable", "suspected," "questionable," "rule out," "compatible with," "consistent with," or "working diagnosis" or other similar terms indicating uncertainty. Rather, code the condition(s) to the highest degree of certainty for that encounter/visit, such as symptoms, signs, abnormal test results, or other reason for the visit.

Please note: This differs from the coding practices used by short-term, acute care, long-term care and psychiatric hospitals.

I. Chronic diseases

Chronic diseases treated on an ongoing basis may be coded and reported as many times as the patient receives treatment and care for the condition(s)

J. Code all documented conditions that coexist

Code all documented conditions that coexist at the time of the encounter/visit, and require or affect patient care treatment or management. Do not code conditions that were previously treated and no longer exist. However, history codes (categories Z80- Z87) may be used as secondary codes if the historical condition or family history has an impact on current care or influences treatment.

K. Patients receiving diagnostic services only

For patients receiving diagnostic services only during an encounter/visit, sequence first the diagnosis, condition, problem, or other reason for encounter/visit shown in the medical record to be chiefly responsible for the outpatient services provided during the encounter/visit. Codes for other diagnoses (e.g., chronic conditions) may be sequenced as additional diagnoses.

For encounters for routine laboratory/radiology testing in the absence of any signs, symptoms, or associated diagnosis, assign Z01.89, Encounter for other specified special examinations. If routine testing is performed during the same encounter as a test to evaluate a sign, symptom, or diagnosis, it is appropriate to assign both the Z code and the code describing the reason for the non-routine test.

For outpatient encounters for diagnostic tests that have been interpreted by a physician, and the final report is available at the time of coding, code any confirmed or definitive diagnosis(es) documented in the interpretation. Do not code related signs and symptoms as additional diagnoses.

Please note: This differs from the coding practice in the hospital inpatient setting regarding abnormal findings on test results.

L. Patients receiving therapeutic services only

For patients receiving therapeutic services only during an encounter/visit, sequence first the diagnosis, condition, problem, or other reason for encounter/visit shown in the medical record to be chiefly responsible for the outpatient services provided during the encounter/visit. Codes for other diagnoses (e.g., chronic conditions) may be sequenced as additional diagnoses.

The only exception to this rule is that when the primary reason for the admission/encounter is chemotherapy or radiation therapy, the appropriate Z code for the service is listed first, and the diagnosis or problem for which the service is being performed listed second.

M. Patients receiving preoperative evaluations only

For patients receiving preoperative evaluations only, sequence first a code from subcategory Z01.81, Encounter for pre-procedural examinations, to describe the pre-op consultations. Assign a code for the condition to describe the reason for the surgery as an additional diagnosis. Code also any findings related to the pre-op evaluation.

N. Ambulatory surgery

For ambulatory surgery, code the diagnosis for which the surgery was performed. If the postoperative diagnosis is known to be different from the preoperative diagnosis at the time the diagnosis is confirmed, select the postoperative diagnosis for coding, since it is the most definitive.

O. Routine outpatient prenatal visits

See Section I.C.15. Routine outpatient prenatal visits.

P. Encounters for general medical examinations with abnormal findings

The subcategories for encounters for general medical examinations, Z00.0- and encounter for routine child health examination, Z00.12-, provide codes for with and without abnormal findings. Should a general medical examination result in an abnormal finding, the code for general medical examination with abnormal finding should be assigned as the first-listed diagnosis. An examination with abnormal findings refers to a condition/diagnosis that is newly identified or a change in severity of a chronic condition (such as uncontrolled hypertension, or an acute exacerbation of chronic obstructive pulmonary disease) during a routine physical examination. A secondary code for the abnormal finding should also be coded.

Q. Encounters for routine health screenings

See Section I.C.21. Factors influencing health status and contact with health services, Screening

Appendix I

Refer to the complete guidelines on FindACode.com

Notes:

Notes

Appendix C. Provider Documentation Guides

Introduction

This section contains a selection of *Provider Documentation Guides (PDGs)™* which were explained and introduced in Chapter 2 – Provider Documentation Training. *PDGs* are simply summaries of all the pertinent information a provider or coder might need to make sure a diagnosis is documented in a manner that allows for correct coding and reporting. ICD-10-CM codes are highly specific, and as such, have more specific criteria. All medical coding is derived from the information healthcare providers document in the medical record. A thorough understanding of the coding rules and options are vital to avoid negative post-payment audits.

These *PDGs* can help in the following ways:

- Use them for inservice training with providers and staff.
- Use them to identify the commonly reported codes for your specialty.
- Use them to avoid unspecified codes through proper documentation.

The following items are all included in each Provider Documentation Guide:

1. The condition (i.e., diagnosis), including, the ICD-10-CM code or code range
2. Helpful information (e.g., terminology, what to document, list for the provider, and notes for the coder)
3. Applicable instructional notes/guidelines and indicator(s) at the chapter and block levels
4. Information conveyed by each character level with instructional notes, guidelines, and indicators applicable at the category and subcategory levels

If a particular condition is not found in this section, build a *PDG* by hand by looking up the code in The Tabular List and recording the relevant information on a worksheet.

Resource: Access thousands of additional *PDGs* with an add-on subscription to your Find-A-Code account.

Contents — Provider Documentation Guides

Migraine without Aura

ICD-1Ø-CM: G43.ØØ1 - G43.Ø19

What to Document

3rd Character: Type of disorder
4th Character: Type of migraine
5th Character: Intractable or not intractable
6th Character: With or without status migrainosus

Document:
- Adverse effect, if applicable, to identify drug

Chapter Guidelines

6. Diseases of the nervous system (GØØ-G99)

Excludes2:
certain conditions originating in the perinatal period (PØ4-P96)
certain infectious and parasitic diseases (AØØ-B99)
complications of pregnancy, childbirth and the puerperium (OØØ-O9A)
congenital malformations, deformations, and chromosomal abnormalities (QØØ-Q99)
endocrine, nutritional and metabolic diseases (EØØ-E88)
injury, poisoning and certain other consequences of external causes (SØØ-T88)
neoplasms (CØØ-D49)
symptoms, signs and abnormal clinical and laboratory findings, not elsewhere classified (RØØ-R94)
See Guidelines: 1;C.2Ø.a.1

EPISODIC AND PAROXYSMAL DISORDERS (G4Ø-G47)

3rd Character

Document: Type of disorder

G4Ø- Epilepsy and recurrent seizures
G43- Migraine
G44- Other headache syndromes
G45- Transient cerebral ischemic attacks and related syndromes
G46- Vascular syndromes of brain in cerebrovascular diseases
G47- Sleep disorders

4th Character

Document: Type of migraine

Notes:
the following terms are to be considered equivalent to intractable: pharmacoresistant (pharmacologically resistant), treatment resistant, refractory (medically) and poorly controlled
Use additional code for adverse effect, if applicable, to identify drug (T36-T5Ø with fifth or sixth character 5)
Excludes1:
headache NOS (R51.9)
lower half migraine (G44.ØØ)
Excludes2:
headache syndromes (G44.-)
Indicator(s): RxØ5: 166

G43.Ø- Migraine without aura
Including: Common migraine
Excludes1:
chronic migraine without aura (G43.7-)

G43.1- Migraine with aura
Including: Basilar migraine, Classical migraine, Migraine equivalents, Migraine preceded or accompanied by transient focal neurological phenomena, Migraine triggered seizures, Migraine with acute-onset aura, Migraine with aura without headache (migraine equivalents), Migraine with prolonged aura, Migraine with typical aura, Retinal migraine
Code Also
any associated seizure (G4Ø.-, R56.9)
Excludes1:
persistent migraine aura (G43.5-, G43.6-)

G43.4- Hemiplegic migraine
Including: Familial, Sporadic

G43.5- Persistent migraine aura without cerebral infarction

G43.6- Persistent migraine aura with cerebral infarction
Code Also
the type of cerebral infarction (I63.-)

G43.7- Chronic migraine without aura
Including: Transformed migraine
Excludes1:
migraine without aura (G43.Ø-)

G43.8- Other migraine

G43.9- Migraine, unspecified

G43.A- Cyclical vomiting
Excludes1:
cyclical vomiting syndrome unrelated to migraine (R11.15)

G43.B- Ophthalmoplegic migraine

G43.C- Periodic headache syndromes in child or adult

G43.D- Abdominal migraine

Migraine without Aura (continued)

5th Character

Document: Intractable or not intractable

Including: Common migraine
Excludes1:
chronic migraine without aura (G43.7-)

G43.ØØ- Migraine without aura, not intractable
Including: without mention of refractory migraine

G43.Ø1- Migraine without aura, intractable
Including: with refractory migraine

6th Character

Document: With or without status migrainosus

Applies to: G43.ØØ-

Including: without mention of refractory migraine

1 With status migrainosus

9 Without status migrainosus
Including: without aura NOS

Applies to: G43.Ø1-

Including: without aura with refractory migraine

1 With status migrainosus

9 Without status migrainosus

7th Character

N/A

Tension-Type Headache

ICD-10-CM: G44.201 - G44.229

What to Document

3rd Character: Type of disorder
4th Character: Type of headache
5th Character: Chronic or episodic
6th Character: Intractable or not intractable

Terminology:
Intractable: In this context, means that the headache is not easily relieved or cured
Episodic: Last 30 minutes to a week and occur less than 15 days out of the month. Frequent episodic tension headaches can turn into chronic tension headaches.
Chronic: Lasts hours and may be continuous and last more than 15 days a month for at least three months

Chapter Guidelines

6. Diseases of the nervous system (G00-G99)

Excludes2:
certain conditions originating in the perinatal period (P04-P96)
certain infectious and parasitic diseases (A00-B99)
complications of pregnancy, childbirth and the puerperium (O00-O9A)
congenital malformations, deformations, and chromosomal abnormalities (Q00-Q99)
endocrine, nutritional and metabolic diseases (E00-E88)
injury, poisoning and certain other consequences of external causes (S00-T88)
neoplasms (C00-D49)
symptoms, signs and abnormal clinical and laboratory findings, not elsewhere classified (R00-R94)
See Guidelines: 1;C.20.a.1

EPISODIC AND PAROXYSMAL DISORDERS (G40-G47)

3rd Character

Document: Type of disorder

G40- Epilepsy and recurrent seizures
G43- Migraine
G44- Other headache syndromes
G45- Transient cerebral ischemic attacks and related syndromes
G46- Vascular syndromes of brain in cerebrovascular diseases
G47- Sleep disorders

4th Character

Document: Type of headache

Excludes1:
headache NOS (R51.9)
Excludes2:
atypical facial pain (G50.1)
headache due to lumbar puncture (G97.1)
migraines (G43.-)
trigeminal neuralgia (G50.0)

G44.0- Cluster headaches and other trigeminal autonomic cephalgias (TAC)
G44.1 Vascular headache, not elsewhere classified
Excludes2:
cluster headache (G44.0)
complicated headache syndromes (G44.5-)
drug-induced headache (G44.4-)
migraine (G43.-)
other specified headache syndromes (G44.8-)
post-traumatic headache (G44.3-)
tension-type headache (G44.2-)
G44.2- Tension-type headache
G44.3- Post-traumatic headache
G44.4- Drug-induced headache, not elsewhere classified
Including: Medication overuse headache
Use additional code for adverse effect, if applicable, to identify drug (T36-T50 with fifth or sixth character 5)
G44.5- Complicated headache syndromes
G44.8- Other specified headache syndromes
Excludes2:
headache with orthostatic or positional component, not elsewhere classified (R51.0)

5th Character

Document: Chronic or episodic

G44.20- Tension-type headache, unspecified
G44.21- Episodic tension-type headache
G44.22- Chronic tension-type headache

Tension-Type Headache (continued)

6th Character

Document: Intractable or not intractable

Applies to: G44.2Ø-

1 Intractable

9 Not intractable

Including: Tension headache NOS

Applies to: G44.21-

1 Intractable

9 Not intractable

Including: Episodic tension-type headache NOS

Applies to: G44.22-

1 Intractable

9 Not intractable

Including: Chronic tension-type headache NOS

7th Character

N/A

Post-Traumatic Headache

ICD-10-CM: G44.301 - G44.329

What to Document

3rd Character: Type of disorder
4th Character: Type of headache
5th Character: Acute vs chronic
6th Character: Intractable or not intractable

Terminology:
Intractable: In this context, means that the headache is not easily relieved or cured
Chronic: Having more than 15 headache days in a month, 8 or more which are migrainous, for a 3 month time span

Chapter Guidelines

6. Diseases of the nervous system (G00-G99)

Excludes2:
certain conditions originating in the perinatal period (P04-P96)
certain infectious and parasitic diseases (A00-B99)
complications of pregnancy, childbirth and the puerperium (O00-O9A)
congenital malformations, deformations, and chromosomal abnormalities (Q00-Q99)
endocrine, nutritional and metabolic diseases (E00-E88)
injury, poisoning and certain other consequences of external causes (S00-T88)
neoplasms (C00-D49)
symptoms, signs and abnormal clinical and laboratory findings, not elsewhere classified (R00-R94)
See Guidelines: 1;C.20.a.1

EPISODIC AND PAROXYSMAL DISORDERS (G40-G47)

3rd Character

Document: Type of disorder

G40- Epilepsy and recurrent seizures
G43- Migraine
G44- Other headache syndromes
G45- Transient cerebral ischemic attacks and related syndromes
G46- Vascular syndromes of brain in cerebrovascular diseases
G47- Sleep disorders

4th Character

Document: Type of headache

Excludes1:
headache NOS (R51.9)
Excludes2:
atypical facial pain (G50.1)
headache due to lumbar puncture (G97.1)
migraines (G43.-)
trigeminal neuralgia (G50.0)

G44.0- Cluster headaches and other trigeminal autonomic cephalgias (TAC)
G44.1 Vascular headache, not elsewhere classified
Excludes2:
cluster headache (G44.0)
complicated headache syndromes (G44.5-)
drug-induced headache (G44.4-)
migraine (G43.-)
other specified headache syndromes (G44.8-)
post-traumatic headache (G44.3-)
tension-type headache (G44.2-)

G44.2- Tension-type headache
G44.3- Post-traumatic headache
G44.4- Drug-induced headache, not elsewhere classified
Including: Medication overuse headache
Use additional code for adverse effect, if applicable, to identify drug (T36-T50 with fifth or sixth character 5)

G44.5- Complicated headache syndromes
G44.8- Other specified headache syndromes
Excludes2:
headache with orthostatic or positional component, not elsewhere classified (R51.0)

5th Character

Document: Acute vs chronic

G44.30- Post-traumatic headache, unspecified
G44.31- Acute post-traumatic headache
G44.32- Chronic post-traumatic headache

Post-Traumatic Headache (continued)

6th Character

Document: Intractable or not intractable

Applies to: G44.3Ø-

1 Intractable

9 Not intractable

Including: Post-traumatic headache NOS

Applies to: G44.31-

1 Intractable

9 Not intractable

Including: Acute post-traumatic headache NOS

Applies to: G44.32-

1 Intractable

9 Not intractable

Including: Chronic post-traumatic headache NOS

7th Character

N/A

See Appendix A — Coding Reference Tables for lists of the ICD-10-CM Tabular indicators, HAC categories, and HCC codes.

Nerve Root and Plexus Disorders

ICD-1Ø-CM: G54.Ø - G54.9

What to Document

3rd Character: Type of nerve disorder
4th Character: Specified nerve root/plexus disorder

Terminology:
Neuralgic amyotrophy: Episodes of pain that occur in the shoulder and arm with atrophy of the muscles of the affected areas

Chapter Guidelines

6. Diseases of the nervous system (GØØ-G99)

Excludes2:
certain conditions originating in the perinatal period (PØ4-P96)
certain infectious and parasitic diseases (AØØ-B99)
complications of pregnancy, childbirth and the puerperium (OØØ-O9A)
congenital malformations, deformations, and chromosomal abnormalities (QØØ-Q99)
endocrine, nutritional and metabolic diseases (EØØ-E88)
injury, poisoning and certain other consequences of external causes (SØØ-T88)
neoplasms (CØØ-D49)
symptoms, signs and abnormal clinical and laboratory findings, not elsewhere classified (RØØ-R94)
See Guidelines: *1;C.2Ø.a.1*

NERVE, NERVE ROOT AND PLEXUS DISORDERS (G5Ø-G59)

Excludes1:
current traumatic nerve, nerve root and plexus disorders - see Injury, nerve by body region
neuralgia NOS (M79.2)
neuritis NOS (M79.2)
peripheral neuritis in pregnancy (O26.82-)
radiculitis NOS (M54.1-)

3rd Character

Document: Type of nerve disorder

G5Ø- Disorders of trigeminal nerve
G51- Facial nerve disorders
G52- Disorders of other cranial nerves
G53 Cranial nerve disorders in diseases classified elsewhere
G54- Nerve root and plexus disorders
G55 Nerve root and plexus compressions in diseases classified elsewhere
G56- Mononeuropathies of upper limb
G57- Mononeuropathies of lower limb
G58- Other mononeuropathies
G59 Mononeuropathy in diseases classified elsewhere

4th Character

Document: Specified nerve root/plexus disorder

Excludes1:
current traumatic nerve root and plexus disorders - see nerve injury by body region
intervertebral disc disorders (M5Ø-M51)
neuralgia or neuritis NOS (M79.2)
neuritis or radiculitis brachial NOS (M54.13)
neuritis or radiculitis lumbar NOS (M54.16)
neuritis or radiculitis lumbosacral NOS (M54.17)
neuritis or radiculitis thoracic NOS (M54.14)
radiculitis NOS (M54.1Ø)
radiculopathy NOS (M54.1Ø)
spondylosis (M47.-)

Applies to: G54.-

Ø Brachial plexus
Including: Thoracic outlet syndrome

1 Lumbosacral plexus

2 Cervical root, NEC

3 Thoracic root, NEC

4 Lumbosacral root, NEC

5 Neuralgic amyotrophy
Including: Parsonage-Aldren-Turner syndrome, Shoulder-girdle neuritis
Excludes1:
neuralgic amyotrophy in diabetes mellitus (EØ8-E13 with .44)

6 Phantom limb syndrome with pain
Indicator(s): *CMS22: 189 | CMS23: 189 | CMS24: 189 | ESRD21: 189 | HHSØ4: 254 | HHSØ5: 254*

7 Phantom limb syndrome without pain
Including: Phantom limb syndrome NOS
Indicator(s): *CMS22: 189 | CMS23: 189 | CMS24: 189 | ESRD21: 189 | HHSØ4: 254 | HHSØ5: 254*

8 Other

9 Unspecified

5th Character

N/A

6th Character

N/A

7th Character

N/A

Pain in Joint

ICD-1Ø-CM: M25.5Ø - M25.579

What to Document

3rd Character: Type of joint disorder
5th Character: Anatomic site
6th Character: Laterality

Document:
- Any external cause, if applicable

Chapter Guidelines

13. Diseases of the musculoskeletal system and connective tissue (MØØ-M99)

Notes:
Use an external cause code following the code for the musculoskeletal condition, if applicable, to identify the cause of the musculoskeletal condition
Excludes2:
arthropathic psoriasis (L4Ø.5-)
certain conditions originating in the perinatal period (PØ4-P96)
certain infectious and parasitic diseases (AØØ-B99)
compartment syndrome (traumatic) (T79.A-)
complications of pregnancy, childbirth and the puerperium (OØØ-O9A)
congenital malformations, deformations, and chromosomal abnormalities (QØØ-Q99)
endocrine, nutritional and metabolic diseases (EØØ-E88)
injury, poisoning and certain other consequences of external causes (SØØ-T88)
neoplasms (CØØ-D49)
symptoms, signs and abnormal clinical and laboratory findings, not elsewhere classified (RØØ-R94)
See Guidelines: 1;C.13.a-b | 1;C.2Ø.a.1

ARTHROPATHIES (MØØ-M25)

Includes:
Disorders affecting predominantly peripheral (limb) joints

OTHER JOINT DISORDERS (M2Ø-M25)

Excludes2:
joints of the spine (M4Ø-M54)

3rd Character

Document: Type of joint disorder

M2Ø- Acquired deformities of fingers and toes
M21- Other acquired deformities of limbs
M22- Disorder of patella
M23- Internal derangement of knee
M24- Other specific joint derangements
M25- Other joint disorder, not elsewhere classified

4th Character

Excludes2:
abnormality of gait and mobility (R26.-)
acquired deformities of limb (M2Ø-M21)
calcification of bursa (M71.4-)
calcification of shoulder (joint) (M75.3)
calcification of tendon (M65.2-)
difficulty in walking (R26.2)
temporomandibular joint disorder (M26.6-)

M25.Ø- Hemarthrosis
Excludes1:
current injury - see injury of joint by body region
hemophilic arthropathy (M36.2)

M25.1- Fistula of joint

M25.2- Flail joint

M25.3- Other instability of joint
Excludes1:
instability of joint secondary to old ligament injury (M24.2-)
instability of joint secondary to removal of joint prosthesis (M96.8-)
Excludes2:
spinal instabilities (M53.2-)

M25.4- Effusion of joint
Excludes1:
hydrarthrosis in yaws (A66.6)
intermittent hydrarthrosis (M12.4-)
other infective (teno)synovitis (M65.1-)

M25.5- Pain in joint
Excludes2:
pain in hand (M79.64-)
pain in fingers (M79.64-)
pain in foot (M79.67-)
pain in limb (M79.6-)
pain in toes (M79.67-)

M25.6- Stiffness of joint, not elsewhere classified
Excludes1:
ankylosis of joint (M24.6-)
contracture of joint (M24.5-)

M25.7- Osteophyte

M25.8- Other specified joint disorders

M25.9 Joint disorder, unspecified

Pain in Joint (continued)

5th Character

Document: Anatomic site
Reminder: All final codes are in **BOLD**

Excludes2:
pain in hand (M79.64-)
pain in fingers (M79.64-)
pain in foot (M79.67-)
pain in limb (M79.6-)
pain in toes (M79.67-)

M25.5Ø Pain in unspecified joint
M25.51- Pain in shoulder
M25.52- Pain in elbow
M25.53- Pain in wrist
M25.54- Pain in joints of hand
M25.55- Pain in hip
M25.56- Pain in knee
M25.57- Pain in ankle and joints of foot
M25.59 Pain in other specified joint

6th Character

Document: Laterality

Applies to: M25.51-, M25.52-, M25.53-, M25.55-, M25.56-, M25.57-

1 Right
2 Left
9 Unspecified

Applies to: M25.54-

1 Right
2 Left
9 Unspecified
Including: Pain in joints of hand NOS

7th Character

N/A

Stiffness of Joint, NEC

ICD-1Ø-CM: M25.6Ø - M25.676

What to Document

4th Character: Type of joint disorder
5th Character: Anatomic site
6th Character: Laterality

Document:
- Any external cause, if applicable

Chapter Guidelines

13. Diseases of the musculoskeletal system and connective tissue (MØØ-M99)

Notes:
Use an external cause code following the code for the musculoskeletal condition, if applicable, to identify the cause of the musculoskeletal condition

Excludes2:
arthropathic psoriasis (L4Ø.5-)
certain conditions originating in the perinatal period (PØ4-P96)
certain infectious and parasitic diseases (AØØ-B99)
compartment syndrome (traumatic) (T79.A-)
complications of pregnancy, childbirth and the puerperium (OØØ-O9A)
congenital malformations, deformations, and chromosomal abnormalities (QØØ-Q99)
endocrine, nutritional and metabolic diseases (EØØ-E88)
injury, poisoning and certain other consequences of external causes (SØØ-T88)
neoplasms (CØØ-D49)
symptoms, signs and abnormal clinical and laboratory findings, not elsewhere classified (RØØ-R94)

See Guidelines: 1;C.13.a-b | 1;C.2Ø.a.1

ARTHROPATHIES (MØØ-M25)

Includes:
Disorders affecting predominantly peripheral (limb) joints

OTHER JOINT DISORDERS (M2Ø-M25)

Excludes2:
joints of the spine (M4Ø-M54)

3rd Character

M2Ø- Acquired deformities of fingers and toes
M21- Other acquired deformities of limbs
M22- Disorder of patella
M23- Internal derangement of knee
M24- Other specific joint derangements
M25- Other joint disorder, not elsewhere classified

4th Character

Document: Type of joint disorder

Excludes2:
abnormality of gait and mobility (R26.-)
acquired deformities of limb (M2Ø-M21)
calcification of bursa (M71.4-)
calcification of shoulder (joint) (M75.3)
calcification of tendon (M65.2-)
difficulty in walking (R26.2)
temporomandibular joint disorder (M26.6-)

M25.Ø- Hemarthrosis
Excludes1:
current injury - see injury of joint by body region
hemophilic arthropathy (M36.2)

M25.1- Fistula of joint

M25.2- Flail joint

M25.3- Other instability of joint
Excludes1:
instability of joint secondary to old ligament injury (M24.2-)
instability of joint secondary to removal of joint prosthesis (M96.8-)
Excludes2:
spinal instabilities (M53.2-)

M25.4- Effusion of joint
Excludes1:
hydrarthrosis in yaws (A66.6)
intermittent hydrarthrosis (M12.4-)
other infective (teno)synovitis (M65.1-)

M25.5- Pain in joint
Excludes2:
pain in hand (M79.64-)
pain in fingers (M79.64-)
pain in foot (M79.67-)
pain in limb (M79.6-)
pain in toes (M79.67-)

M25.6- Stiffness of joint, not elsewhere classified
Excludes1:
ankylosis of joint (M24.6-)
contracture of joint (M24.5-)

M25.7- Osteophyte

M25.8- Other specified joint disorders

M25.9 Joint disorder, unspecified

Stiffness of Joint, NEC (continued)

5th Character

Document: Anatomic site
Reminder: All final codes are in **BOLD**

Excludes1:
ankylosis of joint (M24.6-)
contracture of joint (M24.5-)

M25.60 Stiffness of unspecified joint, not elsewhere classified
M25.61- Stiffness of shoulder, not elsewhere classified
M25.62- Stiffness of elbow, not elsewhere classified
M25.63- Stiffness of wrist, not elsewhere classified
M25.64- Stiffness of hand, not elsewhere classified
M25.65- Stiffness of hip, not elsewhere classified
M25.66- Stiffness of knee, not elsewhere classified
M25.67- Stiffness of ankle and foot, not elsewhere classified
M25.69 Stiffness of other specified joint, not elsewhere classified

6th Character

Document: Laterality

Applies to: M25.61-, M25.62-, M25.63-, M25.64-, M25.65-, M25.66-

1 Right
2 Left
9 Unspecified

Applies to: M25.67-

1 Right ankle
2 Left ankle
3 Unspecified ankle
4 Right foot
5 Left foot
6 Unspecified foot

7th Character

N/A

Juvenile and Adolescent Idiopathic Scoliosis

ICD-1Ø-CM: M41.112 - M41.129

What to Document

3rd Character: Type of deforming dorsopathy
4th Character: Type of scoliosis
5th Character: Juvenile idiopathic or adolescent
6th Character: Spinal region

Document:
- Any external cause, if applicable

Terminology:
Adolescent idiopathic scoliosis: Abnormal side-to-side curvature of the spine that develops with no known cause; occurs in late childhood/adolescence
Juvenile idiopathic scoliosis: Abnormal side-to-side curvature of the spine that develops with no known cause; occurs in early childhood

Chapter Guidelines

13. Diseases of the musculoskeletal system and connective tissue (MØØ-M99)

Notes:
Use an external cause code following the code for the musculoskeletal condition, if applicable, to identify the cause of the musculoskeletal condition

Excludes2:
arthropathic psoriasis (L4Ø.5-)
certain conditions originating in the perinatal period (PØ4-P96)
certain infectious and parasitic diseases (AØØ-B99)
compartment syndrome (traumatic) (T79.A-)
complications of pregnancy, childbirth and the puerperium (OØØ-O9A)
congenital malformations, deformations, and chromosomal abnormalities (QØØ-Q99)
endocrine, nutritional and metabolic diseases (EØØ-E88)
injury, poisoning and certain other consequences of external causes (SØØ-T88)
neoplasms (CØØ-D49)
symptoms, signs and abnormal clinical and laboratory findings, not elsewhere classified (RØØ-R94)

See Guidelines: 1;C.13.a-b | 1;C.2Ø.a.1

DORSOPATHIES (M4Ø-M54)

DEFORMING DORSOPATHIES (M4Ø-M43)

3rd Character

Document: Type of deforming dorsopathy

M4Ø- Kyphosis and lordosis
M41- Scoliosis
M42- Spinal osteochondrosis
M43- Other deforming dorsopathies

4th Character

Document: Type of scoliosis

Includes:
kyphoscoliosis

Excludes1:
congenital scoliosis NOS (Q67.5)
congenital scoliosis due to bony malformation (Q76.3)
postural congenital scoliosis (Q67.5)
kyphoscoliotic heart disease (I27.1)

Excludes2:
postprocedural scoliosis (M96.-)

M41.Ø- Infantile idiopathic scoliosis
M41.1- Juvenile and adolescent idiopathic scoliosis
M41.2- Other idiopathic scoliosis
M41.3- Thoracogenic scoliosis
M41.4- Neuromuscular scoliosis
Including: Scoliosis secondary to cerebral palsy, Friedreich's ataxia, poliomyelitis and other neuromuscular disorders
Code Also
underlying condition
M41.5 Other secondary scoliosis
Code first underlying disease
M41.8- Other forms of scoliosis
M41.9 Scoliosis, unspecified

5th Character

Document: Juvenile idiopathic or adolescent

M41.11- Juvenile idiopathic scoliosis
M41.12- Adolescent scoliosis

See Appendix A — Coding Reference Tables for lists of the ICD-10-CM Tabular indicators, HAC categories, and HCC codes.

Juvenile and Adolescent Idiopathic Scoliosis (continued)

6th Character

Document: Spinal region

Applies to: M41.11-

2 Cervical region
3 Cervicothoracic region
4 Thoracic region
5 Thoracolumbar region
6 Lumbar region
7 Lumbosacral region
9 Site unspecified

Applies to: M41.12-

2 Idiopathic, cervical region
3 Idiopathic, cervicothoracic region
4 Idiopathic, thoracic region
5 Idiopathic, thoracolumbar region
6 Idiopathic, lumbar region
7 Idiopathic, lumbosacral region
9 Idiopathic, site unspecified

7th Character

N/A

Spondylolisthesis

ICD-1Ø-CM: M43.1Ø - M43.19

What to Document

4th Character: Type of dorsopathy
5th Character: Anatomic region

Document:
- Any external cause, if applicable

Terminology:
Spondylolisthesis: When a vertebrae slides forward onto the one beneath it

Chapter Guidelines

13. Diseases of the musculoskeletal system and connective tissue (MØØ-M99)

Notes:
Use an external cause code following the code for the musculoskeletal condition, if applicable, to identify the cause of the musculoskeletal condition

Excludes2:
arthropathic psoriasis (L4Ø.5-)
certain conditions originating in the perinatal period (PØ4-P96)
certain infectious and parasitic diseases (AØØ-B99)
compartment syndrome (traumatic) (T79.A-)
complications of pregnancy, childbirth and the puerperium (OØØ-O9A)
congenital malformations, deformations, and chromosomal abnormalities (QØØ-Q99)
endocrine, nutritional and metabolic diseases (EØØ-E88)
injury, poisoning and certain other consequences of external causes (SØØ-T88)
neoplasms (CØØ-D49)
symptoms, signs and abnormal clinical and laboratory findings, not elsewhere classified (RØØ-R94)

See Guidelines: *1;C.13.a-b | 1;C.2Ø.a.1*

DORSOPATHIES (M4Ø-M54)

DEFORMING DORSOPATHIES (M4Ø-M43)

3rd Character

M4Ø- Kyphosis and lordosis
M41- Scoliosis
M42- Spinal osteochondrosis
M43- Other deforming dorsopathies

4th Character

Document: Type of dorsopathy

Excludes1:
congenital spondylolysis and spondylolisthesis (Q76.2)
hemivertebra (Q76.3-Q76.4)
Klippel-Feil syndrome (Q76.1)
lumbarization and sacralization (Q76.4)
platyspondylisis (Q76.4)
spina bifida occulta (Q76.Ø)
spinal curvature in osteoporosis (M8Ø.-)
spinal curvature in Paget's disease of bone [osteitis deformans] (M88.-)

M43.Ø- Spondylolysis
Excludes1:
congenital spondylolysis (Q76.2)
spondylolisthesis (M43.1)

M43.1- Spondylolisthesis
Excludes1:
acute traumatic of lumbosacral region (S33.1)
acute traumatic of sites other than lumbosacral- code to Fracture, vertebra, by region
congenital spondylolisthesis (Q76.2)

M43.2- Fusion of spine
Including: Ankylosis of spinal joint
Excludes1:
ankylosing spondylitis (M45.Ø-)
congenital fusion of spine (Q76.4)
Excludes2:
arthrodesis status (Z98.1)
pseudoarthrosis after fusion or arthrodesis (M96.Ø)

M43.3 Recurrent atlantoaxial dislocation with myelopathy

M43.4 Other recurrent atlantoaxial dislocation

M43.5- Other recurrent vertebral dislocation
Excludes1:
biomechanical lesions NEC (M99.-)

M43.6 Torticollis
Excludes1:
congenital (sternomastoid) torticollis (Q68.Ø)
current injury - see Injury, of spine, by body region
ocular torticollis (R29.891)
psychogenic torticollis (F45.8)
spasmodic torticollis (G24.3)
torticollis due to birth injury (P15.2)

M43.8- Other specified deforming dorsopathies
Excludes2:
kyphosis and lordosis (M4Ø.-)
scoliosis (M41.-)

M43.9 Deforming dorsopathy, unspecified
Including: Curvature of spine NOS

 See Appendix A — Coding Reference Tables for lists of the ICD-10-CM Tabular indicators, HAC categories, and HCC codes.

Spondylolisthesis (continued)

5th Character

Document: Anatomic region

Excludes1:
acute traumatic of lumbosacral region (S33.1)
acute traumatic of sites other than lumbosacral- code to Fracture, vertebra, by region
congenital spondylolisthesis (Q76.2)

Applies to: M43.1-

Ø Site unspecified
1 Occipito-atlanto-axial region
2 Cervical region
3 Cervicothoracic region
4 Thoracic region
5 Thoracolumbar region
6 Lumbar region
7 Lumbosacral region
8 Sacral and sacrococcygeal region
9 Multiple sites in spine

6th Character

N/A

7th Character

N/A

Torticollis

ICD-1Ø-CM: M43.6 - M43.6

What to Document

3rd Character: Type of dorsopathy
4th Character: Type and location

Document:
- Any external cause, if applicable

Terminology:
Torticollis: A contraction of the neck that pulls the head to one side, resulting in a tilt

Chapter Guidelines

13. Diseases of the musculoskeletal system and connective tissue (MØØ-M99)

Notes:
Use an external cause code following the code for the musculoskeletal condition, if applicable, to identify the cause of the musculoskeletal condition
Excludes2:
arthropathic psoriasis (L4Ø.5-)
certain conditions originating in the perinatal period (PØ4-P96)
certain infectious and parasitic diseases (AØØ-B99)
compartment syndrome (traumatic) (T79.A-)
complications of pregnancy, childbirth and the puerperium (OØØ-O9A)
congenital malformations, deformations, and chromosomal abnormalities (QØØ-Q99)
endocrine, nutritional and metabolic diseases (EØØ-E88)
injury, poisoning and certain other consequences of external causes (SØØ-T88)
neoplasms (CØØ-D49)
symptoms, signs and abnormal clinical and laboratory findings, not elsewhere classified (RØØ-R94)
See Guidelines: 1;C.13.a-b | 1;C.2Ø.a.1

DORSOPATHIES (M4Ø-M54)

DEFORMING DORSOPATHIES (M4Ø-M43)

3rd Character

Document: Type of dorsopathy

M4Ø- Kyphosis and lordosis
M41- Scoliosis
M42- Spinal osteochondrosis
M43- Other deforming dorsopathies

4th Character

Document: Type and location

Excludes1:
congenital spondylolysis and spondylolisthesis (Q76.2)
hemivertebra (Q76.3-Q76.4)
Klippel-Feil syndrome (Q76.1)
lumbarization and sacralization (Q76.4)
platyspondylisis (Q76.4)
spina bifida occulta (Q76.Ø)
spinal curvature in osteoporosis (M8Ø.-)
spinal curvature in Paget's disease of bone [osteitis deformans] (M88.-)

Applies to: M43.-

6 Torticollis
Excludes1:
congenital (sternomastoid) torticollis (Q68.Ø)
current injury - see Injury, of spine, by body region
ocular torticollis (R29.891)
psychogenic torticollis (F45.8)
spasmodic torticollis (G24.3)
torticollis due to birth injury (P15.2)

5th Character

N/A

6th Character

N/A

7th Character

N/A

See Appendix A — Coding Reference Tables for lists of the ICD-10-CM Tabular indicators, HAC categories, and HCC codes.

Other Spondylosis with Radiculopathy

ICD-10-CM: M47.2Ø - M47.28

What to Document

3rd Character: Type of spondylopathy
4th Character: Type of spondylosis
5th Character: Anatomic region

Document:
- Any external cause, if applicable

Terminology:
Spondylopathy: A disorder in the spine
Spondylosis: Degeneration of the spine

Chapter Guidelines

13. Diseases of the musculoskeletal system and connective tissue (MØØ-M99)

Notes:
Use an external cause code following the code for the musculoskeletal condition, if applicable, to identify the cause of the musculoskeletal condition
Excludes2:
arthropathic psoriasis (L4Ø.5-)
certain conditions originating in the perinatal period (PØ4-P96)
certain infectious and parasitic diseases (AØØ-B99)
compartment syndrome (traumatic) (T79.A-)
complications of pregnancy, childbirth and the puerperium (OØØ-O9A)
congenital malformations, deformations, and chromosomal abnormalities (QØØ-Q99)
endocrine, nutritional and metabolic diseases (EØØ-E88)
injury, poisoning and certain other consequences of external causes (SØØ-T88)
neoplasms (CØØ-D49)
symptoms, signs and abnormal clinical and laboratory findings, not elsewhere classified (RØØ-R94)
See Guidelines: 1;C.13.a-b | 1;C.2Ø.a.1

DORSOPATHIES (M4Ø-M54)

SPONDYLOPATHIES (M45-M49)

3rd Character

Document: Type of spondylopathy

M45- Ankylosing spondylitis
M46- Other inflammatory spondylopathies
M47- Spondylosis
M48- Other spondylopathies
M49- Spondylopathies in diseases classified elsewhere

4th Character

Document: Type of spondylosis

Includes:
arthrosis or osteoarthritis of spine
degeneration of facet joints

M47.Ø- Anterior spinal and vertebral artery compression syndromes
M47.1- Other spondylosis with myelopathy
Including: Spondylogenic compression of spinal cord
Excludes1:
vertebral subluxation (M43.3-M43.5X9)
M47.2- Other spondylosis with radiculopathy
M47.8- Other spondylosis
M47.9 Spondylosis, unspecified

5th Character

Document: Anatomic region

Applies to: M47.2-

Ø Site unspecified
1 Occipito-atlanto-axial region
2 Cervical region
3 Cervicothoracic region
4 Thoracic region
5 Thoracolumbar region
6 Lumbar region
7 Lumbosacral region
8 Sacral and sacrococcygeal region

6th Character

N/A

7th Character

N/A

Other Spondylosis

ICD-1Ø-CM: M47.811 - M47.899

What to Document

3rd Character: Type of spondylopathy
4th Character: Type of spondylosis
6th Character: Anatomic region

Document:
- Any external cause, if applicable

Terminology:
Spondylopathy: A disorder in the spine
Myelopathy: A disorder of the spinal cord
Radiculopathy: The disorder of a nerve root

Chapter Guidelines

13. Diseases of the musculoskeletal system and connective tissue (MØØ-M99)

Notes:
Use an external cause code following the code for the musculoskeletal condition, if applicable, to identify the cause of the musculoskeletal condition

Excludes2:
arthropathic psoriasis (L4Ø.5-)
certain conditions originating in the perinatal period (PØ4-P96)
certain infectious and parasitic diseases (AØØ-B99)
compartment syndrome (traumatic) (T79.A-)
complications of pregnancy, childbirth and the puerperium (OØØ-O9A)
congenital malformations, deformations, and chromosomal abnormalities (QØØ-Q99)
endocrine, nutritional and metabolic diseases (EØØ-E88)
injury, poisoning and certain other consequences of external causes (SØØ-T88)
neoplasms (CØØ-D49)
symptoms, signs and abnormal clinical and laboratory findings, not elsewhere classified (RØØ-R94)

See Guidelines: 1;C.13.a-b | 1;C.2Ø.a.1

DORSOPATHIES (M4Ø-M54)

SPONDYLOPATHIES (M45-M49)

3rd Character

Document: Type of spondylopathy

M45- Ankylosing spondylitis
M46- Other inflammatory spondylopathies
M47- Spondylosis
M48- Other spondylopathies
M49- Spondylopathies in diseases classified elsewhere

4th Character

Document: Type of spondylosis

Includes:
arthrosis or osteoarthritis of spine
degeneration of facet joints

M47.Ø- Anterior spinal and vertebral artery compression syndromes
M47.1- Other spondylosis with myelopathy
Including: Spondylogenic compression of spinal cord
Excludes1:
vertebral subluxation (M43.3-M43.5X9)
M47.2- Other spondylosis with radiculopathy
M47.8- Other spondylosis
M47.9 Spondylosis, unspecified

5th Character

M47.81- Spondylosis without myelopathy or radiculopathy
M47.89- Other spondylosis

6th Character

Document: Anatomic region

Applies to: M47.81-, M47.89-

1 Occipito-atlanto-axial region
2 Cervical region
3 Cervicothoracic region
4 Thoracic region
5 Thoracolumbar region
6 Lumbar region
7 Lumbosacral region
8 Sacral and sacrococcygeal region
9 Site unspecified

7th Character

N/A

Spinal Stenosis

ICD-1Ø-CM: M48.ØØ - M48.Ø8

What to Document

4th Character: Type of spondylopathy
5th Character: Anatomic region
6th Character: With/without neurogenic claudication

Document:
- Any external cause, if applicable

Terminology:
Spinal stenosis: The narrowing of the spinal column and other openings of the spine, causing nerve root and spinal compression
Spondylopathy: A disorder in the spine
Neurogenic claudication: Leg pain and weakness due to nerve compression in the spine

Chapter Guidelines

13. Diseases of the musculoskeletal system and connective tissue (MØØ-M99)

Notes:
Use an external cause code following the code for the musculoskeletal condition, if applicable, to identify the cause of the musculoskeletal condition
Excludes2:
arthropathic psoriasis (L4Ø.5-)
certain conditions originating in the perinatal period (PØ4-P96)
certain infectious and parasitic diseases (AØØ-B99)
compartment syndrome (traumatic) (T79.A-)
complications of pregnancy, childbirth and the puerperium (OØØ-O9A)
congenital malformations, deformations, and chromosomal abnormalities (QØØ-Q99)
endocrine, nutritional and metabolic diseases (EØØ-E88)
injury, poisoning and certain other consequences of external causes (SØØ-T88)
neoplasms (CØØ-D49)
symptoms, signs and abnormal clinical and laboratory findings, not elsewhere classified (RØØ-R94)
See Guidelines: 1;C.13.a-b | 1;C.2Ø.a.1

DORSOPATHIES (M4Ø-M54)

SPONDYLOPATHIES (M45-M49)

3rd Character

M45- Ankylosing spondylitis
M46- Other inflammatory spondylopathies
M47- Spondylosis
M48- Other spondylopathies
M49- Spondylopathies in diseases classified elsewhere

4th Character

Document: Type of spondylopathy

M48.Ø- Spinal stenosis
Including: Caudal stenosis

M48.1- Ankylosing hyperostosis [Forestier]
Including: Diffuse idiopathic skeletal hyperostosis [DISH]

M48.2- Kissing spine

M48.3- Traumatic spondylopathy

M48.4- Fatigue fracture of vertebra
Including: Stress fracture of vertebra
Excludes1:
pathological fracture NOS (M84.4-)
pathological fracture of vertebra due to neoplasm (M84.58)
pathological fracture of vertebra due to other diagnosis (M84.68)
pathological fracture of vertebra due to osteoporosis (M8Ø.-)
traumatic fracture of vertebrae (S12.Ø-S12.3-, S22.Ø-, S32.Ø-)
The appropriate 7th character is to be added to each code from subcategory M48.4:
A - initial encounter for fracture
D - subsequent encounter for fracture with routine healing
G - subsequent encounter for fracture with delayed healing
S - sequela of fracture

M48.5- Collapsed vertebra, not elsewhere classified
Including: Collapsed vertebra NOS, Compression fracture of vertebra NOS, Wedging of vertebra NOS
Excludes1:
current injury - see Injury of spine, by body region
fatigue fracture of vertebra (M48.4)
pathological fracture of vertebra due to neoplasm (M84.58)
pathological fracture of vertebra due to other diagnosis (M84.68)
pathological fracture of vertebra due to osteoporosis (M8Ø.-)
pathological fracture NOS (M84.4-)
stress fracture of vertebra (M48.4-)
traumatic fracture of vertebra (S12.-, S22.-, S32.-)
The appropriate 7th character is to be added to each code from subcategory M48.5:
A - initial encounter for fracture
D - subsequent encounter for fracture with routine healing
G - subsequent encounter for fracture with delayed healing
S - sequela of fracture
Indicator(s): *CC (7th A) | CMS22: 169 (7th A) | CMS23: 169 (7th A) | CMS24: 169 (7th A) | RxØ5: 87 (7th A) | ESRD21: 169 (7th A) | HHSØ4: 226 (7th A) | HHSØ5: 226 (7th A)*

M48.8- Other specified spondylopathies
Including: Ossification of posterior longitudinal ligament
Indicator(s): *CMS22: 4Ø | CMS23: 4Ø | CMS24: 4Ø | RxØ5: 84 | ESRD21: 4Ø | HHSØ4: 56 | HHSØ5: 56*

M48.9 Spondylopathy, unspecified

Spinal Stenosis (continued)

5th Character

Document: Anatomic region
Reminder: All final codes are in **BOLD**

Including: Caudal stenosis

M48.ØØ Spinal stenosis, site unspecified
M48.Ø1 Spinal stenosis, occipito-atlanto-axial region
M48.Ø2 Spinal stenosis, cervical region
M48.Ø3 Spinal stenosis, cervicothoracic region
M48.Ø4 Spinal stenosis, thoracic region
M48.Ø5 Spinal stenosis, thoracolumbar region
M48.Ø6- Spinal stenosis, lumbar region
M48.Ø7 Spinal stenosis, lumbosacral region
M48.Ø8 Spinal stenosis, sacral and sacrococcygeal region

6th Character

Document: With/without neurogenic claudication

Applies to: M48.Ø6-

1 Without neurogenic claudication
Including: Spinal stenosis, lumbar region NOS

2 With neurogenic claudication

7th Character

N/A

Cervical Disc Disorder with Myelopathy

ICD-1Ø-CM: M5Ø.ØØ - M5Ø.Ø3

What to Document

3rd Character: Dorsopathy and spinal region
4th Character: Type of cervical disc disorder
5th Character: Cervical region
6th Character: Level

Document:
- Any external cause, if applicable

Terminology:
Myelopathy: Disorder of the spine

Chapter Guidelines

13. Diseases of the musculoskeletal system and connective tissue (MØØ-M99)

Notes:
Use an external cause code following the code for the musculoskeletal condition, if applicable, to identify the cause of the musculoskeletal condition

Excludes2:
arthropathic psoriasis (L4Ø.5-)
certain conditions originating in the perinatal period (PØ4-P96)
certain infectious and parasitic diseases (AØØ-B99)
compartment syndrome (traumatic) (T79.A-)
complications of pregnancy, childbirth and the puerperium (OØØ-O9A)
congenital malformations, deformations, and chromosomal abnormalities (QØØ-Q99)
endocrine, nutritional and metabolic diseases (EØØ-E88)
injury, poisoning and certain other consequences of external causes (SØØ-T88)
neoplasms (CØØ-D49)
symptoms, signs and abnormal clinical and laboratory findings, not elsewhere classified (RØØ-R94)

See Guidelines: *1;C.13.a-b | 1;C.2Ø.a.1*

DORSOPATHIES (M4Ø-M54)

OTHER DORSOPATHIES (M5Ø-M54)

Excludes1:
current injury - see injury of spine by body region
discitis NOS (M46.4-)

3rd Character

Document: Dorsopathy and spinal region

M5Ø- Cervical disc disorders
M51- Thoracic, thoracolumbar, and lumbosacral intervertebral disc disorders
M53- Other and unspecified dorsopathies, not elsewhere classified
M54- Dorsalgia

4th Character

Document: Type of cervical disc disorder

Includes:
cervicothoracic disc disorders with cervicalgia
cervicothoracic disc disorders

M5Ø.Ø- Cervical disc disorder with myelopathy
M5Ø.1- Cervical disc disorder with radiculopathy
Excludes2:
brachial radiculitis NOS (M54.13)
M5Ø.2- Other cervical disc displacement
M5Ø.3- Other cervical disc degeneration
M5Ø.8- Other cervical disc disorders
M5Ø.9- Cervical disc disorder, unspecified

5th Character

Document: Cervical region
Reminder: All final codes are in **BOLD**

M5Ø.ØØ Cervical disc disorder with myelopathy, unspecified cervical region
M5Ø.Ø1 Cervical disc disorder with myelopathy, high cervical region
Including: C2-C3, C3-C4
M5Ø.Ø2- Cervical disc disorder with myelopathy, mid-cervical region
M5Ø.Ø3 Cervical disc disorder with myelopathy, cervicothoracic region
Including: C7-T1 disc disorder with myelopathy

Cervical Disc Disorder with Myelopathy (continued)

6th Character

Document: Level

Applies to: M5Ø.Ø2-

Ø Unspecified level

1 At C4-C5 level
 Including: C4-C5 disc disorder

2 At C5-C6 level
 Including: C5-C6 disc disorder

3 At C6-C7 level
 Including: C6-C7 disc disorder

7th Character

N/A

Other Cervical Disc Displacement

ICD-1Ø-CM: M5Ø.2Ø - M5Ø.23

What to Document

3rd Character: Type of dorsopathy
4th Character: Type of cervical disc disorder
5th Character: Anatomic region
6th Character: Level

Document:
- Any external cause, if applicable

Chapter Guidelines

13. Diseases of the musculoskeletal system and connective tissue (MØØ-M99)

Notes:
Use an external cause code following the code for the musculoskeletal condition, if applicable, to identify the cause of the musculoskeletal condition

Excludes2:
arthropathic psoriasis (L4Ø.5-)
certain conditions originating in the perinatal period (PØ4-P96)
certain infectious and parasitic diseases (AØØ-B99)
compartment syndrome (traumatic) (T79.A-)
complications of pregnancy, childbirth and the puerperium (OØØ-O9A)
congenital malformations, deformations, and chromosomal abnormalities (QØØ-Q99)
endocrine, nutritional and metabolic diseases (EØØ-E88)
injury, poisoning and certain other consequences of external causes (SØØ-T88)
neoplasms (CØØ-D49)
symptoms, signs and abnormal clinical and laboratory findings, not elsewhere classified (RØØ-R94)

See Guidelines: 1;C.13.a-b | 1;C.2Ø.a.1

DORSOPATHIES (M4Ø-M54)

OTHER DORSOPATHIES (M5Ø-M54)

Excludes1:
current injury - see injury of spine by body region
discitis NOS (M46.4-)

3rd Character

Document: Type of dorsopathy

M5Ø- Cervical disc disorders
M51- Thoracic, thoracolumbar, and lumbosacral intervertebral disc disorders
M53- Other and unspecified dorsopathies, not elsewhere classified
M54- Dorsalgia

4th Character

Document: Type of cervical disc disorder

Includes:
cervicothoracic disc disorders with cervicalgia
cervicothoracic disc disorders

M5Ø.Ø- Cervical disc disorder with myelopathy
M5Ø.1- Cervical disc disorder with radiculopathy
Excludes2:
brachial radiculitis NOS (M54.13)
M5Ø.2- Other cervical disc displacement
M5Ø.3- Other cervical disc degeneration
M5Ø.8- Other cervical disc disorders
M5Ø.9- Cervical disc disorder, unspecified

5th Character

Document: Anatomic region
Reminder: All final codes are in **BOLD**

M5Ø.2Ø Other cervical disc displacement, unspecified cervical region
M5Ø.21 Other cervical disc displacement, high cervical region
Including: C2-C3, C3-C4
M5Ø.22- Other cervical disc displacement, mid-cervical region
M5Ø.23 Other cervical disc displacement, cervicothoracic region
Including: C7-T1 cervical disc displacement

6th Character

Document: Level

Applies to: M5Ø.22-

Ø Unspecified level
1 C4-C5 level
Including: C4-C5 cervical disc displacement
2 C5-C6 level
Including: C5-C6 cervical disc displacement
3 C6-C7 level
Including: C6-C7 cervical disc displacement

7th Character

N/A

Other Cervical Disc Degeneration

ICD-1Ø-CM: M5Ø.3Ø - M5Ø.33

What to Document

3rd Character: Type of dorsopathy
4th Character: Type of cervical disc disorder
5th Character: Cervical region
6th Character: Level

Document:
- Any external cause, if applicable

Chapter Guidelines

13. Diseases of the musculoskeletal system and connective tissue (MØØ-M99)

<u>*Notes:*</u>
Use an external cause code following the code for the musculoskeletal condition, if applicable, to identify the cause of the musculoskeletal condition
<u>*Excludes2:*</u>
arthropathic psoriasis (L4Ø.5-)
certain conditions originating in the perinatal period (PØ4-P96)
certain infectious and parasitic diseases (AØØ-B99)
compartment syndrome (traumatic) (T79.A-)
complications of pregnancy, childbirth and the puerperium (OØØ-O9A)
congenital malformations, deformations, and chromosomal abnormalities (QØØ-Q99)
endocrine, nutritional and metabolic diseases (EØØ-E88)
injury, poisoning and certain other consequences of external causes (SØØ-T88)
neoplasms (CØØ-D49)
symptoms, signs and abnormal clinical and laboratory findings, not elsewhere classified (RØØ-R94)
<u>*See Guidelines:*</u> *1;C.13.a-b | 1;C.2Ø.a.1*

DORSOPATHIES (M4Ø-M54)

OTHER DORSOPATHIES (M5Ø-M54)

<u>*Excludes1:*</u>
current injury - see injury of spine by body region
discitis NOS (M46.4-)

3rd Character

Document: Type of dorsopathy

M5Ø- Cervical disc disorders
M51- Thoracic, thoracolumbar, and lumbosacral intervertebral disc disorders
M53- Other and unspecified dorsopathies, not elsewhere classified
M54- Dorsalgia

4th Character

Document: Type of cervical disc disorder

<u>*Includes:*</u>
cervicothoracic disc disorders with cervicalgia
cervicothoracic disc disorders

M5Ø.Ø- Cervical disc disorder with myelopathy
M5Ø.1- Cervical disc disorder with radiculopathy
<u>*Excludes2:*</u>
brachial radiculitis NOS (M54.13)
M5Ø.2- Other cervical disc displacement
M5Ø.3- Other cervical disc degeneration
M5Ø.8- Other cervical disc disorders
M5Ø.9- Cervical disc disorder, unspecified

5th Character

Document: Cervical region
Reminder: All final codes are in **BOLD**

M5Ø.3Ø Other cervical disc degeneration, unspecified cervical region
M5Ø.31 Other cervical disc degeneration, high cervical region
Including: C2-C3, C3-C4
M5Ø.32- Other cervical disc degeneration, mid-cervical region
M5Ø.33 Other cervical disc degeneration, cervicothoracic region
Including: C7-T1 cervical disc degeneration

6th Character

Document: Level

Applies to: M5Ø.32-

Ø Unspecified level
1 C4-C5 level
Including: C4-C5 cervical disc degeneration
2 C5-C6 level
Including: C5-C6 cervical disc degeneration
3 C6-C7 level
Including: C6-C7 cervical disc degeneration

7th Character

N/A

Thoracic, Thoracolumbar, and Lumbosacral Intervertebral Disc Disorders

ICD-1Ø-CM: M51.Ø4 - M51.9

What to Document

3rd Character: Type of dorsopathy
4th Character: Type of intervertebral disc disorder
5th Character: Spinal region

Document:
- Any external cause, if applicable

Terminology:
Schmorl's nodes: Protrusion of the nucleus pulposus through the vertebral body into the adjacent vertebrae; common to the thoracic and lumbar spines, can cause inflammation and back pain

Chapter Guidelines

13. Diseases of the musculoskeletal system and connective tissue (MØØ-M99)

Notes:
Use an external cause code following the code for the musculoskeletal condition, if applicable, to identify the cause of the musculoskeletal condition

Excludes2:
arthropathic psoriasis (L4Ø.5-)
certain conditions originating in the perinatal period (PØ4-P96)
certain infectious and parasitic diseases (AØØ-B99)
compartment syndrome (traumatic) (T79.A-)
complications of pregnancy, childbirth and the puerperium (OØØ-O9A)
congenital malformations, deformations, and chromosomal abnormalities (QØØ-Q99)
endocrine, nutritional and metabolic diseases (EØØ-E88)
injury, poisoning and certain other consequences of external causes (SØØ-T88)
neoplasms (CØØ-D49)
symptoms, signs and abnormal clinical and laboratory findings, not elsewhere classified (RØØ-R94)

See Guidelines: *1;C.13.a-b | 1;C.2Ø.a.1*

DORSOPATHIES (M4Ø-M54)

OTHER DORSOPATHIES (M5Ø-M54)

Excludes1:
current injury - see injury of spine by body region
discitis NOS (M46.4-)

3rd Character

Document: Type of dorsopathy

M5Ø- Cervical disc disorders
M51- Thoracic, thoracolumbar, and lumbosacral intervertebral disc disorders
M53- Other and unspecified dorsopathies, not elsewhere classified
M54- Dorsalgia

4th Character

Document: Type of intervertebral disc disorder
Reminder: All final codes are in **BOLD**

Excludes2:
cervical and cervicothoracic disc disorders (M5Ø.-)
sacral and sacrococcygeal disorders (M53.3)

M51.Ø- Thoracic, thoracolumbar and lumbosacral intervertebral disc disorders with myelopathy

M51.1- Thoracic, thoracolumbar and lumbosacral intervertebral disc disorders with radiculopathy
Including: Sciatica due to intervertebral disc disorder
Excludes1:
lumbar radiculitis NOS (M54.16)
sciatica NOS (M54.3)

M51.2- Other thoracic, thoracolumbar and lumbosacral intervertebral disc displacement
Including: Lumbago due to displacement of intervertebral disc

M51.3- Other thoracic, thoracolumbar and lumbosacral intervertebral disc degeneration

M51.4- Schmorl's nodes

M51.8- Other thoracic, thoracolumbar and lumbosacral intervertebral disc disorders

M51.9 Unspecified thoracic, thoracolumbar and lumbosacral intervertebral disc disorder

M51.A- Other lumbar and lumbosacral annulus fibrosus disc defects

Thoracic, Thoracolumbar, and Lumbosacral Intervertebral Disc Disorders (continued)

5th Character

Document: Spinal region

Applies to: M51.Ø-

4 Thoracic region
5 Thoracolumbar region
6 Lumbar region

Applies to: M51.1-, M51.2-, M51.3-, M51.4-, M51.8-

4 Thoracic region
5 Thoracolumbar region
6 Lumbar region
7 Lumbosacral region

Applies to: M51.A

Ø lumbar region, unspecified size
Code first , if applicable, lumbar disc herniation (M51.06, M51.16, M51.26)

1 lumbar region, small
Code first, if applicable, lumbar disc herniation (M51.06, M51.16, M51.26)

2 lumbar region, large
Code first, if applicable, lumbar disc herniation (M51.06, M51.16, M51.26)

3 lumbosacral region, unspecified size
Code first, if applicable, lumbosacral disc herniation (M51.170 M51.27)

4 lumbosacral region, small
Code first, if applicable, lumbosacral disc herniation (M51.170 M51.27)

5 lumbosacral region, large
Code first, if applicable, lumbosacral disc herniation (M51.170 M51.27)

6th Character

N/A

7th Character

N/A

See Appendix A — Coding Reference Tables for lists of the ICD-10-CM Tabular indicators, HAC categories, and HCC codes.

Cervicocranial and Cervicobrachial Syndromes

ICD-1Ø-CM: M53.Ø - M53.1

What to Document

3rd Character: Type of dorsopathy

Document:
- Any external cause, if applicable

Chapter Guidelines

13. Diseases of the musculoskeletal system and connective tissue (MØØ-M99)

Notes:

Use an external cause code following the code for the musculoskeletal condition, if applicable, to identify the cause of the musculoskeletal condition

Excludes2:

arthropathic psoriasis (L4Ø.5-)
certain conditions originating in the perinatal period (PØ4-P96)
certain infectious and parasitic diseases (AØØ-B99)
compartment syndrome (traumatic) (T79.A-)
complications of pregnancy, childbirth and the puerperium (OØØ-O9A)
congenital malformations, deformations, and chromosomal abnormalities (QØØ-Q99)
endocrine, nutritional and metabolic diseases (EØØ-E88)
injury, poisoning and certain other consequences of external causes (SØØ-T88)
neoplasms (CØØ-D49)
symptoms, signs and abnormal clinical and laboratory findings, not elsewhere classified (RØØ-R94)

See Guidelines: *1;C.13.a-b | 1;C.2Ø.a.1*

DORSOPATHIES (M4Ø-M54)

OTHER DORSOPATHIES (M5Ø-M54)

Excludes1:

current injury - see injury of spine by body region
discitis NOS (M46.4-)

3rd Character

Document: Type of dorsopathy

M5Ø- Cervical disc disorders

M51- Thoracic, thoracolumbar, and lumbosacral intervertebral disc disorders

M53- Other and unspecified dorsopathies, not elsewhere classified

M54- Dorsalgia

4th Character

Reminder: All final codes are in **BOLD**

Applies to: M53.-

Ø Cervicocranial syndrome

Including: Posterior cervical sympathetic syndrome

1 Cervicobrachial syndrome

Excludes2:

cervical disc disorder (M5Ø.-)
thoracic outlet syndrome (G54.Ø)

5th Character

N/A

6th Character

N/A

7th Character

N/A

Spinal Instabilities

ICD-1Ø-CM: M53.2X1 - M53.2X9

What to Document

4th Character: Type of dorsopathy
6th Character: Spinal region

Document:
- Cause of the musculoskeletal condition, if applicable

Chapter Guidelines

13. Diseases of the musculoskeletal system and connective tissue (MØØ-M99)

Notes:
Use an external cause code following the code for the musculoskeletal condition, if applicable, to identify the cause of the musculoskeletal condition
Excludes2:
arthropathic psoriasis (L4Ø.5-)
certain conditions originating in the perinatal period (PØ4-P96)
certain infectious and parasitic diseases (AØØ-B99)
compartment syndrome (traumatic) (T79.A-)
complications of pregnancy, childbirth and the puerperium (OØØ-O9A)
congenital malformations, deformations, and chromosomal abnormalities (QØØ-Q99)
endocrine, nutritional and metabolic diseases (EØØ-E88)
injury, poisoning and certain other consequences of external causes (SØØ-T88)
neoplasms (CØØ-D49)
symptoms, signs and abnormal clinical and laboratory findings, not elsewhere classified (RØØ-R94)
See Guidelines: 1;C.13.a-b | 1;C.2Ø.a.1

DORSOPATHIES (M4Ø-M54)

OTHER DORSOPATHIES (M5Ø-M54)

Excludes1:
current injury - see injury of spine by body region
discitis NOS (M46.4-)

3rd Character

M5Ø- Cervical disc disorders
M51- Thoracic, thoracolumbar, and lumbosacral intervertebral disc disorders
M53- Other and unspecified dorsopathies, not elsewhere classified
M54- Dorsalgia

4th Character

Document: Type of dorsopathy

M53.Ø Cervicocranial syndrome
Including: Posterior cervical sympathetic syndrome

M53.1 Cervicobrachial syndrome
Excludes2:
cervical disc disorder (M5Ø.-)
thoracic outlet syndrome (G54.Ø)

M53.2- Spinal instabilities

M53.3 Sacrococcygeal disorders, not elsewhere classified
Including: Coccygodynia

M53.8- Other specified dorsopathies

M53.9 Dorsopathy, unspecified

5th Character

M53.2X- Spinal instabilities

6th Character

Document: Spinal region

Applies to: M53.2X-

1 Occipito-atlanto-axial region
2 Cervical region
3 Cervicothoracic region
4 Thoracic region
5 Thoracolumbar region
6 Lumbar region
7 Lumbosacral region
8 Sacral and sacrococcygeal region
9 Site unspecified

7th Character

N/A

Radiculopathy

ICD-1Ø-CM: M54.1Ø - M54.18

What to Document

3rd Character: Type of dorsopathy
4th Character: Type of dorsalgia
5th Character: Spinal region

Document:
- Any external cause, if applicable

Terminology:
Radiculopathy: Disease affecting a nerve root, causing pain, muscle weakness, numbness, and poor muscular control

Chapter Guidelines

13. Diseases of the musculoskeletal system and connective tissue (MØØ-M99)

Notes:
Use an external cause code following the code for the musculoskeletal condition, if applicable, to identify the cause of the musculoskeletal condition

Excludes2:
arthropathic psoriasis (L4Ø.5-)
certain conditions originating in the perinatal period (PØ4-P96)
certain infectious and parasitic diseases (AØØ-B99)
compartment syndrome (traumatic) (T79.A-)
complications of pregnancy, childbirth and the puerperium (OØØ-O9A)
congenital malformations, deformations, and chromosomal abnormalities (QØØ-Q99)
endocrine, nutritional and metabolic diseases (EØØ-E88)
injury, poisoning and certain other consequences of external causes (SØØ-T88)
neoplasms (CØØ-D49)
symptoms, signs and abnormal clinical and laboratory findings, not elsewhere classified (RØØ-R94)

See Guidelines: 1;C.13.a-b | 1;C.2Ø.a.1

DORSOPATHIES (M4Ø-M54)

OTHER DORSOPATHIES (M5Ø-M54)

Excludes1:
current injury - see injury of spine by body region
discitis NOS (M46.4-)

3rd Character

Document: Type of dorsopathy

M5Ø- Cervical disc disorders
M51- Thoracic, thoracolumbar, and lumbosacral intervertebral disc disorders
M53- Other and unspecified dorsopathies, not elsewhere classified
M54- Dorsalgia

4th Character

Document: Type of dorsalgia

Excludes1:
psychogenic dorsalgia (F45.41)

M54.Ø- Panniculitis affecting regions of neck and back
Excludes1:
lupus panniculitis (L93.2)
panniculitis NOS (M79.3)
relapsing [Weber-Christian] panniculitis (M35.6)

M54.1- Radiculopathy
Including: Brachial, Lumbar, Lumbosacral, Thoracic neuritis or radiculitis NOS; Radiculitis NOS
Excludes1:
neuralgia and neuritis NOS (M79.2)
radiculopathy with cervical disc disorder (M5Ø.1)
radiculopathy with lumbar and other intervertebral disc disorder (M51.1-)
radiculopathy with spondylosis (M47.2-)

M54.2 Cervicalgia
Excludes1:
cervicalgia due to intervertebral cervical disc disorder (M5Ø.-)
See Guidelines: 1;C.6.b.1.b

M54.3- Sciatica
Excludes1:
lesion of sciatic nerve (G57.Ø)
sciatica due to intervertebral disc disorder (M51.1-)
sciatica with lumbago (M54.4-)

M54.4- Lumbago with sciatica
Excludes1:
lumbago with sciatica due to intervertebral disc disorder (M51.1-)

M54.5- Low back pain

M54.6 Pain in thoracic spine
Excludes1:
pain in thoracic spine due to intervertebral disc disorder (M51.-)

M54.8- Other dorsalgia
Excludes1:
dorsalgia in thoracic region (M54.6)
low back pain (M54.5-)

M54.9 Dorsalgia, unspecified
Including: Backache NOS, Back pain NOS

Radiculopathy (continued)

5th Character

Document: Spinal region

Including: Brachial, Lumbar, Lumbosacral, Thoracic neuritis or radiculitis NOS; Radiculitis NOS

Excludes1:

neuralgia and neuritis NOS (M79.2)
radiculopathy with cervical disc disorder (M5Ø.1)
radiculopathy with lumbar and other intervertebral disc disorder (M51.1-)
radiculopathy with spondylosis (M47.2-)

Applies to: M54.1-

Ø Site unspecified
1 Occipito-atlanto-axial region
2 Cervical region
3 Cervicothoracic region
4 Thoracic region
5 Thoracolumbar region
6 Lumbar region
7 Lumbosacral region
8 Sacral and sacrococcygeal region

6th Character

N/A

7th Character

N/A

Cervicalgia

ICD-1Ø-CM: M54.2 - M54.2

What to Document

3rd Character: Type of dorsopathy
4th Character: Type of dorsalgia

Document:
- Any external cause, if applicable

Terminology:
Dorsalgia: Back pain
Cervicalgia: Neck pain

Chapter Guidelines

13. Diseases of the musculoskeletal system and connective tissue (MØØ-M99)

Notes:
Use an external cause code following the code for the musculoskeletal condition, if applicable, to identify the cause of the musculoskeletal condition

Excludes2:
arthropathic psoriasis (L4Ø.5-)
certain conditions originating in the perinatal period (PØ4-P96)
certain infectious and parasitic diseases (AØØ-B99)
compartment syndrome (traumatic) (T79.A-)
complications of pregnancy, childbirth and the puerperium (OØØ-O9A)
congenital malformations, deformations, and chromosomal abnormalities (QØØ-Q99)
endocrine, nutritional and metabolic diseases (EØØ-E88)
injury, poisoning and certain other consequences of external causes (SØØ-T88)
neoplasms (CØØ-D49)
symptoms, signs and abnormal clinical and laboratory findings, not elsewhere classified (RØØ-R94)

See Guidelines: 1;C.13.a-b | 1;C.2Ø.a.1

DORSOPATHIES (M4Ø-M54)

OTHER DORSOPATHIES (M5Ø-M54)

Excludes1:
current injury - see injury of spine by body region
discitis NOS (M46.4-)

3rd Character

Document: Type of dorsopathy

M5Ø- Cervical disc disorders
M51- Thoracic, thoracolumbar, and lumbosacral intervertebral disc disorders
M53- Other and unspecified dorsopathies, not elsewhere classified
M54- Dorsalgia

4th Character

Document: Type of dorsalgia

Excludes1:
psychogenic dorsalgia (F45.41)

Applies to: M54.-

2 Cervicalgia

Excludes1:
cervicalgia due to intervertebral cervical disc disorder (M5Ø.-)

See Guidelines: 1;C.6.b.1.b

5th Character

N/A

6th Character

N/A

7th Character

N/A

Sciatica

ICD-1Ø-CM: M54.3Ø - M54.32

What to Document

3rd Character: Type of dorsopathy
4th Character: Type of dorsalgia
5th Character: Laterality

Document:
- Any external cause, if applicable

Terminology:
Dorsalgia: Back pain
Sciatica: Pain that radiates along the sciatic nerve

Chapter Guidelines

13. Diseases of the musculoskeletal system and connective tissue (MØØ-M99)

Notes:
Use an external cause code following the code for the musculoskeletal condition, if applicable, to identify the cause of the musculoskeletal condition
Excludes2:
arthropathic psoriasis (L4Ø.5-)
certain conditions originating in the perinatal period (PØ4-P96)
certain infectious and parasitic diseases (AØØ-B99)
compartment syndrome (traumatic) (T79.A-)
complications of pregnancy, childbirth and the puerperium (OØØ-O9A)
congenital malformations, deformations, and chromosomal abnormalities (QØØ-Q99)
endocrine, nutritional and metabolic diseases (EØØ-E88)
injury, poisoning and certain other consequences of external causes (SØØ-T88)
neoplasms (CØØ-D49)
symptoms, signs and abnormal clinical and laboratory findings, not elsewhere classified (RØØ-R94)
See Guidelines: 1;C.13.a-b | 1;C.2Ø.a.1

DORSOPATHIES (M4Ø-M54)

OTHER DORSOPATHIES (M5Ø-M54)

Excludes1:
current injury - see injury of spine by body region
discitis NOS (M46.4-)

3rd Character

Document: Type of dorsopathy

M5Ø- Cervical disc disorders

M51- Thoracic, thoracolumbar, and lumbosacral intervertebral disc disorders

M53- Other and unspecified dorsopathies, not elsewhere classified

M54- Dorsalgia

4th Character

Document: Type of dorsalgia

Excludes1:
psychogenic dorsalgia (F45.41)

M54.Ø- Panniculitis affecting regions of neck and back
Excludes1:
lupus panniculitis (L93.2)
panniculitis NOS (M79.3)
relapsing [Weber-Christian] panniculitis (M35.6)

M54.1- Radiculopathy
Including: Brachial, Lumbar, Lumbosacral, Thoracic neuritis or radiculitis NOS; Radiculitis NOS
Excludes1:
neuralgia and neuritis NOS (M79.2)
radiculopathy with cervical disc disorder (M5Ø.1)
radiculopathy with lumbar and other intervertebral disc disorder (M51.1-)
radiculopathy with spondylosis (M47.2-)

M54.2 Cervicalgia
Excludes1:
cervicalgia due to intervertebral cervical disc disorder (M5Ø.-)
See Guidelines: 1;C.6.b.1.b

M54.3- Sciatica
Excludes1:
lesion of sciatic nerve (G57.Ø)
sciatica due to intervertebral disc disorder (M51.1-)
sciatica with lumbago (M54.4-)

M54.4- Lumbago with sciatica
Excludes1:
lumbago with sciatica due to intervertebral disc disorder (M51.1-)

M54.5- Low back pain

M54.6 Pain in thoracic spine
Excludes1:
pain in thoracic spine due to intervertebral disc disorder (M51.-)

M54.8- Other dorsalgia
Excludes1:
dorsalgia in thoracic region (M54.6)
low back pain (M54.5-)

M54.9 Dorsalgia, unspecified
Including: Backache NOS, Back pain NOS

Sciatica (continued)

5th Character

Document: Laterality

Excludes1:
lesion of sciatic nerve (G57.Ø)
sciatica due to intervertebral disc disorder (M51.1-)
sciatica with lumbago (M54.4-)

Applies to: M54.3-

Ø Unspecified side
1 Right side
2 Left side

6th Character

N/A

7th Character

N/A

Lumbago with Sciatica

ICD-1Ø-CM: M54.4Ø - M54.42

What to Document

3rd Character: Type of dorsopathy
4th Character: Type of dorsalgia
5th Character: Laterality

Document:
- Any external cause, if applicable

Terminology:
Dorsalgia: Back pain
Lumbago: Pain in the muscles and joints of the lower back
Sciatica: Compression of a spinal nerve root, often due to intervertebral disc degeneration, causing pain in the back, hip, and leg

Chapter Guidelines

13. Diseases of the musculoskeletal system and connective tissue (MØØ-M99)

Notes:
Use an external cause code following the code for the musculoskeletal condition, if applicable, to identify the cause of the musculoskeletal condition

Excludes2:
arthropathic psoriasis (L4Ø.5-)
certain conditions originating in the perinatal period (PØ4-P96)
certain infectious and parasitic diseases (AØØ-B99)
compartment syndrome (traumatic) (T79.A-)
complications of pregnancy, childbirth and the puerperium (OØØ-O9A)
congenital malformations, deformations, and chromosomal abnormalities (QØØ-Q99)
endocrine, nutritional and metabolic diseases (EØØ-E88)
injury, poisoning and certain other consequences of external causes (SØØ-T88)
neoplasms (CØØ-D49)
symptoms, signs and abnormal clinical and laboratory findings, not elsewhere classified (RØØ-R94)

See Guidelines: 1;C.13.a-b | 1;C.2Ø.a.1

DORSOPATHIES (M4Ø-M54)

OTHER DORSOPATHIES (M5Ø-M54)

Excludes1:
current injury - see injury of spine by body region
discitis NOS (M46.4-)

3rd Character

Document: Type of dorsopathy

M5Ø- Cervical disc disorders

M51- Thoracic, thoracolumbar, and lumbosacral intervertebral disc disorders

3rd Character (continued)

M53- Other and unspecified dorsopathies, not elsewhere classified

M54- Dorsalgia

4th Character

Document: Type of dorsalgia

Excludes1:
psychogenic dorsalgia (F45.41)

M54.Ø- Panniculitis affecting regions of neck and back

Excludes1:
lupus panniculitis (L93.2)
panniculitis NOS (M79.3)
relapsing [Weber-Christian] panniculitis (M35.6)

M54.1- Radiculopathy

Including: Brachial, Lumbar, Lumbosacral, Thoracic neuritis or radiculitis NOS; Radiculitis NOS

Excludes1:
neuralgia and neuritis NOS (M79.2)
radiculopathy with cervical disc disorder (M5Ø.1)
radiculopathy with lumbar and other intervertebral disc disorder (M51.1-)
radiculopathy with spondylosis (M47.2-)

M54.2 Cervicalgia

Excludes1:
cervicalgia due to intervertebral cervical disc disorder (M5Ø.-)

See Guidelines: 1;C.6.b.1.b

M54.3- Sciatica

Excludes1:
lesion of sciatic nerve (G57.Ø)
sciatica due to intervertebral disc disorder (M51.1-)
sciatica with lumbago (M54.4-)

M54.4- Lumbago with sciatica

Excludes1:
lumbago with sciatica due to intervertebral disc disorder (M51.1-)

M54.5- Low back pain

M54.6 Pain in thoracic spine

Excludes1:
pain in thoracic spine due to intervertebral disc disorder (M51.-)

M54.8 Other dorsalgia

Excludes1:
dorsalgia in thoracic region (M54.6)
low back pain (M54.5-)

M54.9 Dorsalgia, unspecified

Including: Backache NOS, Back pain NOS

Lumbago with Sciatica (continued)

5th Character

Document: Laterality

Excludes1:
lumbago with sciatica due to intervertebral disc disorder (M51.1-)

Applies to: M54.4-

Ø Unspecified side
1 Right side
2 Left side

6th Character

N/A

7th Character

N/A

Low Back Pain

ICD-1Ø-CM: M54.5Ø - M54.59

What to Document

3rd Character: Type of dorsopathy
4th Character: Type of dorsalgia
5th Character: Further specification

Document:
- Any external cause, if applicable

Terminology:
Dorsalgia: Back pain
Vertebrogenic: arising in a vertebra or in the vertebral column

Chapter Guidelines

13. Diseases of the musculoskeletal system and connective tissue (MØØ-M99)

Notes:
Use an external cause code following the code for the musculoskeletal condition, if applicable, to identify the cause of the musculoskeletal condition

Excludes2:
arthropathic psoriasis (L4Ø.5-)
certain conditions originating in the perinatal period (PØ4-P96)
certain infectious and parasitic diseases (AØØ-B99)
compartment syndrome (traumatic) (T79.A-)
complications of pregnancy, childbirth and the puerperium (OØØ-O9A)
congenital malformations, deformations, and chromosomal abnormalities (QØØ-Q99)
endocrine, nutritional and metabolic diseases (EØØ-E88)
injury, poisoning and certain other consequences of external causes (SØØ-T88)
neoplasms (CØØ-D49)
symptoms, signs and abnormal clinical and laboratory findings, not elsewhere classified (RØØ-R94)

See Guidelines: *1;C.13.a-b | 1;C.2Ø.a.1*

DORSOPATHIES (M4Ø-M54)

OTHER DORSOPATHIES (M5Ø-M54)

Excludes1:
current injury - see injury of spine by body region
discitis NOS (M46.4-)

3rd Character

Document: Type of dorsopathy

M5Ø- Cervical disc disorders
M51- Thoracic, thoracolumbar, and lumbosacral intervertebral disc disorders
M53- Other and unspecified dorsopathies, not elsewhere classified
M54- Dorsalgia

4th Character

Document: Type of dorsalgia

Excludes1:
psychogenic dorsalgia (F45.41)

M54.Ø- Panniculitis affecting regions of neck and back
M54.1- Radiculopathy
M54.2 Cervicalgia
M54.3- Sciatica
M54.4- Lumbago with sciatica
M54.5- Low back pain
M54.6 Pain in thoracic spine
M54.8- Other dorsalgia
M54.9 Dorsalgia, unspecified

5th Character

Document: Further specification

Applies to: M54.5-

Ø Unspecified
Including: Loin pain, Lumbago NOS

1 Vertebrogenic
Including: Low back vertebral endplate

9 Other

6th Character

N/A

7th Character

N/A

C

Appendix C. Chiropractic PDGs

Pain in Thoracic Spine

ICD-10-CM: M54.6 - M54.6

What to Document

3rd Character: Type of dorsopathy
4th Character: Type of dorsalgia

Document:
- Any external cause, if applicable

Terminology:
Dorsalgia: Back pain

Chapter Guidelines

13. Diseases of the musculoskeletal system and connective tissue (MØØ-M99)

Notes:
Use an external cause code following the code for the musculoskeletal condition, if applicable, to identify the cause of the musculoskeletal condition

Excludes2:
arthropathic psoriasis (L4Ø.5-)
certain conditions originating in the perinatal period (PØ4-P96)
certain infectious and parasitic diseases (AØØ-B99)
compartment syndrome (traumatic) (T79.A-)
complications of pregnancy, childbirth and the puerperium (OØØ-O9A)
congenital malformations, deformations, and chromosomal abnormalities (QØØ-Q99)
endocrine, nutritional and metabolic diseases (EØØ-E88)
injury, poisoning and certain other consequences of external causes (SØØ-T88)
neoplasms (CØØ-D49)
symptoms, signs and abnormal clinical and laboratory findings, not elsewhere classified (RØØ-R94)

See Guidelines: *1;C.13.a-b | 1;C.2Ø.a.1*

DORSOPATHIES (M4Ø-M54)

OTHER DORSOPATHIES (M5Ø-M54)

Excludes1:
current injury - see injury of spine by body region
discitis NOS (M46.4-)

3rd Character

Document: Type of dorsopathy

M5Ø- Cervical disc disorders

M51- Thoracic, thoracolumbar, and lumbosacral intervertebral disc disorders

M53- Other and unspecified dorsopathies, not elsewhere classified

M54- Dorsalgia

4th Character

Document: Type of dorsalgia

Excludes1:
psychogenic dorsalgia (F45.41)

Applies to: M54.-

6 Pain in thoracic spine

Excludes1:
pain in thoracic spine due to intervertebral disc disorder (M51.-)

5th Character

N/A

6th Character

N/A

7th Character

N/A

Other Specified Disorders of Muscle

ICD-1Ø-CM: M62.81 - M62.89

What to Document

4th Character: Type of muscle disorder
5th Character: Other specifications
6th Character: Anatomic site

Document:
- Any external cause, if applicable
- Any underlying disease, if applicable, such as: disorders of myoneural junction and muscle disease in diseases classified elsewhere, other and unspecified myopathies, primary disorders of muscles

Terminology:
Rhabdomyolysis Muscle tissue breakdown that releases harmful contents into the body
Sarcopenia: Degeneration of muscle mass and strength in relation to aging

Chapter Guidelines

13. Diseases of the musculoskeletal system and connective tissue (MØØ-M99)

Notes:
Use an external cause code following the code for the musculoskeletal condition, if applicable, to identify the cause of the musculoskeletal condition
Excludes2:
arthropathic psoriasis (L4Ø.5-)
certain conditions originating in the perinatal period (PØ4-P96)
certain infectious and parasitic diseases (AØØ-B99)
compartment syndrome (traumatic) (T79.A-)
complications of pregnancy, childbirth and the puerperium (OØØ-O9A)
congenital malformations, deformations, and chromosomal abnormalities (QØØ-Q99)
endocrine, nutritional and metabolic diseases (EØØ-E88)
injury, poisoning and certain other consequences of external causes (SØØ-T88)
neoplasms (CØØ-D49)
symptoms, signs and abnormal clinical and laboratory findings, not elsewhere classified (RØØ-R94)
See Guidelines: *1;C.13.a-b | 1;C.2Ø.a.1*

SOFT TISSUE DISORDERS (M6Ø-M79)

DISORDERS OF MUSCLES (M6Ø-M63)

Excludes1:
dermatopolymyositis (M33.-)
muscular dystrophies and myopathies (G71-G72)
myopathy in amyloidosis (E85.-)
myopathy in polyarteritis nodosa (M3Ø.Ø)
myopathy in rheumatoid arthritis (MØ5.32)
myopathy in scleroderma (M34.-)
myopathy in Sjögren's syndrome (M35.Ø3)
myopathy in systemic lupus erythematosus (M32.-)

3rd Character

M6Ø- Myositis
M61- Calcification and ossification of muscle
M62- Other disorders of muscle
M63- Disorders of muscle in diseases classified elsewhere

4th Character

Document: Type of muscle disorder

Excludes1:
alcoholic myopathy (G72.1)
cramp and spasm (R25.2)
drug-induced myopathy (G72.Ø)
myalgia (M79.1-)
stiff-man syndrome (G25.82)
Excludes2:
nontraumatic hematoma of muscle (M79.81)

M62.Ø- Separation of muscle (nontraumatic)
Including: Diastasis of muscle
Excludes1:
diastasis recti complicating pregnancy, labor and delivery (O71.8)
traumatic separation of muscle- see strain of muscle by body region

M62.1- Other rupture of muscle (nontraumatic)
Excludes1:
traumatic rupture of muscle - see strain of muscle by body region
Excludes2:
rupture of tendon (M66.-)

M62.2- Nontraumatic ischemic infarction of muscle
Excludes1:
compartment syndrome (traumatic) (T79.A-)
nontraumatic compartment syndrome (M79.A-)
traumatic ischemia of muscle (T79.6)
rhabdomyolysis (M62.82)
Volkmann's ischemic contracture (T79.6)

M62.3 Immobility syndrome (paraplegic)

M62.4- Contracture of muscle
Including: Tendon (sheath)
Excludes1:
contracture of joint (M24.5-)

Other Specified Disorders of Muscle (continued)

4th Character (continued)

M62.5- Muscle wasting and atrophy, not elsewhere classified

Including: Disuse atrophy NEC

Excludes1:

neuralgic amyotrophy (G54.5)
progressive muscular atrophy (G12.29)
sarcopenia (M62.84)

Excludes2:

pelvic muscle wasting (N81.84)

M62.8- Other specified disorders of muscle

Excludes2:

nontraumatic hematoma of muscle (M79.81)

M62.9 Disorder of muscle, unspecified

5th Character

Document: Other specifications

Reminder: All final codes are in **BOLD**

Excludes2:

nontraumatic hematoma of muscle (M79.81)

M62.81 Muscle weakness (generalized)

Excludes1:

muscle weakness in sarcopenia (M62.84)

M62.82 Rhabdomyolysis

Excludes1:

traumatic rhabdomyolysis (T79.6)

M62.83- Muscle spasm

M62.84 Sarcopenia

Including: Age-related sarcopenia

Code First:

underlying disease, if applicable, such as:
disorders of myoneural junction and muscle disease in diseases classified elsewhere (G73.-)
other and unspecified myopathies (G72.-)
primary disorders of muscles (G71.-)

M62.89 Other specified disorders of muscle

Including: Muscle (sheath) hernia

6th Character

Document: Anatomic site

Applies to: M62.83-

Ø Back

1 Calf

Including: Charley-horse

8 Other

7th Character

N/A

Pain in Limb

ICD-1Ø-CM: M79.6Ø1 - M79.676

What to Document

4th Character: Type of soft tissue disorder
5th Character: Anatomic site
6th Character: Laterality

Document:
- Laterality
- Any external cause, if applicable

Chapter Guidelines

13. Diseases of the musculoskeletal system and connective tissue (MØØ-M99)

Notes:
Use an external cause code following the code for the musculoskeletal condition, if applicable, to identify the cause of the musculoskeletal condition

Excludes2:
arthropathic psoriasis (L4Ø.5-)
certain conditions originating in the perinatal period (PØ4-P96)
certain infectious and parasitic diseases (AØØ-B99)
compartment syndrome (traumatic) (T79.A-)
complications of pregnancy, childbirth and the puerperium (OØØ-O9A)
congenital malformations, deformations, and chromosomal abnormalities (QØØ-Q99)
endocrine, nutritional and metabolic diseases (EØØ-E88)
injury, poisoning and certain other consequences of external causes (SØØ-T88)
neoplasms (CØØ-D49)
symptoms, signs and abnormal clinical and laboratory findings, not elsewhere classified (RØØ-R94)

See Guidelines: 1;C.13.a-b | 1;C.2Ø.a.1

SOFT TISSUE DISORDERS (M6Ø-M79)

OTHER SOFT TISSUE DISORDERS (M7Ø-M79)

3rd Character

M7Ø- Soft tissue disorders related to use, overuse and pressure
M71- Other bursopathies
M72- Fibroblastic disorders
M75- Shoulder lesions
M76- Enthesopathies, lower limb, excluding foot
M77- Other enthesopathies
M79- Other and unspecified soft tissue disorders, not elsewhere classified

4th Character

Document: Type of soft tissue disorder

Excludes1:
psychogenic rheumatism (F45.8)
soft tissue pain, psychogenic (F45.41)

M79.Ø Rheumatism, unspecified
Excludes1:
fibromyalgia (M79.7)
palindromic rheumatism (M12.3-)

M79.1- Myalgia
Including: Myofascial pain syndrome
Excludes1:
fibromyalgia (M79.7)
myositis (M6Ø.-)

M79.2 Neuralgia and neuritis, unspecified
Excludes1:
brachial radiculitis NOS (M54.1)
lumbosacral radiculitis NOS (M54.1)
mononeuropathies (G56-G58)
radiculitis NOS (M54.1)
sciatica (M54.3-M54.4)

M79.3 Panniculitis, unspecified
Excludes1:
lupus panniculitis (L93.2)
neck and back panniculitis (M54.Ø-)
relapsing [Weber-Christian] panniculitis (M35.6)

M79.4 Hypertrophy of (infrapatellar) fat pad

M79.5 Residual foreign body in soft tissue
Excludes1:
foreign body granuloma of skin and subcutaneous tissue (L92.3)
foreign body granuloma of soft tissue (M6Ø.2-)

M79.6- Pain in limb, hand, foot, fingers and toes
Excludes2:
pain in joint (M25.5-)

M79.7 Fibromyalgia
Including: Fibromyositis, Fibrositis, Myofibrositis

M79.8- Other specified soft tissue disorders

M79.9 Soft tissue disorder, unspecified

M79.A- Nontraumatic compartment syndrome
Code First:
if applicable, associated postprocedural complication
Excludes1:
compartment syndrome NOS (T79.A-)
fibromyalgia (M79.7)
nontraumatic ischemic infarction of muscle (M62.2-)
traumatic compartment syndrome (T79.A-)

See Appendix A — Coding Reference Tables for lists of the ICD-10-CM Tabular indicators, HAC categories, and HCC codes.

Pain in Limb (continued)

5th Character

Document: Anatomic site

Excludes2:
pain in joint (M25.5-)

M79.6Ø- Pain in limb, unspecified
M79.62- Pain in upper arm
Including: Pain in axillary region
M79.63- Pain in forearm
M79.64- Pain in hand and fingers
M79.65- Pain in thigh
M79.66- Pain in lower leg
M79.67- Pain in foot and toes

6th Character

Document: Laterality

Applies to: M79.6Ø-

1 Right arm
Including: Pain in right upper limb NOS
2 Left arm
Including: Pain in left upper limb NOS
3 Unspecified arm
Including: Pain in upper limb NOS
4 Right leg
Including: Pain in right lower limb NOS
5 Left leg
Including: Pain in left lower limb NOS
6 Unspecified leg
Including: Pain in lower limb NOS
9 Unspecified limb
Including: Pain in limb NOS

Applies to: M79.62-

Including: Pain in axillary region

1 Right
2 Left
9 Unspecified

Applies to: M79.63-, M79.65-, M79.66-

1 Right
2 Left
9 Unspecified

6th Character (continued)

Applies to: M79.64-

1 Right hand
2 Left hand
3 Unspecified hand
4 Right finger(s)
5 Left finger(s)
6 Unspecified finger(s)

Applies to: M79.67-

1 Right foot
2 Left foot
3 Unspecified foot
4 Right toe(s)
5 Left toe(s)
6 Unspecified toe(s)

7th Character

N/A

Biomechanical Lesions, NEC

ICD-1Ø-CM: M99.ØØ - M99.9

What to Document

4th Character: Type of lesion
5th Character: Anatomic region

Document:
- Any external cause, if applicable

Notes:
If the condition can be classified elsewhere, this category should not be used

Terminology:
Somatic dysfunction: Impaired or altered function of related components of the somatic (body framework) system: skeletal, arthrodial and myofascial structures, and their related vascular, lymphatic, and neural elements.
Stenosis: Narrowing of a passage in the body.

Chapter Guidelines

13. Diseases of the musculoskeletal system and connective tissue (MØØ-M99)

Notes:
Use an external cause code following the code for the musculoskeletal condition, if applicable, to identify the cause of the musculoskeletal condition

Excludes2:
arthropathic psoriasis (L4Ø.5-)
certain conditions originating in the perinatal period (PØ4-P96)
certain infectious and parasitic diseases (AØØ-B99)
compartment syndrome (traumatic) (T79.A-)
complications of pregnancy, childbirth and the puerperium (OØØ-O9A)
congenital malformations, deformations, and chromosomal abnormalities (QØØ-Q99)
endocrine, nutritional and metabolic diseases (EØØ-E88)
injury, poisoning and certain other consequences of external causes (SØØ-T88)
neoplasms (CØØ-D49)
symptoms, signs and abnormal clinical and laboratory findings, not elsewhere classified (RØØ-R94)

See Guidelines: 1;C.13.a-b | 1;C.2Ø.a.1

M99 BIOMECHANICAL LESIONS, NOT ELSEWHERE CLASSIFIED (M99) (M99-M99)

3rd Character

M99- Biomechanical lesions, not elsewhere classified

4th Character

Document: Type of lesion
Reminder: All final codes are in **BOLD**

Notes:
This category should not be used if the condition can be classified elsewhere.

M99.Ø- Segmental and somatic dysfunction
M99.1- Subluxation complex (vertebral)
M99.2- Subluxation stenosis of neural canal
M99.3- Osseous stenosis of neural canal
M99.4- Connective tissue stenosis of neural canal
M99.5- Intervertebral disc stenosis of neural canal
M99.6- Osseous and subluxation stenosis of intervertebral foramina
M99.7- Connective tissue and disc stenosis of intervertebral foramina
M99.8- Other biomechanical lesions
M99.9 Biomechanical lesion, unspecified

5th Character

Document: Anatomic region

Applies to: M99.Ø-, M99.2-, M99.3-, M99.4-, M99.5-, M99.6-, M99.7-, M99.8-

Ø Head region
1 Cervical region
2 Thoracic region
3 Lumbar region
4 Sacral region
5 Pelvic region
6 Lower extremity
7 Upper extremity
8 Rib cage region
9 Abdomen and other regions

Biomechanical Lesions, NEC (continued)

5th Character (continued)

Applies to: M99.1-

Ø Head region

Indicator(s): HAC: Ø5

1 Cervical region

Indicator(s): HAC: Ø5

2 Thoracic region

3 Lumbar region

4 Sacral region

5 Pelvic region

6 Lower extremity

7 Upper extremity

8 Rib cage region

Indicator(s): HAC: Ø5

9 Abdomen and other regions

6th Character

N/A

7th Character

N/A

Sprain of Ligaments of Cervical Spine

ICD-1Ø-CM: S13.4XXA - S13.4XXS

What to Document

3rd Character: Type of injury
4th Character: Subluxation/dislocation, rupture, or sprain
7th Character: Episode of care

Document:
- Any external cause, if applicable
- Any retained foreign body, if applicable
- Any associated open wound

Terminology:
Strain: A strain is tear or damage to contractile tissues, such as muscles and tendons
Sprain: A sprain is a tear or damage to non contractile tissue, such as ligaments

Chapter Guidelines

19. Injury, poisoning and certain other consequences of external causes (SØØ-T88)

Notes:
Use secondary code(s) from Chapter 2Ø, External causes of morbidity, to indicate cause of injury. Codes within the T section that include the external cause do not require an additional external cause code
Use additional code to identify any retained foreign body, if applicable (Z18.-)
Excludes1:
birth trauma (P1Ø-P15)
obstetric trauma (O7Ø-O71)
Notes:
The chapter uses the S-section for coding different types of injuries related to single body regions and the T-section to cover injuries to unspecified body regions as well as poisoning and certain other consequences of external causes.
See Guidelines: 1;C.15.m | 1;C.19.a-b | 1;C.2Ø.a.1

INJURIES TO THE NECK (S1Ø-S19)

Includes:
injuries of nape
injuries of supraclavicular region
injuries of throat
Excludes2:
burns and corrosions (T2Ø-T32)
effects of foreign body in esophagus (T18.1)
effects of foreign body in larynx (T17.3)
effects of foreign body in pharynx (T17.2)
effects of foreign body in trachea (T17.4)
frostbite (T33-T34)
insect bite or sting, venomous (T63.4)
See Guidelines: 1;C.19.b

3rd Character

Document: Type of injury

S1Ø- Superficial injury of neck
S11- Open wound of neck
S12- Fracture of cervical vertebra and other parts of neck
S13- Dislocation and sprain of joints and ligaments at neck level
S14- Injury of nerves and spinal cord at neck level
S15- Injury of blood vessels at neck level
S16- Injury of muscle, fascia and tendon at neck level
S17- Crushing injury of neck
S19- Other specified and unspecified injuries of neck

4th Character

Document: Subluxation/dislocation, rupture, or sprain

Includes:
avulsion of joint or ligament at neck level
laceration of cartilage, joint or ligament at neck level
sprain of cartilage, joint or ligament at neck level
traumatic hemarthrosis of joint or ligament at neck level
traumatic rupture of joint or ligament at neck level
traumatic subluxation of joint or ligament at neck level
traumatic tear of joint or ligament at neck level
Code Also
any associated open wound
Excludes2:
strain of muscle or tendon at neck level (S16.1)
The appropriate 7th character is to be added to each code from category S13
A - initial encounter
D - subsequent encounter
S - sequela
Indicator(s): POAEx (7th D/S)

S13.Ø- Traumatic rupture of cervical intervertebral disc
Excludes1:
rupture or displacement (nontraumatic) of cervical intervertebral disc NOS (M5Ø.-)

S13.1- Subluxation and dislocation of cervical vertebrae
Code Also
any associated:
open wound of neck (S11.-)
spinal cord injury (S14.1-)
Excludes2:
fracture of cervical vertebrae (S12.Ø-S12.3-)
Indicator(s): CC (7th A) | HAC: Ø5 (7th A)

Sprain of Ligaments of Cervical Spine (continued)

4th Character (continued)

S13.2- Dislocation of other and unspecified parts of neck
Indicator(s): *CC (7th A) | HAC: Ø5 (7th A)*

S13.4- Sprain of ligaments of cervical spine
Including: Anterior longitudinal (ligament), cervical; atlanto-axial, atlanto-occipital joints; Whiplash injury

S13.5- Sprain of thyroid region
Including: Cricoarytenoid, cricothyroid (joint) (ligament); thyroid cartilage

S13.8- Sprain of joints and ligaments of other parts of neck

S13.9- Sprain of joints and ligaments of unspecified parts of neck

5th Character

Including: Anterior longitudinal (ligament), cervical; atlanto-axial, atlanto-occipital joints; Whiplash injury

S13.4X-

6th Character

X-

7th Character

Document: Episode of care

Applies to: S13.4XX-

A Initial encounter

D Subsequent encounter

S Sequela

Injury of Muscle, Fascia, and Tendon at Neck Level

ICD-1Ø-CM: S16.1XXA - S16.9XXS

What to Document

3rd Character: Type of neck injury
4th Character: Other specifications of injury
7th Character: Episode of care

Document:
- Any external cause, if applicable
- Any retained foreign body, if applicable
- Any associated open wound

Terminology:
Strain: A strain is tear or damage to contractile tissues, such as muscles and tendons
Sprain: A sprain is a tear or damage to non contractile tissue such as ligaments

Chapter Guidelines

19. Injury, poisoning and certain other consequences of external causes (SØØ-T88)

Notes:
Use secondary code(s) from Chapter 2Ø, External causes of morbidity, to indicate cause of injury. Codes within the T section that include the external cause do not require an additional external cause code
Use additional *code to identify any retained foreign body, if applicable (Z18.-)*
Excludes1:
birth trauma (P1Ø-P15)
obstetric trauma (O7Ø-O71)
Notes:
The chapter uses the S-section for coding different types of injuries related to single body regions and the T-section to cover injuries to unspecified body regions as well as poisoning and certain other consequences of external causes.
See Guidelines: *1;C.15.m | 1;C.19.a-b | 1;C.2Ø.a.1*

INJURIES TO THE NECK (S1Ø-S19)

Includes:
injuries of nape
injuries of supraclavicular region
injuries of throat
Excludes2:
burns and corrosions (T2Ø-T32)
effects of foreign body in esophagus (T18.1)
effects of foreign body in larynx (T17.3)
effects of foreign body in pharynx (T17.2)
effects of foreign body in trachea (T17.4)
frostbite (T33-T34)
insect bite or sting, venomous (T63.4)
See Guidelines: *1;C.19.b*

3rd Character

Document: Type of neck injury

S1Ø- Superficial injury of neck
S11- Open wound of neck
S12- Fracture of cervical vertebra and other parts of neck
S13- Dislocation and sprain of joints and ligaments at neck level
S14- Injury of nerves and spinal cord at neck level
S15- Injury of blood vessels at neck level
S16- Injury of muscle, fascia and tendon at neck level
S17- Crushing injury of neck
S19- Other specified and unspecified injuries of neck

4th Character

Document: Other specifications of injury

Code Also
any associated open wound (S11.-)
Excludes2:
sprain of joint or ligament at neck level (S13.9)
The appropriate 7th character is to be added to each code from category S16
A - initial encounter
D - subsequent encounter
S - sequela
Indicator(s): *POAEx (7th D/S)*

S16.1- Strain of muscle, fascia and tendon at neck level
S16.2- Laceration of muscle, fascia and tendon at neck level
S16.8- Other specified injury of muscle, fascia and tendon at neck level
S16.9- Unspecified injury of muscle, fascia and tendon at neck level

5th Character

Note: 5th character X applies to all

S16.1X-

6th Character

X-

C

Appendix C. Chiropractic PDGs

Injury of Muscle, Fascia, and Tendon at Neck Level (continued)

7th Character

Document: Episode of care

Applies to: S16.1XX-, S16.2XX-, S16.8XX-, S16.9XX-

A Initial encounter

D Subsequent encounter

S Sequela

Sprain of Ligaments of Thoracic Spine

ICD-1Ø-CM: S23.3XXA - S23.3XXS

What to Document

3rd Character: Type of injury
4th Character: Subluxation/dislocation, rupture, or sprain
7th Character: Episode of care

Document:
- Any external cause, if applicable
- Any retained foreign body, if applicable
- Any associated open wound

Terminology:
Strain: A strain is tear or damage to contractile tissues, such as muscles and tendons
Sprain: A sprain is a tear or damage to non contractile tissue such as ligaments

Chapter Guidelines

19. Injury, poisoning and certain other consequences of external causes (SØØ-T88)

Notes:
Use secondary code(s) from Chapter 2Ø, External causes of morbidity, to indicate cause of injury. Codes within the T section that include the external cause do not require an additional external cause code
Use additional code to identify any retained foreign body, if applicable (Z18.-)
Excludes1:
birth trauma (P1Ø-P15)
obstetric trauma (O7Ø-O71)
Notes:
The chapter uses the S-section for coding different types of injuries related to single body regions and the T-section to cover injuries to unspecified body regions as well as poisoning and certain other consequences of external causes.
See Guidelines: 1;C.15.m | 1;C.19.a-b | 1;C.2Ø.a.1

INJURIES TO THE THORAX (S2Ø-S29)

Includes:
injuries of breast
injuries of chest (wall)
injuries of interscapular area
Excludes2:
burns and corrosions (T2Ø-T32)
effects of foreign body in bronchus (T17.5)
effects of foreign body in esophagus (T18.1)
effects of foreign body in lung (T17.8)
effects of foreign body in trachea (T17.4)
frostbite (T33-T34)
injuries of axilla
injuries of clavicle
injuries of scapular region
injuries of shoulder
insect bite or sting, venomous (T63.4)
See Guidelines: 1;C.19.b

3rd Character

Document: Type of injury

S2Ø- Superficial injury of thorax
S21- Open wound of thorax
S22- Fracture of rib(s), sternum and thoracic spine
S23- Dislocation and sprain of joints and ligaments of thorax
S24- Injury of nerves and spinal cord at thorax level
S25- Injury of blood vessels of thorax
S26- Injury of heart
S27- Injury of other and unspecified intrathoracic organs
S28- Crushing injury of thorax, and traumatic amputation of part of thorax
S29- Other and unspecified injuries of thorax

4th Character

Document: Subluxation/dislocation, rupture, or sprain

Includes:
avulsion of joint or ligament of thorax
laceration of cartilage, joint or ligament of thorax
sprain of cartilage, joint or ligament of thorax
traumatic hemarthrosis of joint or ligament of thorax
traumatic rupture of joint or ligament of thorax
traumatic subluxation of joint or ligament of thorax
traumatic tear of joint or ligament of thorax
Code Also
any associated open wound
Excludes2:
dislocation, sprain of sternoclavicular joint (S43.2, S43.6)
strain of muscle or tendon of thorax (S29.Ø1-)
The appropriate 7th character is to be added to each code from category S23
A - initial encounter
D - subsequent encounter
S - sequela
Indicator(s): POAEx (7th D/S)

S23.Ø- Traumatic rupture of thoracic intervertebral disc
Excludes1:
rupture or displacement (nontraumatic) of thoracic intervertebral disc NOS (M51.- with fifth character 4)

C

Appendix C. Chiropractic PDGs

Sprain of Ligaments of Thoracic Spine (continued)

4th Character (continued)

S23.1- Subluxation and dislocation of thoracic vertebra

Code Also
any associated:
open wound of thorax (S21.-)
spinal cord injury (S24.Ø-, S24.1-)
Excludes2:
fracture of thoracic vertebrae (S22.Ø-)

S23.2- Dislocation of other and unspecified parts of thorax

S23.3- Sprain of ligaments of thoracic spine

S23.4- Sprain of ribs and sternum

S23.8- Sprain of other specified parts of thorax

S23.9- Sprain of unspecified parts of thorax

5th Character

S23.3X-

6th Character

X-

7th Character

Document: Episode of care

Applies to: S23.3XX-

A Initial encounter

D Subsequent encounter

S Sequela

Sprain of Ligaments of Lumbar Spine

ICD-1Ø-CM: S33.5XXA - S33.5XXS

What to Document

3rd Character: Type of injury
4th Character: Type and anatomic site
7th Character: Episode of care

Document:
- External cause, if applicable
- Any retained foreign body, if applicable
- Any associated open wound

Terminology:
Strain: A strain is tear or damage to contractile tissues, such as muscles and tendons
Sprain: A sprain is a tear or damage to non contractile tissue such as ligaments

Chapter Guidelines

19. Injury, poisoning and certain other consequences of external causes (SØØ-T88)

Notes:
Use secondary code(s) from Chapter 2Ø, External causes of morbidity, to indicate cause of injury. Codes within the T section that include the external cause do not require an additional external cause code
Use additional *code to identify any retained foreign body, if applicable (Z18.-)*
Excludes1:
birth trauma (P1Ø-P15)
obstetric trauma (O7Ø-O71)
Notes:
The chapter uses the S-section for coding different types of injuries related to single body regions and the T-section to cover injuries to unspecified body regions as well as poisoning and certain other consequences of external causes.
See Guidelines: *1;C.15.m | 1;C.19.a-b | 1;C.2Ø.a.1*

INJURIES TO THE ABDOMEN, LOWER BACK, LUMBAR SPINE, PELVIS AND EXTERNAL GENITALS (S3Ø-S39)

Includes:
injuries to the abdominal wall
injuries to the anus
injuries to the buttock
injuries to the external genitalia
injuries to the flank
injuries to the groin
Excludes2:
burns and corrosions (T2Ø-T32)
effects of foreign body in anus and rectum (T18.5)
effects of foreign body in genitourinary tract (T19.-)
effects of foreign body in stomach, small intestine and colon (T18.2-T18.4)
frostbite (T33-T34)
insect bite or sting, venomous (T63.4)
See Guidelines: *1;C.19.b*

3rd Character

Document: Type of injury

S3Ø- Superficial injury of abdomen, lower back, pelvis and external genitals
S31- Open wound of abdomen, lower back, pelvis and external genitals
S32- Fracture of lumbar spine and pelvis
S33- Dislocation and sprain of joints and ligaments of lumbar spine and pelvis
S34- Injury of lumbar and sacral spinal cord and nerves at abdomen, lower back and pelvis level
S35- Injury of blood vessels at abdomen, lower back and pelvis level
S36- Injury of intra-abdominal organs
S37- Injury of urinary and pelvic organs
S38- Crushing injury and traumatic amputation of abdomen, lower back, pelvis and external genitals
S39- Other and unspecified injuries of abdomen, lower back, pelvis and external genitals

4th Character

Document: Type and anatomic site

Includes:
avulsion of joint or ligament of lumbar spine and pelvis
laceration of cartilage, joint or ligament of lumbar spine and pelvis
sprain of cartilage, joint or ligament of lumbar spine and pelvis
traumatic hemarthrosis of joint or ligament of lumbar spine and pelvis
traumatic rupture of joint or ligament of lumbar spine and pelvis
traumatic subluxation of joint or ligament of lumbar spine and pelvis
traumatic tear of joint or ligament of lumbar spine and pelvis
Code Also
any associated open wound
Excludes1:
nontraumatic rupture or displacement of lumbar intervertebral disc NOS (M51.-)
obstetric damage to pelvic joints and ligaments (O71.6)
Excludes2:
dislocation and sprain of joints and ligaments of hip (S73.-)
strain of muscle of lower back and pelvis (S39.Ø1-)
The appropriate 7th character is to be added to each code from category S33
A - initial encounter
D - subsequent encounter
S - sequela
Indicator(s): *POAEx (7th D/S)*

C

Appendix C. Chiropractic PDGs

 See Appendix A — Coding Reference Tables for lists of the ICD-10-CM Tabular indicators, HAC categories, and HCC codes.

Sprain of Ligaments of Lumbar Spine (continued)

4th Character (continued)

S33.Ø- Traumatic rupture of lumbar intervertebral disc

Excludes1:

rupture or displacement (nontraumatic) of lumbar intervertebral disc NOS (M51.- with fifth character 6)

S33.1- Subluxation and dislocation of lumbar vertebra

Code Also

any associated:

open wound of abdomen, lower back and pelvis (S31)

spinal cord injury (S24.Ø, S24.1-, S34.Ø-, S34.1-)

Excludes2:

fracture of lumbar vertebrae (S32.Ø-)

S33.2- Dislocation of sacroiliac and sacrococcygeal joint

S33.3- Dislocation of other and unspecified parts of lumbar spine and pelvis

S33.4- Traumatic rupture of symphysis pubis

S33.5- Sprain of ligaments of lumbar spine

S33.6- Sprain of sacroiliac joint

S33.8- Sprain of other parts of lumbar spine and pelvis

S33.9- Sprain of unspecified parts of lumbar spine and pelvis

5th Character

S33.5X-

6th Character

X-

7th Character

Document: Episode of care

Applies to: S33.5XX-

A Initial encounter

D Subsequent encounter

S Sequela

Sprain of Sacroiliac Joint

ICD-1Ø-CM: S33.6XXA - S33.6XXS

What to Document

3rd Character: Type of Injury
4th Character: Dislocation/subluxation, sprain, or rupture, and anatomic site
7th Character: Episode of care

Document:
- Any external cause, if applicable
- Any retained foreign body, if applicable
- Any associated open wound

Terminology:
Sprain: A tear or stretch of non-contractile tissue at a joint, such as ligaments
Strain: A strain is tear or damage to contractile tissues, such as muscles and tendons

Chapter Guidelines

19. Injury, poisoning and certain other consequences of external causes (SØØ-T88)

Notes:
Use secondary code(s) from Chapter 2Ø, External causes of morbidity, to indicate cause of injury. Codes within the T section that include the external cause do not require an additional external cause code
Use additional *code to identify any retained foreign body, if applicable (Z18.-)*
Excludes1:
birth trauma (P1Ø-P15)
obstetric trauma (O7Ø-O71)
Notes:
The chapter uses the S-section for coding different types of injuries related to single body regions and the T-section to cover injuries to unspecified body regions as well as poisoning and certain other consequences of external causes.
See Guidelines: *1;C.15.m | 1;C.19.a-b | 1;C.2Ø.a.1*

INJURIES TO THE ABDOMEN, LOWER BACK, LUMBAR SPINE, PELVIS AND EXTERNAL GENITALS (S3Ø-S39)

Includes:
injuries to the abdominal wall
injuries to the anus
injuries to the buttock
injuries to the external genitalia
injuries to the flank
injuries to the groin
Excludes2:
burns and corrosions (T2Ø-T32)
effects of foreign body in anus and rectum (T18.5)
effects of foreign body in genitourinary tract (T19.-)
effects of foreign body in stomach, small intestine and colon (T18.2-T18.4)
frostbite (T33-T34)
insect bite or sting, venomous (T63.4)
See Guidelines: *1;C.19.b*

3rd Character

Document: Type of Injury

- S3Ø- Superficial injury of abdomen, lower back, pelvis and external genitals
- S31- Open wound of abdomen, lower back, pelvis and external genitals
- S32- Fracture of lumbar spine and pelvis
- S33- Dislocation and sprain of joints and ligaments of lumbar spine and pelvis
- S34- Injury of lumbar and sacral spinal cord and nerves at abdomen, lower back and pelvis level
- S35- Injury of blood vessels at abdomen, lower back and pelvis level
- S36- Injury of intra-abdominal organs
- S37- Injury of urinary and pelvic organs
- S38- Crushing injury and traumatic amputation of abdomen, lower back, pelvis and external genitals
- S39- Other and unspecified injuries of abdomen, lower back, pelvis and external genitals

4th Character

Document: Dislocation/subluxation, sprain, or rupture, and anatomic site

Includes:
avulsion of joint or ligament of lumbar spine and pelvis
laceration of cartilage, joint or ligament of lumbar spine and pelvis
sprain of cartilage, joint or ligament of lumbar spine and pelvis
traumatic hemarthrosis of joint or ligament of lumbar spine and pelvis
traumatic rupture of joint or ligament of lumbar spine and pelvis
traumatic subluxation of joint or ligament of lumbar spine and pelvis
traumatic tear of joint or ligament of lumbar spine and pelvis
Code Also
any associated open wound
Excludes1:
nontraumatic rupture or displacement of lumbar intervertebral disc NOS (M51.-)
obstetric damage to pelvic joints and ligaments (O71.6)
Excludes2:
dislocation and sprain of joints and ligaments of hip (S73.-)
strain of muscle of lower back and pelvis (S39.Ø1-)
The appropriate 7th character is to be added to each code from category S33
A - initial encounter
D - subsequent encounter
S - sequela
Indicator(s): *POAEx (7th D/S)*

C

Appendix C. Chiropractic PDGs

Sprain of Sacroiliac Joint (continued)

4th Character (continued)

S33.Ø- Traumatic rupture of lumbar intervertebral disc

Excludes1:
rupture or displacement (nontraumatic) of lumbar intervertebral disc NOS (M51.- with fifth character 6)

S33.1- Subluxation and dislocation of lumbar vertebra

Code Also
any associated:
open wound of abdomen, lower back and pelvis (S31)
spinal cord injury (S24.Ø, S24.1-, S34.Ø-, S34.1-)
Excludes2:
fracture of lumbar vertebrae (S32.Ø-)

S33.2- Dislocation of sacroiliac and sacrococcygeal joint

S33.3- Dislocation of other and unspecified parts of lumbar spine and pelvis

S33.4- Traumatic rupture of symphysis pubis

S33.5- Sprain of ligaments of lumbar spine

S33.6- Sprain of sacroiliac joint

S33.8- Sprain of other parts of lumbar spine and pelvis

S33.9- Sprain of unspecified parts of lumbar spine and pelvis

5th Character

S33.6X-

6th Character

X-

7th Character

Document: Episode of care

Applies to: S33.6XX-

A Initial encounter

D Subsequent encounter

S Sequela

Injury of Muscle, Fascia, and Tendon of Abdomen, Lower Back, and Pelvis

ICD-1Ø-CM: S39.ØØ1A - S39.Ø93S

What to Document

5th Character: Type of injury
6th Character: Anatomic site
7th Character: Episode of care

Document:
- External cause, if any
- Any retained foreign body, if applicable
- Any associated open wound

Chapter Guidelines

19. Injury, poisoning and certain other consequences of external causes (SØØ-T88)

Notes:
Use secondary code(s) from Chapter 2Ø, External causes of morbidity, to indicate cause of injury. Codes within the T section that include the external cause do not require an additional external cause code
Use additional code to identify any retained foreign body, if applicable (Z18.-)
Excludes1:
birth trauma (P1Ø-P15)
obstetric trauma (O7Ø-O71)
Notes:
The chapter uses the S-section for coding different types of injuries related to single body regions and the T-section to cover injuries to unspecified body regions as well as poisoning and certain other consequences of external causes.
See Guidelines: 1;C.15.m | 1;C.19.a-b | 1;C.2Ø.a.1

INJURIES TO THE ABDOMEN, LOWER BACK, LUMBAR SPINE, PELVIS AND EXTERNAL GENITALS (S3Ø-S39)

Includes:
injuries to the abdominal wall
injuries to the anus
injuries to the buttock
injuries to the external genitalia
injuries to the flank
injuries to the groin
Excludes2:
burns and corrosions (T2Ø-T32)
effects of foreign body in anus and rectum (T18.5)
effects of foreign body in genitourinary tract (T19.-)
effects of foreign body in stomach, small intestine and colon (T18.2-T18.4)
frostbite (T33-T34)
insect bite or sting, venomous (T63.4)
See Guidelines: 1;C.19.b

3rd Character

S3Ø- Superficial injury of abdomen, lower back, pelvis and external genitals
S31- Open wound of abdomen, lower back, pelvis and external genitals
S32- Fracture of lumbar spine and pelvis
S33- Dislocation and sprain of joints and ligaments of lumbar spine and pelvis
S34- Injury of lumbar and sacral spinal cord and nerves at abdomen, lower back and pelvis level
S35- Injury of blood vessels at abdomen, lower back and pelvis level
S36- Injury of intra-abdominal organs
S37- Injury of urinary and pelvic organs
S38- Crushing injury and traumatic amputation of abdomen, lower back, pelvis and external genitals
S39- Other and unspecified injuries of abdomen, lower back, pelvis and external genitals

4th Character

Code Also
any associated open wound (S31.-)
Excludes2:
sprain of joints and ligaments of lumbar spine and pelvis (S33.-)
The appropriate 7th character is to be added to each code from category S39
A - initial encounter
D - subsequent encounter
S - sequela
Indicator(s): POAEx (7th D/S)

S39.Ø- Injury of muscle, fascia and tendon of abdomen, lower back and pelvis
S39.8- Other specified injuries of abdomen, lower back, pelvis and external genitals
S39.9- Unspecified injury of abdomen, lower back, pelvis and external genitals

See Appendix A — Coding Reference Tables for lists of the ICD-10-CM Tabular indicators, HAC categories, and HCC codes.

Injury of Muscle, Fascia, and Tendon of Abdomen, Lower Back, and Pelvis (continued)

5th Character

Document: Type of injury

S39.ØØ- Unspecified injury of muscle, fascia and tendon of abdomen, lower back and pelvis

S39.Ø1- Strain of muscle, fascia and tendon of abdomen, lower back and pelvis

S39.Ø2- Laceration of muscle, fascia and tendon of abdomen, lower back and pelvis

S39.Ø9- Other injury of muscle, fascia and tendon of abdomen, lower back and pelvis

6th Character

Document: Anatomic site

Note: The sixth characters identifying whether the injury applies to the abdomen, lower back, or pelvis should be applied to any of the subcategories listed in the 5th character section above.

1- Abdomen

2- Lower back

3- Pelvis

7th Character

Document: Episode of care

Applies to: S39.ØØ1-, S39.ØØ2-, S39.ØØ3-, S39.Ø11-, S39.Ø12-, S39.Ø13-, S39.Ø21-, S39.Ø22-, S39.Ø23-, S39.Ø91-, S39.Ø92-, S39.Ø93-

A Initial encounter

D Subsequent encounter

S Sequela

Notes: